I0066454

Clinical Gastroenterology and Hepatology

Clinical Gastroenterology and Hepatology

Editor: Phillip Lawson

FOSTER ACADEMICS

www.fosteracademics.com

www.fosteracademics.com

FOSTER ACADEMICS

Cataloging-in-Publication Data

Clinical gastroenterology and hepatology / edited by Phillip Lawson.
p. cm.
Includes bibliographical references and index.
ISBN 978-1-63242-654-3
1. Gastroenterology. 2. Hepatology. 3. Digestive organs--Diseases. I. Lawson, Phillip.
RC801 .C55 2019
616.33--dc23

© Foster Academics, 2019

Foster Academics,
118-35 Queens Blvd., Suite 400,
Forest Hills, NY 11375, USA

ISBN 978-1-63242-654-3 (Hardback)

This book contains information obtained from authentic and highly regarded sources. Copyright for all individual chapters remain with the respective authors as indicated. All chapters are published with permission under the Creative Commons Attribution License or equivalent. A wide variety of references are listed. Permission and sources are indicated; for detailed attributions, please refer to the permissions page and list of contributors. Reasonable efforts have been made to publish reliable data and information, but the authors, editors and publisher cannot assume any responsibility for the validity of all materials or the consequences of their use.

Trademark Notice: Registered trademark of products or corporate names are used only for explanation and identification without intent to infringe.

Contents

Preface IX

Chapter 1 **The Effects of Extra Virgin Olive Oil on Alanine Aminotransferase, Aspartate Aminotransferase and Ultrasonographic Indices of Hepatic Steatosis in Nonalcoholic Fatty Liver Disease Patients Undergoing Low Calorie Diet** 1
Farzad Shidfar, Samaneh Sadat Bahrololumi, Saeid Doaei, Assieh Mohammadzadeh, Maryam Gholamalizadeh and Ali Mohammadimanesh

Chapter 2 **A Contemporary Review of the Treatment Landscape and the Role of Predictive and Prognostic Biomarkers in Pancreatic Adenocarcinoma** 8
Irene S. Yu and Winson Y. Cheung

Chapter 3 **Preoperative Thrombocytopenia may Predict Poor Surgical Outcome after Extended Hepatectomy** 18
Mohammad Golriz, Omid Ghamarnejad, Elias Khajeh, Mohammadsadegh Sabagh, Markus Mieth, Katrin Hoffmann, Alexis Ulrich, Thilo Hackert, Karl Heinz Weiss, Peter Schirmacher, Markus W. Büchler and Arianeb Mehrabi

Chapter 4 **Management Strategies and Outcomes for Hyponatremia in Cirrhosis in the Hyponatremia Registry** 29
Samuel H. Sigal, Alpesh Amin, Joseph A. Chiodo III and Arun Sanyal

Chapter 5 **Laparoscopic versus Open Surgery for Hepatocellular Carcinoma** 37
Ke Chen, Yu Pan, Bin Zhang, Xiao-long Liu, Hendi Maher and Xue-yong Zheng

Chapter 6 **Body Composition in Crohn's Disease and Ulcerative Colitis: Correlation with Disease Severity and Duration** 52
Dawesh P. Yadav, Saurabh Kedia, Kumble Seetharama Madhusudhan, Sawan Bopanna, Sandeep Goyal, Saransh Jain, Naval K. Vikram, Raju Sharma, Govind K. Makharia and Vineet Ahuja

Chapter 7 **Thromboembolic Events Secondary to Endoscopic Cyanoacrylate Injection: Can we Foresee any Red Flags?** 60
Yujen Tseng, Lili Ma, Tiancheng Luo, Xiaoqing Zeng, Yichao Wei, Ling Li, Pengju Xu and Shiyao Chen

Chapter 8 **Low Total Dose of Anti-Human T-Lymphocyte Globulin (ATG) Guarantees a Good Glomerular Filtration Rate after Liver Transplant in Recipients with Pretransplant Renal Dysfunction** 70
Cristina Dopazo, Ramón Charco, Mireia Caralt, Elizabeth Pando, José Luis Lázaro, Concepción Gómez-Gavara, Lluis Castells and Itxarone Bilbao

Chapter 9 **Efficacy and Safety of Immunosuppressive Therapy for PBC–AIH Overlap Syndrome Accompanied by Decompensated Cirrhosis** 77
Xiaoli Fan, Yongjun Zhu, Ruoting Men, Maoyao Wen, Yi Shen, Changli Lu and Li Yang

Chapter 10 **A Systematic Review of the Efficacy and Safety of Fecal Microbiota Transplant for *Clostridium difficile* Infection in Immunocompromised Patients** 85
Oluwaseun Shogbesan, Dilli Ram Poudel, Samjeris Victor, Asad Jehangir, Opeyemi Fadahunsi, Gbenga Shogbesan and Anthony Donato

Chapter 11 **Choice of Allograft in Patients Requiring Intestinal Transplantation** 95
Genevieve Huard, Thomas Schiano, Jang Moon and Kishore Iyer

Chapter 12 **Transcriptome Analysis of Porcine PBMCs Reveals the Immune Cascade Response and Gene Ontology Terms Related to Cell Death and Fibrosis in the Progression of Liver Failure** 105
YiMin Zhang, Li Shao, Ning Zhou, JianZhou Li, Yu Chen, Juan Lu, Jie Wang, ErMei Chen, ZhongYang Xie and LanJuan Li

Chapter 13 **Choosing an Animal Model for the Study of Functional Dyspepsia** 113
Yang Ye, Xue-Rui Wang, Yang Zheng, Jing-Wen Yang, Na-Na Yang, Guang-Xia Shi and Cun-Zhi Liu

Chapter 14 **Alpha-Fetoprotein as a Predictive Marker for Patients with Hepatitis B-Related Acute-on-Chronic Liver Failure** 126
Xiaoping Wang, Caifei Shen, Jianjiang Yang, Xianjun Yang, Sen Qin, Haijun Zeng, Xiaoling Wu, Shanhong Tang and Weizheng Zeng

Chapter 15 **48-Week Outcome after Cessation of Nucleos(t)ide Analogue Treatment in Chronic Hepatitis B Patient and the Associated Factors with Relapse** 132
Wen-xiong Xu, Qian Zhang, Xiang Zhu, Chao-shuang Lin, You-ming Chen, Hong Deng, Yong-yu Mei, Zhi-xin Zhao, Dong-ying Xie, Zhi-liang Gao, Chan Xie and Liang Peng

Chapter 16 **The Value of Ozone in CT-Guided Drainage of Multiloculated Pyogenic Liver Abscesses** 142
Bing Li, Chuan Liu, Lang Wang, Yang Li, Yong Du, Chuan Zhang, Xiao-xue Xu and Han Feng Yang

Chapter 17 **Portal Hypertensive Polyposis in Advanced Liver Cirrhosis: The Unknown Entity?** 148
David Kara, Anna Hüsing-Kabar, Hartmut Schmidt, Inga Grünewald, Gursimran Chandhok, Miriam Maschmeier and Iyad Kabar

Chapter 18 **The Expanding Role of Systemic Therapy in the Management of Hepatocellular Carcinoma** 155
Omar Abdel-Rahman and Winson Y. Cheung

Chapter 19 **Immunotherapy in Advanced Gastric Cancer: An Overview of the Emerging Strategies** 159
Helena Magalhães, Mário Fontes-Sousa and Manuela Machado

Chapter 20 **Analysis of the Patient Information Quality and Readability on Esophagogastroduodenoscopy (EGD) on the Internet** 167
P. Priyanka, Yousaf B. Hadi and G. J. Reynolds

Chapter 21 **Dynamic Changes of the Frequency of Classic and Inflammatory Monocytes Subsets and Natural Killer Cells in Chronic Hepatitis C Patients Treated by Direct-Acting Antiviral Agents** 175
Gang Ning, Yi-ting Li, You-ming Chen, Ying Zhang, Ying-fu Zeng and Chao-shuang Lin

Chapter 22 **Evaluation of Adrenal Function in Nonhospitalized Patients with Cirrhosis** 183
Maryam Moini, Mitra Yazdani Sarvestani, Mesbah Shams and Masood Nomovi

Chapter 23 **The Relationship between Gender, Severity of Disease, Treatment Type and Employment Outcome in Patients with Inflammatory Bowel Disease in Israel** 189
Timna Naftali, Adi Eindor-Abarbanel, Nahum Ruhimovich, Ariella Bar-Gil Shitrit, Fabiana Sklerovsky-Benjaminov, Fred Konikoff, Shay Matalon, Haim Shirin, Yael Milgrom, Tomer Ziv-Baran and Efrat Broide

Chapter 24 **Laparoscopy-Assisted versus Open Hepatectomy for Live Liver Donor** 194
Bin Zhang, Yu Pan, Ke Chen, Hendi Maher, Ming-Yu Chen, He-Pan Zhu, Yi-Bin Zhu, Yi Dai, Jiang Chen and Xiu-jun Cai

Chapter 25 **Normal Uptake of ^{11}C-Acetate in Pancreas, Liver, Spleen and Suprarenal Gland in PET** 206
Bogdan Malkowski, Pawel Wareluk, Tomasz Gorycki, Katarzyna Skrobisz and Michal Studniarek

Chapter 26 **Bone Loss Prevention of Bisphosphonates in Patients with Inflammatory Bowel Disease** 210
Yan Hu, Xiaoting Chen, Xiaojing Chen, Shuang Zhang, Tianyan Jiang, Jing Chang and Yanhong Gao

Chapter 27 **New Insights in Genetic Cholestasis: From Molecular Mechanisms to Clinical Implications** 221
Eva Sticova, Milan Jirsa and Joanna PawBowska

Chapter 28 **"Fatal Gastrointestinal and Peritoneal Ischemic Disease" of Unknown Cause** 233
Jilcha Diribi Feyisa, Melka Kenea, Efrem Gashaw, Eskezyiaw Agedew Getahun, Barry Leon Hicks and Hailemichael Desalegn

Chapter 29 **Nonalcoholic Fatty Liver Disease Cirrhosis: A Review of Its Epidemiology, Risk Factors, Clinical Presentation, Diagnosis, Management and Prognosis** 237
Bei Li, Chuan Zhang and Yu-Tao Zhan

Chapter 30 **The Prevalence of Hjortsjo Crook Sign of Right Posterior Sectional Bile Duct and Bile Duct Anatomy in ERCP** 244
Hanan M. Alghamdi, Afnan F. Almuhanna, Bander F. Aldhafery, Raed M. AlSulaiman, Ahmed Almarhabi and Abdulaziz AlQurain

Chapter 31 **Current Perspectives Regarding Stem Cell-based Therapy for Liver Cirrhosis** 248
Kyeong-Ah Kwak, Hyun-Jae Cho, Jin-Young Yang and Young-Seok Park

Chapter 32 **The Effect of Prucalopride on Small Bowel Transit Time in Hospitalized Patients Undergoing Capsule Endoscopy** 267
Majid Alsahafi, Paula Cramer, Nazira Chatur and Fergal Donnellan

Permissions

List of Contributors

Index

Preface

The branch of medicine focused on the functioning of the digestive system and the diverse disorders related to it is called gastroenterology. All diseases related to the internal organs from mouth to anus, along the alimentary canal are studied under gastroenterology. Hepatology is a sub-field of gastroenterology. It is concerned with the study of organs like, liver, gallbladder, pancreas and bile ducts. Hepatitis and fatty liver disease are two of the most common liver diseases. The inflammation of the liver tissue is called hepatitis, whereas, fatty liver disease is the condition where excess fat builds up in the liver. Different approaches, evaluations, methodologies and advanced studies on clinical gastroenterology and hepatology have been included in this book. It presents researches and studies performed by experts across the globe. This book is appropriate for students seeking detailed information in this area as well as for doctors and experts.

This book is a comprehensive compilation of works of different researchers from varied parts of the world. It includes valuable experiences of the researchers with the sole objective of providing the readers (learners) with a proper knowledge of the concerned field. This book will be beneficial in evoking inspiration and enhancing the knowledge of the interested readers.

In the end, I would like to extend my heartiest thanks to the authors who worked with great determination on their chapters. I also appreciate the publisher's support in the course of the book. I would also like to deeply acknowledge my family who stood by me as a source of inspiration during the project.

Editor

1

The Effects of Extra Virgin Olive Oil on Alanine Aminotransferase, Aspartate Aminotransferase, and Ultrasonographic Indices of Hepatic Steatosis in Nonalcoholic Fatty Liver Disease Patients Undergoing Low Calorie Diet

Farzad Shidfar,[1] Samaneh Sadat Bahrololumi,[1] Saeid Doaei,[2,3] Assieh Mohammadzadeh,[4] Maryam Gholamalizadeh,[5] and Ali Mohammadimanesh[6]

[1] *Department of Nutrition, School of Public Health, Iran University of Medical Sciences, Tehran, Iran*
[2] *Natural Products and Medicinal Plants Research Center, North Khorasan University of Medical Sciences, Bojnurd, Iran*
[3] *Department of Public Health, School of Health, North Khorasan University of Medical Sciences, Bojnurd, Iran*
[4] *Department of Nutrition Sciences, Student Research Committee, Ahvaz Jundishapur University of Medical Sciences, Ahvaz, Iran*
[5] *Student Research Committee, Cancer Research Center, Shahid Beheshti University of Medical Sciences, Tehran, Iran*
[6] *Student Counseling Center, Hamadan University of Medical Sciences, Hamadan, Iran*

Correspondence should be addressed to Samaneh Sadat Bahrololumi; sama.ss74@yahoo.com

Academic Editor: Branka Filipović

Background. Coronary artery disease is the most common cause of death in the patients with nonalcoholic fatty liver disease (NAFLD). Studies have shown that there is a strong relation between the increase in the aminotransferase levels and fat accumulation in the liver with cardiovascular complications, independent of all aspects of the metabolic syndrome. This study aimed to examine the effect of virgin olive oil on alanine aminotransferase (ALT) and aspartate aminotransferase (AST) and the severity of steatosis in the NAFLD patients undergoing a weight-loss diet. *Methods.* This clinical trial was carried out on 50 patients with nonalcoholic fatty liver (mean age of 45.91 ± 9.61 years, mean BMI of 29.7 ± 0.58 Kg/m^2) and the subjects were randomly assigned to the olive oil group (receiving the equivalent of 20% of their total daily energy requirement from olive oil) or the control group (with normal consumption of oil) for 12 weeks. All the patients received a hypocaloric diet during the study. At the beginning and the end of the study, the serum levels of ALT and AST and liver steatosis were measured. *Findings.* A significant decrease in the level of ALT enzymes was observed in the control group at the end of the study ($P = 0.004$). In the olive oil group, both enzymes decreased compared to baseline measurements ($P < 0.01$). There were significant differences in the ALT and AST levels between the two groups ($P < 0.02$). The severity of liver steatosis did not change significantly during the study. *Conclusion.* The consumption of a low calorie diet enriched with olive oil, along with slight weight reduction, reinforces the desired effects of weight loss in improving the levels of the hepatic enzymes.

1. Introduction

At present, nonalcoholic fatty liver disease (NAFLD) is the most common cause of elevated serum aminotransferase [1]. In fact, elevated serum alanine aminotransferase (ALT) not only is a consequence of the NAFLD but also predicts the progression of the disease [2]. Recent findings point out that NAFLD may be linked to an increased risk of cardiovascular disease (CVD), which is the most common cause of overall mortality [3, 4]. Many long-term follow-up studies of NAFLD found a strong link between mortality related to the coronary artery disease and NAFLD. Another common reason for mortality in the NAFLD patients is hepatic failure, especially in those with nonalcoholic steatohepatitis (NASH) [5–7]. The increased levels of the liver enzymes including ALT, aspartate aminotransferase (AST), and γ-glutamyl transferase (GGT) are the markers of NAFLD and the occurrence of CVD events in both nondiabetic subjects and the patients with type

2 diabetes [8]. Studies have also shown that ALT predicts cardiovascular events, early carotid atherosclerosis [9, 10]. This suggests that NAFLD is associated with coronary heart disease (CHD), independent of the other features of the metabolic syndrome. The studies showed that the prevalence of NAFLD in Iran was relatively high and the people with NAFLD had a higher risk of 10-year CVD events than the individuals without NAFLD [4, 11].

Animal models and human studies suggest that the dietary factors play a key role in the progression of NAFLD. In particular, the amount and type of dietary fat can affect fatty infiltration and lipid peroxidation in NAFLD [12, 13]. There is little research on the effects of the type of dietary fat in NAFLD [14]. Recently, the Mediterranean diet has received attention as a diet that prevents NAFLD and cardiovascular disease. It is known that olive oil, which is rich in the monounsaturated fatty acids (MUFAs), is responsible for the major part of the beneficial effects of the Mediterranean diet [15–17].

Animal studies indicated that olive oil consumption leads to an increase in the release of the triglycerides from the liver and a decrease in the flux of free fatty acids (FFAs) from the peripheral adipose tissue back to the liver [18]. In rats, a diet rich in olive oil led to the remission of hepatic steatosis [19]. In other animal studies, liver damage was found to be decreased in rats receiving olive oil, compared to those given polyunsaturated oil [20]. However, the role of MUFA or olive oil in human NAFLD is yet to be demonstrated.

Some human studies have been conducted on the effects of a high-fat diet (40%) on the serum ALT enzyme and the severity of steatosis in patients with type 2 diabetes [21, 22].

There is only one study on the effects of olive oil in patients with NAFLD who were given a low-fat diet (20% fats) [23]. In this study no significant changes were found in the ALT and AST levels.

Considering the high prevalence of NAFLD in Iran, we have tried to examine the effects of extra virgin olive oil in a normal fat diet (30%) on the serum levels of the ALT and AST enzymes and on the severity of steatosis in the NAFLD patients on a weight-loss diet.

2. Materials and Methods

2.1. The Subjects. This clinical trial was carried out on 50 patients (19 women and 31 men) with nonalcoholic fatty liver in Tehran, Iran. The mean age was 45.91 ± 9.61 years, and the mean BMI was 29.7 ± 0.58 Kg/m^2. The clinical inclusion criteria were the increase of the AST and ALT enzymes (U/L < 30 in men and <20 in women), the elimination of all other causes for the increase in the liver enzymes (other liver diseases), age of 20–65 years, BMI of 25–40 kg/m^2, no use of hepatotoxic medicines, no history of $\geq$30 gr/d alcohol consumption, no CVD, no diabetes, no pregnancy or breast feeding, no smoking, no consumption of mineral and multivitamins supplements, no consumption of olive products, and lipid-lowering medicines in the last three months. All the subjects gave their informed consent in writing. The trial was approved by the TUMS Research Ethical Committee and was registered in the Iranian website for clinical trials (http://www.irct.ir, code: IRCT201111022709N20).

2.2. Sample Size. The sample size was calculated based on the only published paper in this area at the time of this study, which showed that a modified Mediterranean diet (rich in olive oil) caused a reduction in the ALT levels in obese patients with type 2 diabetes [21]. To determine the outcome with type one (α) and type two errors (β) of 0.05 and 0.20 (power = 80%) and 10% dropouts, 25 subjects in each group were recruited.

2.3. The Study Design. The study was a randomized, single-blind trial. The patients were randomly chosen by the qualified experts. The sample was recruited from the visiting patients in the gastroenterology ward of Imam Khomeini's Training and Treatment Hospital in Tehran, Iran. Then, the necessary briefing and the aims of the study were given to the subjects, and they were requested not to use olive oil for 10 days before starting the study. Then, the patients were divided into two groups by using the method of random allocation. The olive oil group received the hypocaloric diet enriched with olive oil (20% of total energy intake) while the control group received the hypocaloric diet with normal fat. None of the participants know about the other group and alternative treatment.

2.3.1. Experimental Design for the Weight-Loss Diet. At the beginning of the study, the weight-loss diet was set with an objective of 5% weight reduction during three months of the study. The daily energy intake recommendations were 50% carbohydrates, 20% protein, and 30% fats for both groups. First, the energy required by each individual was calculated on the basis of their age, weight, and height and the gram quantity of each macronutrient was estimated based on the information. Then, the personalized diet was set, and different food groups and the food-exchanging table were explained to the subjects.

In this diet, 20% of the total fat (30%) was allocated to olive oil or the usual culinary fat, for the olive oil group and the control group, respectively. The remaining 10% of the required daily amount of fat was provided from the other nutrition groups such as dairy, meats, and nuts. Necessary training was given to the patients in the olive oil group for the correct way of consumption of the olive oil at the beginning of the study. The patients in both groups were asked not to change the advised diet and their level of physical activities.

2.3.2. The Preparation Method for Olive Oil. The virgin olive oil used in this study belonged to the Eteka brand (Roudbar, Iran), affiliated to the Khoramshahr Extraction oil company. The required oil dosage was allocated and supplied to each patient every week. In order to reduce the bias in the consumption amount of oil, identical measuring mugs were given to each patient with the required oil amount printed on it.

Table 1: Demographic characteristics of the study subjects.

Variables	Groups		P value
	Olive oil (n = 25)	Control (n = 28)[††]	
Sex			
Male	13 (61.9%)	13 (61.9%)	0.993**
Female	8 (38.1%)	9 (40.9%)	
Age (Year)	46.14 ± 8.44	45.68 ± 10.8	0.87*
Disease duration (Year)	7.16 ± 2.4	6.91 ± 2.7	0.72*
Type of oil			0.83**
Nonhydrogenated oil[†]	15 (71.4%)	16 (73.76%)	
Hydrogenated oil	2 (9.5%)	3 (13.6%)	
Both	4 (9.1%)	3 (13/6%)	

*P value reported based on Independent Sample t-test; **P value reported based on Chi-Square test. Quantitative data represented as mean ± SD or median (min-max). Qualitative data reported as frequency (percentage). †In all of the patients using nonhydrogenated oil was sunflower oil. ††Was given usual daily consuming oil.

2.4. Measurements

2.4.1. Demographic Data. The demographic questionnaires were completed by interview. The height was measured by using the stadiometer attached to the scale with an accuracy of 0.5 cm without shoes; the weight was also measured by the Seca scale, with an accuracy of 0.5 kg, in the fasting state, and with minimum clothing without shoes. The waist circumference was measured by using the strip meter, with an accuracy of 0.5 cm, with minimum clothing in the standing position at the beginning and the end of the study. The body mass index (BMI) was calculated using weight in kg divided by meters squared. All the patients' medical and drug history were recorded. The level of physical activities was evaluated by using the physical activity international questionnaire.

2.4.2. Dietary Intake. The food record questionnaires were completed over three days (two normal days and one holiday) at the beginning and at the end of the study to estimate the consumption of energy, carbohydrates, protein, fat, vitamins C and E, beta carotene, zinc, selenium, and fiber. The nutrition information was analyzed with the Nutritionist IV software.

2.4.3. Biochemical Assessment. From each patient, 10 cc venous blood sample was taken from the vein in the left arm, after 12–14-hour fasting. The blood samples were taken with the patients in the sitting position, in the Laboratory of Imam Khomeini's Training and Treatment Center, Tehran, Iran. The blood serum was immediately separated using the centrifuge in the 3000th (temperature of 4°C) cycle. The AST and ALT hepatic enzymes in the samples were measured immediately with the enzymatic colorimetric method.

2.4.4. Ultrasound Imaging of the Liver. The severity of the steatosis was measured with an ultrasound in the afternoon, eight hours after a light breakfast. The liver ultrasound was carried out with a 3.5-MHz curvilinear probe by a radiologist. The patients were classified into three groups based on the fat accumulation in their livers, that is, slight, moderate, and severe degrees.

2.5. Statistical Analysis. The Statistical Package for the Social Sciences software (version 20, SPSS Inc., Chicago, IL, USA) was used to analyze the data. The Kolmogorov-Smirnov test was carried out to test the normality of the distribution. All variables were reported as mean ± standard deviation (SD). The Chi-Square's test and the independent t-test was used for analysing the variables such as physical activity, the type of medicines consumed, the type of edible oil used, and the severity of steatosis between two groups. Within each group, the comparisons were done by the paired-sample t-test and by the McNemar's test variables. A $P < 0.05$ was considered statistically significant.

3. Results

3.1. Demographic Data. Out of the 50 NAFLD patients who participated in this study, 4 patients were eliminated from the olive oil group and 3 patients were removed from the control group. A total of 43 patients completed the trial. The mean age of the subjects was 46.14 ± 8.44 and 45.68 ± 10.8 in the olive oil group and in the control group, respectively. Moreover, the mean BMI in the olive oil group was 29.64 ± 3.93 and in the control group was 29.9 ± 3.77 kg/m^2. There were no significant differences in gender, age, duration of disease (Table 1), weight, BMI, and waist circumstance (Table 2) between the two groups at the beginning and the end of the study. Given the energy limitation imposed at the beginning of the study, a significant weight reduction of 3.45 kg (4.33%) was observed in the olive oil group and a weight reduction of 2.89 kg (3.54%) was seen in the control group at the end of the study (P < 0/001) (Table 2).

As shown in Table 3, there was a significant decreased intake in total energy, carbohydrates, proteins, fat, PUFA, and saturated fatty acids (SFA) in each group and a significant difference in the poly unsaturated fatty acids (PUFA) and the monounsaturated fatty acids (MUFA) intake between the two groups (P < 0/001).

3.2. AST and ALT Levels and the Severity of Steatosis. There was no significant difference at the beginning of the study in the serum AST and ALT levels between the two groups. At the

Table 2: Anthropometric measurements at baseline and the end of study.

Variables	Groups		P value
	Olive oil (n = 25)	control (n = 28)	
W at baseline (cm)	79.65 ± 11	81.65 ± 13.6	0.58*
W at end-of-trial (cm)	76.2 ± 10.1	78.7 ± 12.9	0.47*
P value	<0.001**	<0.001**	
BMI at baseline (kg/m^2)	29.64 ± 3.93	29.9 ± 3.77	
BMI at end-of-trial (kg/m^2)	28.4 ± 3.91	29.13 ± 3.8	0.81*
P value	<0.001**	<0.001**	0.68*
WC at baseline (cm)	103.8 ± 10.81	104.18 ± 10.62	0.92*
WC at end-of-trial (cm)	100.61 ± 10.1	102.13 ± 10.2	0.63*
P value	<0.001**	<0.001**	

*P value reported based on Independent Sample t-test; **P value reported based on Paired t-test. Quantitative data represented as mean ± SD or median (min-max). W = weight, BMI = body mass index, and WC = waist circumference.

end of the study, a significant decrease was seen in the ALT and AST levels in the olive oil group ($P < 0.01$), compared to the control group. Moreover, there was a significant difference in both enzymes between the two groups at the end of the study ($P < 0.05$). Although the intragroup liver fat assessment revealed an improvement in both groups (more in the olive oil), there was no significant statistical difference in steatosis between the two groups at the end of the study (Table 4).

4. Discussion

In the present study, there was a significant decrease in weight and the ALT and AST levels observed at the end of the study, in both the olive oil group and the control group. Moreover, decrease in the ALT and AST levels in the olive oil group was significantly higher than the control group.

Weight reduction is the first treatment line in the patients suffering from nonalcoholic fatty liver and can motivate the improvement of steatosis and the aminotransferase levels [24]. One study has observed that 5% of weight decrease is enough to decrease the serum's ALT value and to improve steatosis, while a minimum of 9% weight loss is necessary for a significant improvement of NASH [25]. Another study indicated that the patients with more than 7% of their base weight reduction experienced significant improvement in steatosis, inflammation, and the score of NASH tissue activity compared to the patients whose weight loss is less than 7% [26]. Moreover, a weight-loss diet with a goal of 8% initial weight decrease in obese women for a period of 3 to 6 months showed that the effect of weight loss on the improvement of steatosis depends on the rate of weight loss and the initial content of liver fat [27]. In our research, none of the patients had a high or severe steatosis at the beginning of the study and the weight loss was less than 7% in both groups at the end of the study.

Dietary components, particularly the type and the amount of fats, are crucial for liver fat accumulation and are responsible for 15% of the liver fat content. The dietary fats can exert their role in liver steatosis both directly and indirectly (via its influence on adipose tissues) [28]. The studies carried out in this field are limited to the survey of the effects of the modified Mediterranean diet with high fat content and MUFA and its comparison to a low-fat diet in the patients with insulin resistance.

Our research is the first study that has surveyed the effects of the MUFA (from olive oil source) in a diet with normal fat content (30%) administered to the patients with nonalcoholic fatty liver. In one study a balanced-fat diet rich in olive oil rather than sunflower oil after one month leading to a decrease in steatosis and the hepatic enzymes in rats was observed. In human, one study reported that a high-fat (45%) and high-MUFA diet lead to the decrease of the ALT enzymes [21]. These findings are in concurrence with our study. In another study, the patients with NAFLD in the intervention group received a high-MUFA diet (olive oil or canola) for six months [23]. The total content of fat in their diet was 20% of the daily energy intake. Contrary to our study, the daily consumption of 20 g of olive oil had no effect on the serum aminotransferase. The low-fat diet in this study could be a reason for the significant decrease in steatosis. However, the improvement in liver fat content was not adequate for a significant decrease in the aminotransferases.

In a study in the patients with type 2 diabetes it was observed that the percentage of liver fat content in the MUFA-receiving groups with or without exercise had a significant decrease as compared to the groups receiving carbohydrate (CHO) with or without exercise [22].

The beneficial effects of the MUFAs on the hepatic fat content can be explained by the more rapid oxidization of the MUFAs than the saturated fatty acids in the postprandial phase. The more favorable MUFAs deposit in the adipose tissue rather than in the liver following a diet rich in MUFAs may help avoid fat deposition in the liver [29]. In addition, a high-MUFA diet stimulates the activity of lipoprotein lipase more than a diet rich in saturated fats that leads to increase in clearance of circulating triglyceride-rich lipoproteins [30]. In addition to type, the amount of fat also plays a role in the pathogenesis and, probably, in the treatment of fatty liver as well. In our study, the amount of MUFA was less than 20%.

On the other hand, recent studies on nutritional genomics supported a key role of gene-diet interaction in NAFLD development [31]. For example, it is suggested that the obesity-associated (FTO) gene levels in the liver are involved

TABLE 3: Dietary intake of study participants, at baseline and after intervention.

Variables	Groups	Before Mean ± SD	After Mean ± SD	P value■
Energy (Kcal/day)	Olive oil	2613.8 ± 662.3	1756.5 ± 538	<0.001
	Control	2449.2 ± 723.2	1695 ± 527.1	0.001
	P value*	0.44	0.7	
Protein (g/day)	Olive oil	79.5 ± 24.28	63.92 ± 23.8	0.001
	Control	82.68 ± 23.18	61.5 ± 22.13	0.005
	P value*	0.69	0.74	
Carbohydrates (g/day)	Olive oil	374.16 ± 79.1	252.5 ± 53.7	0.004
	Control	334.1 ± 62.6	246.6 ± 49.3	0.005
	P value*	0.22	0.832	
FAT (g/day)	Olive oil	92.41 ± 55.38	57.3 ± 23.18	0.001
	Control	86.03 ± 36.64	55.33 ± 20.1	<0.001
	P value*	0.58	0.59	
SFA (g/day)	Olive oil	23.94 ± 9.5	13.67 ± 8.18	0.003
	Control	28.93 ± 8.45	14.03 ± 6.09	0.001
	P value*	0.411	0.870	
MUFA (g/day)	Olive oil	24.95 ± 9.28	29.27 ± 10.76	0.47
	Control	23.53 ± 10.81	†13.45 ± 6.56	0.19
	P value*	0.873	<0.001	
PUFA (g/day)	Olive oil	37.88 ± 14.63	12.43 ± 4.36	0.002
	Control	32.52 ± 11.8	†26.3 ± 8.4	0.003
	P value*	0.275	<0.001	
Fiber (g/day)	Olive oil	12.49 ± 5.8	10.94 ± 6.5	0.333
	Control	13.4 ± 5.32	11.69 ± 6.23	0.291
	P value*	0.595	0.070	
Beta-carotene (μg/d)	Olive oil	245/7 ± 57.28	226.68 ± 30.76	0.234
	Control	239.23 ± 95.81	218.82 ± 72.54	0.171
	P value	0.708	0.895	
Vitamin E (mg/day)	Olive oil	5.1 ± 3.5	2.53 ± 2.64	0.174
	Control	4.31 ± 3.1	2.16 ± 1.79	0.122
	P value*	0.634	0.587	
Vitamin C (mg/day)	Olive oil	61.25 ± 42.95	70.95 ± 32.95	0.621
	Control	63.9 ± 22.72	68.05 ± 32.51	0.404
	P value*	0.863	0.761	
Selenium (mg/day)	Olive oil	0.09 ± 0.04	0.07 ± 0.04	0.134
	Control	0.13 ± 0.17	0.12 ± 0.12	0.823
	P value*	0.366	0.277	
Zinc (mg/day)	Olive oil	7.04 ± 4.62	10.94 ± 6.5	0.895
	Control	8/04 ± 4.9	11.69 ± 6.23	0.767
	P value*	0.711	0.615	

*P value reported based on Independent Sample t-test; ■P value reported based on Paired t-test; SFAs = saturated fatty acids, PUFAs = polyunsaturated fatty acids, and MUFAs = monounsaturated fatty acids.

in oxidative stress and lipid deposition, which characterize NAFLD [32]. The level of FTO gene expression is related to the level of dietary macronutrients [33]. Interestingly, the FTO genotype can affect the success of lifestyle interventions in the prevention and treatment of obesity [34].

Moreover, the observed difference may be related to the method of measuring the fatty contents [35]. The NMR (Nuclear Magnetic Resonance) or the spectroscopic golden standard method is used for measuring the existing fat percentage in the liver. It has high precision and accuracy and is considered as the strength of the mentioned study, as described by the researcher. However, in our study, ultrasonography was used because of its cost effectiveness and prevalence. This method has some limitations, including the fact that the results obtained by it depend on the mastery and expertise skills of the operator and the detecting sensitivity

Table 4: Aminotransferase and severity of steatosis at the start and the end of study.

Variables	Groups	Before Mean ± SD	After Mean ± SD	
				P value■
ALT (IU/dl)	Olive oil	48 ± 12.9	35.71 ± 11.33	<0.001
	Control	50.82 ± 10.37	46.18 ± 10.26	0.004
	P value*	0.43	0.003	
AST (IU/dl)	Olive oil	34.53 ± 5.3	26.1 ± 5.4	<0.001
	Control	34.68 ± 8.9	32.28 ± 2.2	0.25
	P value*	0.94	0.002	
				P value©
Steatosis *N*(%)				
Slight	Olive oil	10 (47.61%)	15 (71.42%)	0.008
Moderate		11 (52.38%)	6 (28.57%)	
Severe		0	0	
Slight	Control	7 (31.81%)	10 (45.46%)	0.17
Moderate		15 (68.18%)	12 (54.54%)	
Severe		0	0	
	P value**	0.23	0.13	

**P* value reported based on Paired Sample *t*-test. ■*P* value reported based on Independent Sample *t*-test. ©*P* value reported based on McNemar. ***P* value reported based on Chi-Square. $P < 0.05$: significant.

of ultrasonography decreases with a degree of fat infiltration less than 30% [2]. Considering the low grade of steatosis in our patients, in contrast to the Nigma study where the patients had higher liver fat, the use of ultrasonography may prevent the obtaining of accurate information on the changes of liver steatosis. Another limitation of this study was sample size and short follow-up duration. A larger group of patients and longer follow-up period are needed to confirm the results.

5. Conclusion

In conclusion, the results of this study suggest that normal fat percentage (30%) in a diet containing olive oil (consumption the equivalent of 20% of total calorie intake from virgin olive oil) along with slight weight loss (approximately 5%) reinforces the desired effects of weight loss in improving the levels of the ALT and AST enzymes.

Acknowledgments

This paper is derived from the M.S. thesis of Samaneh Sadat Bahrololumi, submitted to Tehran University of Medical Sciences, Tehran, Iran (Code: 15369). This paper was supported by the Khoramshahr Oil Company. The authors would like to thank Javad Salimi, head of the oil factory of Ganjeh, Roudbar, and Aboozar Falahzadeh, head of the oil factory laboratory.

References

[1] C. D. Byrne, R. Olufad, K. D. Bruce, F. R. Cagampang, and M. H. Ahmed, "Metabolic disturbances in non-alcoholic fatty liver disease," *Clinical Science*, vol. 116, no. 7, pp. 539–564, 2009.

[2] M. Obika and H. Noguchi, "Diagnosis and evaluation of nonalcoholic fatty liver disease," *Journal of Diabetes Research*, vol. 2012, Article ID 145754, 12 pages, 2012.

[3] B. Baharvand-Ahmadi, K. Sharifi, and M. Namdari, "Prevalence of non-alcoholic fatty liver disease in patients with coronary artery disease," *ARYA Atherosclerosis*, vol. 12, no. 4, pp. 201–205, 2016.

[4] N. Motamed, B. Rabiee, H. Poustchi et al., "Non-alcoholic fatty liver disease (NAFLD) and 10-year risk of cardiovascular diseases," *Clinics and Research in Hepatology and Gastroenterology*, vol. 41, no. 1, pp. 31–38, 2017.

[5] N. Rafiq and Z. M. Younossi, "Nonalcoholic fatty liver disease: a practical approach to evaluation and management," *Clinics in Liver Disease*, vol. 13, no. 2, pp. 249–266, 2009.

[6] J. P. Ong, A. Pitts, and Z. M. Younossi, "Increased overall mortality and liver-related mortality in non-alcoholic fatty liver disease," *Journal of Hepatology*, vol. 49, no. 4, pp. 608–612, 2008.

[7] J. P. Ong and Z. M. Younossi, "Epidemiology and natural history of NAFLD and NASH," *Clinics in Liver Disease*, vol. 11, no. 1, pp. 1-16, 2007.

[8] K. G. Tolman, V. Fonseca, M. H. Tan, and A. Dalpiaz, "Narrative review: Hepatobiliary disease in type 2 diabetes mellitus," *Annals of Internal Medicine*, vol. 141, no. 12, pp. 946–956, 2004.

[9] J. Shen, J. Zhang, J. Wen, Q. Ming, and Y. Xu, "Correlation of serum alanine aminotransferase and aspartate aminotransferase with coronary heart disease," *International Journal of Clinical and Experimental Medicine*, vol. 8, no. 3, pp. 4399–4404, 2015.

[10] R. K. Schindhelm, J. M. Dekker, G. Nijpels et al., "Alanine aminotransferase predicts coronary heart disease events: a 10-year follow-up of the hoorn study," *Atherosclerosis*, vol. 191, no. 2, pp. 391–396, 2007.

[11] I. Moghaddasifar, K. B. Lankarani, M. Moosazadeh et al., "Prevalence of non-alcoholic fatty liver disease and its related factors in Iran," *International Journal of Organ Transplantation Medicine*, vol. 7, no. 3, pp. 149–160, 2016.

[12] O. Molendi-Coste, V. Legry, and I. A. Leclercq, "Dietary lipids and NAFLD: suggestions for improved nutrition," *Acta Gastro-Enterologica Belgica*, vol. 73, no. 4, pp. 431–436, 2010.

[13] R. Buettner, K. G. Parhofer, M. Woenckhaus et al., "Defining high-fat-diet rat models: metabolic and molecular effects of different fat types," *Molecular Endocrinology*, vol. 36, no. 3, pp. 485–501, 2006.

[14] S. Zelber-Sagi, V. Ratziu, and R. Oren, "Nutrition and physical activity in NAFLD: an overview of the epidemiological evidence," *World Journal of Gastroenterology*, vol. 17, no. 29, pp. 3377–3389, 2011.

[15] M. C. Ryan, C. Itsiopoulos, T. Thodis et al., "The Mediterranean diet improves hepatic steatosis and insulin sensitivity in individuals with non-alcoholic fatty liver disease," *Journal of Hepatology*, vol. 59, no. 1, pp. 138–143, 2013.

[16] N. Assy, F. Nassar, G. Nasser, and M. Grosovski, "Olive oil consumption and non-alcoholic fatty liver disease," *World Journal of Gastroenterology*, vol. 15, no. 15, pp. 1809–1815, 2009.

[17] S. Zelber-Sagi, F. Salomone, and L. Mlynarsky, "The Mediterranean dietary pattern as the diet of choice for non-alcoholic fatty liver disease: evidence and plausible mechanisms," *Liver International*, vol. 37, no. 7, pp. 936–949, 2017.

[18] O. Hussein, M. Grosovski, E. Lasri, S. Svalb, U. Ravid, and N. Assy, "Monounsaturated fat decreases hepatic lipid content in non-alcoholic fatty liver disease in rats," *World Journal of Gastroenterology*, vol. 13, no. 3, pp. 361–368, 2007.

[19] R. Hernández, E. Martínez-Lara, A. Cañuelo et al., "Steatosis recovery after treatment with a balanced sunflower of olive oil-based diet: Involvement of perisinusoidal stellate cells," *World Journal of Gastroenterology*, vol. 11, no. 47, pp. 7480–7485, 2005.

[20] B. Szende, F. Timár, and B. Hargitai, "Olive oil decreases liver damage in rats caused by carbon tetrachloride (CCl4)," *Experimental and Toxicologic Pathology*, vol. 46, no. 4-5, pp. 355–359, 1994.

[21] A. Fraser, R. Abel, D. A. Lawlor, D. Fraser, and A. Elhayany, "A modified Mediterranean diet is associated with the greatest reduction in alanine aminotransferase levels in obese type 2 diabetes patients: Results of a quasi-randomised controlled trial," *Diabetologia*, vol. 51, no. 9, pp. 1616–1622, 2008.

[22] L. Bozzetto, A. Prinster, G. Annuzzi et al., "Liver fat is reduced by an isoenergetic MUFA diet in a controlled randomized study in type 2 diabetic patients," *Diabetes Care*, vol. 35, no. 7, pp. 1429–1435, 2012.

[23] P. Nigam, S. Bhatt, A. Misra et al., "Effect of a 6-month intervention with cooking oils containing a high concentration of monounsaturated fatty acids (olive and canola oils) compared with control oil in male asian indians with nonalcoholic fatty liver disease," *Diabetes Technology & Therapeutics*, vol. 16, no. 4, pp. 255–261, 2014.

[24] B. P. Lam and Z. M. Younossi, "Treatment regimens for non-alcoholic fatty liver disease," *Annals of Hepatology*, vol. 8, supplement 1, pp. S51–S59, 2009.

[25] S. A. Harrison, W. Fecht, E. M. Brunt, and B. A. Neuschwander-Tetri, "Orlistat for overweight subjects with nonalcoholic steatohepatitis: a randomized, prospective trial," *Hepatology*, vol. 49, no. 1, pp. 80–86, 2009.

[26] K. Promrat, D. E. Kleiner, H. M. Niemeier et al., "Randomized controlled trial testing the effects of weight loss on nonalcoholic steatohepatitis," *Hepatology*, vol. 51, no. 1, pp. 121–129, 2010.

[27] M. Tiikkainen, R. Bergholm, S. Vehkavaara et al., "Effects of identical weight loss on body composition and features of insulin resistance in obese women with high and low liver fat content," *Diabetes*, vol. 52, no. 3, pp. 701–707, 2003.

[28] K. L. Donnelly, C. I. Smith, S. J. Schwarzenberg, J. Jessurun, M. D. Boldt, and E. J. Parks, "Sources of fatty acids stored in liver and secreted via lipoproteins in patients with nonalcoholic fatty liver disease," *The Journal of Clinical Investigation*, vol. 115, no. 5, pp. 1343–1351, 2005.

[29] J. P. DeLany, M. M. Windhauser, C. M. Champagne, and G. A. Bray, "Differential oxidation of individual dietary fatty acids in humans," *American Journal of Clinical Nutrition*, vol. 72, no. 4, pp. 905–911, 2000.

[30] A. A. Rivellese, R. Giacco, G. Annuzzi et al., "Effects of monounsaturated vs. saturated fat on postprandial lipemia and adipose tissue lipases in type 2 diabetes," *Clinical Nutrition*, vol. 27, no. 1, pp. 133–141, 2008.

[31] P. Dongiovanni and L. Valenti, "A nutrigenomic approach to non-alcoholic fatty liver disease," *International Journal of Molecular Sciences*, vol. 18, no. 7, article 1534, 2017.

[32] J. Guo, W. Ren, A. Li et al., "Fat mass and obesity-associated gene enhances oxidative stress and lipogenesis in nonalcoholic fatty liver disease," *Digestive Diseases and Sciences*, vol. 58, no. 4, pp. 1004–1009, 2013.

[33] S. Doaei, N. Kalantari, N. K. Mohammadi, G. A. Tabesh, and M. Gholamalizadeh, "Macronutrients and the FTO gene expression in hypothalamus; a systematic review of experimental studies," *Indian Heart Journal*, vol. 69, no. 2, pp. 277–281, 2017.

[34] N. Kalantari, S. Doaei, N. Keshavarz-Mohammadi, M. Gholamalizadeh, and N. Pazan, "Review of studies on the fat mass and obesity-associated (FTO) gene interactions with environmental factors affecting on obesity and its impact on lifestyle interventions," *ARYA Atherosclerosis*, vol. 12, no. 6, pp. 281–290, 2016.

[35] X. Ma, N. S. Holalkere, R. A. Kambadakone, M. Mino-Kenudson, P. F. Hahn, and D. V. Sahani, "Imaging-based quantification of hepatic fat: methods and clinical applications," *RadioGraphics*, vol. 29, no. 5, pp. 1253–1277, 2009.

2

A Contemporary Review of the Treatment Landscape and the Role of Predictive and Prognostic Biomarkers in Pancreatic Adenocarcinoma

Irene S. Yu[1] and Winson Y. Cheung[2]

[1]*Division of Medical Oncology, Department of Medicine, British Columbia Cancer Agency, University of British Columbia, Vancouver, BC, Canada*
[2]*Section of Medical Oncology, Department of Oncology, Tom Baker Cancer Centre, University of Calgary, Calgary, AB, Canada*

Correspondence should be addressed to Winson Y. Cheung; winson.cheung@ahs.ca

Academic Editor: Kiran L. Sharma

Pancreatic cancer continues to represent one of the leading causes of cancer-related morbidity and mortality in the developed world. Over the past decade, novel systemic therapy combination regimens have contributed to clinically meaningful and statistically significant improvements in overall survival as compared to conventional monotherapy. However, the prognosis for most patients remains guarded secondary to the advanced stages of disease at presentation. There is growing consensus that outcomes can be further optimized with the use of predictive and prognostic biomarkers whereby the former can be enriching for patients who would benefit from therapies and the latter can inform decision-making regarding the need and timing of advanced care planning. One of the challenges of current biomarkers is the lack of standardization across clinical practices such that comparability between jurisdictions can be difficult or even impossible. This inconsistency can impede widespread implementation of their use. In this review article, we provide a comprehensive overview of the contemporary treatment options for pancreatic cancer and we offer some insights into the existing landscape and future directions of biomarker development for this disease.

1. Background

In Canada, pancreatic cancer represents the fourth leading cause of cancer-related mortality [1]. In 2017 alone, 5,500 Canadians were diagnosed with the disease, and 4,800 of these cases resulted in death [1]. It is further projected that the number of deaths will surpass that of breast cancer in the near future [2]. Among all cancers, pancreatic cancer carries the lowest five-year overall survival rate at less than 10% [1, 3], owing largely to the advanced stage of disease at the time of diagnosis. While surgery remains the only curative modality, greater than 60% of patients with pancreatic cancer are considered unresectable at presentation [1]. Without appropriate treatments, median overall survival is estimated to be only 3 to 5 months [4]. Pancreatic tumors are classified into exocrine and endocrine subtypes. The former category constitutes approximately 90% of pancreatic malignancies and it also carries significantly worse prognosis than the latter. Advances in systemic therapies for unresectable disease in the past decade have helped to improve outcomes, but further progress is required since the prognosis for the majority of cases continues to be guarded. There is significant interest and an emerging body of evidence to support the development and use of biomarkers to help risk-stratify patients based on their outcomes and to identify subpopulations that may benefit from specific therapies. In this review article, we offer a comprehensive and contemporary review of the treatment landscape and the role of predictive and prognostic biomarkers in the setting of pancreatic cancers.

2. History of Systemic Therapies

In the 1950s, fluoropyrimidine-based chemotherapy was the mainstay of treatment for unresectable pancreatic adenocarcinoma (PDAC) [5]. Multiple studies have evaluated different 5-fluorouracil (5-FU) combinations, including pairing it with anthracyclines, platinums, vinca alkaloids, alkylating agents, and mitomycin. However, none of these studies showed an improvement in overall survival (OS) when compared to 5-FU alone [6, 7]. In 1997, Burris III et al. demonstrated that gemcitabine was superior to 5-FU in conferring "clinical benefit," which was defined as better appetite, less weight loss, and lower need for pain control. Gemcitabine was also associated with a modest improvement in median OS from 4.41 months to 5.65 months ($p = 0.0025$) [8]. Because of this finding, gemcitabine was approved as the preferred first-line therapy. Subsequent trials examining various gemcitabine combinations, such as with capecitabine, platinum agents, irinotecan, and pemetrexed [9–13], failed to extend survival further.

For patients with good performance status, however, Cunningham et al. showed a trend towards improvement in OS (7.1 versus 6.2 months, $p = 0.08$) and 12-month progression-free survival (PFS) (13.9 versus 8.4%, $p = 0.004$) with the use of gemcitabine plus capecitabine [9]. A post hoc analysis by Herrmann et al. supported this observation, where high functioning patients (KPS 90–100%) had statistically improved OS (10.1 versus 7.4 months, $p = 0.014$) [14]. Of note, uptake of this combination has not been high, possibly because of worse toxicities.

Likewise, a phase III National Cancer Institute of Canada randomized controlled trial investigated the addition of erlotinib to gemcitabine and also found a statistically significant improvement in OS (6.24 versus 5.91 months, $p = 0.023$) and PFS (3.75 versus 3.55 months, $p = 0.004$) [15]. This combination was approved, but the additional survival benefit of only 0.33 months in the context of excess adverse effects and significant increase in costs to the healthcare system have limited the widespread adoption of this regimen in most countries [16]. Hence, gemcitabine monotherapy remained for a long time the primary standard of care for unresectable PDAC.

3. Recent Therapeutic Advances

In the past decade, several landmark trials in the treatment of advanced PDAC have been published, renewing optimism for this disease. The PRODIGE 4 (ACCORD 11) phase II/III trial randomized 342 patients with untreated metastatic PDAC to single agent gemcitabine versus FOLFIRINOX. Median OS (11.1 months versus 6.8 months, $p < 0.001$) and PFS (6.4 versus 3.3 months, $p < 0.001$) were significantly higher in the FOLFIRINOX group although there were increased rates of grade 3/4 toxicities [17]. This landmark study altered the treatment landscape since FOLFIRINOX represented the first regimen to provide a survival benefit of over 4 months compared to gemcitabine. However, the administration of multiagent chemotherapy requires a good performance status, which proved to be challenging in this patient population where the majority can be significantly frail and debilitated by the aggressive biology that is typically associated with pancreatic cancer.

One reason why PDAC has been resistant to most conventional chemotherapy choices is that there is dense desmoplastic stroma surrounding the pancreas, which is perceived to impede chemotherapy delivery [18]. Efforts to overcome this include increasing the bioavailability of chemotherapy to the tumor site. An example of this is the use of nab-paclitaxel, which represents an albumin-bound formulation of paclitaxel. Nab-paclitaxel has shown antitumor activity in different malignancies that overexpress the albumin-binding protein SPARC, including cancers of the breast, lung, and skin [19–21]. In the phase I/II trial by Von Hoff et al., nab-paclitaxel combined with gemcitabine showed a median OS of 12.2 months and a 1-year survival rate of 48% [22]. The subsequent phase III MPACT study randomized 861 patients to nab-paclitaxel plus gemcitabine versus gemcitabine alone. The addition of nab-paclitaxel improved both median OS (8.5 versus 6.7 months, $p < 0.001$) and PFS (5.5 versus 3.7 months, $p < 0.001$) [23]. Tumor response rates were also higher for the combination (23% versus 7%, $p < 0.001$). Cumulative toxicities of the doublet regimen were higher, namely, in terms of myelosuppression (38 versus 27%) and peripheral neuropathy (17 versus 1%). Despite these limitations, the combination of gemcitabine and nab-paclitaxel became another first-line option for patients, particularly for the many patients who were deemed to be ineligible or unfit to receive the more potent FOLFIRINOX.

With the recent introduction of FOLFIRINOX and gemcitabine plus nab-paclitaxel into the treatment paradigm, there is growing interest in developing second-line therapies. The NAPOLI trial compared the novel agent nanoliposomal irinotecan (MM-398) versus 5-FU/leucovorin versus nanoliposomal irinotecan plus 5-FU/leucovorin in patients who failed first-line gemcitabine. MM-398 is a formulation in which irinotecan is encapsulated into liposomal-based nanoparticles, with the goal of prolonging the active drug circulation time. The authors concluded that combination nanoliposomal irinotecan plus 5-FU/leucovorin significantly improved median OS (6.1 versus 4.2 months, $p = 0.012$) and PFS (3.1 versus 1.5 months, $p = 0.0001$) compared to 5-FU/leucovorin alone [24]. Single agent nanoliposomal irinotecan did not significantly improve outcomes. Based on these results, nanoliposomal irinotecan in combination with 5-FU/leucovorin has recently been approved for second-line treatment of patients who experience disease progression or intolerance to gemcitabine.

4. The Need for Biomarkers

Currently, either FOLFIRINOX or gemcitabine plus nab-paclitaxel is used in the first-line treatment setting for advanced PDAC. Most clinicians will base their treatment selection on a number of factors, including comorbidities, performance status, and patient preference. However, the decision can be frequently difficult since there are very few tools that can accurately predict response to the chosen therapy. Likewise, the prognosis of patients can vary to some degree and treatment selection can be influenced by the patients' anticipated lifespan. Thus, there is a growing need to explore predictive and prognostic biomarkers to aid in the personalized treatment of PDAC. This will become increasingly relevant as more therapeutic options are developed and introduced.

The National Cancer Institute defines a biomarker as "a biological molecule found in blood, other body fluids, or tissues that is a sign of normal or abnormal process, or of a condition or disease" [25]. Biomarkers encompass a variety of molecules, including peptides, proteins, nucleic acids, and antibodies. Multiple clinical uses of biomarkers in oncology have been described. A biomarker is defined as predictive if the treatment effect varies for biomarker-positive patients compared to biomarker-negative patients [26]. In contrast, prognostic biomarkers provide information on a likely cancer outcome independent of treatment received and can be applied even in the absence of any treatment [26]. Currently, there are no FDA-approved predictive or prognostic biomarkers for PDAC even though there is a significant clinical need to identify and validate these to define subpopulations of patients that will likely benefit from a specific therapy or patients that may require an urgent intervention to avoid negative outcomes.

5. Landscape of Predictive Biomarkers

5.1. Microsatellite Instability. Microsatellite instability (MSI) is a hypermutable phenotype with a predisposition to genetic mutations due to a deficient mismatch repair (dMMR) system. The literature has supported the use of MSI status as a predictive and prognostic biomarker in colorectal cancer (CRC). MSI-high (MSI-H) patients are shown to not derive benefit from adjuvant 5-FU [27, 28]. They also have lower rates of recurrence, delayed time to recurrence, and improved survival compared to their proficient MMR counterparts [29]. Approximately 15% of CRC tumors are dMMR; this contrasts the less than 1% of sporadic PDAC [30, 31]. More recently, MSI status has been utilized to predict response to immunotherapy agents in the treatment of metastatic CRC. Both pembrolizumab and nivolumab achieved significant objective response and disease control rates [32–34] and have been approved for use after failing conventional chemotherapy in metastatic CRC with dMMR. Ipilimumab was evaluated in a phase II trial for unresectable PDAC, but it failed to show tumor response in 27 patients [35], but patients were not explicitly tested for MMR status. Recently, the indication for pembrolizumab has been extended to all MSI-H unresectable or metastatic solid tumors after progression on conventional therapies, including PDAC. This decision was based on the study by Le et al., which enrolled 86 patients with 12 different tumor types and included some PDAC cases. Objective radiographic responses were achieved in 46 (53%) patients, and complete responses were seen in 18 (21%) patients; median PFS and OS were not reached in the latest publication [36]. There were 8 (9%) pancreatic cases; 5 (62%) patients showed an objective response rate and 6 (75%) showed disease control. Despite the small sample size, this presents an appealing option for the treatment of dMMR PDAC, underscoring that further studies are warranted. However, the small proportion of pancreatic tumors that are MSI-H in the general population will likely limit the impact of this biomarker.

5.2. BRCA Mutations. BRCA1/2 are tumor suppressor genes involved in the repair of double-stranded DNA breaks via homologous recombination. Defective BRCA genes lead to the use of alternative low-fidelity repair pathways and have been associated with the development of multiple malignancies including breast, ovarian, prostate, and pancreatic cancers [37–40]. The Breast Cancer Linkage Consortium estimated the overall relative risk of PDAC to be 2.26 and 3.51 higher than the general population for BRCA1 and BRCA2 mutation carriers, respectively [41, 42]. There is a growing body of evidence for BRCA's role as a predictive biomarker for response to platinum agents and poly(ADP-ribose) polymerase (PARP) inhibitors. Platinum agents cause cross-linking of DNA to induce double-stranded DNA breaks, which are ineffectively repaired in those with a BRCA mutation. PARP aids in the repair of single-stranded DNA breaks and nucleoside base damage; PARP inhibition leads to the transformation of single-stranded breaks into double-stranded breaks. Similarly, this is hypothesized to be cytotoxic in cells with defective BRCA repair mechanisms.

The addition of platinum agents to gemcitabine has previously been reported to be ineffective in extending survival compared to gemcitabine alone in multiple studies [10, 43, 44]. Sonnenblick et al. described the use of cisplatin plus gemcitabine in a PDAC patient with a BRCA2 1153 insertion T mutation. There was initial progression on gemcitabine monotherapy, but the addition of cisplatin resulted in a complete radiographic and serologic (CA19-9) response [45]. A retrospective review by Lowery et al. studied 15 patients with BRCA mutations and locally advanced or metastatic PDAC; five of six patients receiving first-line platinum chemotherapy showed partial or complete response by RECIST criteria [46]. Subsequently, Golan et al. performed a review with 71 patients with BRCA mutations and observed a superior OS for those with stage III/IV disease treated with platinum compared to nonplatinum chemotherapy (22 versus 9 months, $p = 0.039$) [47].

Similarly, Fogelman et al. illustrated a case where iniparib, a PARP-1 inhibitor, was used in combination with gemcitabine in a patient with a known BRCA mutation. The patient initially had her disease resected followed by adjuvant chemoradiation; subsequently, her disease recurrence was treated with 3 cycles of iniparib plus gemcitabine and achieved complete pathologic response [48]. A phase II trial by Kaufman et al. enrolled a spectrum of BRCA1/2-associated cancers to investigate the safety and efficacy of the PARP inhibitor olaparib; 23 PDAC cases were included. A response rate of 22% was demonstrated in heavily pretreated patients with metastatic PDAC, with an average of two prior lines of treatment [49]. Median OS and PFS were 9.8 and 4.6 months, respectively [49].

Domchek et al. presented RUCAPANC at the 2016 ASCO Annual Meeting, which included 19 BRCA-mutated patients treated with rucaparib. Objective response rate was 11% and disease control rate (defined as partial response or stable disease > 12 weeks) was 32% [50]. There was a suggestion that individuals less heavily pretreated derived more benefit as all responders only received one prior line of chemotherapy.

With the growing evidence for the role of platinum agents and PARP inhibitors in this patient subgroup, the National Comprehensive Cancer Network (NCCN) has recommended consideration of a first-line platinum-based regimen for advanced PDAC in the setting of a BRCA mutation [51]. The ongoing phase III POLO trial is investigating the effectiveness of maintenance olaparib monotherapy after platinum therapy and may provide further direction on the use of PARP inhibitors in PDAC.

5.3. SPARC. Secreted protein acidic and rich in cysteine (SPARC), also known as osteonectin, is an albumin-binding protein involved in mediating interactions between cells and their extracellular environment during morphogenesis, tissue remodeling, and angiogenesis [52]. SPARC is frequently upregulated in tumor tissue and it is implicated to play a role in cancer development and growth. In PDAC, SPARC is hypothesized to facilitate the effective uptake of nab-paclitaxel. In a phase I/II trial by Von Hoff et al. investigating the safety and efficacy of gemcitabine plus nab-paclitaxel, SPARC levels were also evaluated. SPARC status was available for thirty-six patients who were divided into high- and low-level SPARC groups; a higher median OS was observed in the high SPARC cohort (17.8 versus 8.1 months, $p = 0.0431$) [22]. SPARC found in pancreatic stromal tissue correlated with OS but not SPARC derived from tumor cells. Nab-paclitaxel markedly depleted tumor stroma, while significantly enhancing intratumoral gemcitabine concentrations by 2.8-fold. Overall, nab-paclitaxel was thought to target stromal SPARC to incite an antidesmoplastic response to effectively deliver gemcitabine to the tumor site.

In a post hoc analysis, Hidalgo et al. explored the relationship between SPARC and clinical outcomes using data from the phase III MPACT trial. Contrary to prior evidence, SPARC levels from the stroma, tumor epithelium, and plasma were not found to be predictive of the overall response rate to nab-paclitaxel and gemcitabine [53]. Currently, PDAC samples are not routinely sent for SPARC testing and further studies are required to better characterize the role of SPARC as a predictive biomarker for response to nab-paclitaxel and gemcitabine. Unfortunately, there is a lack of standardization in grading SPARC expressivity, which may have influenced the seemingly contradictory study findings.

5.4. Human ENT1. Human equilibrative nucleoside transporter 1 (hENT1) aids in the movement of nucleosides across the cell membrane for nucleotide synthesis via the salvage pathway. Both gemcitabine and 5-FU are nucleoside analogues. Thus, nucleoside transporter expression levels may influence their uptake into tumor cells. Mohelnikova-Duchonova et al. demonstrated that PDAC cell lines have decreased levels of hENT1 mRNA compared to nonmalignant pancreatic tissue [54], which may contribute to the intrinsic chemorefractory nature of PDAC. In vitro studies have shown that increased hENT1 expression can play a role in intratumoral gemcitabine and 5-FU levels, although findings have been conflicting and other intracellular processes may be at play [55, 56]. Prior studies have shown signals whereby high levels of hENT1 in PDAC tumors that were treated with adjuvant gemcitabine predicted longer survival [57, 58], but the same did not apply to 5-FU treated patients [59]. Neoptolemos et al. investigated the therapeutic predictability of hENT1 utilizing tumor samples from the adjuvant ESPAC1/3 trials; 352 patients who received either gemcitabine or 5-FU were included. Survival between the two groups was similar, but the low-hENT1 gemcitabine group had lower survival compared to the high-hENT1 cohort (17.1 versus 26.2 months, $p = 0.002$) [60]. There was no survival benefit between low- and high-hENT1 expression groups in patients who received 5-FU.

The data on the use of hENT1 as a biomarker in the metastatic setting have been less robust. Giovannetti et al. demonstrated that high-hENT1 expression was associated with significantly longer median OS (22.34 versus 12.42 months, $p < 0.001$) and disease-free survival (DFS) (20.43 versus 9.26 months, $p < 0.05$) in those who received gemcitabine, but the patient population was heterogenous with approximately 50% of patients having stage III/IV disease [61]. In a large phase II study conducted by Poplin et al., no difference in OS was observed between the low-hENT1 and the high-hENT1 groups who received gemcitabine [62]. Overall, hENT1 testing is limited to the clinical trial setting, but it may play a role in identifying patients who will derive benefit from adjuvant gemcitabine therapy; less evidence is available for the palliative setting.

5.5. Human CNT3. Human concentrative nucleoside transporter 3 (hCNT3) is another cell membrane transporter that assists in the uptake of gemcitabine intracellularly against the concentration gradient. There is less evidence to support the predictive value of hCNT3 expression in estimating response to adjuvant gemcitabine compared to hENT1. Maréchal et al. studied tumor blocks from 45 PDAC patients treated with adjuvant chemoradiation consisting of gemcitabine. The high-hCNT3 group had longer median OS, which was not reached during the follow-up period, versus 12.6 months in the low-hCNT3 group; three-year survival was also higher in the high-hCNT3 group (54.6% versus 26.1%, $p = 0.028$) [63]. In a combined analysis, 15 identified patients with both high hCNT3 and hENT1 levels had longer median OS compared to those with either high hCNT3 or hENT1 levels and those with low levels of both transporters (median OS not reached versus 18.7 months versus 12.2 months, $p < 0.0001$). There may be an emerging role in combining the various nucleoside transporters as a panel of biomarkers; these will require validation in future studies.

6. Landscape of Prognostic Biomarkers

6.1. CA19-9. CA19-9 is the most widely utilized biomarker in PDAC; it is a cell surface protein derived from the Lewis blood group antigen, which is expressed in 90 to 95% of the general population. Previous studies have mainly focused on the hypothetical role of CA19-9 in cancer screening with an estimated sensitivity and specificity of 78% and 82%, respectively [64]. ASCO guidelines currently recommend against using CA19-9 as a screening biomarker [65] as increased levels can be seen in nonpancreatic malignancies in addition to other benign conditions. Kim et al. assessed more than 70,000 asymptomatic patients with serum CA19-9 levels and abdominal ultrasound imaging. Using the cutoff value of 37 U/ml, the positive predictive value was 0.9% with only 4 cases of pancreatic cancer diagnosed [66]. Like with other biomarkers, endeavors to improve the positive predictive value of CA19-9 using higher thresholds would compromise the sensitivity of the test.

Using CA19-9 as a prognostic marker has been studied in both preoperative and postoperative settings. Ferrone et al. demonstrated that preoperative CA19-9 levels are strongly associated with final pathologic staging, with higher median CA19-9 values correlating with more advanced stages of disease [67]. In a retrospective study of patients with potentially resectable disease undergoing diagnostic laparoscopy, Maithel et al. identified a cutoff value of 130 U/ml for which levels above were predictive of occult metastatic disease by imaging. Unresectable disease was identified in 26% and 11% of patients with CA19-9 levels ≥ 130 U/ml and < 130 U/ml, respectively [68]. Hartwig et al. reviewed more than 1500 patients who underwent surgery and found the degree of preoperative CA19-9 elevation correlated with tumor resectability and survival rates. Comparing the low CA19-9 (<37 U/ml) versus high CA19-9 (≥4000 U/ml) cohorts, resectability was 80% versus 38% and median OS was 28.5 versus 14.4 months, respectively [69]. This is supported by Montgomery et al. who described a median OS of 34 versus 16 months using the preoperative threshold of 1052 U/ml [70]. In the postoperative setting, greater median survival has been shown in those with low postoperative CA19-9 levels (36.8 versus 14.6 months, $p < 0.0001$), using 37 U/ml as the threshold [69]. Similarly, Ferrone et al. observed that both an absolute decrease in CA19-9 and a cutoff of < 200 U/ml were predictive of overall survival [67].

Overall, CA19-9 is clinically used for serial monitoring after potentially curative surgery and for those on systemic therapy for unresectable disease, with the goals of detecting recurrence and assessing disease response. One limitation to the above studies is the variability in CA19-9 thresholds. Efforts to standardize the cutoff values used should be one of the emphases in future studies. CA19-9 levels generally correlate with the burden of disease and thus CA19-9 levels have also shown promise in aiding clinicians in the preoperative evaluation for resectability.

6.2. Clinical Factors (Nodal Status, Overall Stage, and Surgical Margins). For individuals who have undergone resection of their PDAC, studies have shown that lymph node metastasis is associated with worse prognosis, although data are conflicting [71–75]. This may be due to the bias of incomplete lymphadenectomy at the time of surgery or the nature of the histopathologic examination. Kang et al. investigated both the lymph node ratio and the absolute lymph node number as potential prognostic biomarkers in 398 patients who underwent surgery for PDAC. Median OS was significantly higher in those without lymph node metastasis compared to one lymph node involvement (25.4 versus 17.3 months, $p = 0.001$) [76]. In patients with N1 nodal status, the lymph node ratio and number of lymph nodes did not significantly affect prognosis. Tomlinson et al. determined that at least 15 lymph nodes are required to accurately stage node negative PDAC [77]. Other studies have evaluated the location of lymph node metastasis as a potential prognostic marker. In particular, para-aortic lymph nodes have received attention as they are considered "extraregional." A meta-analysis by Paiella et al. found that para-aortic lymph node metastases were associated with increased mortality, regardless of regional nodal status (HR 1.85, $p < 0.001$) [78]. The authors suggested that intraoperative frozen section of para-aortic lymph nodes should be examined and taken into consideration prior to proceeding to pancreaticoduodenectomy. This is presently not the standard of practice as a staging laparoscopy and peritoneal cytology examination are often performed instead. Given the high perioperative morbidity and mortality of the procedure, identifying patients who may not derive significant benefit from surgery would have significant utility.

Overall disease stage remains the most important prognostic factor in PDAC. This was validated in the study of Bilimoria et al. who restaged over 121,000 patients from the National Cancer Database using the AJCC 6th edition guidelines in order to assess the predictive ability of the staging system on survival. For all patients, there was 5-year survival discrimination by stage ($p < 0.0001$). In patients who underwent surgery, the stage of disease predicted 5-year survival: 31.4% for stage IA, 27.2% for stage IB, 15.7% for stage IIA, 7.7% for stage IIB, 6.8% for stage III, and 2.8% for stage IV [79].

Studies have also evaluated whether surgical margin status is an independent prognostic factor for survival. Results are conflicting. The definition of an incomplete microscopic resection has been inconsistent, varying from presence of tumor cells at the surface of the resection margin versus within 1.0 mm of the margin. A large study by Yeo et al. showed that a negative resection margin is a strong predictor of long-term survival, but pancreatoduodenectomy specimens examined in the study included other pathologies in addition to PDAC [80]. Konstantinidis et al. demonstrated that patients undergoing R0 resections have improved median OS compared to R1 resections (23 versus 14 months, $p < 0.001$) [81]. However, the survival benefit of an R0 resection is lost when a tumor is found within 1 mm of the surgical margin. Subsequently, Chang et al. studied the volume of residual disease by stratifying margins by 0.5 mm increments and found that a margin clearance of 1.5 mm is important for long-term survival [82]. They suggested that margins less than this threshold may require further adjuvant locoregional therapies. Overall, evidence of a positive margin decreases survival but the consensus on the definition of a negative margin remains variable and requires special attention when interpreting studies.

6.3. DNA Methylation. DNA hypermethylation is an epigenetic mechanism that leads to the addition of a methyl (CH_3) residue on cytosines preceding guanosines (CpGs). It is well known that hypermethylation within promoter regions of tumor suppressor genes can lead to inactivation and contribute to oncogenesis [83]. A literature review by Henriksen et al. did not identify a hypermethylated gene that can be used on its own as a diagnostic marker for pancreatic cancer due to insufficient power [84]. Based on this study, they selected a 28-gene panel and examined promoter hypermethylation from cell-free DNA as a potential diagnostic marker. The authors found a significant difference in the mean number of methylated genes between the PDAC and control groups (8.41 versus 4.74, $p < 0.001$); their diagnostic prediction model had a sensitivity of 76% and specificity of 83% [85]. Recently, the same group utilized the panel of genes to explore the relationship between DNA methylation and stage of disease. The number of hypermethylated genes was similar for stages I–III and higher for stage IV (7 versus 10). However, their prediction model differentiated stage I-II from stage III-IV disease with a sensitivity of 73% and specificity of 80% [86]. The numbers are not ideal for clinical use but this represents a promising potential for blood-based prognostic markers. More recently, there is emerging interest in investigating DNA methylation to predict survival. Yokoyama et al. examined the effect of MUC1/4 gene methylation status on overall survival. Mucins (MUC) are transmembrane proteins that are overexpressed in different cancers and have been linked to poorer prognosis. The authors found that low methylation of MUC 1 and/or MUC 4 correlated with decreased overall survival in PDAC [87]. Additional research to identify relevant hypermethylated genes in PDAC is anticipated, especially since they may also serve as potential targets for therapeutic intervention.

6.4. BRCA. Unlike breast cancer, the data on using BRCA mutational status as a prognostic factor in pancreatic cancer is not well established in the literature. A recent retrospective analysis by Golan et al. included 25 cases of resected BRCA-associated PDAC and found no difference in median OS and DFS between cases and controls. There was a trend towards increased DFS in BRCA-positive patients who received a platinum agent (39.1 versus 12.4 months, $p = 0.255$) [88]. Recently, a study was published investigating polymorphisms in tumor suppressor genes to explore any effects on survival. Zhu et al. identified a specific BRCA1 missense variant that is associated with a poorer prognosis (median OS 7.5 months versus 6.7 months) [89]. Despite this, there is not enough evidence at this time to support the use of BRCA as a prognosticator of outcomes, with the exception of its potential utility in predicting response to platinum and PARP inhibitor therapies.

6.5. SPARC. The role of SPARC in carcinogenesis is complex and variable for different tumor sites. The lack of SPARC expression in CRC is a poor prognostic factor [90] whereas high SPARC expression in breast, melanoma, and gastric cancers is associated with worse outcomes [91–93]. For PDAC, Infante et al. reported that peritumoral SPARC expression was associated with worse prognosis when compared to the lack of SPARC expression (median survival 15 versus 30 months, $p < 0.001$) [94]. The expression of SPARC in tumor cells did not significantly affect prognosis. On the contrary, Miyoshi et al. explored the relationship between pancreatic tumor SPARC mRNA levels and prognosis; they described a higher 5-year survival for the low SPARC mRNA group compared to the high SPARC mRNA group (22.48% versus 0%, $p < 0.0001$) [95]. One limitation is that the specimens that were dissected may have included stromal tissue, as microdissection was not employed. Thus, the prognostic value of tumor SPARC expression remains uncertain.

7. Future Directions

There are emerging studies in the literature that are beginning to evaluate a combination of biomarkers in a panel fashion in an effort to improve the clinical value of these tests. This is particularly true in PDAC screening where there is hope that patients can be diagnosed at a much earlier stage. For instance, Zhang et al. demonstrated that CA19-9 combined with CA242 was associated with a higher sensitivity (89%) without a concomitant decrease in specificity (75%) [96]. Similarly, Brand et al. studied different circulating proteins from patients with PDAC, those with benign pancreatic disease, and healthy controls. The authors identified the combination of CA19-9, intercellular adhesion molecule 1, and osteoprotegerin to have the highest sensitivity and specificity for discriminating PDAC from healthy controls (sensitivity 88%, specificity 90%) [97]. This concept has also been extended to the prognostic setting. Kim et al. studied the combination of postoperative CEA and CA19-9 and found that patients with normal postoperative CEA levels have a longer survival even in the setting of elevated CA19-9 levels (19.1 versus 9.3 months, $p = 0.004$) [98]. In the metastatic setting, Park et al. risk-stratified patients based on performance status and certain bloodwork parameters (hemoglobin, white blood cell count, and CEA). Based on these factors, survival was found to be 11.7, 6.2, and 1.3 months for the low-, intermediate-, and high-risk groups, respectively ($p < 0.001$) [99]. Further investigations into the potential role of predictive or prognostic biomarker panels will likely improve the sensitivity and specificity of prediction and prognostication.

8. Conclusions

Despite advances in treatments, the prognosis of patients diagnosed with pancreatic cancer continues to be poor, due largely to the advanced stages of disease at presentation and the aggressive biology that frequently results in poor performance status and intolerance to available therapies. In order to optimize the selection of the right patients for the right therapies, there are significant efforts to develop more precise strategies which can identify subgroups of patients that will benefit from chosen treatments and those that have a limited prognosis and in whom treatments would be futile. The ultimate goal is to better tailor therapy to the individual in a move towards personalized medicine. While there have been significant gains in biomarker discovery and validation, there is still a significant gap in translating these advances from the research laboratory to the clinical bedside. One major barrier to the widespread use and implementation of existing biomarkers is the lack of standardization across jurisdictions. A collaborative and consensus-driven approach to future biomarker development may facilitate more rapid and consistent adoption of biomarkers into routine clinical practice and optimize the care that is delivered to PDAC patients.

References

[1] Canadian Cancer Society's Advisory Committee on Cancer Statistics, *Canadian Cancer Statistics*, Canadian Cancer Society, Toronto, Canada, 2017.

[2] J. Ferlay, C. Partensky, and F. Bray, "More deaths from pancreatic cancer than breast cancer in the EU by 2017," *Acta Oncologica*, vol. 55, no. 9-10, pp. 1158–1160, 2016.

[3] S. Fung, T. Forte, R. Rahal, J. Niu, and H. Bryant, "Provincial rates and time trends in pancreatic cancer outcomes," *Current Oncology*, vol. 20, no. 5, pp. 279–281, 2013.

[4] R. Wilkowski, M. Wolf, and V. Heinemann, "Primary advanced unresectable pancreatic cancer," *Recent Results in Cancer Research*, vol. 177, no. 1, pp. 79–93, 2008.

[5] A. Teague, K. H. Lim, and A. Wang Gillam, "Advanced pancreatic adenocarcinoma: A review of current treatment strategies and developing therapies," *Therapeutic Advances in Medical Oncology*, vol. 7, no. 2, pp. 68–84, 2015.

[6] S. A. Cullinan, C. G. Moertel, T. R. Fleming et al., "A Comparison of Three Chemotherapeutic Regimens in the Treatment of Advanced Pancreatic and Gastric Carcinoma: Fluorouracil vs Fluorouracil and Doxorubicin vs Fluorouracil, Doxorubicin, and Mitomycin," *Journal of the American Medical Association*, vol. 253, no. 14, pp. 2061–2067, 1985.

[7] S. Cullinan, C. G. Moertel, H. S. Wieand et al., "A phase III trial on the therapy of advanced pancreatic carcinoma evaluations of the mallinson regimen and combined 5-fluorouracil, doxorubicin, and cisplatin," *Cancer*, vol. 65, no. 10, pp. 2207–2212, 1990.

[8] H. A. Burris III, M. J. Moore, J. Andersen et al., "Improvements in survival and clinical benefit with gemcitabine as first-line therapy for patients with advanced pancreas cancer: a randomized trial," *Journal of Clinical Oncology*, vol. 15, no. 6, pp. 2403–2413, 1997.

[9] D. Cunningham, I. Chau, D. D. Stocken et al., "Phase III randomized comparison of gemcitabine versus gemcitabine plus capecitabine in patients with advanced pancreatic cancer," *Journal of Clinical Oncology*, vol. 27, no. 33, pp. 5513–5518, 2009.

[10] G. Colucci, R. Labianca, F. Di Costanzo et al., "Randomized phase III trial of gemcitabine plus cisplatin compared with single-agent gemcitabine as first-line treatment of patients with advanced pancreatic cancer: the GIP-1 study," *Journal of Clinical Oncology*, vol. 28, no. 10, pp. 1645–1651, 2010.

[11] E. Poplin, Y. Feng, J. Berlin et al., "Phase III, randomized study of gemcitabine and oxaliplatin versus gemcitabine (fixed-dose rate infusion) compared with gemcitabine (30-minute infusion) in patients with pancreatic carcinoma E6201: a trial of the Eastern Cooperative Oncology Group," *Journal of Clinical Oncology*, vol. 27, no. 23, pp. 3778–3785, 2009.

[12] G. P. Stathopoulos, K. Syrigos, G. Aravantinos et al., "A multicenter phase III trial comparing irinotecan-gemcitabine (IG) with gemcitabine (G) monotherapy as first-line treatment in patients with locally advanced or metastatic pancreatic cancer," *British Journal of Cancer*, vol. 95, no. 5, pp. 587–592, 2006.

[13] H. Oettle, D. Richards, R. K. Ramanathan et al., "A phase III trial of pemetrexed plus gemcitabine versus gemcitabine in patients with unresectable or metastatic pancreatic cancer," *Annals of Oncology*, vol. 16, no. 10, pp. 1639–1645, 2005.

[14] R. Herrmann, G. Bodoky, T. Ruhstaller et al., "Gemcitabine plus capecitabine compared with gemcitabine alone in advanced pancreatic cancer: a randomized, multicenter, phase III trial of the Swiss Group for Clinical Cancer Research and the Central European Cooperative Oncology Group," *Journal of Clinical Oncology*, vol. 25, no. 16, pp. 2212–2217, 2007.

[15] M. J. Moore, D. Goldstein, J. Hamm et al., "Erlotinib plus gemcitabine compared with gemcitabine alone in patients with advanced pancreatic cancer: a phase III trial of the National Cancer Institute of Canada Clinical Trials Group," *Journal of Clinical Oncology*, vol. 25, no. 15, pp. 1960–1966, 2007.

[16] R. A. Miksad, L. Schnipper, and M. Goldstein, "Does a statistically significant survival benefit of erlotinib plus gemcitabine for advanced pancreatic cancer translate into clinical significance and value?" *Journal of Clinical Oncology*, vol. 25, no. 28, pp. 4506-4507, 2007.

[17] T. Conroy, F. Desseigne, and M. Ychou, "FOLFIRINOX versus gemcitabine for metastatic pancreatic cancer," *The New England Journal of Medicine*, vol. 364, no. 19, pp. 1817–1825, 2011.

[18] J. Long, Y. Zhang, X. Yu et al., "Overcoming drug resistance in pancreatic cancer," *Expert Opinion on Therapeutic Targets*, vol. 15, no. 7, pp. 817–828, 2011.

[19] W. J. Gradishar, S. Tjulandin, N. Davidson et al., "Phase III trial of nanoparticle albumin-bound paclitaxel compared with polyethylated castor oil-based paclitaxel in women with breast cancer," *Journal of Clinical Oncology*, vol. 23, no. 31, pp. 7794–7803, 2005.

[20] M. A. Socinski, I. N. Bondarenko, N. A. Karaseva et al., "Survival results of a randomized, phase 3 trial of nab-paclitaxel and carboplatin compared with cremophor-based paclitaxel and carboplatin as first-line therapy in advanced non-small cell lung cancer," *Journal of Clinical Oncology*, vol. 28, no. 18, 2010.

[21] E. M. Hersh, S. J. O'Day, A. Ribas et al., "A phase 2 clinical trial of nab-Paclitaxel in previously treated and chemotherapy-naive patients with metastatic melanoma," *Cancer*, vol. 116, no. 1, pp. 155–163, 2010.

[22] D. D. Von Hoff, R. K. Ramanathan, M. J. Borad et al., "Gemcitabine plus *nab*-paclitaxel is an active regimen in patients with advanced pancreatic cancer: a phase I/II trial," *Journal of Clinical Oncology*, vol. 29, no. 34, pp. 4548–4554, 2011.

[23] D. D. Von Hoff, T. Ervin, F. P. Arena et al., "Increased survival in pancreatic cancer with nab-paclitaxel plus gemcitabine," *The New England Journal of Medicine*, vol. 369, no. 18, pp. 1691–1703, 2013.

[24] A. Wang-Gillam, C.-P. Li, G. Bodoky et al., "Nanoliposomal irinotecan with fluorouracil and folinic acid in metastatic pancreatic cancer after previous gemcitabine-based therapy (NAPOLI-1): A global, randomised, open-label, phase 3 trial," *The Lancet*, vol. 387, no. 10018, pp. 545–557, 2016.

[25] N. L. Henry and D. F. Hayes, "Cancer biomarkers," *Molecular Oncology*, vol. 6, no. 2, pp. 140–146, 2012.

[26] K. V. Ballman, "Biomarker: Predictive or prognostic?" *Journal of Clinical Oncology*, vol. 33, no. 33, pp. 3968–3971, 2015.

[27] S. Popat, R. Hubner, and R. S. Houlston, "Systematic review of microsatellite instability and colorectal cancer prognosis," *Journal of Clinical Oncology*, vol. 23, no. 3, pp. 609–618, 2005.

[28] D. J. Sargent, S. Marsoni, G. Monges et al., "Defective mismatch repair as a predictive marker for lack of efficacy of fluorouracil-based adjuvant therapy in colon cancer," *Journal of Clinical Oncology*, vol. 28, no. 20, pp. 3219–3226, 2010.

[29] F. A. Sinicrope, N. R. Foster, S. N. Thibodeau et al., "DNA mismatch repair status and colon cancer recurrence and survival in clinical trials of 5-fluorouracil-based adjuvant therapy," *Journal of the National Cancer Institute*, vol. 103, no. 11, pp. 863–875, 2011.

[30] L. Laghi, S. Beghelli, A. Spinelli et al., "Irrelevance of Microsatellite Instability in the Epidemiology of Sporadic Pancreatic Ductal Adenocarcinoma," *PLoS ONE*, vol. 7, no. 9, Article ID e46002, 2012.

[31] J. L. Humphris, A. M. Patch, K. Nones et al., "Hypermutation in pancreatic cancer," *Gastroenterology*, vol. 152, no. 1, pp. 68–74, 2017.

[32] D. T. Le, "Programmed death-1 blockade in mismatch repair deficient colorectal cancer," *Journal of Clinical Oncology*, vol. 34, no. 29, pp. 3502–3510, 2016.

[33] D. T. Le, J. N. Uram, H. Wang et al., "PD-1 blockade in tumors with mismatch-repair deficiency," *The New England Journal of Medicine*, vol. 372, no. 26, pp. 2509–2520, 2015.

[34] M. J. Overman, R. McDermott, J. L. Leach et al., "Nivolumab in patients with metastatic DNA mismatch repair-deficient or microsatellite instability-high colorectal cancer (CheckMate 142): An open-label, multicentre, phase 2 study," *The Lancet Oncology*, 2017.

[35] R. E. Royal, C. Levy, K. Turner et al., "Phase 2 trial of single agent ipilimumab (Anti-CTLA-4) for locally advanced or metastatic pancreatic adenocarcinoma," *Journal of Immunotherapy*, vol. 33, no. 8, pp. 828–833, 2010.

[36] D. T. Le, J. N. Durham, K. N. Smith et al., "Mismatch repair deficiency predicts response of solid tumors to PD-1 blockade," *Science*, vol. 357, no. 6349, pp. 409–413, 2017.

[37] Y. Miki, J. Swensen, D. Shattuck-Eidens et al., "A strong candidate for the breast and ovarian cancer susceptibility gene *BRCA1*," *Science*, vol. 266, no. 5182, pp. 66–71, 1994.

[38] D. Ford, D. F. Easton, D. T. Bishop, S. A. Narod, and D. E. Goldgar, "Risks of cancer in BRCA1-mutation carriers," *The Lancet*, vol. 343, no. 8899, pp. 692–695, 1994.

[39] R. Wooster, G. Bignell, J. Lancaster et al., "Identification of the breast cancer susceptibility gene *BRCA2*," *Nature*, vol. 378, no. 6559, pp. 789–792, 1995.

[40] J. B. Greer and D. C. Whitcomb, "Role of BRCA1 and BRCA2 mutations in pancreatic cancer," *Gut*, vol. 56, no. 5, pp. 601–605, 2007.

[41] D. Thompson and D. F. Easton, "Cancer incidence in BRCA1 mutation carriers," *Journal of the National Cancer Institute*, vol. 94, no. 18, pp. 1358–1365, 2002.

[42] The Breast Cancer Linkage Consortium, "Cancer risks in BRCA2 mutation carriers," *Journal of the National Cancer Institute*, vol. 91, no. 15, pp. 1310–1316, 1999.

[43] V. Heinemann, D. Quietzsch, F. Gieseler et al., "Randomized phase III trial of gemcitabine plus cisplatin compared with gemcitabine alone in advanced pancreatic cancer," *Journal of Clinical Oncology*, vol. 24, no. 24, pp. 3946–3952, 2006.

[44] G. Colucci, F. Giuliani, V. Gebbia et al., "Gemcitabine alone or with cisplatin for the treatment of patients with locally advanced and/or metastatic pancreatic carcinoma: A prospective, randomized phase III study of the Gruppo Oncologico dell'Italia Meridionale," *Cancer*, vol. 94, no. 4, pp. 902–910, 2002.

[45] A. Sonnenblick, L. Kadouri, L. Appelbaum et al., "Complete remission, in BRCA2 mutation carrier with metastatic pancreatic adenocarcinoma, treated with cisplatin based therapy," *Cancer Biology & Therapy*, vol. 12, no. 3, pp. 165–168, 2011.

[46] M. A. Lowery, D. P. Kelsen, Z. K. Stadler et al., "An emerging entity: pancreatic adenocarcinoma associated with a known brca mutation: clinical descriptors, treatment implications, and future directions," *The Oncologist*, vol. 16, no. 10, pp. 1397–1402, 2011.

[47] T. Golan, Z. S. Kanji, R. Epelbaum et al., "Overall survival and clinical characteristics of pancreatic cancer in BRCA mutation carriers," *British Journal of Cancer*, vol. 111, no. 6, pp. 1132–1138, 2014.

[48] D. R. Fogelman, R. A. Wolff, S. Kopetz et al., "Evidence for the efficacy of iniparib, a PARP-1 inhibitor, in BRCA2-associated pancreatic cancer," *Anticancer Reseach*, vol. 31, no. 4, pp. 1417–1420, 2011.

[49] B. Kaufman, R. Shapira-Frommer, R. K. Schmutzler et al., "Olaparib monotherapy in patients with advanced cancer and a germline BRCA1/2 mutation," *Journal of Clinical Oncology*, vol. 33, no. 3, pp. 244–250, 2015.

[50] S. M. Domchek, A. E. Hendifar, R. R. McWilliams et al., "RUCA-PANC: An open-label, phase 2 trial of the PARP inhibitor rucaparib in patients (pts) with pancreatic cancer (PC) and a known deleterious germline or somatic BRCA mutation," *Journal of Clinical Oncology*, vol. 34, no. 15, 2016.

[51] M. A. Tempero, M. P. Malafa, M. Al-Hawary et al., "Pancreatic adenocarcinoma, version 2.2017: Clinical practice guidelines in Oncology," *JNCCN — Journal of the National Comprehensive Cancer Network*, vol. 15, no. 8, pp. 1028–1061, 2017.

[52] J. L. Lindner, S. Loibl, C. Denkert et al., "Expression of secreted protein acidic and rich in cysteine (SPARC) in breast cancer and response to neoadjuvant chemotherapy," *Annals of Oncology*, vol. 26, no. 1, pp. 95–100, 2015.

[53] M. Hidalgo, C. Plaza, M. Musteanu et al., "SPARC expression did not predict efficacy of nab-paclitaxel plus gemcitabine or gemcitabine alone for metastatic pancreatic cancer in an exploratory analysis of the phase III MPACT trial," *Clinical Cancer Research*, vol. 21, no. 21, pp. 4811–4818, 2015.

[54] B. Mohelnikova-Duchonova, V. Brynychova, V. Hlavac et al., "The association between the expression of solute carrier transporters and the prognosis of pancreatic cancer," *Cancer Chemotherapy and Pharmacology*, vol. 72, no. 3, pp. 669–682, 2013.

[55] R. Mori, T. Ishikawa, Y. Ichikawa et al., "Human equilibrative nucleoside transporter 1 is associated with the chemosensitivity of gemcitabine in human pancreatic adenocarcinoma and biliary tract carcinoma cells," *Oncology Reports*, vol. 17, no. 5, pp. 1201–1205, 2007.

[56] M. Tsujie, S. Nakamori, S. Nakahira et al., "Human equilibrative nucleoside transporter 1, as a predictor of 5-fluorouracil resistance in human pancreatic cancer," *Anticancer Reseach*, vol. 27, no. 4 B, pp. 2241–2249, 2007.

[57] R. Maréchal, J.-B. Bachet, J. R. MacKey et al., "Levels of gemcitabine transport and metabolism proteins predict survival times of patients treated with gemcitabine for pancreatic adenocarcinoma," *Gastroenterology*, vol. 143, no. 3, pp. 664–e6, 2012.

[58] N. Nakagawa, Y. Murakami, K. Uemura et al., "Combined analysis of intratumoral human equilibrative nucleoside transporter 1 (hENT1) and ribonucleotide reductase regulatory subunit M1 (RRM1) expression is a powerful predictor of survival in patients with pancreatic carcinoma treated with adjuvant

gemcitabine-based chemotherapy after operative resection," *Surgery*, vol. 153, no. 4, pp. 565–575, 2013.

[59] J. J. Farrell, H. Elsaleh, M. Garcia et al., "Human Equilibrative Nucleoside Transporter 1 Levels Predict Response to Gemcitabine in Patients With Pancreatic Cancer," *Gastroenterology*, vol. 136, no. 1, pp. 187–195, 2009.

[60] J. P. Neoptolemos, W. Greenhalf, P. Ghaneh et al., "HENT1 tumor levels to predict survival of pancreatic ductal adenocarcinoma patients who received adjuvant gemcitabine and adjuvant 5FU on the ESPAC trials," *Journal of Clinical Oncology*, vol. 31, no. 15, 2013.

[61] E. Giovannetti, M. Del Tacca, V. Mey et al., "Transcription analysis of human equilibrative nucleoside transporter-1 predicts survival in pancreas cancer patients treated with gemcitabine," *Cancer Research*, vol. 66, no. 7, pp. 3928–3935, 2006.

[62] E. Poplin, H. Wasan, L. Rolfe et al., "Randomized, multicenter, phase ii study of co-101 versus gemcitabine in patients with metastatic pancreatic ductal adenocarcinoma: Including a prospective evaluation of the role of hENT1 in gemcitabine or CO-101 sensitivity," *Journal of Clinical Oncology*, vol. 31, no. 35, pp. 4453–4461, 2013.

[63] R. Maréchal, J. R. Mackey, R. Lai et al., "Human equilibrative nucleoside transporter 1 and human concentrative nucleoside transporter 3 predict survival after adjuvant gemcitabine therapyin resected pancreatic adenocarcinoma," *Clinical Cancer Research*, vol. 15, no. 8, pp. 2913–2919, 2009.

[64] K. E. Poruk, D. Z. Gay, K. Brown et al., "The clinical utility of CA 19-9 in pancreatic Adenocarcinoma: Diagnostic and prognostic updates," *Current Molecular Medicine*, vol. 13, no. 3, pp. 340–351, 2013.

[65] G. Y. Locker, S. Hamilton, J. Harris et al., "ASCO 2006 update of recommendations for the use of tumor markers in gastrointestinal cancer," *Journal of Clinical Oncology*, vol. 24, no. 33, pp. 5313–5327, 2006.

[66] J.-E. Kim, K. T. Lee, J. K. Lee, S. W. Paik, J. C. Rhee, and K. W. Choi, "Clinical usefulness of carbohydrate antigen 19-9 as a screening test for pancreatic cancer in an asymptomatic population," *Journal of Gastroenterology and Hepatology*, vol. 19, no. 2, pp. 182–186, 2004.

[67] C. R. Ferrone, D. M. Finkelstein, S. P. Thayer, A. Muzikansky, C. Fernandez-Del Castillo, and A. L. Warshaw, "Perioperative CA19-9 levels can predict stage and survival in patients with resectable pancreatic adenocarcinoma," *Journal of Clinical Oncology*, vol. 24, no. 18, pp. 2897–2902, 2006.

[68] S. K. Maithel, S. Maloney, C. Winston et al., "Preoperative CA 19-9 and the yield of staging laparoscopy in patients with radiographically resectable pancreatic adenocarcinoma," *Annals of Surgical Oncology*, vol. 15, no. 12, pp. 3512–3520, 2008.

[69] W. Hartwig, O. Strobel, U. Hinz et al., "CA19-9 in potentially resectable pancreatic cancer: Perspective to adjust surgical and perioperative therapy," *Annals of Surgical Oncology*, vol. 20, no. 7, pp. 2188–2196, 2013.

[70] R. C. Montgomery, J. P. Hoffman, L. B. Riley, A. Rogatko, J. A. Ridge, and B. L. Eisenberg, "Prediction of recurrence and survival by post-resection CA 19-9 values in patients with adenocarcinoma of the pancreas," *Annals of Surgical Oncology*, vol. 4, no. 7, pp. 551–556, 1997.

[71] M. F. Brennan, M. W. Kattan, D. Klimstra, and K. Conlon, "Prognostic nomogram for patients undergoing resection for adenocarcinoma of the pancreas," *Annals of Surgery*, vol. 240, no. 2, pp. 293–298, 2004.

[72] J. M. Winter, J. L. Cameron, K. A. Campbell et al., "1423 Pancreaticoduodenectomies for pancreatic cancer: a single-institution experience," *Journal of Gastrointestinal Surgery*, vol. 10, no. 9, pp. 1199–1211, 2006.

[73] J. E. Lim, M. W. Chien, and C. C. Earle, "Prognostic factors following curative resection for pancreatic adenocarcinoma: a population-based, linked database analysis of 396 patients," *Annals of Surgery*, vol. 237, no. 1, pp. 74–85, 2003.

[74] T. A. Sohn, C. J. Yeo, J. L. Cameron et al., "Resected adenocarcinoma of the pancreas—616 patients: results, outcomes, and prognostic indicators," *Journal of Gastrointestinal Surgery*, vol. 4, no. 6, pp. 567–579, 2000.

[75] C. Sperti, M. Gruppo, M. Valmasoni et al., "Para-aortic node involvement is not an independent predictor of survival after resection for pancreatic cancer," *World Journal of Gastroenterology*, vol. 23, no. 24, pp. 4399–4406, 2017.

[76] M. J. Kang, J.-Y. Jang, Y. R. Chang, W. Kwon, W. Jung, and S.-W. Kim, "Revisiting the concept of lymph node metastases of pancreatic head cancer: Number of metastatic lymph nodes and lymph node ratio according to N stage," *Annals of Surgical Oncology*, vol. 21, no. 5, pp. 1545–1551, 2014.

[77] J. S. Tomlinson, S. Jain, D. J. Bentrem et al., "Accuracy of staging node-negative pancreas cancer a potential quality measure," *JAMA Surgery*, vol. 142, no. 8, pp. 767–773, 2007.

[78] S. Paiella, M. Sandini, L. Gianotti, G. Butturini, R. Salvia, and C. Bassi, "The prognostic impact of para-aortic lymph node metastasis in pancreatic cancer: A systematic review and meta-analysis," *European Journal of Surgical Oncology*, vol. 42, no. 5, pp. 616–624, 2016.

[79] K. Y. Bilimoria, D. J. Bentrem, C. Y. Ko et al., "Validation of the 6th edition AJCC pancreatic cancer staging system: Report from the National Cancer Database," *Cancer*, vol. 110, no. 4, pp. 738–744, 2007.

[80] C. J. Yeo, J. L. Cameron, T. A. Sohn et al., "Six hundred fifty consecutive pancreaticoduodenectomies in the 1990s: pathology, complications, and outcomes," *Annals of Surgery*, vol. 226, no. 3, pp. 248–260, 1997.

[81] I. T. Konstantinidis, A. L. Warshaw, J. N. Allen et al., "Pancreatic ductal adenocarcinoma: is there a survival difference for R1 resections versus locally advanced unresectable tumors? What is a "true" R0 resection?" *Annals of Surgery*, vol. 257, no. 4, pp. 731–736, 2013.

[82] D. K. Chang, A. L. Johns, and N. D. Merrett, "Margin clearence and outcome in resected pancreatic cancer," *Journal of Clinical Oncology*, vol. 27, no. 17, pp. 2855–2862, 2009.

[83] M. Kulis and M. Esteller, "DNA methylation and cancer," *Advances in Genetics*, vol. 70, pp. 27–56, 2010.

[84] S. D. Henriksen, P. H. Madsen, A. C. Larsen et al., "Promoter hypermethylation in plasma-derived cell-free DNA as a prognostic marker for pancreatic adenocarcinoma staging," *International Journal of Cancer*, 2017.

[85] S. D. Henriksen, P. H. Madsen, H. Krarup, and O. Thorlacius-Ussing, "DNA hypermethylation as a blood-based marker for pancreatic cancer: A literature review," *Pancreas*, vol. 44, no. 7, pp. 1036–1045, 2015.

[86] S. D. Henriksen, P. H. Madsen, A. C. Larsen et al., "Cell-free DNA promoter hypermethylation in plasma as a diagnostic marker for pancreatic adenocarcinoma," *Clinical Epigenetics*, vol. 8, no. 1, article no. 117, 2016.

[87] S. Yokoyama, M. Higashi, S. Kitamoto et al., "Aberrant methylation of MUC1 and MUC4 promoters are potential prognostic

biomarkers for pancreatic ductal adenocarcinomas," *Oncotarget*, vol. 7, no. 27, pp. 42553–42565, 2016.

[88] T. Golan, T. Sella, E. M. O'Reilly et al., "Overall survival and clinical characteristics of BRCA mutation carriers with stage I/II pancreatic cancer," *British Journal of Cancer*, vol. 116, no. 6, pp. 694–702, 2017.

[89] Y. Zhu, K. Zhai, J. Ke et al., "BRCA1 missense polymorphisms are associated with poor prognosis of pancreatic cancer patients in a Chinese population," *Oncotarget* , vol. 8, no. 22, 2017.

[90] E. Yang, J. K. Hyun, H. K. Kwi, H. Rhee, K. K. Nam, and H. Kim, "Frequent inactivation of SPARC by promoter hypermethylation in colon cancers," *International Journal of Cancer*, vol. 121, no. 3, pp. 567–575, 2007.

[91] C. Jones, A. Mackay, A. Grigoriadis et al., "Expression profiling of purified normal human luminal and myoepithelial breast cells: identification of novel prognostic markers for breast cancer," *Cancer Research*, vol. 64, no. 9, pp. 3037–3045, 2004.

[92] C.-S. Wang, K.-H. Lin, S.-L. Chen, Y.-F. Chan, and S. Hsueh, "Overexpression of SPARC gene in human gastric carcinoma and its clinic-pathologic significance," *British Journal of Cancer*, vol. 91, no. 11, pp. 1924–1930, 2004.

[93] D. Massi, A. Franchi, L. Borgognoni, U. M. Reali, and M. Santucci, "Osteonectin expression correlates with clinical outcome in thin cutaneous malignant melanomas," *Human Pathology*, vol. 30, no. 3, pp. 339–344, 1999.

[94] J. R. Infante, H. Matsubayashi, N. Sato et al., "Peritumoral fibroblast SPARC expression and patient outcome with resectable pancreatic adenocarcinoma," *Journal of Clinical Oncology*, vol. 25, no. 3, pp. 319–325, 2007.

[95] K. Miyoshi, N. Sato, K. Ohuchida, K. Mizumoto, and M. Tanaka, "SPARC mRNA expression as a prognostic marker for pancreatic adenocarcinoma patients," *Anticancer Reseach*, vol. 30, no. 3, pp. 867–872, 2010.

[96] Y. Zhang, J. Yang, H. Li, Y. Wu, H. Zhang, and W. Chen, "Tumor markers CA19-9, CA242 and CEA in the diagnosis of pancreatic cancer: A meta-analysis," *International Journal of Clinical and Experimental Medicine*, vol. 8, no. 7, pp. 11683–11691, 2015.

[97] R. E. Brand, B. M. Nolen, H. J. Zeh et al., "Serum biomarker panels for the detection of pancreatic cancer," *Clinical Cancer Research*, vol. 17, no. 4, pp. 805–816, 2011.

[98] J. Kim, Y. S. Lee, I. K. Hwang et al., "Postoperative carcinoembryonic antigen as a complementary tumor marker of carbohydrate antigen 19-9 in pancreatic ductal adenocarcinoma," *Journal of Korean Medical Science*, vol. 30, no. 3, pp. 259–263, 2015.

[99] H. S. Park, H. S. Lee, J. S. Park et al., "Prognostic scoring index for patients with metastatic pancreatic adenocarcinoma," *Cancer Research and Treatment*, vol. 48, no. 4, pp. 1253–1263, 2016.

3

Preoperative Thrombocytopenia May Predict Poor Surgical Outcome after Extended Hepatectomy

Mohammad Golriz,[1,2] Omid Ghamarnejad,[1] Elias Khajeh,[1] Mohammadsadegh Sabagh,[1] Markus Mieth,[1] Katrin Hoffmann,[1,2] Alexis Ulrich,[1] Thilo Hackert,[1] Karl Heinz Weiss,[2,3] Peter Schirmacher,[2,4] Markus W. Büchler,[1] and Arianeb Mehrabi[1,2]

[1] *Department of General, Visceral, and Transplantation Surgery, University of Heidelberg, Heidelberg, Germany*
[2] *Liver Cancer Center Heidelberg (LCCH), Heidelberg, Germany*
[3] *Department of Gastroenterology and Hepatology, University of Heidelberg, Heidelberg, Germany*
[4] *Institute of Pathology, University of Heidelberg, Heidelberg, Germany*

Correspondence should be addressed to Arianeb Mehrabi; arianeb.mehrabi@med.uni-heidelberg.de

Academic Editor: Tatsuo Kanda

Background. It is a novel idea that platelet counts may be associated with postoperative outcome following liver surgery. This may help in planning an extended hepatectomy (EH), which is a surgical procedure with high morbidity and mortality. *Aim.* The aim of this study was to evaluate the predictive potential of platelet counts on the outcome of EH in patients without portal hypertension, splenomegaly, or cirrhosis. *Methods.* A series of 213 consecutive patients underwent EH (resection of ≥ five liver segments) between 2001 and 2016. The association of preoperative platelet counts with posthepatectomy liver failure (PHLF), morbidity (based on Clavien-Dindo classification), and 30-day mortality was evaluated using multivariate analysis. *Results.* PHLF was detected in 26.3% of patients, major complications in 26.8%, and 30-day mortality in 11.3% of patients. Multivariate analysis revealed that the preoperative platelet count is an independent predictor of PHLF (odds ratio [OR] 4.4, 95% confidence interval [CI] 1.3–15.0, p=0.020) and 30-day mortality (OR 4.4, 95% CI 1.1–18.8, p=0.043). *Conclusions.* Preoperative platelet count is associated with PHLF and mortality following extended liver resection. This association was independent of other related parameters. Prospective studies are needed to evaluate the predictive role and to determine the impact of preoperative correction of platelet count on postoperative outcomes after EH.

1. Introduction

Extended hepatectomy (EH) is the only curative treatment for large primary or bilobar metastatic hepatic malignancies that improves long-term survival [1, 2]. Surgical developments, better patient selection, and improvements in perioperative care have increased the number of EH procedures being performed [3, 4]. However, the rate of postoperative morbidity is high following EH, especially posthepatectomy liver failure (PHLF) [5, 6]. Preoperative predictive factors of PHLF may play an important role in assessing the risk of post-EH morbidity and mortality.

Several studies have evaluated different predictive factors for PHLF and other postoperative clinical outcomes [7–12]. Recently, the association of the perioperative (preoperative or immediate postoperative) platelet count with PHLF and postoperative mortality has been investigated [13–16]. However, findings have been controversial; some studies have shown a negative association between perioperative platelet counts and postoperative morbidity and mortality, while findings from other studies have indicated no association [13, 15, 17]. Although low platelet count is related to intraoperative poor outcome such as bleeding, it may have a direct impact on posthepatectomy outcomes by promoting liver regeneration and lowering the risk of PHLF. To the best of our knowledge, the association between preoperative platelet count and postoperative outcome has not been investigated exclusively in EH, which has a higher postoperative morbidity and mortality compared with minor hepatectomy.

The aim of this study was to investigate the association of the preoperative platelet count and postoperative clinical outcomes following EH in patients without portal hypertension, splenomegaly, or cirrhosis. To do this, we investigated the effect of preoperative thrombocytopenia on PHLF, morbidity, and mortality after EH.

2. Patients and Methods

2.1. Study Population. We investigated all patients who underwent liver resection to treat primary, metastatic, or benign liver disease at the department of General, Visceral, and Transplantation Surgery at the University of Heidelberg between October 2001 and September 2016. All patients were followed up until September 2017. Only patients who underwent EH were included in the study. EH was defined as resection of five or more hepatic segments based on the Brisbane 2000 classification [18]. Patients under 18 years old and patients who underwent a two-stage hepatectomy (portal vein embolization or associated liver partition and portal vein ligation for staged hepatectomy) were excluded. At the end, a total of 213 patients were included in our study. Furthermore, preoperative imaging reports, intraoperative flowmetry, and postoperative histopathological examinations were screened to assess splenomegaly, portal hypertension, and cirrhosis, respectively. Demographic and baseline clinical characteristics, as well as data on the surgical procedure and perioperative course, were prospectively collected and analyzed. This study was approved by the independent ethics committee of the University of Heidelberg. All procedures were conducted in accordance with the most recent revision of the Declaration of Helsinki.

2.2. Definition and Classification of Postoperative Outcomes. PHLF was diagnosed and graded (grade A, B, or C) according to the proposed definition by the International Study Group of Liver Surgery (ISGLS) [19]. Briefly, PHLF was defined as an increased international normalized ratio (INR), the need for coagulation factors to maintain normal INR, and hyperbilirubinemia on or after postoperative day 5. Hyperbilirubinemia was defined as a serum bilirubin concentration greater than 1 mg/dl and increased INR was defined as an INR greater than 1.2. In patients with preoperative hyperbilirubinemia or increased INR, PHLF was defined as an increase in serum bilirubin levels or INR on or after postoperative day 5.

The severity of postoperative morbidities were classified as grade I to V based on the Clavien-Dindo classification [20]. Grade I and II morbidities were defined as minor and grade III and IV morbidities were defined as major. Postoperative mortality was defined as all-cause death occurring within the first 30 days after surgery.

2.3. Preoperative Evaluations. All preoperative clinical evaluations including medical history, physical examination, and laboratory findings were recorded. All patients underwent cross-sectional contrast-enhanced computed tomography or magnetic resonance imaging of the chest, abdomen, and pelvis to assess the resectability of the tumor and to plan the hepatectomy. The preoperative platelet count was measured on the day of surgery and thrombocytopenia was defined as a platelet count $<150 \times 10^9$/L.

2.4. Statistical Analysis. Statistical analysis was performed using IBM SPSS Statistics for Windows, Version 22.0 (IBM Corp. Released 2013. Armonk, NY). Categorical data were presented as frequencies and proportions, and continuous data were presented as means ± standard deviations. Categorical data were compared using chi-square test of association or Fisher's exact test. Continuous data were compared using Student's t-test. Univariate and multivariate logistic regression analyses were performed to determine independent preoperative predictive factors of PHLF, major morbidity, and 30-day mortality. Variables with a p value <0.1 from the univariate analysis were included in the multivariate regression analysis. Results of univariate and multivariate analyses were reported as odds ratio (OR) with 95% confidence interval (CI). If thrombocytopenia was confirmed in the multivariate analysis, a comparison between patients with platelet counts $<150 \times 10^9$/L and platelet counts $\geq 150 \times 10^9$/L was performed. One-year and three-year patient survival were analyzed using the Kaplan-Meier method. Patients who were lost to follow up were censored. The mean patient survival in the two groups was compared using the log-rank test. A two-sided p value less than 0.05 was considered significant in all analyses.

3. Results

The mean age of patients was 60.8±11.7 years and 50.7% were female. Primary hepatic malignancy was the most common indication for EH (57.7% of patients), and 35.8% of patients received preoperative systemic chemotherapy. PHLF was detected in 26.3% of patients, major complications (grade III–IV) in 26.8% of patients, and 30-day mortality in 11.3% of patients. Detailed patient demographics and clinical data are shown in Table 1.

Seventeen patients (8.0%) had a preoperative platelet count of $<150 \times 10^9$/L (mean platelet count=122.3±22.3 x 10^9 per L), and the remaining 196 (92.0%) patients had a preoperative platelet count of $\geq 150 \times 10^9$/L (mean platelet count=315.5±114.0 x 10^9 per L). Baseline characteristics and clinical outcome of the patients with preoperative thrombocytopenia are shown in Table 2. Nine of 17 patients (52.9%) with preoperative platelet count $<150 \times 10^9$/L were diagnosed with primary liver malignancy (cholangiocarcinoma). Furthermore, preoperative imaging, intraoperative flowmetry, and postoperative histopathological examinations revealed no splenomegaly, portal hypertension, or cirrhosis in the thrombocytopenia group. There were only seven patients with Child-Pugh score A cirrhosis in platelet count $\geq 150 \times 10^9$/L group. The postoperative intensive care unit (ICU) stay was longer in the preoperative platelet count $<150 \times 10^9$/L group (16.7 ± 9.5 days versus 8.0 ± 14.5 days, p=0.017).

TABLE 1: Clinicopathologic characteristics of patients who underwent extended hepatectomy.

Variables	Total (n = 213)
Age (years)	60.8 ±11.7
Gender	
Female/male	108/105
BMI (kg/m^2)	25.53 ± 4.44
ASA score	
Class 1	4 (2.5%)
Class 2	76 (46.9%)
Class 3	82 (50.6%)
Cirrhosis	
Yes	7 (3.2%)
Indication of extended hepatectomy	
Benign liver disease	9 (4.2%)
Primary malignancy	123 (57.7%)
Cholangiocarcinoma	105 (85.4)
Hepatocellular carcinoma	18 (14.6%)
Metastatic disease	81 (38.0%)
Preoperative chemotherapy	
Yes	73 (35.8%)
Preoperative platelet count (x 10^9/L)	
Mean (SD)	300.1 ± 121.5
Intraoperative blood loss (ml)	1638.21 ± 1535.49
Transfusion of RBC	
Patient	60 (31.1%)
Unit	1.52 ± 3.34
Transfusion of FFP	
Patient	44 (22.8%)
Unit	1.43 ± 3.64
Operation time (min)	293.78 ± 115.15
PHLF [a]	56 (26.3%)
Grade A	16 (28.6%)
Grade B	14 (25.0%)
Grade C	26 (46.4%)
Major morbidity [b]	57 (26.8%)
ICU stay (days)	8.14 ± 13.47
Hospitalization (days)	23.43 ± 16.68
30-day mortality	24 (11.3%)

BMI: body mass index; ASA: American Society of Anesthesiologists; SD: standard deviation; RBC: red blood cells; FFP: fresh-frozen plasma; PHLF: posthepatectomy liver failure; ICU: intensive care unit.
[a] Based on the ISGLS definition.
[b] Grades III and IV based on the Clavien-Dindo classification.

Furthermore, in the group with platelet count of <150 x 10^9/L PHLF, major complications and 30-day mortality were detected in 58.8%, 35.3%, and 35.3% of patients, respectively (Table 2).

3.1. Predictive Value of Preoperative Platelet Count. To investigate the impact of the preoperative platelet count on postoperative outcomes including PHLF, morbidity, and 30-day mortality, we performed univariate and multivariate regression analysis. Univariate analysis (Table 3(a)) revealed that patients with a preoperative platelet count of <150 x 10^9/L are significantly more at risk of PHLF (OR 4.7, 95% CI 1.7–12.9, p=0.003). According to univariate analysis, indication of EH, intraoperative blood loss, transfusion of red

TABLE 2: Clinicopathologic characteristics of patients with a preoperative platelet count of <150 x 10^9/L.

Variables	Total (n = 17)
Age (years)	63.1 ±12.5
Gender	
Female/male	8/9
BMI (kg/m^2)	25.08 ± 3.88
ASA score	
Class 1	0 (0.0%)
Class 2	8 (57.1%)
Class 3	6 (42.9%)
Cirrhosis	
Yes	0 (0.0%)
Indication of extended hepatectomy	
Benign liver disease	2 (11.8%)
Primary malignancy	9 (52.9%)
Cholangiocarcinoma	9 (100%)
Hepatocellular carcinoma	0 (0.0%)
Metastatic disease	6 (35.3%)
Preoperative chemotherapy	
Yes	5 (29.4%)
Preoperative platelet count (x 10^9/L)	
Mean (SD)	122.3 ± 22.3
Intraoperative blood loss (ml)	3352.94 ± 2019.32
Transfusion of RBC	
Patient	8 (50.0%)
Unit	4.38 ± 6.26
Transfusion of FFP	
Patient	9 (56.3%)
Unit	4.31 ± 5.91
Operation time (min)	381.29 ± 136.05
PHLF [a]	10 (58.8%)
Grade A	0 (0.0%)
Grade B	2 (20.0%)
Grade C	8 (80.0%)
Major morbidity [b]	6 (35.3%)
ICU stay (days)	16.65 ± 9.50
Hospitalization (days)	30.18 ± 15.20
30-day mortality	6 (35.3%)

BMI: body mass index; ASA: American Society of Anesthesiologists; SD: standard deviation; RBC: red blood cells; FFP: fresh-frozen plasma; PHLF: posthepatectomy liver failure; ICU: intensive care unit.

[a] Based on the ISGLS definition.

[b] Grades III and IV based on the Clavien-Dindo classification.

blood cells or fresh frozen plasma, and operation time also had a significant impact on PHLF. In contrast, multivariate regression only revealed preoperative thrombocytopenia as an independent preoperative predictor of PHLF (OR 4.4, 95% CI 1.3–15.0, p=0.020).

According to multivariate analysis, patient age (OR 1.1, 95% CI 1.0–1.1, p=0.001), metastatic liver disease (OR 2.4, 95% CI 1.1–5.1, p=0.026), and operation time (OR 1.2, 95% CI 1.0–1.5, p=0.042) independently predicted major postoperative morbidities (Table 3(b)). Postoperative major

TABLE 3: Univariate and multivariate analysis of predictive factors of PHLF, major morbidity, and 30-day mortality after extended hepatectomy.

(a) PHLF

Variables	Univariate OR	Univariate 95% CI	Univariate *p*	Multivariate OR	Multivariate 95% CI	Multivariate *p*
Age	1.015	0.988–1.043	0.280			
Gender	0.963	0.523–1.772	0.902			
BMI (kg/m^2)	0.989	0.914–1.071	0.793			
ASA score	1.429	0.743–2.751	0.285			
Indication of extended hepatectomy						
Benign liver disease	Reference	Reference	Reference	Reference	Reference	Reference
Primary malignancy	1.367	0.256–7.290	0.714	0.810	0.120–5.470	0.828
Metastatic disease	2.306	1.159–4.591	0.017	1.897	0.806–4.463	0.141
Preoperative chemotherapy	1.679	0.723–3.896	0.228			
Platelet count <150 x 10^9/L	4.658	1.678–12.929	0.003	4.351	1.266–14.953	0.020
Intraoperative blood loss (L)	1.159	1.036–1.297	0.010	0.884	0.615–1.271	0.506
Intraoperative RBC/FFP transfusion	2.617	1.343–5.098	0.005	2.226	0.859–5.769	0.099
Operation time (hour)	1.264	1.076–1.484	0.004	1.167	0.961–1.417	0.120

(b) Major morbidity

Variables	Univariate OR	Univariate 95% CI	Univariate p	Multivariate OR	Multivariate 95% CI	Multivariate p
Age	1.036	1.010–1.062	0.006	1.050	1.020–1.083	0.001
Gender	1.148	0.669–1.969	0.617			
BMI (kg/m^2)	1.011	0.944–1.083	0.758			
ASA score	1.329	0.752–2.346	0.328			
Indication of extended hepatectomy						
Benign liver disease	Reference	Reference	Reference	Reference	Reference	Reference
Primary malignancy	2.017	0.497–8.187	0.326	1.347	0.195–9.291	0.762
Metastatic disease	3.331	1.827–6.072	<0.001	2.387	1.111–5.127	0.026
Preoperative chemotherapy	0.626	0.274–1.428	0.266			
Platelet count <150 x 10^9/L	10.427	2.321–46.845	0.002	4.923	0.922–26.296	0.062
Intraoperative blood loss (L)	1.365	1.181–1.577	<0.001	1.309	0.863–1.985	0.206
Intraoperative RBC/FFP transfusion	2.880	1.555–5.336	0.001	1.285	0.491–3.363	0.610
Operation time (hour)	1.431	1.215–1.685	<0.001	1.237	1.007–1.520	0.042

(c) 30-day mortality

Variables	Univariate			Multivariate		
	OR	95% CI	p	OR	95% CI	p
Age	1.038	0.997–1.082	0.073	1.038	0.994–1.085	0.094
Gender	1.720	0.718–4.124	0.224			
BMI (kg/m^2)	1.032	0.928–1.147	0.564			
ASA score	1.179	0.504–2.762	0.704			
Indication of extended hepatectomy						
Benign liver disease	Reference	Reference	Reference	Reference	Reference	Reference
Primary malignancy	2.406	0.239–24.220	0.456	1.784	0.078–40.796	0.717
Metastatic disease	3.517	1.150–10.754	0.027	3.460	0.856–13.980	0.081
Preoperative chemotherapy	0.570	0.126–2.568	0.464			
Platelet count <150 x 10^9/L	5.394	1.784–16.311	0.003	4.430	1.055–18.777	0.043
Intraoperative blood loss (L)	1.342	1.085–1.659	0.007	1.166	0.753–1.805	0.492
Intraoperative RBC/FFP transfusion	3.216	1.295–7.986	0.012	1.604	0.435–5.921	0.478
Operation time (hour)	1.261	1.023–1.555	0.030	1.093	0.839–1.425	0.509

OR: odds ratio; CI: confidence interval; BMI: body mass index; ASA: American Society of Anesthesiologists; RBC: red blood cells; FFP: fresh-frozen plasma.

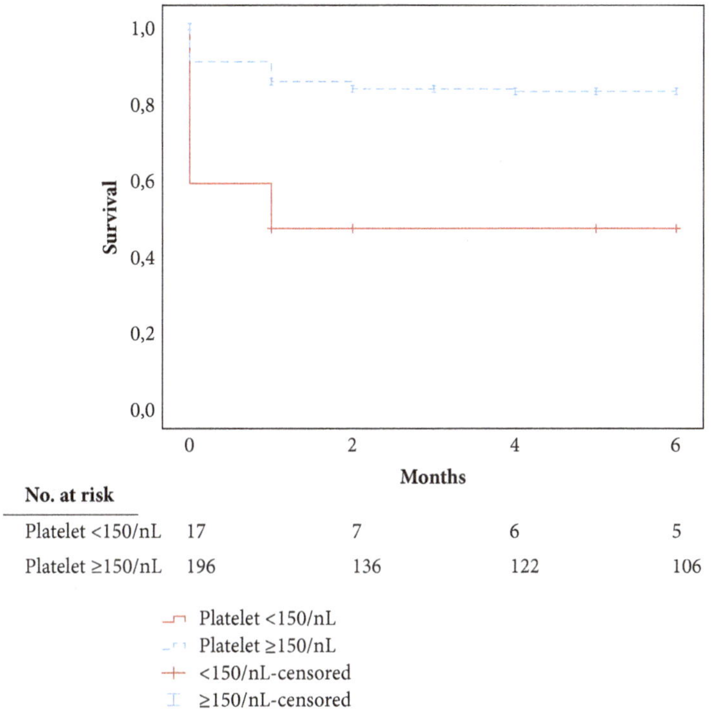

FIGURE 1: Six-month patient survival plot: significantly lower survival rates in patients with low preoperative platelet counts (<150 x 10^9/L) compared with normal preoperative platelet counts (≥150) (log-rank test p<0.001).

morbidities were fivefold higher in patients with a preoperative platelet count <150 x 10^9/L, but this difference was not significant (OR 4.9, 95% CI 0.9–26.3, p=0.062). Furthermore, multivariate analysis showed that postoperative 30-day mortality was fourfold higher in patients with thrombocytopenia compared with normal platelet counts (Table 3(c)) (OR 4.4, 95% CI 1.1–18.8, p=0.043).

After excluding patients with underlying cirrhosis (n = 7), we repeated univariate and multivariate analysis of PHLF, major morbidity and 30-day mortality. As presented in Supplementary Table S1, multivariate analysis demonstrated that PHLF (OR 5.7, 95% CI 2.6–12.8, p<0.001) and 30-day mortality (OR 5.9, 95% CI 1.3–27.1, p=0.021) were sixfold higher in patients with thrombocytopenia compared with those with normal platelet counts.

3.2. Patient Survival. The six-month survival rate was 80.1%±2.8% in our cohort. Patients with a preoperative platelet count <150 x 10^9/L had a significantly lower six-month survival rate than patients with a preoperative platelet count ≥150 x 10^9/L (Figure 1, 47.1%±12.1% versus 83.0%±2.8%, log-rank p<0.001).

4. Discussion

PHLF is a severe and potentially lethal complication after liver resection and is responsible for more than 60% of mortalities after EH [21, 22]. The high rate of mortality and morbidity following EH is a major concern in field of hepatobiliary surgery. Although low platelet count is associated with increased blood loss and longer operation time, it has been shown that low platelet counts can independently diminish postoperative liver regeneration and increase the risk of PHLF as well mortality [13, 23]. Recently, the effect of perioperative (preoperative or immediate postoperative) platelet counts on posthepatectomy morbidity and mortality has been investigated [13, 16, 24–28]. However, these studies investigated the predictive role of platelet count in all types of liver resection (minor, major, and extended) and did not distinguish between the different types of resection. PHLF and mortality rates are higher after EH, therefore we believe that the post-EH outcome is more clinically important and that the predictive role of platelet counts should be investigated separately following EH. To do this, we assessed the association of platelet counts and postoperative outcomes in a homogeneous subgroup of liver resection patients who underwent EH.

We demonstrated that a low preoperative platelet count is a predictive factor of PHLF and higher mortality after EH. In our series of EHs, the odds of development of PHLF and 30-day mortality in patients with low platelet counts were more than 4 and 6 fold higher than patients with normal platelet count, respectively. Moreover, our results showed that long-term survival was lower in patients with low platelet count than patients with normal platelet count. These findings indicate that a low platelet count independently predicts short- and long-term outcomes after EH. We selected a cut-off value of 150 x 10^9/L for platelet counts because this is the minimum normal platelet count in our center and in most clinical settings.

In agreement with our findings, Alkozai et al. [9] reported a fourfold higher 90-day mortality rate after liver resection in colorectal metastasis patients with thrombocytopenia. They also reported delayed postoperative recovery of liver function in patients with low platelet count. However, in their study only 40% of patients underwent liver resection with remnant liver volume of <35%. Others have also shown that perioperative thrombocytopenia affects PHLF, morbidity, and mortality rates [24, 28]. Similar to our study, Venkat et al. [15], Maithel et al. [25], and Margonis et al. [26] evaluated the effect of perioperative platelet counts on PHLF and/or mortality with a cut-off value of 150 x 10^9/L. Although these studies were not consistent in the platelet cut-off levels and type of liver resection they investigated, each has shown that platelet count (100 x 10^9/L or 150 x 10^9/L) is associated with posthepatectomy outcomes. In contrast, some authors have reported no significant association between perioperative platelet count and posthepatectomy outcomes [23, 29]. However, in these studies the platelet count was used as a continuous variable in univariate and/or multivariable analyses. In this regard, it is important to know that the exponentiated coefficient of a continuous predictor in logistic regression is the OR of a one-unit increase in the predictor. A one-unit change in platelet count is not clinically meaningful, which may explain why these authors did not find platelet counts to have significant predictive value.

The predictive role of platelets on PHLF and postoperative mortality may be explained by various mechanisms. One proposed mechanism is the direct promotion of liver regeneration by platelets [30]. This was first suggested by Tomikawa et al. [31] in 1996, who showed that platelets promote liver regeneration after resection by upregulating hepatocyte growth factor. Recent studies have shown that platelets secrete several bioactive factors including serotonin, vascular endothelial growth factor, platelet-derived growth factor, and tumor necrosis factors (TNF-α and TNF-β) to promote liver regeneration in a "direct way" [23, 32, 33]. Another possible mechanism is the "indicative role" of platelets for liver regeneration, which has been described by the parallel regulation of platelet production and liver regeneration by similar factors. Thrombopoietin and interleukin 6 regulate megakaryocyte maturation and platelet production, and can predict the postoperative patient outcome and trigger liver regeneration after hepatectomy [29, 34]. The risk of intra- and postoperative bleeding is increased in patients with thrombocytopenia. This increased blood loss can lead to additional hypoxic liver damage and therefore impaired hepatocyte function/regeneration. This could also explain PHLF and mortality in patients with thrombocytopenia. Surprisingly, Tomimaru and colleagues [14] showed that the platelet count is a better predictor of PHLF in hepatocellular carcinoma patients than the indocyanine green clearance test.

Furthermore, the association between low preoperative platelet count and high portal vein pressure suggests an alternative mechanism [25]. Low platelet counts in patients with liver disease may be secondary to the increased portal vein pressure and subsequent hypersplenism and increased thrombocyte sequestration in the spleen. Indeed, platelet counts can predict PHLF as an accurate and precise surrogate of the portal vein pressure. However, in our study none of the patients in the thrombocytopenia group had splenomegaly, portal hypertension, or cirrhosis. In addition, we performed a subgroup analysis in noncirrhotic patients to reveal the direct association of platelet count with PHLF and mortality.

The retrospective design is a limitation of the present study. However, platelet counts, other laboratory measurements, morbidity, and mortality of all consecutive patients were all recorded prospectively during the study period. To minimize potential bias and estimate the independent effect of the platelet count as accurately as possible, we controlled factors that are known to affect post-EH morbidity and mortality. These potentially confounding factors included age, gender, BMI, American Society of Anesthesiologists (ASA) score, indication of EH, intraoperative blood loss and transfusion, and operation time using univariate and multivariate regression analyses. Therefore, we evaluated the predictive role of platelet count independent of these factors. Cirrhosis is also associated with low platelet count so may confound the effect of thrombocytopenia on posthepatectomy outcome [35]. Therefore, we performed a subgroup analysis after exclusion of patients with cirrhosis.

5. Conclusions

In conclusion, preoperative thrombocytopenia seems to be a reliable predictor of PHLF and increased mortality after EH. This predictive role is independent of other related parameters, including age, cause of hepatectomy, intraoperative blood loss, and duration of surgery. Further randomized studies are required to evaluate the impact of increasing the preoperative platelet count (exogenous platelet infusion versus treatment of the underlying disease) on improving the postoperative outcomes after EH in patients with thrombocytopenia.

Disclosure

This paper was (1) poster presentation at the annual meeting of the German Association for the Study of the Liver (GASL) on January 27, 2018, in Hamburg, Germany (Golriz, M., O. Ghamarnejad, E. Khajeh et al. Preoperative thrombocytopenia may predict poor surgical outcome after extended hepatectomy. Zeitschrift für Gastroenterologie 56, no. 01 (2018): A4-59.), and (2) poster presentation at the 135th congress of the Deutsche Gesellschaft für Chirurgie (DGCH) on April 18, 2018, in Berlin, Germany (Golriz, M., O. Ghamarnejad, E. Khajeh et al. Preoperative thrombocytopenia may predict poor surgical outcome after extended hepatectomy. Innov Surg Sci 2018; 3, (Suppl 1): s1–s231). This research did not receive any specific grant from funding agencies in the public, commercial, or not-for-profit sectors.

References

[1] J.-N. Vauthey, T. M. Pawlik, E. K. Abdalla et al., "Is Extended Hepatectomy for Hepatobiliary Malignancy Justified?" *Annals of Surgery*, vol. 239, no. 5, pp. 722–732, 2004.

[2] P.-A. Clavien, H. Petrowsky, M. L. DeOliveira, and R. Graf, "Strategies for safer liver surgery and partial liver transplantation," *The New England Journal of Medicine*, vol. 356, no. 15, pp. 1545–1559, 2007.

[3] M. H. Squires, N. L. Lad, S. B. Fisher et al., "Value of primary operative drain placement after major hepatectomy: A multi-institutional analysis of 1,041 patients," *Journal of the American College of Surgeons*, vol. 220, no. 4, pp. 396–402, 2015.

[4] R. T. Poon, S. T. Fan, C. M. Lo et al., "Improving perioperative outcome expands the role of hepatectomy in management of benign and malignant hepatobiliary diseases: Analysis of 1222 consecutive patients from a prospective database," *Annals of Surgery*, vol. 240, no. 4, pp. 698–710, 2004.

[5] J. Belghiti, K. Hiramatsu, S. Benoist, P. P. Massault, A. Sauvanet, and O. Farges, "Seven hundred forty-seven hepatectomies in the 1990s: an update to evaluate the actual risk of liver resection," *Journal of the American College of Surgeons*, vol. 191, no. 1, pp. 38–46, 2000.

[6] J. T. Mullen, D. Ribero, S. K. Reddy et al., "Hepatic insufficiency and mortality in 1,059 noncirrhotic patients undergoing major hepatectomy," *Journal of the American College of Surgeons*, vol. 204, no. 5, pp. 854–862, 2007.

[7] N. N. Rahbari, C. Reissfelder, M. Koch et al., "The predictive value of postoperative clinical risk scores for outcome after hepatic resection: A validation analysis in 807 patients," *Annals of Surgical Oncology*, vol. 18, no. 13, pp. 3640–3649, 2011.

[8] J. W. Cheng, P. Zhao, J. B. Liu, X. Liu, and X. L. Wu, "Preoperative aspartate aminotransferase-toplatelet ratio index (APRI) is a predictor on postoperative outcomes of hepatocellular carcinoma," *Medicine (United States)*, vol. 95, no. 48, p. e5486, 2016.

[9] S. Balzan, J. Belghiti, O. Farges et al., "The "50-50 criteria" on postoperative day 5: an accurate predictor of liver failure and death after hepatectomy," *Annals of Surgery*, vol. 242, no. 6, pp. 824–829, 2005.

[10] N. Akamatsu, Y. Sugawara, J. Kanako et al., "Low platelet counts and prolonged prothrombin time early after operation predict the 90 days morbidity and mortality in living-donor liver transplantation," *Annals of Surgery*, vol. 265, no. 1, pp. 166–172, 2017.

[11] H. Zou, Y. Wen, K. Yuan, X.-Y. Miao, L. Xiong, and K.-J. Liu, "Combining albumin-bilirubin score with future liver remnant predicts post-hepatectomy liver failure in HBV-associated HCC patients," *Liver International*, vol. 38, no. 3, pp. 494–502, 2018.

[12] K.-P. Au, S.-C. Chan, K. S.-H. Chok et al., "Child-Pugh Parameters and Platelet Count as an Alternative to ICG Test for Assessing Liver Function for Major Hepatectomy," *HPB Surg*, vol. 2017, 2017.

[13] E. M. Alkozai, M. W. Nijsten, K. P. De Jong et al., "Immediate postoperative low platelet count is associated with delayed liver function recovery after partial liver resection," *Annals of Surgery*, vol. 251, no. 2, pp. 300–306, 2010.

[14] Y. Tomimaru, H. Eguchi, K. Gotoh et al., "Platelet count is more useful for predicting posthepatectomy liver failure at surgery for hepatocellular carcinoma than indocyanine green clearance test," *Journal of Surgical Oncology*, vol. 113, no. 5, pp. 565–569, 2016.

[15] R. Venkat, J. R. Hannallah, R. S. Krouse, and F. B. Maegawa, "Preoperative thrombocytopenia and outcomes of hepatectomy for hepatocellular carcinoma," *Journal of Surgical Research*, vol. 201, no. 2, pp. 498–505, 2016.

[16] A. Mehrabi, M. Golriz, E. Khajeh et al., "Meta-analysis of the prognostic role of perioperative platelet count in posthepatectomy liver failure and mortality," *British Journal of Surgery*, vol. 105, no. 10, pp. 1254–1261, 2018.

[17] P. Starlinger, A. Assinger, S. Haegele et al., "Evidence for serotonin as a relevant inducer of liver regeneration after liver resection in humans," *Hepatology*, vol. 60, no. 1, pp. 257–266, 2014.

[18] J. Belghiti, P.-A. Clavien, E. Gadzijev et al., "The Brisbane 2000 terminology of liver anatomy and resections," *HPB*, vol. 2, no. 3, pp. 333–339, 2000.

[19] N. N. Rahbari, O. J. Garden, R. Padbury et al., "Posthepatectomy liver failure: a definition and grading by the International Study Group of Liver Surgery (ISGLS)," *Surgery*, vol. 149, no. 5, pp. 713–724, 2011.

[20] D. Dindo, N. Demartines, and P. Clavien, "Classification of surgical complications: a new proposal with evaluation in a cohort of 6336 patients and results of a survey," *Annals of Surgery*, vol. 240, no. 2, pp. 205–213, 2004.

[21] M. Donadon, G. Costa, M. Cimino et al., "Safe hepatectomy selection criteria for hepatocellular carcinoma patients:A validation of 336 consecutive hepatectomies. the bilche score," *World Journal of Surgery*, vol. 39, no. 1, pp. 237–243, 2015.

[22] S. Gruttadauria, A. Tropea, D. Pagano et al., "Mini-Invasive Approach Contributes to Expand the Indication for Liver Resection for Hepatocellular Carcinoma Without Increasing the Incidence of Posthepatectomy Liver Failure and Other Perioperative Complications: A Single-Center Analysis," *Journal of Laparoendoscopic & Advanced Surgical Techniques*, vol. 26, no. 6, pp. 439–446, 2016.

[23] J. Cui, E. Heba, C. Hernandez et al., "Magnetic resonance elastography is superior to acoustic radiation force impulse for the Diagnosis of fibrosis in patients with biopsy-proven nonalcoholic fatty liver disease: a prospective study," *Hepatology*, vol. 63, no. 2, pp. 453–461, 2016.

[24] K. Kaneko, Y. Shirai, T. Wakai, N. Yokoyama, K. Akazawa, and K. Hatakeyama, "Low preoperative platelet counts predict a high mortality after partial hepatectomy in patients with hepatocellular carcinoma," *World Journal of Gastroenterology*, vol. 11, no. 37, pp. 5888–5892, 2005.

[25] S. K. Maithel, P. J. Kneuertz, and D. A. Kooby, "Importance of low preoperative platelet count in selecting patients for resection of hepatocellular carcinoma: A multi-institutional analysis," *Journal of the American College of Surgeons*, vol. 212, no. 4, pp. 638–648, 2011.

[26] G. A. Margonis, N. Amini, S. Buettner et al., "Impact of early postoperative platelet count on volumetric liver gain and perioperative outcomes after major liver resection," *British Journal of Surgery*, vol. 103, no. 7, pp. 899–907, 2016.

[27] C. Riediger, J. Bachmann, A. Hapfelmeier, H. Friess, J. Kleeff, and M. W. Mueller, "Low postoperative platelet count is associated with negative outcome after liver resection for hepatocellular carcinoma," *Hepato-Gastroenterology*, vol. 61, no. 133, pp. 1313–1320, 2014.

[28] H.-Q. Wang, J. Yang, J.-Y. Yang, W.-T. Wang, and L.-N. Yan, "Low immediate postoperative platelet count is associated with hepatic insufficiency after hepatectomy," *World Journal of Gastroenterology*, vol. 20, no. 33, pp. 11871–11877, 2014.

[29] S. Haegele, F. Offensperger, D. Pereyra et al., "Deficiency in thrombopoietin induction after liver surgery is associated with postoperative liver dysfunction," *PLoS ONE*, vol. 10, no. 1, 2015.

[30] T. Kurokawa, Y.-W. Zheng, and N. Ohkohchi, "Novel functions of platelets in the liver," *Journal of Gastroenterology and Hepatology*, vol. 31, no. 4, pp. 745–751, 2016.

[31] M. Tomikawa, M. Hashizume, and H. Highashi, "The role of the spleen, platelets, and plasma hepatocyte growth factor activity on hepatic regeneration in rats," *Journal of the American College of Surgeons*, vol. 182, no. 1, pp. 12–16, 1996.

[32] B. Aryal, T. Shimizu, J. Kadono et al., "A switch in the dynamics of intra-platelet VEGF-A from cancer to the later phase of liver regeneration after partial hepatectomy in humans," *PLoS ONE*, vol. 11, no. 3, Article ID e0150446, 2016.

[33] B. Aryal, M. Yamakuchi, and T. Shimizu, "Therapeutic implication of platelets in liver regenerationhopes and hues," *Expert Review of Gastroenterology Hepatology*, vol. no, 2018.

[34] D. Schmidt-Arras and S. Rose-John, "IL-6 pathway in the liver: from physiopathology to therapy," *Journal of Hepatology*, vol. 64, no. 6, pp. 1403–1415, 2016.

[35] N. Afdhal, J. McHutchison, R. Brown et al., "Thrombocytopenia associated with chronic liver disease," *Journal of Hepatology*, vol. 48, no. 6, pp. 1000–1007, 2008.

4

Management Strategies and Outcomes for Hyponatremia in Cirrhosis in the Hyponatremia Registry

Samuel H. Sigal ,[1] Alpesh Amin,[2] Joseph A. Chiodo III,[3] and Arun Sanyal[4]

[1] *Department of Medicine, Montefiore Medical Center and Albert Einstein College of Medicine, Bronx, New York 10467, USA*
[2] *Department of Medicine, University of California, Irvine, California 92868, USA*
[3] *Agile Therapeutics, Inc., Princeton, New Jersey 08540, USA*
[4] *Virginia Commonwealth University Medical Center, Richmond, Virginia 23298, USA*

Correspondence should be addressed to Samuel H. Sigal; ssigal@montefiore.org

Academic Editor: En-Qiang Chen

Aim. Treatment practices and effectiveness in cirrhotic patients with hyponatremia (HN) in the HN Registry were assessed. *Methods.* Characteristics, treatments, and outcomes were compared between patients with HN at admission and during hospitalization. For HN at admission, serum sodium concentration [Na] response was analyzed until correction to > 130 mmol/L, switch to secondary therapy, or discharge or death with sodium ≤ 130 mmol/L. *Results.* Patients with HN at admission had a lower [Na] and shorter length of stay (LOS) than those who developed HN ($P < 0.001$). Most common initial treatments were isotonic saline (NS, 36%), fluid restriction (FR, 33%), and no specific therapy (NST, 20%). Baseline [Na] was higher in patients treated with NST, FR, or NS versus hypertonic saline (HS) and tolvaptan (Tol) ($P < 0.05$). Treatment success occurred in 39%, 39%, 52%, 78%, and 81% of patients with NST, FR, NS, HS, and Tol, respectively. Relapse occurred in 55% after correction and was associated with increased LOS (9 versus 6 days, $P < 0.001$). 34% admitted with HN were discharged with HN corrected. *Conclusions.* Treatment approaches for HN were variable and frequently ineffective. Success was greatest with HS and Tol. Relapse of HN is associated with increased LOS.

1. Introduction

Dilutional hyponatremia (HN) is a frequent consequence of severe portal hypertension in cirrhosis. It is the result of severe vasodilation, leading to increased arginine vasopressin (AVP) release and consequent water retention [1, 2]. HN is especially common in the hospitalized patient [3] and is associated with severe ascites, hepatic encephalopathy (HE), and impaired renal function. In a retrospective study of 20,000 patients, HN was predictive of worsening disease, mortality, a higher 30-day readmission rate [4], and a 1.74-day increase in average hospital length of stay (LOS).

Management options for HN include discontinuation of diuretics, fluid restriction (FR), and administration of isotonic saline (NS), hypertonic saline (HS), or a vasopressin-receptor antagonist (or "vaptan"). FR is usually the first treatment used but is limited by patient adherence. Administration of NS and HS is problematic as they exacerbate fluid overload and ascites. Vaptans block the actions of AVP at vasopressin-2 receptors in cells of the renal collecting duct and provide a targeted approach to treatment in patients with inappropriately elevated AVP levels [5, 6]. There are currently two FDA-approved vaptans: conivaptan (Cumberland Pharmaceuticals, Inc., Nashville, Tennessee, USA) is a dual vasopressin-1A/2-receptor antagonist available for IV use, and tolvaptan (TO; Otsuka Pharmaceutical Co., Ltd., Tokyo, Japan) is an oral selective vasopressin-2-receptor antagonist [5, 6]. Both are indicated for euvolemic and hypervolemic HN. Cirrhosis was initially an approved indication for TO but was subsequently removed due to the development of hepatocellular injury during an investigational study of its use in autosomal dominant polycystic kidney disease [7].

The effectiveness of treatment strategies and impact on LOS for hospitalized cirrhotic patients with HN have not been previously reported. The HN Registry (NCT01240668) is an observational, multicenter, real-world study of patients hospitalized with euvolemic or hypervolemic HN. The objectives were to obtain clinical characteristics of patients and assess treatment practices, effectiveness, and resource utilization using LOS as a surrogate. The results of the entire population have previously been published [8]. In that report, the management and response of all patients with HN regardless of underlying condition were reported with only mention of the percentage of patients with cirrhosis. This analysis specifically assessed the subpopulation of patients with cirrhosis.

2. Materials and Methods

2.1. Study Design. Data from cirrhotic patients enrolled in the HN Registry [8] without concomitant nephrotic proteinuria, severe cardiomyopathy (ejection fraction <50%), or severe azotemia (creatinine ≥3.0 mg/dL) were entered in a database that included clinical characteristics, laboratory results, volume of fluid intake and output over each 24-hour period (if available), amount of FR, treatment with IV NS and HS, diuretics, medications used to treat HN, paracentesis, and LOS [8]. Severity of ascites and hepatic encephalopathy (HE) were recorded, and Child-Pugh scores, MELD, and MELD-Na scores were calculated [9]. Patients were classified as having HN diagnosed at the time of hospital admission versus hospital-acquired HN and categorized as mild ([Na^+] > 125–130 mmol/L), moderate (120–125 mmol/L), and severe (< 120 mmol/L).

Initial treatment for HN was recorded. FR was based on an order by the treating physician. NS treatment was defined as administration of > 500 ml NS over a 24-hour period. No specified therapy (NST) was defined as observation for ≥2 days without a specific treatment. Patients who received NS, HS, or TO alone or in conjunction with FR were combined. A 1-day gap of no therapy between 2 treatment episodes constituted the end of initial treatment except for patients receiving TO in which case a 1-day gap was permitted. The study was exclusively observational, and treatment was solely determined by the treating physician.

Response to therapy for patients admitted with HN was assessed daily. On each day, patients were categorized based on HN severity and achievement of a treatment endpoint (correction to [Na^+] > 130 mmol/L, increase in [Na^+] ≥ 5 mmol/L from baseline, switch to another therapy, discharge with persistent HN, or death or transfer to hospice with persistent HN). The first [Na^+] obtained on the day after treatment was discontinued and was then used as the end-of-therapy value. Patients in whom [Na^+] corrected to > 130 mmol/L with initial therapy were assessed for relapse of HN during the subsequent hospitalization. Patients who were switched by the treating physician to a different treatment were assessed and reclassified based on second treatment provided in the same manner as that for the initial therapy.

At hospital discharge, final [Na^+] and disposition (discharge home with corrected or persistent HN, and mortality [hospital death or transfer to hospice]) were recorded, and LOS was determined. For patients in whom discharge was delayed due to nonmedical reasons, the additional days were not included in LOS if documented as such in the clinical record.

2.2. Statistical Analysis. Clinical characteristics, initial and final [Na^+], hospital mortality, and median LOS of patients with HN at hospital admission versus those who developed HN during hospitalization were compared. The relationship between HN severity and the various clinical parameters, LOS, and hospital mortality were assessed for patients admitted with HN.

Characteristics were compared among the various treatment groups. Cumulative endpoint outcomes were recorded for Days 1–5 and final outcomes at the end of primary treatment. The percentage of patients with initial [Na] < 125 in whom the level increased by ≥ 5 mmol/L on Days 2 and 3 and at the end of therapy was assessed. For patients with moderate or severe HN, the percentage of patients with an increase in [Na^+] ≥ 5 mmol/L was assessed on Days 2 and 3 and end of treatment. A similar analysis was performed for patients who received a secondary therapy. For patients in whom [Na^+] corrected to >130 mmol/L with initial therapy, characteristics and LOS were compared between patients who did and did not experience a relapse.

Descriptive statistics for continuous variables consisted of median number of observations and interquartile range (IQR). Frequency counts and percentages were obtained for categorical variables. Statistical comparisons of continuous variables were performed using nonparametric tests such as the Wilcoxon rank-sum test. Comparisons of categorical variables were performed using chi-square tests for association. Statistical significance for the tests was defined at the 5% level ($P < 0.05$).

2.3. Internal Review Board Approval. Approval was sought from the local research ethics review board at each site using either informed consent or a waiver of consent.

3. Results

3.1. Patient Characteristics. Of the 3087 patients who satisfied the inclusion and exclusion criteria, 650 (21%) had cirrhosis and 595 met the criteria for the current analysis. Baseline characteristics are presented in Table 1. HN was associated with advanced liver disease and severe portal hypertension (Table 2). HN was present in 518 patients (87%) on admission and developed during hospitalization in 77 (13%). Patients with HN on admission had lower initial [Na^+], higher blood urea nitrogen (BUN), and MELD-Na score ($P < 0.05$; Table 2). More than half of the patients had large-volume ascites (Supplemental Table 1). Patients with moderate (25%; $P <$ 0.05) or severe HN (28%; $P < 0.05$) more commonly had overt HE than those with mild HN (17%).

3.2. Initial HN Treatment. The most common initial therapies were NS (36%), FR (33%), NST (20%), TO (5%), and HS (2%; Supplemental Table 2). A variety of other therapies (e.g., salt tablets and conivaptan) and combinations were administered to 22 patients (4%). Initial [Na^+] in the NST group was higher than in the other groups ($P < 0.05$). Initial [Na^+] in the FR

Table 1: Baseline demographic characteristics.

	All Patients[i] (N = 3,087)	Cirrhosis (n = 630)
Age distribution, n (%)[a]		
≤50 y	479 (16)	190 (30)
51–64 y	937 (30)	339 (54)
65–74 y	587 (19)	81 (13)
≥75 y	1,084 (35)	20 (3)
Men, n (%)[b]	1,558 (51)	419 (67)
Race distribution: US only, n (%)[a]		
White	1,927 (74)	455 (72)
African-American	309 (12)	58 (9)
Asian	57 (2)	13 (2)
Other	154 (6)	53 (9)
Unknown	149 (6)	51 (8)
Mean initial [Na+] ± SD, mEq/L[c]	123.6 ± 5.5	124.1 ± 5.0
Mean initial BUN ± SD, mg/dL[a]	20.8 ± 16.8	25.5 ± 18.8
Mean initial creatinine ± SD, mg/dL[d]	1.1 ± 0.73	1.28 ± 0.85
Initial BUN:creatinine ratio[a]	19.4 ± 9.4	19.8 ± 8.6
Prior HN, n (%)[a,e]		
Yes	909 (29)	240 (38)
No	1,176 (38)	178 (28)
Unknown	1,001 (32)	212 (34)
HN at admission, n (%)[f]		
Yes	2,532 (82)	549 (87)
No	531 (17)	81 (13)
Unknown	24 (1)	0 (0)
Primary physician specialty, n (%)		
Nephrologist	104 (3)	8 (1)
Endocrinologist	108 (4)	0
Cardiologist	321 (10)	7 (1)
Hepatologist	260 (8)	246 (39)
Oncologist	111 (4)	11 (2)
Generalist	1,844 (60)	315 (50)
Other	338 (11)	43 (7)
HN subspecialist consulted, n (%)[g,h]		
No	1989 (64)	501 (80)
Yes	1,096 (36)	129 (21)

Abbreviations: BUN, blood urea nitrogen; CHF, congestive heart failure; HN, hyponatremia; [Na^+], sodium concentration; SD, standard deviation; SIADH, syndrome of inappropriate antidiuretic hormone secretion.

[a]SIADH vs CHF and cirrhosis, and CHF vs cirrhosis: P <0.001.

[b]SIADH vs CHF: P = 0.79; and SIADH and CHF vs cirrhosis: P <0.001.

[c]SIADH vs CHF and cirrhosis: P <0.001; CHF vs cirrhosis: P = 0.01.

[d]SIADH vs CHF and cirrhosis: P <0.001; and CHF vs cirrhosis: P = 0.05.

[e]HN during previous hospital admission in prior 12 months.

[f]Data missing for 24 patients in All, 19 in SIADH, and 4 in CHF populations; SIADH vs CHF: P = 0.04; SIADH vs cirrhosis: P = 0.001; and CHF vs cirrhosis: P <0.001.

[g]SIADH vs CHF and cirrhosis: P <0.001; and CHF vs cirrhosis: P = 0.01.

[h]HN specialist defined as nephrologist or endocrinologist.

[i]Includes 171 patients without a diagnosis of SIADH, cirrhosis, or CHF.

TABLE 2: Clinical characteristics of cirrhosis patients admitted with HN subdivided by hyponatremia severity.

	Total N = 518	[Na+], mmol/L <120 n = 106	≥120–≤125 n = 202	>125–≤130 n = 210
Median age, y	56	54	56	57
Male/female, n	345/173	73/33	130/72	142/68
BUN, mg/dL	20.0 (19.0)	18.0 (20.5)	21.0 (20.0)	19.0 (17.0)
Cr, mg/dL	1.0 (0.6)	1.0 (0.7)	1.1 (0.7)	1.0 (0.6)
BUN:Cr ratio	18.9 (10.4)	19.0 (12.0)	19.8 (11.6)	18.0 (9.1)
Alb, g/dL	2.5 (0.8)	2.6 (1.1)	2.5 (0.8)	2.4 (0.6)
Tbili, μmol/L	4.3 (7.4)	4.3 (7.2)	4.5 (6.9)	4.3 (7.6)
INR, s	1.7 (0.6)	1.6 (0.5)	1.7 (0.7)	1.7 (0.7)
Severe ascites, n (%)	284 (55)	53 (50)	124 (61)	107 (51)
Severe HE, n (%)[a]	116 (22)	30 (28)	51 (25)	35 (17)
C-P score	11.0 (3.0)	10.5 (3.0)	11.0 (3.0)	10.0 (3.0)
MELD score	20.2 (9.7)	18.7 (9.0)	20.8 (8.0)	20.2 (10.4)
MELD-Na score	27.3 (6.3)	26.7 (5.6)	28.0 (5.0)	26.3 (7.6)

[a] $P < 0.01$.

Values for blood urea nitrogen (BUN), creatinine (Cr), BUN:Cr ratio, albumin (Alb), total bilirubin (Tbili), international normalized ratio (INR), and Child-Pugh (CP), Model for End-Stage Liver Disease (MELD), and MELD-NA scores are median (interquartile range). HE, hepatic encephalopathy; HN, hyponatremia.

group was higher than in the HS and TO groups (both $P < 0.05$). [Na^+] increased at greater rates in the FR versus NST group ($P = 0.03$), NS versus NST and FR groups ($P < 0.05$), and HS and TO versus NST and FR groups ($P < 0.05$ for all). Median length of treatment for NST, FR, and TO was 3 days and 2 days for NS and HS. It is important to note that the goal of this observational study was to demonstrate the current state of treatment management of hypervolemic HN in various real-world hospital settings. The duration of therapy and the treatment choice were determined by the treating physician as indicated in the clinical chart.

Figure 1 presents the response to initial treatment by various HN categories at Days 1–5. The percentages of patients with moderate or severe HN were significantly higher in the HS (82%) and TO (78%) groups than in the NS (65%) and FR (63%) groups, which, in turn, were higher than in the NST group (32%; all $P < 0.05$). Patients in the HS or TO groups more frequently improved into more less severe HN or treatment success categories than in those treated with NST, FR, or NS.

Table 3 presents the percentages of patients with moderate or severe HN in which [Na^+] increased by ≥ 5 mmol/L at Days 2 and 3 and at final outcome. In the NST and FR groups, 27% of patients achieved this endpoint at Day 2 and 33% and 36%, respectively, at Day 3. Higher percentages achieved this endpoint in the NS versus NST and FR groups at Day 2 ($P = 0.08$ and $= 0.02$, respectively) and Day 3 ($P = 0.08$ and < 0.01). There was a more rapid response in the HS versus NST and FR groups (Days 2 and 3, $P < 0.03$ for both) and TO versus NST and FR groups (Day 2 [$P = 0.15$ and 0.07, respectively] and Day 3 [$P < 0.01$ for both]). The percentages of patients with treatment success were significantly higher in the TO versus NST, FR, and NS groups, and HS versus FR group (all $P < 0.05$).

Of patients admitted to the hospital with HN, 151 (29%) were not receiving diuretic therapy prior to hospital admission. Among these patients, 34 (23%) received ≥ 1 dose of a diuretic during initial HN therapy. Of 367 patients (71%) who received diuretics prior to hospital admission, 287 (78%) received ≥ 1 dose of a diuretic during initial HN therapy.

3.3. Secondary HN Treatment. A second therapy was provided to 275 patients. The secondary HN treatments based on initial therapy, and the characteristics and outcomes by secondary treatment group are presented in Supplemental Tables 4 and 5. Sodium levels prior to the secondary therapy and response rates are presented in Table 3. In general, the sodium response was similar for a specific therapy regardless of whether it was administered as initial or secondary therapy.

3.4. HN Relapse and Final Outcomes. Of the 110 patients who corrected with initial therapy, 61 (55%) experienced a relapse of HN during the subsequent hospitalization (Table 4). Characteristics, initial and final [Na^+] levels, and LOS until HN correction were comparable between patients who did and did not relapse. The LOS after HN correction (6 versus 2 days) and total LOS (9 versus 6 days) were higher in patients who relapsed versus those patients whose [Na] remained above 130 ($P < 0.05$).

For patients admitted with HN, final median [Na^+] was 129 (IQR 7) mmol/L. Of these patients, 174 (34%) were discharged alive with corrected HN, 292 (56%) were discharged with persistent HN (mild: 203 [39%]; moderate: 84 [16%]; and severe: 5 [1%]), and 49 (10%) died during hospitalization or were discharged to hospice. For patients who developed HN during hospitalization, final median [Na^+] was 130 (IQR 6) mmol/L. Of these patients, 25 (33%) were discharged alive with corrected HN, 39 (51%) were discharged with persistent

TABLE 3: Patients with [Na$^+$] ≥5 mmol/L in response to initial and secondary therapy[a].

	Day 2 Response	Day 3 response	Final response
Initial therapy, n (%)			
NST	9 (27)	11 (33)	13 (39)
FR	29 (27)	38 (36)	42 (39)
NS	54 (45)	61 (51)	62 (52)
HS	7 (78)	7 (78)	7 (78)
TO	10 (48)	15 (71)	17 (81)
Secondary therapy, n (%)			
NST	5 (36)	5 (36)	5 (36)
FR	15 (31)	18 (37)	18 (37)
NS	9 (29)	10 (32)	10 (32)
HS	10 (100)	10 (100)	10 (100)
TO	15 (58)	17 (65)	18 (68)

[a]Patients with initial moderate or severe hyponatremia.
Initial therapy P <0.05 for *Day 2 response*: no specific therapy (NST) vs hypertonic saline (HS), and fluid restriction (FR) vs HS and isotonic saline (NS); *Day 3 response:* NST vs HS and tolvaptan (TO); FR vs HS, NS, and TO: *final response:* NST vs TO, FR vs HS and TO, and NS vs TO.

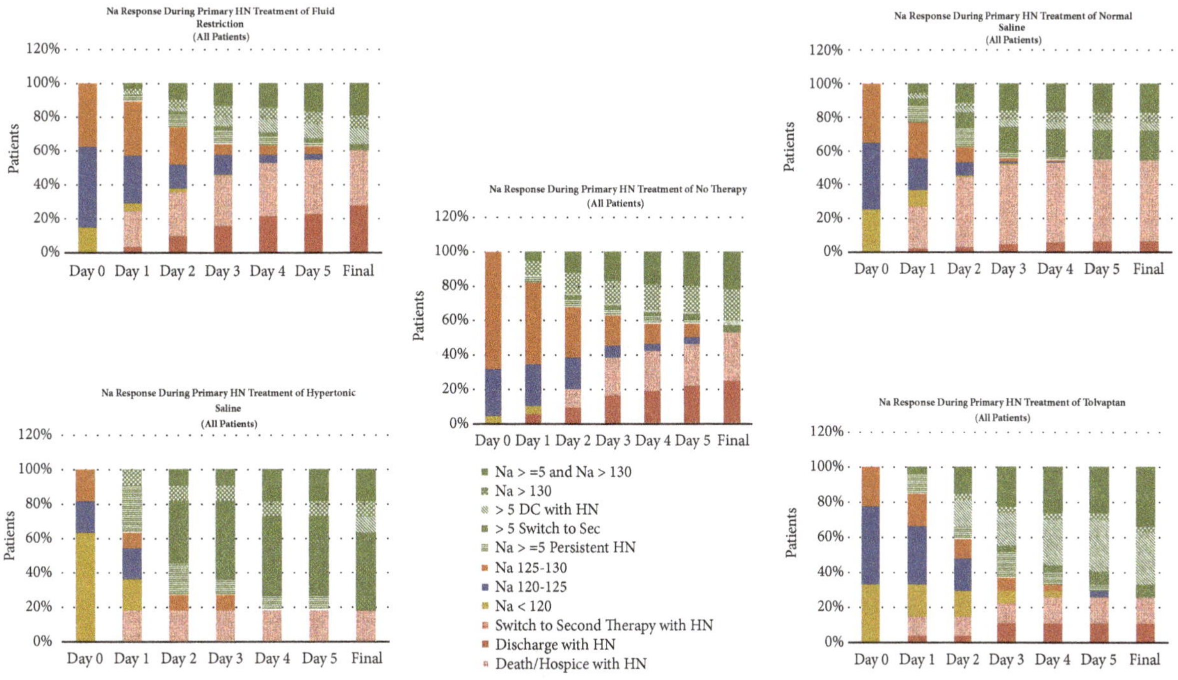

FIGURE 1: Response to primary hyponatremia (HN) treatment by various HN categories. [Na$^+$], sodium concentration; FR, fluid restriction; NS, isotonic saline; NST, no specified therapy; HS, hypertonic saline; TO, tolvaptan; DC, discontinuation.

HN (mild: 31 [40%]; moderate: 8 [10%]; and severe: 0), and 12 (16%) died during hospitalization or were discharged to hospice.

Median (IQR) LOS values for patients admitted with HN and those who developed HN during hospitalization were 6 (5) and 9 (8), respectively (P < 0.05). The distribution of LOS for patients admitted with HN versus those who developed HN during hospitalization is presented in Figure 2. Of patients admitted with HN compared with those who developed HN during hospitalization, 90% versus 75% were discharged by 14 days. Hospital mortality was numerically greater in patients who developed HN during hospitalization than in those admitted with HN but not statistically significant (16% versus 10%; P = 0.25).

4. Discussion

This analysis of the HN Registry—the largest observational study to specifically examine HN in the hospital setting—produced several important findings. There was a

TABLE 4: Patient characteristics and LOS for patients admitted with HN who corrected with initial HN therapy.

	Relapse (n = 61)	No relapse (n = 49)
$[Na^+]$, mmol/L	128.0 (4.0)	127.0 (5.0)
$[Na^+]$ at time of correction, mmol/L[a]	132.0 (2.0)	132.0 (2.0)
BUN, mg/dL	17.0 (17.0)	16.0 (16.0)
Cr, mg/dL	1.0 (0.5)	1.0 (0.9)
BUN:Cr ratio	19.1 (9.6)	17.4 (11.4)
Tbili, μmol/L	4.8 (7.3)	4.3 (6.7)
INR, s	1.8 (0.8)	1.8 (0.5)
Alb, g/doll	2.6 (0.9)	2.8 (0.7)
MELD score at correction	20.9 (6.6)	21.9 (11.3)
LOS, d[a]	9 (6.0)	6 (5.0)
LOS until correction, d	3 (2.0)	3 (1.0)
LOS after correction, d[a]	6 (5.0)	2 (3.0)
Death/ hospice, n (%)	5 (8)	5 (10)

[a] < 0.05.

Values for sodium concentration ($[Na^+]$), $[Na^+]$ at time of correction, blood urea nitrogen (BUN), creatinine (Cr), BUN:CR ratio, total bilirubin (Tbili), albumin (Alb), international normalized ratio (INR), Model for End-Stage Liver Disease (MELD) score at correction, length of stay (LOS), LOS until correction, and LOS after correction are median (interquartile range). HN, hyponatremia.

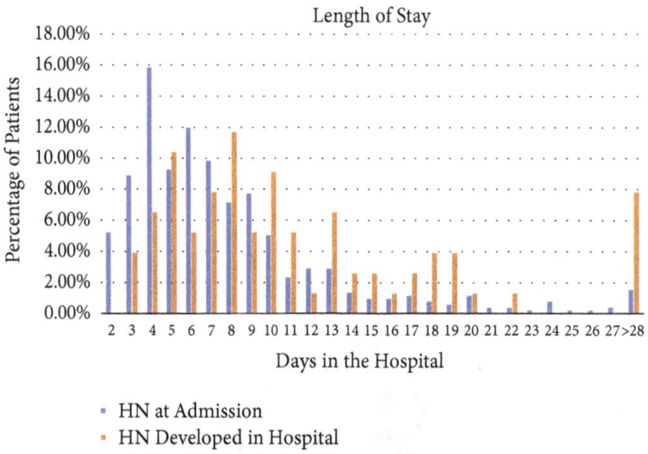

FIGURE 2: The distribution of length of stay (LOS) for patients with hyponatremia (HN) at admission versus those who developed HN during hospitalization.

strong association between HN and advanced cirrhosis with severe portal hypertension as has been previously reported [3]. Large-volume ascites and overt HE were noted in 54% and 22% of patients admitted with HN, respectively. There was not a relationship between the presence of severe ascites and the severity of HN ($p = 0.216$). However, the prevalence of overt HE was related to HN severity.

Treatment approaches were highly variable and frequently ineffective [7]. Twenty percent of patients received NST, and only 34% of the cirrhotic patients admitted to the hospital with HN were discharged with corrected HN. Although FR is recommended in treatment guidelines as initial therapy [10], this is the first study to report outcomes in patients treated with FR in real life practice. The rate of increase in $[Na^+]$ with FR treatment was of limited efficacy and comparable to NST. Of patients with moderate and severe HN, $[Na^+]$ increased by ≥ 5 mmol/L in only 27% and 36% at Days 2 and 3, respectively. These results are in accordance with previous studies that showed a limited or no response with FR [11, 12].

Although not recommended, treatment with NS was the most common initial therapy [13]. Ascites is frequently the reason for hospitalization, and NS can exacerbate its severity and increase the need for invasive procedures, such as paracentesis. It may also exacerbate HN through "a desalination process" in which increased AVP levels lead to water retention and excretion of hypertonic urine [14]. Patients receiving NS had lower $[Na^+]$ than those receiving FR. Although the rate of increase in $[Na^+]$ was greater, its effectiveness was limited: of patients with moderate or severe HN, $[Na^+]$ only increased by ≥ 5 mmol/L in 45% and 51% of patients at Days 2 and 3, respectively.

Correction of HN was most effective with HS and TO. HS is recommended for severe symptomatic HN and was used as initial therapy in 2% of patients [15]. [Na^+] was lowest in patients receiving HS, and 82% had either moderate or severe HN. There are currently no reports on the response to HS in cirrhosis. In this study, HS led to a rapid increase in [Na^+]—an increase ≥ 5 mmol/L by Day 2 in 78% of patients.

TO was used as primary therapy in 5% of patients. The severity of HN was similar to those receiving HS, and 78% patients had either moderate or severe HN. As with HS, [Na^+] rapidly increased but at a slightly more gradual rate. At Day 2, 48% of patients had an increase ≥ 5 mmol/L. However, the percentage at Day 3 was comparable to HS (71% versus 78%; $P = 1.00$). This response rate was comparable to that observed in the cirrhosis population from the SALT1/SALT2 trials in which 40% and 70% of patients treated with TO had an increase ≥ 5 mmol/L at Days 2 and 3, respectively (data on file).

HN is frequent in patients with large-volume ascites [3]. In addition to the nonosmotic release of AVP, the renin-aldosterone system is activated, leading to increased renal sodium reabsorption. Diuretics are the mainstay of treatment of fluid overload but can exacerbate HN by decreasing intravascular volume (leading to increased AVP release) and only blocking sodium reabsorption, leaving continued free-water absorption unopposed [16]. Guidelines recommend tapering and then discontinuing diuretics if HN persists despite FR. However, diuretics were discontinued in only 17% of patients with HN at admission and were initiated in 7% of patients.

HN is associated with increased LOS in hospitalized patients [17–19]. In this study the impact of HN relapse in LOS after initial sodium correction was especially striking. Despite comparable initial Na level, level at correction, and time to correction, LOS was 4 days longer in those in whom HN recurred.

The results of this study are limited by its observational nature and broad definitions. FR was defined only by the physician orders indicated in the chart. NS and diuretic administration were also broadly defined. Albumin administration which is increasingly being used for the treatment of HN and infectious complications were not assessed [20]. In addition, Na levels have recently been reported to increase in response to treatment with midodrine and octreotide in a noncontrolled study [21]. However, the goal of this study was to evaluate treatment practices and outcomes in the real-world setting with the most commonly used approaches. The frequent administration of ineffective and/or nonstandardized therapy that frequently includes NS is not consistent with treatment guidelines. Correction of only 34% of patients at discharge suggests that most physicians do not view correction of HN as a meaningful clinical endpoint. Correction of HN is less important than demonstration of a beneficial impact on clinical endpoints. A question that invariably arises is whether HN is a direct participant in the pathophysiologic process and directly contributes to poor outcomes and increased LOS, or whether it is only a marker of end-stage disease. Preliminary evidence supports a contributory role for HN in hepatic encephalopathy [22]. Finally, treatment of HN with TO has also been shown to shorten LOS in patients with heart failure, syndrome of inappropriate diuretic hormone, and cancer [23, 24].

Determination of the impact of the treatment of HN in patients with cirrhosis will first require standardization of its management with effective therapy. The initial use of FR should be reevaluated, while NS administration should be avoided. Although HS is effective, it is limited by its deleterious impact on fluid overload and need for close monitoring, which frequently requires an intensive-care setting. In addition, the development of tense ascites due to HS administration can aggravate the severity of portal hypertension [23, 24]. Early treatment with TO offers an effective approach that should allow comprehensive assessment of the importance of HN treatment in the hospitalized patient with cirrhosis. Because the FDA-approved indications for TO have removed cirrhosis as an approved population, it is important that treatment with TO in these patients be performed in a carefully controlled manner.

Ethical Approval

The study was reviewed and approved by each site's respective Institutional Review Board.

Authors' Contributions

Samuel H. Sigal participated in data acquisition and analysis and wrote the paper. Alpesh Amin and Arun Sanyal participated in data acquisition and analysis and manuscript preparation. Joseph A. Chiodo III participated in data analysis and manuscript preparation.

Acknowledgments

This work was supported by Otsuka America Pharmaceutical, Inc. Jamie Jarecki-Smith of Clinovative Research provided continuing support for reviewing data entered in preparation for analysis. Statistical analysis was performed by the Mapi™ Group, Lexington, KY, USA, with funding by Otsuka. Editorial assistance was provided by Catherine Fontana and Geoff Marx of BioScience Communications, New York, NY, USA, which was funded by Otsuka.

References

[1] Y. Iwakiri and R. J. Groszmann, "The hyperdynamic circulation of chronic liver diseases: From the patient to the molecule," *Hepatology*, vol. 43, no. 2, pp. S121–S131, 2006.

[2] P. Ginès and M. Guevara, "Hyponatremia in cirrhosis: Pathogenesis, clinical significance, and management," *Hepatology*, vol. 48, no. 3, pp. 1002–1010, 2008.

[3] P. Angeli, F. Wong, H. Watson et al., "Hyponatremia in cirrhosis: Results of a patient population survey," *Hepatology*, vol. 44, no. 6, pp. 1535–1542, 2006.

[4] S. Deitelzweig, A. Amin, R. Christian, K. Friend, J. Lin, and T. J. Lowe, "Hyponatremia-associated healthcare burden among us patients hospitalized for cirrhosis," *Advances in Therapy*, vol. 30, no. 1, pp. 71–80, 2013.

[5] Vaprisol, "Nashville, TN: Cumberland Pharmaceuticals, Inc," 2014.

[6] Samsca, "Tokyo, Japan: Otsuka Pharmaceutical Co, Ltd," 2012.

[7] P. B. Watkins, J. H. Lewis, N. Kaplowitz et al., "Clinical pattern of tolvaptan-associated liver injury in subjects with autosomal dominant polycystic kidney disease: analysis of clinical trials database," *Drug Safety*, vol. 38, no. 11, pp. 1103–1113, 2015.

[8] A. Greenberg, J. G. Verbalis, A. N. Amin et al., "Current treatment practice and outcomes. Report of the hyponatremia registry," *Kidney International*, vol. 88, no. 1, pp. 167–177, 2015.

[9] P. S. Kamath and W. R. Kim, "The model for end-stage liver disease (MELD)," *Hepatology*, vol. 45, no. 3, pp. 797–805, 2007.

[10] J. G. Verbalis, S. R. Goldsmith, A. Greenberg et al., "Diagnosis, evaluation, and treatment of hyponatremia: expert panel recommendations," *American Journal of Medicine*, vol. 126, no. 10, supplement 1, pp. S1–S42, 2013.

[11] F. Wong, A. T. Blei, L. M. Blendis, and P. J. Thuluvath, "A vasopressin receptor antagonist (VPA-985) improves serum sodium concentration in patients with hyponatremia: A multicenter, randomized, placebo-controlled trial," *Hepatology*, vol. 37, no. 1, pp. 182–191, 2003.

[12] A. L. Gerbes, V. Gülberg, P. Ginès et al., "Therapy of hyponatremia in cirrhosis with a vasopressin receptor antagonist: A randomized double-blind multicenter trial," *Gastroenterology*, vol. 124, no. 4, pp. 933–939, 2003.

[13] European Association for the Study of the Liver, "EASL clinical practice guidelines on the management of ascites, spontaneous bacterial peritonitis, and hepatorenal syndrome in cirrhosis," *Journal of Hepatology*, vol. 53, no. 3, pp. 397–417, 2010.

[14] A. Steele, M. Gowrishankar, S. Abrahamson, C. D. Mazer, R. D. Feldman, and M. L. Halperin, "Postoperative hyponatremia despite near-isotonic saline infusion: a phenomenon of desalination," *Annals of Internal Medicine*, vol. 126, pp. 20–25, 1997.

[15] S. John and P. J. Thuluvath, "Hyponatremia in cirrhosis: pathophysiology and management," *World Journal of Gastroenterology*, vol. 21, no. 11, pp. 3197–3205, 2015.

[16] G. Liamis, H. Milionis, and M. Elisaf, "A review of drug-induced hyponatremia," *American Journal of Kidney Diseases*, vol. 52, no. 1, pp. 144–153, 2008.

[17] A. Amin, S. Deitelzweig, R. Christian et al., "Evaluation of incremental healthcare resource burden and readmission rates associated with hospitalized hyponatremic patients in the US," *Journal of Hospital Medicine*, vol. 7, no. 8, pp. 634–639, 2012.

[18] A. Amin, S. Deitelzweig, R. Christian, K. Friend, J. Lin, and T. J. Lowe, "Healthcare resource burden associated with hyponatremia among patients hospitalized for heart failure in the US," *Journal of Medical Economics*, vol. 16, no. 3, pp. 415–420, 2013.

[19] R. Berardi, M. Caramanti, M. Castagnani et al., "Hyponatremia is a predictor of hospital length and cost of stay and outcome in cancer patients," *Supportive Care in Cancer*, vol. 23, no. 10, pp. 3095–3101, 2015.

[20] A. Garioud, J. Cadranel, A. Pauwels et al., "Albumin use in patients with cirrhosis in France: results of the 'ALBU-LIVE' survey: a case for better EASL guidelines diffusions and/or revision," *Journal of Clinical Gastroenterology*, vol. 51, pp. 831–838, 2017.

[21] S. Patel, D. Nguyen, A. Rastogi, M. Nguyen, and M. K. Nguyen, "Treatment of cirrhosis-associated hyponatremia with midodrine and octreotide," *Frontiers in Medicine*, vol. 4, 2017.

[22] V. Ahluwalia, D. M. Heuman, G. Feldman et al., "Correction of hyponatraemia improves cognition, quality of life, and brain oedema in cirrhosis," *Journal of Hepatology*, vol. 62, no. 1, pp. 75–82, 2016.

[23] J. R. Chiong, S. Kim, J. Lin, R. Christian, and J. F. Dasta, "Evaluation of costs associated with tolvaptan-mediated length-of-stay reduction among heart failure patients with hyponatremia in the US, based on the EVEREST trial," *Journal of Medical Economics*, vol. 15, no. 2, pp. 276–284, 2012.

[24] A. K. Salahudeen, N. Ali, M. George, A. Lahoti, and S. Palla, "Tolvaptan in hospitalized cancer patients with hyponatremia: A double-blind, randomized, placebo-controlled clinical trial on efficacy and safety," *Cancer*, vol. 120, no. 5, pp. 744–751, 2014.

5

Laparoscopic versus Open Surgery for Hepatocellular Carcinoma

Ke Chen,[1] Yu Pan,[1] Bin Zhang,[1] Xiao-long Liu,[1] Hendi Maher,[2] and Xue-yong Zheng[1]

[1]*Department of General Surgery, Sir Run Run Shaw Hospital, School of Medicine, Zhejiang University, 3 East Qingchun Road, Hangzhou, Zhejiang 310016, China*
[2]*School of Medicine, Zhejiang University, 866 Yuhangtang Road, Hangzhou, Zhejiang 310058, China*

Correspondence should be addressed to Xue-yong Zheng; 3306053@zju.edu.cn

Academic Editor: Kevork M. Peltekian

Objective. To present a meta-analysis of high-quality case-matched studies comparing laparoscopic (LH) and open hepatectomy (OH) for hepatocellular carcinoma (HCC). *Methods.* Studies published up to September 2017 comparing LH and OH for HCC were identified. Selection of high-quality, nonrandomized comparative studies (NRCTs) with case-matched design was based on a validated tool (Methodological Index for Nonrandomized Studies) since no randomized controlled trials (RCTs) were published. Morbidity, mortality, operation time, blood loss, hospital stay, margin distance, recurrence, and survival outcomes were compared. Subgroup analyses were carried out according to the surgical extension (minor or major hepatectomy). *Results.* Twenty studies with a total of 830 patients (388 in LH and 442 in OH) were identified. For short-term surgical outcomes, LH showed less morbidity (RR = 0.55; 95% CI, 0.47~0.65; $P < 0.01$), less mortality (RR = 0.43; 95% CI, 0.18~1.00; $P = 0.05$), less blood loss (WMD = −93.21 ml, 95% CI, −157.33~−29.09 ml; $P < 0.01$), shorter hospital stay (WMD = −2.86, 95% CI, −3.63~−2.08; $P < 0.01$), and comparable operation time (WMD = 9.15 min; 95% CI: −7.61~25.90, $P = 0.28$). As to oncological outcomes, 5-year overall survival rate was slightly better in LH than OH (HR = 0.66, 95% CI: 0.52~0.84, $P < 0.01$), whereas the 5-year disease-free survival rate was comparable between two groups (HR = 0.88, 95% CI: 0.74~1.06, $P = 0.18$). *Conclusion.* This meta-analysis has highlighted that LH can be safely performed in selective patients and improves surgical outcomes as compared to OH. Given the limitations of study design, especially the limited cases of major hepatectomy, methodologically high-quality comparative studies are needed for further evaluation.

1. Introduction

Although the incidence of hepatocellular carcinoma (HCC) has decreased, HCC is still the fifth most common malignancy and the third leading cause of cancer-related death worldwide [1]. Since laparoscopic hepatectomy (LH) was first reported in 1996 [2, 3], this treatment has been considered a landmark development in the progress of surgical treatment. However, the majority of HCC patients usually have cirrhosis and hypohepatia. Because of this, hepatectomy increases the risk of developing significant postoperative complications including ascites, hepatic failure, encephalopathy, and portal vein thrombosis [4]. There are some controversial aspects of LH for HCC including complications, postoperative recovery, and long-term survival outcomes.

During the last 6 years, a number of meta-analyses that compare LH with open hepatectomy (OH) for HCC have been published [5–8]. Although randomized controlled trials (RCTs) are the most ideal tools for meta-analysis, no RCTs on this topic have been yet conducted. These meta-analyses included the available nonrandomized comparative studies (NRCTs) to overcome the paucity of RCTs. Therefore unreliable results and little strong evidence had been presented. On the other hand, there was evidence that estimates derived from high-quality NRCTs may be similar to those derived from RCTs [9]. Also, when comparing surgical procedures, pooling of high-quality NRCTs could be as accurate as pooling of RCTs [10]. In addition, several comparative studies on this topic have been published in the last 3 years and none of the published meta-analyses included studies published after 2013. Therefore, we performed an updated meta-analysis evaluating all of the available high-quality published trials to compare LH with OH for HCC.

2. Methods

2.1. Systematic Literature Search. Systematic searches of PubMed, Embase, Cochrane Library, and Web of Science were performed to identify articles published up to September 2017. Searches included the terms "laparoscopic," "minimally invasive," "hepatectomy," "liver resection," "hepatocellular carcinoma," and "HCC". All eligible studies in English were retrieved, and their bibliographies were checked for potential relevant publications.

2.2. Eligibility Criteria and Quality Assessment. In order to reduce bias, our meta-analysis synthesized the existing observational studies while strictly limiting inclusion and exclusion criteria. First of all, papers containing any of the following were excluded: (1) studies that included malignant lesions other than HCC, (2) studies focusing on recurrent HCC, (3) studies that included cases of robotic-assisted hepatectomy. Secondly, only studies designed with case-matched analysis were further evaluated and nonmatched studies were excluded. Then, the methodological quality of the eligible nonrandomized comparative studies (NRCTs) was assessed by the Methodological Index for Nonrandomized Studies (MINORS) [11]. In total, 8 items were evaluated, with a maximum score of 16 points. Studies with 12 or more points were considered of high quality and were included in the meta-analysis. Those with less than 12 points were excluded. Besides, if there was overlap between authors or centers, only the higher-quality or more recent literature was selected.

2.3. Data Extraction and Quality Assessment. Two researchers evaluated all the titles and abstracts. Then they assessed the selected full-text articles for eligibility. This work was then reevaluated and confirmed by a senior researcher. The measured outcomes of all eligible publications can be divided into two categories: ① short-term outcomes (operation time, estimated blood loss, transfusion, length of hospital stay, morbidity, and mortality); ② oncological outcomes (tumor size, margin distance, R0 resection, recurrence, and survival). The postoperative morbidity was cataloged according to the Clavien-Dindo classification. Minor complication refers to Grade I and Grade II complications, and major complication includes Grade III to V complications.

2.4. Subgroup Analysis. Because the different levels of hepatectomy can lead to different outcomes, and major hepatectomy is a technically dependent and time-consuming procedure, subgroup analyses were carried out according to surgical extensions. Included studies were assigned to 3 subgroups: minor hepatectomy, mixed hepatectomy, and major hepatectomy.

2.5. Statistical Analysis. The risk ratio (RR) was utilized to analyze the dichotomous variables, and the weighted mean difference (WMD) was utilized to assess the continuous variables. If the study provided medians and ranges instead of means and standard deviations (SDs), we estimated the means and SDs as described by Hozo et al. [12]. Heterogeneity was evaluated by Cochran's Q statistic and Higgins I^2 statistic [13]. If data was not significantly heterogeneous ($P > 0.05$ or $I^2 < 50\%$), the pooled effects were calculated using a fixed model. Otherwise, the pooled effects were calculated using a random model. The hazard ratios (HRs) of a 5-year overall survival rate (OS) and a 5-year disease-free survival rate (DFS) were used with a generic inverse variance meta-analysis. The log HR and its SE were estimated using the method introduced by Tierney et al. [14]. According to the overall morbidity, potential publication bias was determined by carrying out an informal visual inspection of funnel plots. A two-tailed value of $P < 0.05$ was considered significant. All statistical tests were performed with Review Manager version 5.1 (The Cochrane Collaboration, Oxford, England).

3. Results

3.1. Search Results and Baseline Characteristics. The last search was performed on September 20, 2017. A total of 968 potential published articles were initially identified from the search. Of these, 63 articles were selected based on their titles and abstracts, and a full examination of the texts was performed. Further 37 papers were excluded, after being read thoroughly, due to (1) including non-HCC cases ($n = 4$), (2) focusing on recurrent HCC ($n = 3$), (3) robot-assisted hepatectomy ($n = 1$), (4) overlap patient cohorts ($n = 2$), or (5) nonmatched comparative studies ($n = 27$). Then 26 studies were selected for quality assessment, and 6 studies were excluded by a modified MINORS score < 12 [15–20]. Finally, 20 studies were selected for final meta-analysis [21–40]. A flow chart of the search strategies, which contains reasons for excluding studies, is elucidated in Figure 1. The details of the selection process, which included the references of excluded studies and the MINORS assessments of low-quality studies, could be found in Supplementary Materials (available here).

3.2. Study Characteristics. A total of 830 patients were included in the analysis with 388 undergoing LH (46.8%) and 442 undergoing OH (53.2%). The characteristics of these included studies are summarized in Table 1. Studies were well matched in terms of age, gender, ASA classification, body mass index (BMI), tumor size, and surgical extension. Eight studies reported only minor hepatectomy, and three studies focused on major hepatectomy, whereas the remaining nine studies included both minor and major hepatectomy. The majority of studies graded morbidity according to the Clavien-Dindo classification, with the study by Lee et al. being the only exception [24]. The assessments of the NRCTs are illustrated in Table 2. Each trial received more than 12 points (the maximum possible score is 16) and was considered to be of the highest quality (see Supplementary Materials).

Table 1: Basic information of the included literature.

Author	Region	Year	Study period	Sample size LH	Sample size OH	Matching method	Cirrhosis (%) LH	Cirrhosis (%) OH	Surgical extension	Conversion (%)	Clavien-Dindo
Belli et al.	Italy	2007	2000–2004	23	23	CCM	100	100	Minor	4.3	Yes
Tranchart et al.	France	2010	1999–2008	42	42	CCM	73.8	81	Mixed	4.8	Yes
Kim et al.	Korea	2011	2005–2009	26	29	CCM	92.3	86.2	Mixed	E	Yes
Truant et al.	France	2011	2002–2009	36	53	CCM	100	100	Minor	19.4	Yes
Lee et al.	Hong Kong	2011	2004–2010	33	50	CCM	84.8	64	Minor	18.2	NA
Ahn et al.	Korea	2014	2005–2013	51	51	PSM	68.6	66.8	Mixed	9.8	Yes
Kim et al.	Korea	2014	2000–2012	29	29	PSM	62.1	65.5	Minor	E	Yes
Memeo et al.	France	2014	1990–2009	45	45	CCM	100	100	Minor	NA	Yes
Lau et al.	USA	2015	2008–2014	26	26	CCM	80.8	73.1	Mixed	35	Yes
Lee et al.	Canada	2015	2006–2013	43	86	CCM	NA	NA	Mixed	14	Yes
Luo et al.	China	2015	2008–2015	53	53	CCM	100	100	Minor	E	Yes
Takahara et al.	Japan	2015	2000–2010	387	387	PSM	61.7	59.6	Mixed	6.5	Yes
Han et al.	Korea	2015	2004–2013	88	88	PSM	62.5	59.1	Mixed	9.1	Yes
Yoon et al.	Korea	2015	2007–2011	58	174	PSM	NA	NA	Mixed	0	Yes
Cheung et al.	Hong Kong	2016	2002–2015	110	330	PSM	100	100	Mixed	5.5	Yes
Sposito et al.	Italy	2016	2006–2013	43	43	PSM	100	100	Minor	4.7	Yes
Jiang et al.	China	2016	2008–2013	59	59	PSM	100	100	Minor	5.1	Yes
Komatsu et al.	France	2016	2000–2014	38	38	CCM	NA	NA	Major	31.6	Yes
Yoon et al.	Korea	2017	2008–2015	33	33	PSM	100	100	Major	NA	Yes
Xu et al.	China	2017	2015–2017	32	32	PSM	100	100	Major	NA	Yes

CCM: case by case matching; PSM: propensity score matching; E: conversion cases were excluded from the studies; NA: not available.

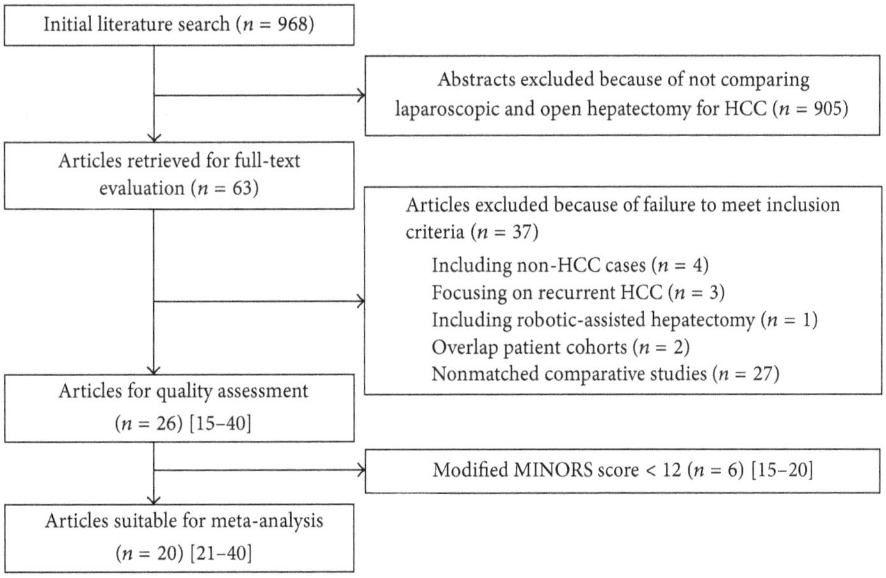

Figure 1: Flow chart of literature search strategies.

3.3. Meta-Analysis of Short-Term Outcomes

3.3.1. Operation Time. Operative time was reported in all studies [21–40]. Statistically significant between-study heterogeneity was identified in all subgroups ($P < 0.01$, $I^2 = 87.2\%$). There was no significant difference between the groups' operation times (Table 3). However, in the subgroup of major hepatectomy, the overall effect size of the mean operation time was significantly longer in LH than that in OH (WMD = 77.93 min, 95% CI: 40.45~115.41, $P < 0.01$).

3.3.2. Intraoperative Blood Loss. Blood loss was available from 17 studies [21, 22, 24–34, 36, 37, 39, 40]. Statistically significant between-study heterogeneity was identified in all subgroups ($P < 0.01$, $I^2 = 88.1\%$). The pooled results showed that LH was associated with less blood loss than OH (Table 3).

TABLE 2: Modified MINORS score of all eligible nonrandomized comparative studies.

Author	①	②	③	④	⑤	⑥	⑦	⑧	Score
Belli et al.	2	2	1	2	2	1	2	1	13
Tranchart et al.	2	2	1	1	2	1	2	2	13
Kim et al.	2	1	1	2	2	2	1	1	12
Truant et al.	2	2	1	1	2	2	1	1	12
Lee et al.	2	2	1	1	2	2	1	1	12
Ahn et al.	2	2	1	1	2	2	2	2	14
Kim et al.	2	1	1	2	2	2	1	1	12
Memeo et al.	2	1	1	1	2	1	2	2	12
Lau et al.	2	1	2	1	2	2	2	1	13
Lee et al.	2	1	1	1	2	2	1	2	12
Luo et al.	2	1	1	1	2	2	2	2	13
Takahara et al.	2	1	1	1	2	2	2	2	13
Han et al.	2	1	1	1	2	2	2	2	13
Yoon et al.	2	1	1	1	2	2	1	2	12
Cheung et al.	2	2	1	1	2	2	2	2	14
Sposito et al.	2	2	1	1	2	2	2	2	14
Jiang et al.	2	1	1	1	2	2	2	2	13
Komatsu et al.	2	1	1	1	2	2	2	1	12
Yoon et al.	2	1	2	2	2	2	2	1	14
Xu et al.	2	2	2	1	2	2	2	1	14

① Consecutive patients, ② prospective data collection, ③ reported endpoints, ④ unbiased outcome evaluation, ⑤ appropriate controls, ⑥ contemporary groups, ⑦ groups equivalent, ⑧ sample size.

However, in the subgroup of major hepatectomy, there was no significant difference between groups (WMD = 3.75 ml, 95% CI: −60.16~67.65, $P = 0.88$).

3.3.3. Blood Transfusion. Fourteen studies recorded perioperative blood transfusion [21–27, 29, 30, 33–35, 37, 39]. There was no evidence of heterogeneity between subgroups ($P = 0.81$, $I^2 = 0\%$). Although none of the subgroups reached a significant difference, the overall pooled data indicated that transfusion rates were lower in LH (RR = 0.73, 95% CI: 0.55~0.96, $P = 0.03$) (Table 3).

3.3.4. Duration of Hospital Stay. The length of hospital stays was pooled for all studies [21–40]. Although statistically significant between-study heterogeneity was identified in each subgroup, there was no evidence of heterogeneity between subgroups ($P = 0.99$, $I^2 = 0\%$). Hospital stays in LH group were shorter than those in OH group (WMD = −2.86 d, 95% CI: −3.63~−2.08, $P < 0.01$) (Table 3).

3.3.5. Morbidity. All studies reported their overall complication rates [21–40]. Because there was no statistical evidence of heterogeneity, the effect sizes of all subgroups were synthesized to generate the overall effect size ($P = 0.91$, $I^2 = 0\%$) (Table 3) (Figure 2). The postoperative morbidity rates were 14.0% (176/1255) in LH and 24.2% (404/1671) in OH. In addition the pooled data showed that LH significantly reduced postoperative complications (RR = 0.55; 95% CI, 0.47~0.65; $P < 0.01$) (Table 3). Moreover, each subgroup also revealed reduced overall morbidity in the LH group (Table 3).

Eighteen studies recorded severe complications [21, 22, 25–40]. Similar to overall morbidity, the results showed that patients in the LH group suffered less severe complications (Table 3). We identified specified complications of ascites, liver failure, and the respiratory system. The results implied that postoperative ascites in patients, regardless of whether they underwent minor or major hepatectomy, was less in LH than in OH (RR = 0.42; 95% CI, 0.31~0.59; $P < 0.01$) (Figure 3(a)). Studies that recorded postoperative liver failure reported a lower incidence of liver failure in LH than in OH with one exception by Xu et al. [39]. The overall pooled data revealed that patients in the LH group were less likely to suffer liver failure than those in the OH group (RR = 0.41; 95% CI, 0.27~0.64; $P < 0.01$) (Figure 3(b)). LH was also associated with a significant reduction in respiratory complications regardless of different surgical extension (RR = 0.43, 95% CI: 0.28~0.64, $P < 0.01$) (Figure 3(c)).

3.3.6. Mortality. Nine studies recorded cases of postoperative death [21, 22, 25, 28–30, 33, 35, 39]. There was no evidence of heterogeneity between subgroups ($P = 0.97$, $I^2 = 0\%$). These studies showed very low incidences of mortality. However, the overall pooled data indicated a more reduced postoperative mortality in LH than that in OH (RR = 0.43; 95% CI, 0.18~1.00; $P = 0.05$) (Table 3).

3.4. Meta-Analysis of Oncological Outcomes

3.4.1. Tumor Size. Only one study did not report tumor size [30]. There was trifling heterogeneity between subgroups, mainly due to the major hepatectomy subgroup ($P = 0.35$, I^2

TABLE 3: Overall outcomes of the meta-analysis.

Outcomes	Studies No.	Sample size LH	OH	Heterogeneity (P, I^2)	Model	Overall effect size	95% CI of overall effect	P
Operation time (min)	20	1255	1671	<0.01, 87%	R	WMD = 9.15	−7.61~25.90	0.28
Minor hepatectomy	8	321	355	<0.01, 78%	R	WMD = 12.04	−5.31~29.39	0.17
Mixed hepatectomy	9	831	1213	<0.01, 83%	R	WMD = −14.28	−40.76~12.21	0.29
Major hepatectomy	3	103	103	0.05, 67%	R	WMD = 77.93	40.45~115.41	**<0.01**
Blood loss (mL)	17	1128	1425	<0.01, 92%	R	WMD = −93.21	−157.33~−29.09	**<0.01**
Minor hepatectomy	7	278	312	0.39, 5%	R	WMD = −76.21	−98.41~−54.01	**<0.01**
Mixed hepatectomy	7	747	1010	0.05, 52%	R	WMD = −212.94	−294.57~−131.31	**<0.01**
Major hepatectomy	3	103	103	0.88, 0%	R	WMD = 3.75	−60.16~67.65	0.88
Transfusion	14	979	1352	0.90, 0%	F	RR = 0.73	0.55~0.96	**0.03**
Minor hepatectomy	4	121	155	0.49, 0%	F	RR = 0.53	0.19~1.45	0.22
Mixed hepatectomy	8	788	1127	0.86, 0%	F	RR = 0.75	0.55~1.01	0.06
Major hepatectomy	2	70	70	0.28, 15%	F	RR = 0.75	0.17~3.25	0.70
Hospital stay (days)	20	1255	1671	<0.01, 80%	R	WMD = −2.86	−3.63~−2.08	**<0.01**
Minor hepatectomy	8	321	355	<0.01, 76%	R	WMD = −2.93	−4.23~−1.63	**<0.01**
Mixed hepatectomy	9	831	1213	0.01, 58%	R	WMD = −2.85	−3.95~−1.76	**<0.01**
Major hepatectomy	3	103	103	0.15, 47%	R	WMD = −2.76	−4.60~−0.92	**<0.01**
Morbidity	20	1255	1671	0.28, 14%	F	RR = 0.55	0.47~0.65	**<0.01**
Minor hepatectomy	8	321	355	0.29, 17%	F	RR = 0.53	0.41~0.69	**<0.01**
Mixed hepatectomy	9	831	1213	0.26, 21%	F	RR = 0.57	0.46~0.72	**<0.01**
Major hepatectomy	3	103	103	0.21, 37%	F	RR = 0.55	0.36~0.83	**<0.01**
Severe complications	18	1196	1476	0.88, 0%	F	RR = 0.51	0.39~0.68	**<0.01**
Minor hepatectomy	7	288	305	0.96, 0%	F	RR = 0.48	0.24~0.96	**0.04**
Mixed hepatectomy	8	805	1068	0.44, 0%	F	RR = 0.54	0.38~0.76	**<0.01**
Major hepatectomy	3	103	103	0.35, 6%	F	RR = 0.42	0.18~1.00	**0.05**
Mortality	9	789	1026	0.88, 0	F	RR = 0.43	0.18~1.00	**0.05**
Minor hepatectomy	3	104	121	0.34, 7	F	RR = 0.39	0.09~1.68	0.21
Mixed hepatectomy	5	653	873	0.84, 0	F	RR = 0.46	0.15~1.43	0.18
Major hepatectomy	1	32	32	Not applicable	F	RR = 0.33	0.01~7.89	0.50
Tumor size (cm)	19	1229	1645	<0.01, 57%	R	WMD = −0.19	−0.41~0.03	0.09
Minor hepatectomy	8	321	355	0.76, 0%	R	WMD = −0.07	−0.26~0.12	0.48
Mixed hepatectomy	8	805	1187	0.50, 0%	R	WMD = −0.09	−0.25~0.07	0.28
Major hepatectomy	3	103	103	<0.01, 92%	R	WMD = −1.77	−4.06~0.53	0.13
Margin distance (cm)	11	501	694	0.14, 47%	R	WMD = 2.61	1.06~4.17	**<0.01**
Minor hepatectomy	5	186	220	0.06, 56%	R	WMD = 2.16	0.15~4.17	**0.03**
Mixed hepatectomy	5	282	441	0.15, 41%	R	WMD = 3.20	0.41~5.99	**0.02**
Major hepatectomy	1	33	33	Not applicable	R	WMD = 5.90	−2.69~14.49	0.18
R0 resection	14	1010	1409	0.70, 0%	F	RR = 1.01	0.99~1.02	0.37
Minor hepatectomy	6	240	257	0.80, 0%	F	RR = 0.98	0.95~1.01	0.23
Mixed hepatectomy	7	738	1120	0.47, 0%	F	RR = 1.01	1.00~1.03	0.13
Major hepatectomy	1	32	32	Not applicable	F	RR = 1.03	0.93~1.15	0.56

WMD: weighted mean difference; RR: risk ratio; F: fixed; R: random.

= 4.2%) (Table 3). Meta-analysis showed that the tumor size of OH was longer than that of LH with a marginal difference (WMD = −0.19 cm; 95% CI: −0.41~−0.03, P = 0.09), which was mainly due to smaller tumors in LH than those in OH in the major hepatectomy subgroup (Table 3).

3.4.2. Margin Distance. Only 11 studies mentioned the distance of the tumor margin [22, 24–29, 31, 34, 38, 40]. Although statistical significant between-study heterogeneity was identified in each subgroup, there was no evidence of heterogeneity between subgroups (P = 0.63, I^2 = 0%). On

Study or subgroup	LH Events	LH Total	OH Events	OH Total	Weight	Risk ratio M-H, fixed, 95% CI	Year
1.8.1 Minor hepatectomy							
Belli et al.	3	23	11	23	3.2%	0.27 [0.09, 0.85]	2007
Truant et al.	9	36	19	53	4.5%	0.70 [0.36, 1.36]	2011
Lee et al.	2	33	12	50	2.8%	0.25 [0.06, 1.06]	2011
Memeo et al.	9	45	20	45	5.9%	0.45 [0.23, 0.88]	2014
Kim et al.	4	29	11	29	3.2%	0.36 [0.13, 1.01]	2014
Luo et al.	16	53	19	53	5.6%	0.84 [0.49, 1.45]	2015
Sposito et al.	8	43	21	43	6.2%	0.38 [0.19, 0.76]	2016
Jiang et al.	12	59	16	59	4.7%	0.75 [0.39, 1.44]	2016
Subtotal (95% CI)		321		355	36.0%	0.53 [0.41, 0.69]	
Total events	63		129				
Heterogeneity: $\chi^2 = 8.45$, df = 7 ($P = 0.29$); $I^2 = 17\%$							
Test for overall effect: $Z = 4.77$ ($P < 0.00001$)							
1.8.2 Mixed hepatectomy							
Tranchart et al.	10	42	18	42	5.3%	0.56 [0.29, 1.06]	2010
Kim et al.	1	26	7	29	1.9%	0.16 [0.02, 1.21]	2011
Ahn et al.	3	51	5	51	1.5%	0.60 [0.15, 2.38]	2014
Takahara et al.	26	387	50	387	14.7%	0.52 [0.33, 0.82]	2015
Han et al.	11	88	18	88	5.3%	0.61 [0.31, 1.22]	2015
Lee et al.	10	43	34	86	6.6%	0.59 [0.32, 1.07]	2015
Lau et al.	14	26	11	26	3.2%	1.27 [0.72, 2.26]	2015
Yoon et al.	5	58	40	174	5.9%	0.38 [0.16, 0.90]	2015
Cheung et al.	10	110	50	330	7.3%	0.60 [0.32, 1.14]	2016
Subtotal (95% CI)		831		1213	51.7%	0.57 [0.46, 0.72]	
Total events	90		233				
Heterogeneity: $\chi^2 = 10.14$, df = 8 ($P = 0.26$); $I^2 = 21\%$							
Test for overall effect: $Z = 4.80$ ($P < 0.00001$)							
1.8.3 Major hepatectomy							
Komatsu et al.	12	38	23	38	6.7%	0.52 [0.31, 0.89]	2016
Xu et al.	10	32	12	32	3.5%	0.83 [0.42, 1.65]	2017
Yoon et al.	1	33	7	33	2.1%	0.14 [0.02, 1.10]	2017
Subtotal (95% CI)		103		103	12.3%	0.55 [0.36, 0.83]	
Total events	23		42				
Heterogeneity: $\chi^2 = 3.16$, df = 2 ($P = 0.21$); $I^2 = 37\%$							
Test for overall effect: $Z = 2.87$ ($P = 0.004$)							
Total (95% CI)		1255		1671	100.0%	0.55 [0.47, 0.65]	
Total events	176		404				
Heterogeneity: $\chi^2 = 22.01$, df = 19 ($P = 0.28$); $I^2 = 14\%$							
Test for overall effect: $Z = 7.28$ ($P < 0.00001$)							
Test for subgroup differences: $\chi^2 = 0.19$, df = 2 ($P = 0.91$), $I^2 = 0\%$							

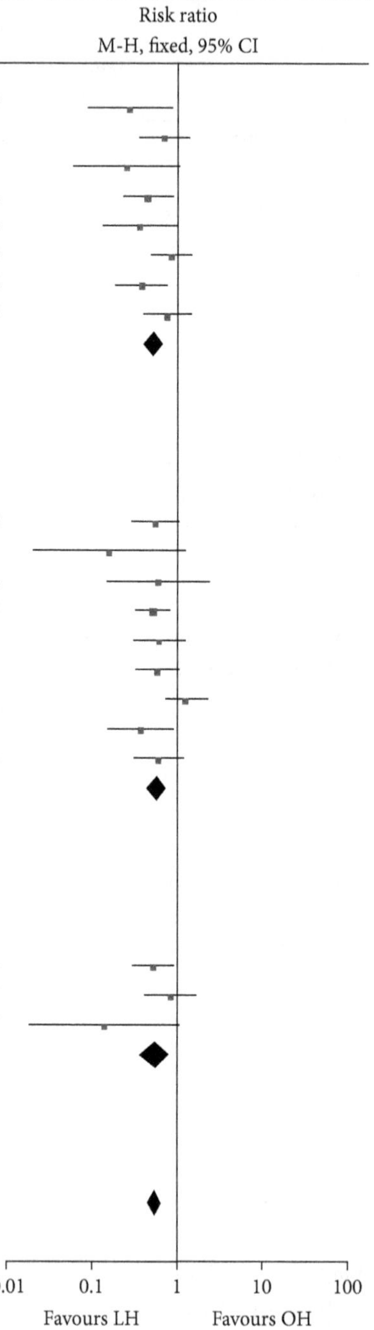

Figure 2: Forest plot of overall morbidity.

pooling the results, the margin distance was longer in the LH group than that in the OH group (WMD = 2.61 cm; 95% CI: 1.06~4.17, $P < 0.01$) (Table 3).

3.4.3. R0 Resection. The R0 resection was reported in 14 studies [21, 23, 24, 27, 29–36, 38, 39]. There was no obvious heterogeneity ($P = 0.18$, $I^2 = 41.8\%$). The pooled estimate for margin distance indicated comparative outcomes between groups (RR = 1.01, 95% CI: 0.99~1.02, $P = 0.37$) (Table 3).

3.4.4. Overall Survival Rate and Disease-Free Survival Rate. Summary of follow-up time, recurrence, and long-term survival rates is listed in Table 4. Nineteen studies reported the detailed long-term outcomes. Among them, the data for 5-year OS rates can be extracted from nine studies and the data for 5-year DFS rates can be extracted from ten studies. The follow-up periods in six studies were less than five years. The survival data of three studies cannot be extracted due to a technical problem with figures. Unfortunately, none of the three major hepatectomy studies can be included in our survival analysis [37, 39, 40]. In all, the pooled 5-year OS rate

Study or subgroup	LH Events	LH Total	OH Events	OH Total	Weight	Risk ratio M-H, fixed, 95% CI	Year
1.10.1 Minor hepatectomy							
Belli et al.	3	23	9	23	8.1%	0.33 [0.10, 1.08]	2007
Lee et al.	0	33	2	50	1.8%	0.30 [0.01, 6.06]	2011
Truant et al.	5	36	12	53	8.7%	0.61 [0.24, 1.59]	2011
Kim et al.	0	29	5	29	4.9%	0.09 [0.01, 1.57]	2014
Memeo et al.	1	45	8	45	7.2%	0.13 [0.02, 0.96]	2014
Luo et al.	3	53	3	53	2.7%	1.00 [0.21, 4.73]	2015
Sposito et al.	6	43	18	43	16.2%	0.33 [0.15, 0.76]	2016
Jiang et al.	2	59	2	59	1.8%	1.00 [0.15, 6.87]	2016
Subtotal (95% CI)		321		355	51.5%	0.39 [0.24, 0.61]	
Total events	20		59				
Heterogeneity: $\chi^2 = 5.66$, df = 7 ($P = 0.58$); $I^2 = 0\%$							
Test for overall effect: $Z = 4.07$ ($P < 0.0001$)							
1.10.2 Mixed hepatectomy							
Tranchart et al.	3	42	11	42	9.9%	0.27 [0.08, 0.91]	2010
Kim et al.	0	26	1	29	1.3%	0.37 [0.02, 8.71]	2011
Ahn et al.	1	51	2	51	1.8%	0.50 [0.05, 5.34]	2014
Takahara et al.	7	387	12	387	10.8%	0.58 [0.23, 1.47]	2015
Lee et al.	7	387	12	387	10.8%	0.58 [0.23, 1.47]	2015
Lau et al.	3	53	3	53	2.7%	1.00 [0.21, 4.73]	2015
Subtotal (95% CI)		946		949	37.3%	0.52 [0.31, 0.86]	
Total events	21		41				
Heterogeneity: $\chi^2 = 1.95$, df = 5 ($P = 0.86$); $I^2 = 0\%$							
Test for overall effect: $Z = 2.52$ ($P = 0.01$)							
1.10.3 Major hepatectomy							
Xu et al.	3	32	10	32	9.0%	0.30 [0.09, 0.99]	2017
Yoon et al.	0	33	2	33	2.2%	0.20 [0.01, 4.01]	2017
Subtotal (95% CI)		65		65	11.2%	0.28 [0.09, 0.85]	
Total events	3		12				
Heterogeneity: $\chi^2 = 0.06$, df = 1 ($P = 0.80$); $I^2 = 0\%$							
Test for overall effect: $Z = 2.25$ ($P = 0.02$)							
Total (95% CI)		1332		1369	100.0%	0.42 [0.31, 0.59]	
Total events	44		112				
Heterogeneity: $\chi^2 = 8.75$, df = 15 ($P = 0.89$); $I^2 = 0\%$							
Test for overall effect: $Z = 5.19$ ($P < 0.00001$)							
Test for subgroup differences: $\chi^2 = 1.32$, df = 2 ($P = 0.52$), $I^2 = 0\%$							

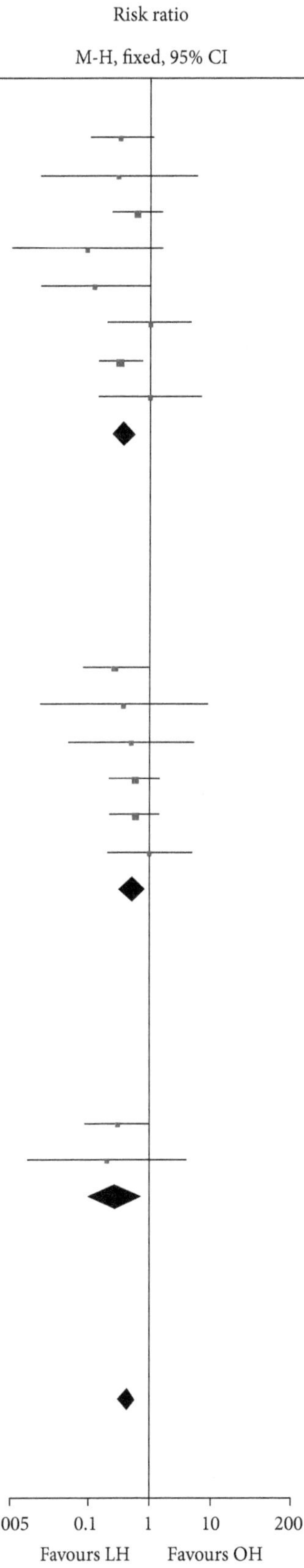

(a)

FIGURE 3: Continued.

Study or subgroup	LH Events	LH Total	OH Events	OH Total	Weight	Risk ratio M-H, fixed, 95% CI	Year
1.11.1 Minor hepatectomy							
Truant et al.	0	36	4	53	5.7%	0.16 [0.01, 2.92]	2011
Memeo et al.	1	45	5	45	7.8%	0.20 [0.02, 1.64]	2014
Luo et al.	1	53	2	53	3.1%	0.50 [0.05, 5.35]	2015
Jiang et al.	0	59	1	59	2.3%	0.33 [0.01, 8.02]	2016
Sposito et al.	0	43	2	43	3.9%	0.20 [0.01, 4.05]	2016
Subtotal (95% CI)		236		253	22.9%	0.25 [0.08, 0.78]	
Total events	2		14				
Heterogeneity: $\chi^2 = 0.52$, df = 4 ($P = 0.97$); $I^2 = 0\%$							
Test for overall effect: $Z = 2.38$ ($P = 0.02$)							
1.11.2 Mixed hepatectomy							
Tranchart et al.	3	42	11	42	17.2%	0.27 [0.08, 0.91]	2010
Takahara et al.	2	387	7	387	11.0%	0.29 [0.06, 1.37]	2015
Han et al.	3	88	8	88	12.5%	0.38 [0.10, 1.37]	2015
Lau et al.	1	53	2	53	3.1%	0.50 [0.05, 5.35]	2015
Cheung et al.	0	110	4	330	3.5%	0.33 [0.02, 6.11]	2016
Subtotal (95% CI)		680		900	47.3%	0.32 [0.16, 0.65]	
Total events	9		32				
Heterogeneity: $\chi^2 = 0.28$, df = 4 ($P = 0.99$); $I^2 = 0\%$							
Test for overall effect: $Z = 3.14$ ($P = 0.002$)							
1.11.3 Major hepatectomy							
Komatsu et al.	6	38	14	38	21.9%	0.43 [0.18, 1.00]	2016
Xu et al.	7	32	5	32	7.8%	1.40 [0.50, 3.95]	2017
Subtotal (95% CI)		70		70	29.7%	0.68 [0.36, 1.28]	
Total events	13		19				
Heterogeneity: $\chi^2 = 3.01$, df = 1 ($P = 0.08$); $I^2 = 87\%$							
Test for overall effect: $Z = 1.18$ ($P = 0.24$)							
Total (95% CI)		986		1223	100.0%	0.41 [0.27, 0.64]	
Total events	24		65				
Heterogeneity: $\chi^2 = 7.19$, df = 11 ($P = 0.78$); $I^2 = 0\%$							
Test for overall effect: $Z = 4.01$ ($P < 0.0001$)							
Test for subgroup differences: $\chi^2 = 3.62$, df = 2 ($P = 0.16$), $I^2 = 44.8\%$							

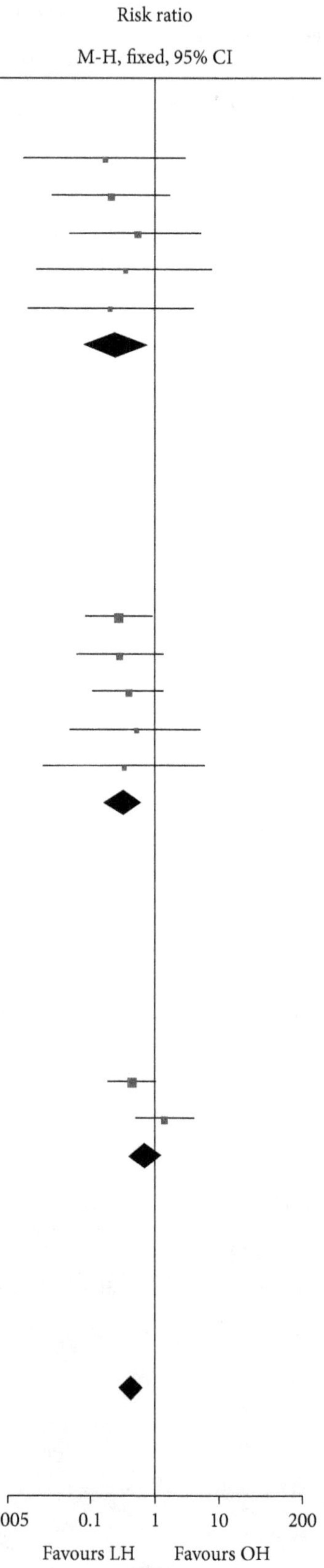

(b)

FIGURE 3: Continued.

Study or subgroup	LH Events	LH Total	OH Events	OH Total	Weight	Risk ratio M-H, fixed, 95% CI	Year
1.12.1 Minor hepatectomy							
Belli et al.	1	23	5	23	6.7%	0.20 [0.03, 1.58]	2007
Lee et al.	1	33	6	50	6.3%	0.25 [0.03, 2.00]	2011
Truant et al.	1	36	3	53	3.2%	0.49 [0.05, 4.53]	2011
Memeo et al.	5	45	8	45	10.6%	0.63 [0.22, 1.76]	2014
Luo et al.	2	53	4	53	5.3%	0.50 [0.10, 2.61]	2015
Jiang et al.	2	59	2	59	2.7%	1.00 [0.15, 6.87]	2016
Sposito et al.	1	43	2	43	2.7%	0.50 [0.05, 5.31]	2016
Subtotal (95% CI)		292		326	37.5%	0.48 [0.25, 0.89]	
Total events	13		30				
Heterogeneity: $\chi^2 = 1.88$, df = 6 ($P = 0.93$); $I^2 = 0\%$							
Test for overall effect: $Z = 2.30$ ($P = 0.02$)							
1.12.2 Mixed hepatectomy							
Tranchart et al.	1	42	4	42	5.3%	0.25 [0.03, 2.14]	2010
Kim et al.	1	26	0	29	0.6%	3.33 [0.14, 78.42]	2011
Takahara et al.	2	387	5	387	6.7%	0.40 [0.08, 2.05]	2015
Han et al.	4	88	6	88	8.0%	0.67 [0.19, 2.28]	2015
Cheung et al.	5	110	40	330	26.6%	0.38 [0.15, 0.93]	2016
Subtotal (95% CI)		653		876	47.2%	0.45 [0.25, 0.83]	
Total events	13		55				
Heterogeneity: $\chi^2 = 2.40$, df = 4 ($P = 0.66$); $I^2 = 0\%$							
Test for overall effect: $Z = 2.55$ ($P = 0.01$)							
1.12.3 Major hepatectomy							
Yoon et al.	0	33	2	33	3.3%	0.20 [0.01, 4.01]	2017
Xu et al.	2	32	9	32	12.0%	0.22 [0.05, 0.95]	2017
Subtotal (95% CI)		65		65	15.3%	0.22 [0.06, 0.80]	
Total events	2		11				
Heterogeneity: $\chi^2 = 0.00$, df = 1 ($P = 0.95$); $I^2 = 0\%$							
Test for overall effect: $Z = 2.29$ ($P = 0.02$)							
Total (95% CI)		1010		1267	100.0%	0.43 [0.28, 0.64]	
Total events	28		96				
Heterogeneity: $\chi^2 = 5.58$, df = 13 ($P = 0.96$); $I^2 = 0\%$							
Test for overall effect: $Z = 4.05$ ($P < 0.0001$)							
Test for subgroup differences: $\chi^2 = 1.17$, df = 2 ($P = 0.56$), $I^2 = 0\%$							

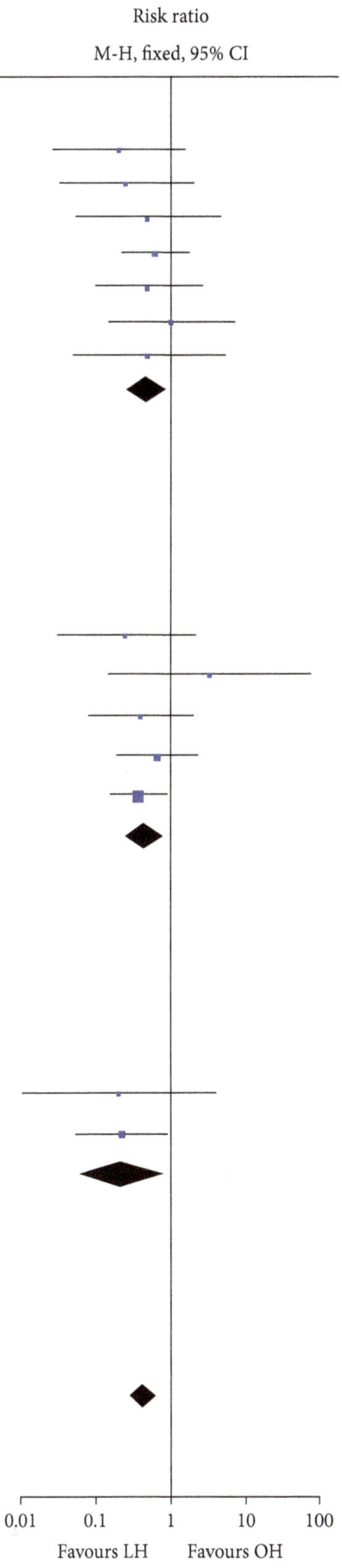

(c)

FIGURE 3: Forest plot of specific complications: (a) ascites, (b) liver failure, (c) respiratory complications.

TABLE 4: Summary of recurrence and long-term survival.

Author	Group	Follow-up	R	Survival (time: month; rate: %)
Tranchart et al.	LH	29.7	10	1, 3, 5 y-DFS: 81.6, 60.9, 45.6; 1, 3, 5 y-OS: 93.1, 74.4, 59.5.
	OH	24.6	12	1, 3, 5 y-DFS: 70.2, 54.3, 37.2; 1, 3, 5 y-OS: 81.8, 73, 47.4.
Kim et al.	LH	21.8	7	MDFS: 13.4; 1 y-DFS: 84.6.
	OH	24.8	10	MDFS: 14.6; 1 y-DFS: 82.8.
Truant et al.	LH	35.7	16	5 y-DFS: 35.5; 5 y-OS: 70.
	OH		23	5 y-DFS: 33.6; 5 y-OS: 46.
Lee et al.	LH	35.4	15	1, 3, 5 y-DFS: 78.8, 51, 45.3; 1, 3, 5 y-OS: 86.9, 81.8, 76.0.
	OH	28.5	19	1, 3, 5 y-DFS: 69.2, 55.9, 55.9; 1, 3, 5 y-OS: 98, 80.6, 76.1.
Ahn et al.	LH	38.6	12	5 y-DFS: 67.8; 5 y-OS: 80.1.
	OH	52.3	21	5 y-DFS: 54.8; 5 y-OS: 85.7.
Kim et al.	LH	47.9	11	MDFS: 15.4; MOS: 47.9; 1, 3, 5 y-DFS: 81.1, 61.7, 54.0; 1, 3, 5 y-OS: 100, 100, 92.2.
	OH	59.5	16	MDFS: 32.6; MOS: 59.5; 1, 3, 5 y-DFS: 78.6, 60.9, 40.1; 1, 3, 5 y-OS: 96.5, 92.2, 87.7.
Memeo et al.	LH	NR	25	1, 5, 10 y-DFS: 80, 19, 0; 1, 5, 10 y-OS: 88, 59, 12.
	OH	NR	28	1, 5, 10 y-DFS: 60, 23, 9; 1, 5, 10 y-OS: 63, 44, 22.
Lee et al.	LH	22.7	NR	1, 3, 5 y-DFS: 60.5, 53.5, 53.5; 1, 3, 5 y-OS: 95.3, 89.7, 89.7.
	OH	44.4	NR	1, 3, 5 y-DFS: 81.5, 66.7, 58.6; 1, 3, 5 y-OS: 93.9, 89.5, 87.3.
Luo et al.	LH	35	20	MDFS: 21.
	OH	37	24	MDFS: 18.
Takahara et al.	LH	46.7	NR	1, 3, 5 y-DFS: 83.7, 58.3, 40.7; 1, 3, 5 y-OS: 95.8, 86.2, 76.8.
	OH	51.7	NR	1, 3, 5 y-DFS: 79.6, 50.4, 39.3; 1, 3, 5 y-OS: 95.8, 84.0, 70.9.
Han et al.	LH	44.0	43	1, 3, 5 y-DFS: 69.7, 52.0, 44.2; 1, 3, 5 y-OS: 91.6, 87.5, 76.4.
	OH	48.7	46	1, 3, 5 y-DFS: 74.7, 49.5, 41.2; 1, 3, 5 y-OS: 93.1, 87.8, 73.2.
Yoon et al.	LH	NR	16	1, 2, 3, 4 y-DFS: 82.0, 63.0, 56.0, 56.0; 1, 2, 3, 4 y-OS: 95.0, 92.0, 86.0, 86.0.
	OH	NR	31	1, 2, 3, 4 y-DFS: 88.0, 79.0, 62.0, 62.0; 1, 2, 3, 4 y-OS: 98.0, 93.0, 84.0, 68.0.
Cheung et al.	LH	34.6	36	MDFS: 66.4; MOS: 136; 1, 3, 5 y-DFS: 87.7, 65.8, 52.2; 1, 3, 5 y-OS: 98.9, 89.8, 83.7.
	OH	46.6	160	MDFS: 52.4; MOS: 120; 1, 3, 5 y-DFS: 75.2, 56.3, 47.9; 1, 3, 5 y-OS: 94, 79.3, and 67.4.
Sposito et al.	LH	39.3	NR	MDFS: 25.5; MOS: 48.8; 3, 5 y-DFS: 41, 25; 3, 5 y-OS: 75, 38.
	OH	44.5	NR	MDFS: 31.7; MOS: 57.8; 3, 5 y-DFS: 44, 11; 3, 5 y-OS: 79, 46.
Jiang et al.	LH	NR	26	MDFS: 17; 5 y-DFS: 44.
	OH	NR	30	MDFS: 15; 5 y-DFS: 40.
Komatsu et al.	LH	24.7	NR	3 y-DFS: 50.3; 3 y-OS: 73.4.
	OH		NR	3 y-DFS: 29.7; 3 y-OS: 69.2.
Yoon et al.	LH	NR	NR	2 y-DFS: 85.1; 2 y-OS: 100.
	OH	NR	NR	2 y-DFS: 83.9; 2 y-OS: 88.8.
Xu et al.	LH	13.8	NR	1, 2 y-DFS: 95.5, 72.9; 1, 2 y-OS: 100, 85.7.
	OH		NR	1, 2 y-DFS: 93.5, 81.5; 1, 2 y-OS: 96.3, 86.7.

Follow-up was shown as median month; R: recurrence; DFS: disease-free survival rate; OS: overall survival rate; MDFS: median disease-free survival time; MOS: median overall survival time; y: year; NR: not reported.

was slightly better in LH than in OH (HR = 0.66, 95% CI: 0.52~0.84, $P < 0.01$) (Figure 4(a)). The 5-year DFS rate was comparable between groups (HR = 0.88, 95% CI: 0.74~1.06, $P = 0.18$) (Figure 4(b)).

3.4.5. Publication Bias. The study by Lau et al. was outside the funnel [30], and the remaining representative plots were distributed symmetrically. We believed such publication bias was acceptable in the studies (Figure 5).

4. Discussion

This meta-analysis selected and summarized high-quality literature that compared the short- and long-term outcomes of LH and OH for the treatment of HCC. All of the studies had case-matched design and were of high quality according to the modified MINORS scale. For short-term surgical outcomes, LH exhibited advantages in terms of blood loss, hospital stay, overall postoperative morbidity, and mortality, whereas no statistically significant differences were identified regarding operation time. As for oncological outcomes, R0 and survival rates of LH were also not inferior to OH.

To date, there have been several meta-analyses comparing LH to OH for HCC [5–8]. The results have demonstrated that LH is comparable to OH regarding the operation time and postoperative mortality and is associated with less blood loss, as well as a shorter hospital stay (Table 5). Previous

Study or subgroup	log[hazard ratio]	SE	Weight	Hazard ratio IV, fixed, 95% CI	Year
1.15.1 Minor hepatectomy					
Truant et al.	−0.75	0.35	11.9%	0.47 [0.24, 0.94]	2011
Lee et al.	0.04	0.5	5.8%	1.04 [0.39, 2.77]	2011
Memeo et al.	−0.48	0.33	13.4%	0.62 [0.32, 1.18]	2014
Kim et al.	−0.62	0.91	1.8%	0.54 [0.09, 3.20]	2014
Subtotal (95% CI)			32.8%	0.61 [0.40, 0.92]	
Heterogeneity: $\chi^2 = 1.70$, df = 3 ($P = 0.64$); $I^2 = 0\%$					
Test for overall effect: $Z = 2.34$ ($P = 0.02$)					
1.15.2 Mixed hepatectomy					
Tranchart et al.	−0.53	0.33	13.4%	0.59 [0.31, 1.12]	2010
Ahn et al.	0.38	0.53	5.2%	1.46 [0.52, 4.13]	2014
Lee et al.	0	0.65	3.4%	1.00 [0.28, 3.58]	2015
Han et al.	−0.21	0.27	20.0%	0.81 [0.48, 1.38]	2015
Cheung et al.	−0.64	0.24	25.3%	0.53 [0.33, 0.84]	2016
Subtotal (95% CI)			67.2%	0.68 [0.51, 0.91]	
Heterogeneity: $\chi^2 = 4.17$, df = 4 ($P = 0.38$); $I^2 = 4\%$					
Test for overall effect: $Z = 2.58$ ($P = 0.010$)					
Total (95% CI)			100.0%	0.66 [0.52, 0.84]	
Heterogeneity: $\chi^2 = 6.07$, df = 8 ($P = 0.64$); $I^2 = 0\%$					
Test for overall effect: $Z = 3.45$ ($P = 0.0006$)					
Test for subgroup differences: $\chi^2 = 0.20$, df = 1 ($P = 0.66$), $I^2 = 0\%$					

Hazard ratio IV, fixed, 95% CI

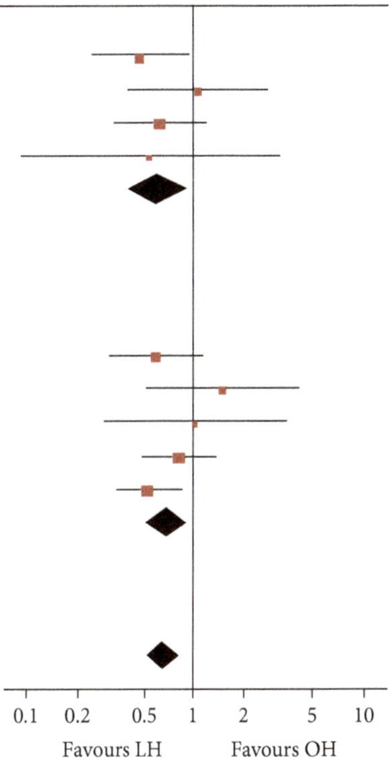

(a)

Study or subgroup	log[hazard ratio]	SE	Weight	Hazard ratio IV, fixed, 95% CI	Year
1.16.1 Minor hepatectomy					
Lee et al.	0.08	0.34	7.3%	1.08 [0.56, 2.11]	2011
Truant et al.	0.15	0.28	10.7%	1.16 [0.67, 2.01]	2011
Memeo et al.	−0.17	0.27	11.5%	0.84 [0.50, 1.43]	2014
Kim et al.	−0.28	0.36	6.5%	0.76 [0.37, 1.53]	2014
Subtotal (95% CI)			36.0%	0.96 [0.71, 1.29]	
Heterogeneity: $\chi^2 = 1.26$, df = 3 ($P = 0.74$); $I^2 = 0\%$					
Test for overall effect: $Z = 0.29$ ($P = 0.77$)					
1.16.2 Mixed hepatectomy					
Tranchart et al.	−0.33	0.29	10.0%	0.72 [0.41, 1.27]	2010
Kim et al.	−0.15	0.43	4.5%	0.86 [0.37, 2.00]	2011
Ahn et al.	−0.38	0.32	8.2%	0.68 [0.37, 1.28]	2014
Han et al.	0	0.4	5.3%	1.00 [0.46, 2.19]	2015
Lee et al.	0.63	0.35	6.9%	1.88 [0.95, 3.73]	2015
Cheung et al.	−0.27	0.17	29.1%	0.76 [0.55, 1.07]	2016
Subtotal (95% CI)			64.0%	0.85 [0.68, 1.06]	
Heterogeneity: $\chi^2 = 6.49$, df = 5 ($P = 0.26$); $I^2 = 23\%$					
Test for overall effect: $Z = 1.45$ ($P = 0.15$)					
Total (95% CI)			100.0%	0.88 [0.74, 1.06]	
Heterogeneity: $\chi^2 = 8.16$, df = 9 ($P = 0.52$); $I^2 = 0\%$					
Test for overall effect: $Z = 1.33$ ($P = 0.18$)					
Test for subgroup differences: $\chi^2 = 0.41$, df = 1 ($P = 0.52$), $I^2 = 0\%$					

Hazard ratio IV, fixed, 95% CI

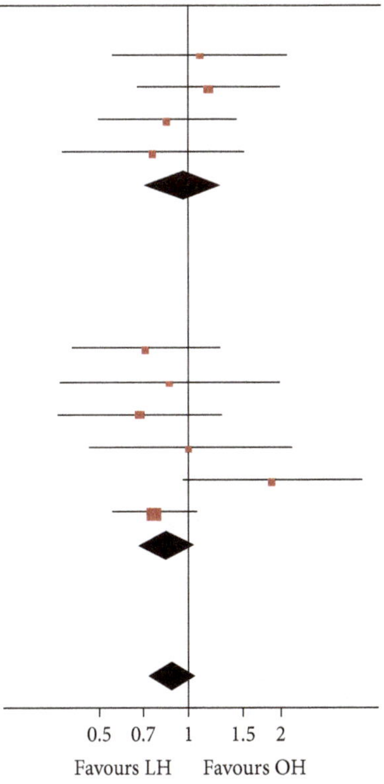

(b)

FIGURE 4: Forest plot of survival rate: (a) 5-year OS, (b) 5-year DFS.

TABLE 5: Previous meta-analyses comparing LH to OH for HCC.

Variables	Zhou	Li	Xiong	Yin
Year	2011	2012	2012	2013
Included studies	10	10	9	15
Total LH numbers	213	244	234	485
Surgical extension	Minor resection	Minor resection	Minor resection	Minor resection
Operation time	NS	NS	NS	NS
Blood loss	Favor LH	Favor LH	Favor LH	Favor LH
Overall morbidity	Favor LH	Favor LH	N/A	Favor LH
Severe complications	N/A	N/A	N/A	N/A
ascites	N/A	N/A	Favor LH	N/A
Liver failure	NS	N/A	Favor LH	N/A
Respiratory complications	NS	N/A	NS	N/A
Mortality	NS	N/A	NS	N/A
Hospital stay	Favor LH	Favor LH	Favor LH	Favor LH
Tumor size	N/A	N/A	N/A	N/A
Margin distance	NS	NS	N/A	NS
R0 resection	N/A	NS	NS	NS
Survival	N/A	N/A	N/A	NS

NS: not significant, N/A: not available.

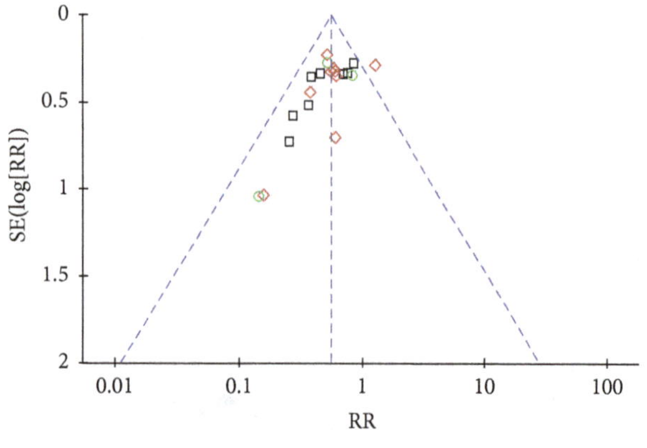

FIGURE 5: Funnel plot of the overall postoperative morbidity.

meta-analyses included all available research [5, 6, 8] but had some limitations. Pooling of low-quality studies could undermine the strength of results, whereas selectively pooling high-quality NRCTs could strengthen the power of results [10]. Patients' characteristics and surgical extension have a major impact on the surgical outcomes of hepatectomy. Previous meta-analyses pooled studies, which did not balance the combined factors of tumor size, location, the severity of cirrhosis, and other underlying liver diseases between LH and OH. These factors would have influenced the decision of surgeons and patients and further influenced the major factors of both short- and long-term outcomes. In addition, previous meta-analyses studied LH confined to minor resection. With the accumulation of surgical techniques, major resection of LH has become more commonly performed, but various efficacy and safety concerns for the procedure are warranted. Furthermore, since the publication of previous meta-analyses, several notable clinical observational studies have become available and some of them are from China, where HCC has the highest prevalence in the world [8, 19]. Therefore, our comprehensive meta-analysis will contribute to a more systematic and objective evaluation of the safety and HCC treatment of LH.

Several previous studies have demonstrated that LH can be feasible and beneficial for minor resections or nonanatomical resections of peripheral HCC. This is in accordance with our study that showed minor resection of LH with similar operation time and less blood loss than OH. However, minor hepatectomy is insufficient for large lesions or those located in posterosuperior liver segments to ensure an adequate resection margin and eliminate intrahepatic recurrence. Major hepatectomy is more frequently performed with a curative intent for multifocal or large size HCC or those with a high propensity to invade the portal vein branches [41–43]. Laparoscopic major hepatectomy is, because of the same steps and principles used in laparotomy, technically demanding. Mobilization of a heavy as well as fragile organ, excisions of bulky parenchyma, and major vascular dissection with its associated risk of major vessel injury are all considered risky under laparoscopy. As expected, the present study revealed longer operation times in laparoscopic major hepatectomy. Furthermore, unlike minor resections, the blood loss of laparoscopic major hepatectomy was not superior to its open counterpart.

Patients with HCC and concurrent cirrhosis tend to have higher incidences of postoperative complications and of greater severity. Therefore, the decreased complications in the LH group should be our most striking finding. In detail, postoperative ascites and liver failure tend to decrease in LH. Postoperative decompensation after hepatectomy occurs more frequently in patients with liver cirrhosis or portal hypertension, even for limited resections. The minimization of surgical incision and the subsequent preservation of abdominal wall circulation and lymphatic flow can explain fewer ascites and liver failure in LH. Moreover, a small incision limits the evacuation of ascites through the wall and decreases the risk of infection, thus facilitating wound healing. Laparoscopic surgery also decreases the manipulation of abdominal organs and exposure of bowels, which will also contribute to reduced ascites. Since refractory ascites and progressive liver insufficiency are major causes of severe postoperative morbidities, reduced severe postoperative morbidities and mortality could be expected. Major surgery was often thought to be unsuitable for those with severely impaired pulmonary function due to a higher risk of postoperative respiratory complications. Hepatectomy involving multiple systems, especially the water and electrolyte balance, is a major risk factor for medical complications. It was observed from the reviewed studies that respiratory complications were the most common medical complications, mainly pulmonary infection, followed by cardiovascular complications. Improved preservation of liver functions in LH maintains enough albumin synthesis and decreases the pleural effusion. The pain caused by large incisions, as well as the use of tension sutures and abdominal bandages after laparotomy, can make it difficult for patients to cough. Earlier postoperative ambulation in the laparoscopic group also helped to reduce respiratory complications and promote the postoperative recovery of gastrointestinal function. In accordance with other laparoscopic surgeries, LH achieved enhanced postoperative recovery. The postoperative hospitalization of LH decreases by more than two days. This can be explained by the milder surgical trauma of LH and subsequent faster bowel recovery. Less postoperative morbidities also contribute to shorter length of hospitalization.

The oncologic results of LH for HCC remain a matter of debate. Adequate surgical margins independently improve the long-term oncological outcomes. Our analysis showed that LH could achieve enough surgical margins (more than 2 cm) as OH. The 5-year OS and DFS also showed that LH was comparable to OH. However, the results warrant prudent interpretation because of the discrepancies among the pooled studies, such as tumor size, tumor number, and status of the vascular invasion. Other biases lie in other factors including preoperative TACE and postoperative adjuvant therapies. Unfortunately, none of the three major hepatectomy studies can be included in our survival analysis. Thus, well-designed RCTs, that balance all potential factors, preferably containing major resection are needed to confirm our results.

In the process of our research and manuscript review, two similar articles by Sotiropoulos et al. were published [44, 45], which also had limitations. Examples include pooling the low-quality studies together, failing to evaluate extension on surgical outcomes, and one paper only investigating studies conducted in Europe [45]. Besides, since these studies were published, several clinical observational studies have become available. Therefore, our comprehensive meta-analysis will contribute to a more systematic and objective evaluation of this subject.

The major limitation of this study was that all included studies are NRCTs and of retrospective design. NRCTs have potential biases that limit an unequivocal conclusion, even though we exclusively included the case-matched studies to minimize the selection biases. Another limitation is the lack of studies on laparoscopic major hepatectomy. The analysis was based on only three pooled studies. Little is known about how these results would hold for a larger sample size, which is particularly important as a fair number of patients with HCC are treated with open major hepatectomy. In addition, data from several studies are extracted using the methods reported by Hozo et al. and Tierney et al., which are not completely accurate and result in bias. Moreover, it is quite possible that surgical teams undertaking research and publishing their results are more experienced and more skillful than others. Publication bias was inevitable since one plot was outside the funnel. The bias would be overcome only with the collection of more reports.

5. Conclusions

This meta-analysis has highlighted that LH can be safely performed in select patients and improves surgical outcomes when compared to OH. The data indicate that laparoscopic minor hepatectomy is acceptable with less blood loss, less postoperative morbidity, shorter hospitalization, and comparable operation times and oncological outcomes. The role of laparoscopic major hepatectomy is promising in terms of decreasing postoperative morbidity and recovery, but the technique also has drawbacks in prolonged operation time. Given the heterogeneity of the patient groups, the limitations of study design, and the small sample size, it is likely that patients have potential to benefit from LH, but further well-designed studies are needed to accurately select them.

Abbreviations

LH:	Laparoscopic hepatectomy
OH:	Open hepatectomy
HCC:	Hepatocellular carcinoma
NRCT:	Nonrandomized comparative study
RCT:	Randomized controlled trial
MINORS:	Methodological Index for Nonrandomized Studies
RR:	Risk ratio
WMD:	Weighted mean difference
SD:	Standard deviation
OS:	Overall survival rate
DFS:	Disease-free survival rate
HR:	Hazard ratio.

Authors' Contributions

Ke Chen designed the study; Yu Pan and Xiao-long Liu collected literature and conducted the analysis of pooled data; Hendi Maher helped to draft the manuscript; Ke Chen and Xue-yong Zheng wrote the manuscript; Xue-yong Zheng proofread and revised the manuscript. All authors have approved the version to be published.

References

[1] L. A. Torre, F. Bray, R. L. Siegel, J. Ferlay, and J. Lortet-Tieulent, "Global cancer statistics, 2012," *CA: A Cancer Journal for Clinicians*, vol. 65, no. 2, pp. 87–108, 2015.

[2] J. S. Azagra, M. Goergen, E. Gilbart, and D. Jacobs, "Laparoscopic anatomical (hepatic) left lateral segmentectomy - Technical aspects," *Surgical Endoscopy*, vol. 10, no. 7, pp. 758–761, 1996.

[3] H. Kaneko, S. Takagi, and T. Shiba, "Laparoscopic partial hepatectomy and left lateral segmentectomy: Technique and results of a clinical series," *Surgery*, vol. 120, no. 3, pp. 468–475, 1996.

[4] A. Kanazawa, T. Tsukamoto, and S. Shimizu, "Impact of laparoscopic liver resection for hepatocellular carcinoma with F4-liver cirrhosis," *Surgical Endoscopy*, vol. 27, no. 7, pp. 2592–2597, 2013.

[5] Y.-M. Zhou, W.-Y. Shao, Y.-F. Zhao, D.-H. Xu, and B. Li, "Meta-analysis of laparoscopic versus open resection for hepatocellular carcinoma," *Digestive Diseases and Sciences*, vol. 56, no. 7, pp. 1937–1943, 2011.

[6] N. Li, Y.-R. Wu, B. Wu, and M.-Q. Lu, "Surgical and oncologic outcomes following laparoscopic versus open liver resection for hepatocellular carcinoma: A meta-analysis," *Hepatology Research*, vol. 42, no. 1, pp. 51–59, 2012.

[7] J.-J. Xiong, K. Altaf, M. A. Javed et al., "Meta-analysis of laparoscopic vs open liver resection for hepatocellular carcinoma," *World Journal of Gastroenterology*, vol. 18, no. 45, pp. 6657–6668, 2012.

[8] Z. Yin, X. Fan, H. Ye, D. Yin, and J. Wang, "Short- and long-term outcomes after laparoscopic and open hepatectomy for hepatocellular carcinoma: a global systematic review and meta-analysis," *Annals of Surgical Oncology*, vol. 20, no. 4, pp. 1203–1215, 2013.

[9] R. R. MacLehose, B. C. Reeves, I. M. Harvey et al., *A systematic review of comparisons of effect sizes derived from randomised and non-randomised studies. Health technology assessment*, vol. 34, Health Technology Assessment, Winchester, England, 2000.

[10] N. S. Abraham, C. J. Byrne, J. M. Young, and M. J. Solomon, "Meta-analysis of well-designed nonrandomized comparative studies of surgical procedures is as good as randomized controlled trials," *Journal of Clinical Epidemiology*, vol. 63, no. 3, pp. 238–245, 2010.

[11] K. Slim, E. Nini, D. Forestier, F. Kwiatkowski, Y. Panis, and J. Chipponi, "Methodological index for non-randomized studies (*Minors*): development and validation of a new instrument," *ANZ Journal of Surgery*, vol. 73, no. 9, pp. 712–716, 2003.

[12] S. P. Hozo, B. Djulbegovic, and I. Hozo, "Estimating the mean and variance from the median, range, and the size of a sample," *BMC Medical Research Methodology*, vol. 5, article 13, 2005.

[13] J. P. T. Higgins, S. G. Thompson, J. J. Deeks, and D. G. Altman, "Measuring inconsistency in meta-analyses," *British Medical Journal*, vol. 327, no. 7414, pp. 557–560, 2003.

[14] J. F. Tierney, L. A. Stewart, D. Ghersi, S. Burdett, and M. R. Sydes, "Practical methods for incorporating summary time-to-event data into meta-analysis," *Trials*, vol. 8, article 16, 2007.

[15] A. Laurent, D. Cherqui, M. Lesurtel et al., "Laparoscopic liver resection for subcapsular hepatocellular carcinoma complicating chronic liver disease," *JAMA Surgery*, vol. 138, no. 7, pp. 763–769, 2003.

[16] E. C. H. Lai, C. N. Tang, J. P. Y. Ha, and M. K. W. Li, "Laparoscopic liver resection for hepatocellular carcinoma ten-year experience in a single center," *JAMA Surgery*, vol. 144, no. 2, pp. 143–147, 2009.

[17] U. Sarpel, M. M. Hefti, J. P. Wisnievsky, S. Roayaie, M. E. Schwartz, and D. M. Labow, "Outcome for patients treated with laparoscopic versus open resection of hepatocellular carcinoma: Case-matched analysis," *Annals of Surgical Oncology*, vol. 16, no. 6, pp. 1572–1577, 2009.

[18] L. Aldrighetti, E. Guzzetti, C. Pulitanò et al., "Case-matched analysis of totally laparoscopic versus open liver resection for HCC: Short and middle term results," *Journal of Surgical Oncology*, vol. 102, no. 1, pp. 82–86, 2010.

[19] B.-S. Hu, K. Chen, H.-M. Tan, X.-M. Ding, and J.-W. Tan, "Comparison of laparoscopic vs open liver lobectomy (segmentectomy) for hepatocellular carcinoma," *World Journal of Gastroenterology*, vol. 17, no. 42, pp. 4725–4728, 2011.

[20] M. Meguro, T. Mizuguchi, M. Kawamoto et al., "Clinical comparison of laparoscopic and open liver resection after propensity matching selection," *Surgery*, vol. 158, no. 3, pp. 573–587, 2015.

[21] G. Belli, C. Fantini, A. D'Agostino et al., "Laparoscopic versus open liver resection for hepatocellular carcinoma in patients with histologically proven cirrhosis: Short- and middle-term results," *Surgical Endoscopy*, vol. 21, no. 11, pp. 2004–2011, 2007.

[22] H. Tranchart, G. Di Giuro, P. Lainas et al., "Laparoscopic resection for hepatocellular carcinoma: A matched-pair comparative study," *Surgical Endoscopy*, vol. 24, no. 5, pp. 1170–1176, 2010.

[23] H. H. Kim, E. K. Park, J. S. Seoung et al., "Liver resection for hepatocellular carcinoma: Case-matched analysis of laparoscopic versus open resection," *Journal of the Korean Surgical Society*, vol. 80, no. 6, pp. 412–419, 2011.

[24] K. F. Lee, C. N. Chong, J. Wong, Y. S. Cheung, J. Wong, and P. Lai, "Long-term results: Of laparoscopic hepatectomy versus open hepatectomy for hepatocellular carcinoma: A case-matched analysis," *World Journal of Surgery*, vol. 35, no. 10, pp. 2268–2274, 2011.

[25] S. Truant, A. F. Bouras, M. Hebbar et al., "Laparoscopic resection vs. open liver resection for peripheral hepatocellular carcinoma in patients with chronic liver disease: A case-matched study," *Surgical Endoscopy*, vol. 25, no. 11, pp. 3668–3677, 2011.

[26] K. S. Ahn, K. J. Kang, Y. H. Kim, T.-S. Kim, and T. J. Lim, "A propensity score-matched case-control comparative study of laparoscopic and open liver resection for hepatocellular carcinoma," *Journal of Laparoendoscopic & Advanced Surgical Techniques*, vol. 24, no. 12, pp. 872–877, 2014.

[27] H. Kim, K.-S. Suh, K.-W. Lee et al., "Long-term outcome of laparoscopic versus open liver resection for hepatocellular carcinoma: A case-controlled study with propensity score matching," *Surgical Endoscopy*, vol. 28, no. 3, pp. 950–960, 2014.

[28] R. Memeo, N. De'Angelis, P. Compagnon et al., "Laparoscopic vs. open liver resection for hepatocellular carcinoma of cirrhotic liver: A case-control study," *World Journal of Surgery*, vol. 38, no. 11, pp. 2919–2926, 2014.

[29] H.-S. Han, A. Shehta, S. Ahn, Y.-S. Yoon, J. Y. Cho, and Y. Choi, "Laparoscopic versus open liver resection for hepatocellular carcinoma: Case-matched study with propensity score matching," *Journal of Hepatology*, vol. 63, no. 3, article no. 5641, pp. 643–650, 2015.

[30] B. Lau, C. Franken, D. Lee, K. Putchakayla, and L. A. DiFronzo, "Short-term outcomes of laparoscopic versus open formal anatomical hepatectomy: A case matched control study," *The American Surgeon*, vol. 81, no. 10, pp. 1097–1100, 2015.

[31] J. J. Lee, J. B. Conneely, and R. L. Smoot, "Laparoscopic versus open liver resection for hepatocellular carcinoma at a North-American Centre: a 2-to-1 matched pair analysis," *HPB: The Official Journal of the International Hepato Pancreato Biliary Association*, vol. 17, no. 4, pp. 304–310, 2015.

[32] L. Luo, H. Zou, Y. Yao, and X. Huang, "Laparoscopic versus open hepatectomy forhepatocellular carcinoma: Short- and long-term outcomes comparison," *International Journal of Clinical and Experimental Medicine*, vol. 8, no. 10, pp. 18772–18778, 2015.

[33] T. Takahara, G. Wakabayashi, T. Beppu et al., "Long-term and perioperative outcomes of laparoscopic versus open liver resection for hepatocellular carcinoma with propensity score matching: A multi-institutional Japanese study," *Journal of Hepato-Biliary-Pancreatic Sciences*, vol. 22, no. 10, pp. 721–727, 2015.

[34] S.-Y. Yoon, K.-H. Kim, D.-H. Jung, A. Yu, and S.-G. Lee, "Oncological and surgical results of laparoscopic versus open liver resection for HCC less than 5 cm: case-matched analysis," *Surgical Endoscopy*, vol. 29, no. 9, pp. 2628–2634, 2015.

[35] T. T. Cheung, W. C. Dai, S. H. Y. Tsang et al., "Pure laparoscopic hepatectomy versus open hepatectomy for hepatocellular carcinoma in 110 patients with liver cirrhosis: A propensity analysis at a single center," *Annals of Surgery*, vol. 264, no. 4, pp. 612–620, 2016.

[36] X. Jiang, L. Liu, Q. Zhang et al., "Laparoscopic versus open hepatectomy for hepatocellular carcinoma: long-term outcomes," *Journal of BUON : official journal of the Balkan Union of Oncology*, vol. 21, no. 1, pp. 135–141, 2016.

[37] S. Komatsu, R. Brustia, C. Goumard, F. Perdigao, O. Soubrane, and O. Scatton, "Laparoscopic versus open major hepatectomy for hepatocellular carcinoma: a matched pair analysis," *Surgical Endoscopy*, vol. 30, no. 5, pp. 1965–1974, 2016.

[38] C. Sposito, C. Battiston, A. Facciorusso et al., "Propensity score analysis of outcomes following laparoscopic or open liver resection for hepatocellular carcinoma," *British Journal of Surgery*, vol. 103, no. 7, pp. 871–880, 2016.

[39] H.-W. Xu, F. Liu, H.-Y. Li, Y.-G. Wei, and B. Li, "Outcomes following laparoscopic versus open major hepatectomy for hepatocellular carcinoma in patients with cirrhosis: a propensity score-matched analysis," *Surgical Endoscopy*, pp. 1–8, 2017.

[40] Y.-I. Yoon, K.-H. Kim, S.-H. Kang et al., "Pure Laparoscopic Versus Open Right Hepatectomy for Hepatocellular Carcinoma in Patients with Cirrhosis," *Annals of Surgery*, vol. 265, no. 5, pp. 856–863, 2017.

[41] D. Dahiya, T.-J. Wu, C.-F. Lee, K.-M. Chan, W.-C. Lee, and M.-F. Chen, "Minor versus major hepatic resection for small hepatocellular carcinoma (HCC) in cirrhotic patients: A 20-year experience," *Surgery*, vol. 147, no. 5, pp. 676–685, 2010.

[42] K. Hasegawa, N. Kokudo, H. Imamura et al., "Prognostic impact of anatomic resection for hepatocellular carcinoma," *Annals of Surgery*, vol. 242, no. 2, pp. 252–259, 2005.

[43] B. H.-H. Lang, R. T.-P. Poon, S.-T. Fan, and J. Wong, "Perioperative and long-term outcome of major hepatic resection for small solitary hepatocellular carcinoma in patients with cirrhosis," *JAMA Surgery*, vol. 138, no. 11, pp. 1207–1213, 2003.

[44] G. C. Sotiropoulos, A. Prodromidou, I. D. Kostakis, and N. Machairas, "Meta-analysis of laparoscopic vs open liver resection for hepatocellular carcinoma," *Updates in Surgery*, vol. 69, no. 3, pp. 291–311, 2017.

[45] G. C. Sotiropoulos, A. Prodromidou, and N. Machairas, "Machairas N: Meta-analysis of laparoscopic vs open liver resection for hepatocellular carcinoma: The European experience," *Journal of BUON : Official Journal of the Balkan Union of Oncology*, vol. 22, no. 5, pp. 1160–1171, 2017.

6

Body Composition in Crohn's Disease and Ulcerative Colitis: Correlation with Disease Severity and Duration

Dawesh P. Yadav,[1] Saurabh Kedia,[1] Kumble Seetharama Madhusudhan,[2] Sawan Bopanna,[1] Sandeep Goyal,[1] Saransh Jain,[1] Naval K. Vikram,[3] Raju Sharma,[2] Govind K. Makharia,[1] and Vineet Ahuja[1]

[1]*Department of Gastroenterology and Human Nutrition, All India Institute of Medical Sciences, New Delhi 110029, India*
[2]*Department of Radiodiagnosis, All India Institute of Medical Sciences, New Delhi 110029, India*
[3]*Department of Medicine, All India Institute of Medical Sciences, New Delhi 110029, India*

Correspondence should be addressed to Vineet Ahuja; vineet.aiims@gmail.com

Academic Editor: Maikel P. Peppelenbosch

Background. Results on body composition in Crohn's disease (CD) and ulcerative colitis (UC) have been heterogeneous and are lacking from Asia. Present study assessed body composition in CD/UC and correlated it with disease severity/duration. *Methods.* Patients of CD/UC following between Dec 2014 and Dec 2015 who consented for bioimpedance analysis for body fat measurement were included. Lean mass and fat-free mass index (FFMI) were calculated with standard formulae. Visceral fat area (VFA), subcutaneous fat area (SCA), and visceral to subcutaneous fat ratio (VF/SC) were evaluated in CD patients on abdominal CT. *Results.* Lean mass in CD ($n = 44$, mean age: 41.2 ± 15.8 years, 73% males) was significantly lower than UC ($n = 53$, mean age: 33.2 ± 11.2 years, 68% males; 44.2 ± 7.8 versus 48.3 ± 8.4 Kg, $p = 0.01$). In both UC/CD, disease severity was associated with nonsignificant decline in BMI (UC: 22.1 ± 4.9 versus 20.2 ± 3.2 versus $19.9 \pm 3.2\,\mathrm{kg/m^2}$, $p = 0.23$; CD: 22.1 ± 4.2 versus 19.9 ± 2.3 versus $19.7 \pm 4.2\,\mathrm{kg/m^2}$, $p = 0.18$) and fat mass (UC: 10.9 ± 8.9 versus 8.1 ± 5.9 versus 5.7 ± 3.6 kg, $p = 0.14$; CD: 11.2 ± 7 versus 7.9 ± 4.4 versus 7.2 ± 5.9 kg, $p = 0.16$), and disease duration was associated with significant decline in FFMI ($p < 0.05$). In CD, disease severity was associated with nonsignificant decline in SCA and increase in VF/SC. *Conclusions.* CD patients have lower lean mass than UC. Body fat decreases with increasing disease severity and fat-free mass decreases with increasing disease duration in both UC/CD.

1. Introduction

There has been a recent rise in the disease burden of inflammatory bowel disease (IBD) in India and other Asian countries and as per a recent report, the overall number of IBD patients in India is second highest in the world after USA [1–3]. This increase will gradually burden the healthcare system and will put increasing pressure on the IBD physician for optimal care of patients. The optimal IBD care dose not only include the control of disease activity with immune based therapies, but also include improvement in quality of life, part of which is compromised by poor nutritional status of the patient which may be caused by low dietary intake, changes in metabolism, increased intestinal protein loss, and nutrient malabsorption [4]. The conventional indices for assessment of nutritional status such as body mass index (BMI) have been suboptimal and therefore require better modalities such as fat mass and fat percentage (for assessment of body fat) and fat-free mass index (FFMI) and lean mass (for assessment of fat-free mass) which can be assessed by bioimpedance analysis or DEXA (dual energy X-Rat absorptiometry) [5, 6]. There are several recent reports which have assessed and compared body composition with these techniques in patients with Ulcerative colitis (UC) as well as Crohn's disease (CD), but the results from these studies have been heterogeneous and inconsistent and very few of these studies are from Asian countries [7–11]. The distribution of body fat is different between Asians and Caucasians and therefore the results from West cannot be extrapolated to Asian patients. Abdominal fat (visceral and subcutaneous fat and visceral to subcutaneous fat ratio) has also studied in IBD and studies have inconsistently linked visceral fat to severity of CD and postoperative recurrence of CD [12–15].

This study was therefore planned to compare body composition between patients of UC and CD, correlate body composition with disease severity and duration in both UC and CD patients, correlate body composition with disease behavior in CD and disease extent in UC, and correlate abdominal fat with disease behavior, severity, and disease duration in CD patients.

2. Materials and Methods

2.1. Patient Population. Adult patients with diagnosis of ulcerative colitis and Crohn's disease attending the inflammatory bowel diseases (IBD) clinic at All India Institute of Medical Sciences, New Delhi, India, from Dec 2014 to Dec 2015, were screened for inclusion in the study. Of these, patients who consented for bioimpedance analysis were included in the study. Written informed consent was obtained from all patients included in the study. Institutional ethics committee approved the study.

2.2. Study Design. In this prospective study, patients with UC and CD were subjected to a uniform clinical evaluation including detailed history and examination, laboratory assessment, endoscopy (UGI endoscopy or colonoscopy as appropriate), and mucosal biopsies. Patient data was collected on their demographics, clinical, endoscopic, histologic, and radiologic features and treatment given and its response. All patients underwent body fat measurement with the bioimpedance machine. In addition, visceral fat area, subcutaneous fat area, and visceral to subcutaneous fat ratio (VF/SC) was evaluated in patients with Crohn's disease with the help of abdominal CT.

2.3. Definitions

2.3.1. Crohn's Disease. The patients were diagnosed as CD on the basis of the European Crohn's and Colitis Organization (ECCO) guidelines, with a combination of clinical, endoscopic, and histological features [16]. The location and behavior of Crohn's disease were classified as per Montreal classification [17]. Severity of CD was measured by Crohn's disease activity index (CDAI) [18].

2.3.2. Ulcerative Colitis. Diagnosis of ulcerative colitis was made on the basis of European Crohn's and Colitis Organization (ECCO) guidelines with a combination of clinical symptoms like bloody diarrhoea and endoscopic appearance and histological findings compatible with ulcerative colitis [19]. Disease activity in UC was measured by Simple Clinical Colitis Activity Index [20] and endoscopic severity was assessed by Baron's endoscopic score [21].

2.3.3. Technique of Measuring Total Body Fat. Total body fat was measured by leg to leg bioimpedance machine (TANITA body composition analyzer, model TBF-215) in patients of ulcerative colitis and Crohn's disease [22]. Subjects were asked to stand barefoot on the metal sole plates of the machine, and age, gender, and height details were entered manually into the system via a keyboard. Body weight and percentage body fat, estimated using the standard built in prediction equations for adults, were displayed on the machine and printed out.

2.3.4. Technique of Measuring Lean Mass and Fat-Free Mass Index. Lean mass was calculated with the following formula:

$$\text{Lean mass} = \text{Body weight} * (1 - (\text{body fat}\%/100)).$$

Fat-free mass index (FFMI) was calculated with the following formula:

$$\text{FFMI} = (\text{Lean mass}/2.2)/((\text{Height in meters})^2 \times 2.20462).$$

2.3.5. Technique of Measuring Visceral Fat. Visceral fat (VF) and subcutaneous fat (SC) area were measured at the level of umbilicus (L4 vertebrae level) with the patient in supine position by multislice CT scanner (Siemens, Erlangen, Germany) in all the patients. The technique used for fat tissue measurements on CT has been standardized and validated [23]. The VF area was defined as all the pixels with adipose tissue attenuation coefficients. The tomographic attenuation of adipose tissue was defined to be between −150 and −50 Hounsfield units. The CT measurement was done by a radiologist blinded to the clinical data.

2.4. Statistical Analysis. Qualitative data was expressed as frequency and percentage. Quantitative data was expressed as mean ± SD if normally distributed and as median (interquartile range) when the data distribution was skewed. BMI, fat percentage, fat mass, lean mass, and FFMI were compared between CD and UC by Student's t-test, and comparison between various UC and CD subgroups according to disease extent, location, and behavior; clinical and endoscopic severity; and steroid requirement and disease duration was done by ANNOVA test. p value of <0.05 was considered as statistically significant. Data was analyzed by using statistical software SPSS, version 20.

3. Results

3.1. Baseline Clinical and Demographic Characteristics. A total of 53 patients with ulcerative colitis and 44 patients with Crohn's disease were enrolled in the study (Table 1). Mean age of the UC and CD patients was 33.2 ± 11.2 years and 41.2 ± 15.8 years, respectively. About two-thirds of patients were males in both the groups. Median duration of symptoms in UC and CD patients was 24 (IQR, 12–48) and 36 (IQR, 18–105) months, respectively. Among the UC patients, 5.6% patients had proctitis, 66% had left sided colitis, and 28.3% had pancolitis. Among CD patients, disease location was L1 in 47.7%, L2 in 22.7%, L3 in 25%, and L4 in 22.7% patients; and disease behavior was inflammatory in 45.7%, stricturing

Table 1: Baseline characteristics of patients of ulcerative colitis and Crohn's disease.

	UC ($N = 53$)	CD ($N = 44$)	p value
Parameters			
Age in years, mean ± SD	33.2 ± 11.2	41.2 ± 15.8	0.01
Sex, male (n, %)	36 (67.9%)	32 (72.7%)	0.61
Duration of symptoms (months), median	24 (12–48)	36 (18–105)	0.15
Haemoglobin, g/dL, mean ± SD	11.8 ± 2.5	10.8 ± 2.9	0.02
Albumin, g/dL, mean ± SD	4.2 ± 0.5	4.0 ± 0.8	0.11
Extent/location of disease	E1: 3 (5.6%) E2: 35 (66%) E3: 15 (28.3%)	L1: 21 (47.7%) L2: 10 (22.7%) L3: 11 (25%) L4: 10 (22.7%)	
Disease behavior		B1: 21 (45.7%) B2: 23 (50%) B3: 2 (4.3%)	
Treatment received			
5-ASA	53 (100)	10 (22.7)	
Steroids	16 (30.2)	29 (65.9)	
Immunomodulators	17 (32.1)	26 (40.9)	
Biologics	0 (0)	0 (0)	

E1: proctitis; E2: left sided colitis; E3: pancolitis; L1: terminal ileum ± caecum; L2: colonic; L3: ileocolonic; L4: proximal small intestine; B1: inflammatory; B2: stricturing; B3: penetrating; p: perianal; ASA: aminosalicylic acid.

in 50% and fistulizing in 4.3% patients. There was significant correlation between subcutaneous fat and fat mass ($r = 0.9$, $p < 0.001$). The treatment details of these patients have been mentioned in Table 1.

3.2. Comparison of Body Composition between CD and UC Patients. There was no significant difference in the mean BMI, fat percentage, and fat mass between CD and UC patients (Table 2). The lean mass in CD patients was significantly lower as compared to UC patients (44.2 ± 7.8 kg versus 48.3 ± 8.4 kg, $p = 0.01$) and though not statistically significant, FFMI was also lower in CD as compared to UC patients (17.2 ± 1.8 versus 17.7 ± 1.9, $p = 0.09$).

Table 2: Comparison of body composition between patients of Crohn's disease and ulcerative colitis.

Parameters	UC ($N = 53$)	CD ($N = 44$)	p value
Body mass index (kg/m^2), mean ± SD	21.1 ± 4.2	20.5 ± 3.7	0.51
Fat percentage, mean ± SD	14.4 ± 9.1	15.6 ± 9.3	0.52
Fat mass in kg, mean ± SD	9.04 ± 7.5	8.7 ± 5.9	0.81
Lean mass in kg, mean ± SD	48.3 ± 8.4	44.2 ± 7.8	0.01
Fat-free mass index (FFMI), mean ± SD	17.7 ± 1.9	17.2 ± 1.8	0.09

3.3. *Effect of Disease Extent, Clinical Disease Severity, Endoscopic Severity, Steroid Requirement, and Disease Duration on Body Composition in Patients of Ulcerative Colitis*

3.3.1. Effect of Disease Extent. There was no effect of disease extent on any of the parameters (BMI, fat percentage, fat mass, lean mass, FFMI) (Table 3).

3.3.2. Effect of Clinical Disease Severity. Of 53 patients, 26 were in clinical remission, 17 had mild disease activity, and 10 had moderate to severe disease activity. There was progressive, though not statistically significant, decline in BMI (22.1 ± 4.9 kg/m^2 versus 20.2 ± 3.2 kg/m^2 versus 19.9 ± 3.2 kg/m^2, $p = 0.23$), fat percentage (16.5 ± 10.2% versus 13.9 ± 8.6% versus 9.7 ± 4.9%, $p = 0.13$), and fat mass (10.9 ± 8.9 kg versus 8.1 ± 5.9 kg versus 5.7 ± 3.6 kg, $p = 0.14$) with increase in disease severity. However, there was no effect of disease severity on lean mass and FFMI (Table 3).

3.3.3. Effect of Endoscopic Severity. Of 53 patients, 7 patients had grade I, 37 had grade II, and 7 patients had grade III disease as per Baron's endoscopic severity. Patients having grade II and III disease had significantly lower BMI (20.3 ± 3.8 kg/m^2 versus 20.8 ± 3 kg/m^2 versus 24.2 ± 5.3 kg/m^2, $p = 0.04$) and lesser body fat percentage (12.3 ± 7.9% versus 14.7 ± 5.8% versus 22.6 ± 11.4%, $p = 0.01$) and fat mass (7.4±5.9 kg versus 8.3±3.7 kg versus 16.3±10.8 kg, $p = 0.004$) as compared to patients having grade I score. However, again there was no effect of endoscopic severity on lean mass and FFMI (Table 3).

TABLE 3: Effect of disease extent, clinical and endoscopic severity, steroid requirement, and disease duration on body fat and lean mass in patients with ulcerative colitis.

	BMI	Fat percentage	Fat mass in kg	Lean mass in kg	FFMI
Disease extent					
E1 ($n = 3$)	21.9 ± 4.5	14.6 ± 9.5	9.4 ± 6.9	48.6 ± 8.4	18.5 ± 2.1
E2 ($n = 35$)	21.3 ± 4.5	15.1 ± 10.1	9.6 ± 8.3	47.3 ± 8.3	17.8 ± 2.1
E3 ($n = 15$)	20.2 ± 3.3	12.8 ± 6.4	7.4 ± 5.1	48.3 ± 8.4	17.5 ± 1.7
p value	0.64	0.73	0.44	0.77	0.72
Disease severity					
Remission ($n = 26$)	22.1 ± 4.9	16.5 ± 10.2	10.9 ± 8.9	49.4 ± 9.3	18.1 ± 2.2
Mild ($n = 17$)	20.2 ± 3.2	13.9 ± 8.6	8.1 ± 5.9	46.5 ± 7.3	17.2 ± 1.9
Moderate to severe ($n = 10$)	19.9 ± 3.2	9.7 ± 4.9	5.7 ± 3.6	48.6 ± 7.8	17.9 ± 1.9
p value	0.23	0.13	0.14	0.54	0.36
*Endoscopic severity**					
Grade I ($n = 7$)	24.2 ± 5.3	22.6 ± 11.4	16.3 ± 10.8	51.9 ± 8.2	18.3 ± 1.6
Grade II ($n = 37$)	20.3 ± 3.8	12.3 ± 7.9	7.4 ± 5.9	47.6 ± 8.5	17.6 ± 2.1
Grade III ($n = 9$)	20.8 ± 3	14.7 ± 5.8	8.3 ± 3.7	47.7 ± 7.9	17.7 ± 1.9
p value	0.04	0.01	0.004	0.37	0.62
Steroid requirement					
None ($n = 14$)	22.1 ± 5.3	16.7 ± 10.9	11.1 ± 10.1	48.1 ± 9.4	17.9 ± 2.0
1/year ($n = 15$)	20.8 ± 3.6	12.8 ± 7.1	7.5 ± 4.6	48.9 ± 8.1	18.0 ± 1.9
>1/year ($n = 24$)	20.6 ± 3.9	14.1 ± 9.2	8.8 ± 7.1	48.1 ± 8.2	17.5 ± 1.9
	0.59	0.50	0.41	0.95	0.62
Disease duration (years)					
<1 year ($n = 9$)	21.4 ± 2.9	14.5 ± 6.1	8.5 ± 4.5	47.6 ± 9.3	18.1 ± 1.7
1–5 years ($n = 20$)	21.9 ± 4.8	15.8 ± 10.6	10.5 ± 8.9	49.4 ± 8.6	18.0 ± 2.0
>5 years ($n = 15$)	17.9 ± 2.3	9.4 ± 6.0	4.9 ± 3.3	45.8 ± 5.5	16.1 ± 1.2
	0.04	0.18	0.13	0.51	0.03

E1: proctitis; E2: left sided colitis; E3: pancolitis; Remission: SCCAI < 3; Mild: SCCAI 3–6; Moderate to severe: SCCAI > 6. *According to Baron's index.

3.3.4. Effect of Steroid Requirement. There was no effect of steroid requirement on any of the parameters (BMI, fat percentage, fat mass, lean mass, FFMI) (Table 3).

3.3.5. Effect of Disease Duration. Among 53 patients, 14 had a disease duration of <1 year, 30 had a disease duration between 1 and 5 years, and 9 patients had disease duration > 5 years. The BMI ($17.9 \pm 2.3\,kg/m^2$ versus $21.4 \pm 2.9\,kg/m^2$ versus $21.9 \pm 4.8\,kg/m^2$, $p = 0.04$) and FFMI (16.1 ± 1.2 versus 18.1 ± 1.7 versus 18.0 ± 2, $p = 0.004$) were significantly lower in patients with disease duration > 5 years as compared to patients with disease duration between 1 and 5 years and disease duration < 1 year. Fat percentage and fat mass also showed a nonsignificant trend towards decline in patients with disease duration > 5 years (Table 3).

3.4. Effect of Disease Behavior, Clinical Disease Severity, and Disease Duration on Body Composition in Patients of Crohn's Disease

3.4.1. Effect of Disease Behavior. There was no effect of disease behavior on any of the parameters (BMI, fat percentage, fat mass, lean mass, FFMI) (Table 4).

3.4.2. Effect of Clinical Disease Severity. Of 44 patients, 14 were in clinical remission, 16 had mild disease activity, and 14 had moderate to severe disease activity. Like patients with UC, there was progressive, though not statistically significant, decline in BMI ($22.1 \pm 4.2\,kg/m^2$ versus $19.9 \pm 2.3\,kg/m^2$ versus $19.7 \pm 4.2\,kg/m^2$, $p = 0.18$), fat percentage (18.3 ± 10% versus 15.6 ± 8.5% versus 12.9 ± 9.4%, $p = 0.32$), and fat mass (11.2 ± 7 kg versus 7.9 ± 4.4 kg versus 7.2 ± 5.9 kg, $p = 0.16$) with increase in disease severity. However, there was no effect of disease severity on lean mass and FFMI (Table 3).

3.4.3. Effect of Disease Duration. Among 44 patients, 9 had a disease duration of <1 year, 20 had a disease duration between 1 and 5 years, and 15 patients had disease duration > 5 years. The lean mass (40.9 ± 6.5 kg versus 43.6 ± 5.7 kg versus 52.3 ± 8.3 kg, $p = 0.001$) and FFMI (16.3±1.4 versus 17.3±0.9 versus 18.6±2.6, $p = 0.003$) were significantly lower in patients with disease duration between 1 and 5 years and disease duration > 5 years as compared to patients with disease duration < 1 year. BMI and fat mass also showed a nonsignificant trend towards decline in patients with disease duration between 1 and 5 years and disease duration > 5 years (Table 4).

TABLE 4: Effect of disease behavior, clinical severity, and disease duration on body composition in patients with Crohn's disease.

	BMI	Fat percentage	Fat mass in kg	Lean mass in kg	FFMI
Disease behavior					
B1 (n = 21)	20.6 ± 4.4	14.8 ± 9.7	8.5 ± 6.9	43.8 ± 8.3	17.2 ± 2.0
B2 and B3 (n = 22 and 1)	20.5 ± 2.9	16.4 ± 9.1	9.1 ± 5.1	44.4 ± 7.7	16.9 ± 1.7
p value	0.82	0.54	0.69	0.79	0.91
Disease severity					
Remission (n = 14)	22.1 ± 4.2	18.3 ± 10.0	11.2 ± 7.0	46.4 ± 7.9	17.7 ± 1.9
Mild (n = 16)	19.9 ± 2.3	15.6 ± 8.5	7.9 ± 4.4	41.8 ± 5.7	16.7 ± 1.2
Moderate to severe (n = 14)	19.7 ± 4.2	12.9 ± 9.4	7.2 ± 5.9	44.6 ± 9.4	16.9 ± 2.3
p value	0.18	0.32	0.16	0.27	0.31
Disease duration (years)					
<1 year (n = 9)	22.5 ± 5.2	15.6 ± 8.6	10.9 ± 7.6	52.3 ± 8.3	18.6 ± 2.6
1–5 years (n = 20)	19.4 ± 3.3	15.1 ± 10.0	7.8 ± 5.8	40.9 ± 6.5	16.3 ± 1.4
>5 years (n = 15)	20.8 ± 2.5	16.2 ± 9.4	8.6 ± 5.1	43.6 ± 5.7	17.3 ± 0.9
p value	0.11	0.95	0.44	0.001	0.003

B1: inflammatory; B2: stricturing; B3: penetrating; Remission: CDAI < 150; Mild: CDAI: 150–220; Moderate to severe: CDAI > 220.

TABLE 5: Effect of disease behavior, clinical severity, and disease duration on visceral and subcutaneous fat area and visceral to subcutaneous fat ratio (VF/SC).

	Visceral fat area	Subcutaneous fat area	VF/SC ratio
Disease behavior			
B1 (n = 21)	93.1 ± 59.2	105.8 ± 79.5	1.32 ± 0.8
B2 and B3 (n = 22 and 1)	114.9 ± 79.2	108.4 ± 68.1	1.28 ± 0.7
p value	0.31	0.91	0.90
Disease severity			
Remission (n = 14)	115.1 ± 54.1	141.04 ± 77.9	0.98 ± 0.4
Mild (n = 16)	97.6 ± 54.9	95.9 ± 58.5	1.37 ± 0.6
Moderate to severe (n = 14)	101.8 ± 99.2	86.2 ± 75.5	1.53 ± 0.9
p value	0.79	0.10	0.09
Disease duration (years)			
<1 year (n = 9)	106.5 ± 60.8	145.3 ± 88.2	1.09 ± 0.5
1–5 years (n = 20)	93.6 ± 84.6	88.4 ± 62.8	1.36 ± 0.8
>5 years (n = 15)	117.8 ± 55.4	109.4 ± 71.3	1.33 ± 0.6
p value	0.61	0.15	0.63

B1: inflammatory; B2: stricturing; B3: penetrating; Remission: CDAI < 150; Mild: CDAI: 150–220; Moderate to severe: CDAI > 220.

3.5. Effect of Disease Behavior, Clinical Disease Severity, and Disease Duration on Abdominal Fat in Patients of Crohn's Disease

3.5.1. Effect of Disease Behavior. There was no difference in visceral and subcutaneous fat area and VF/SC ratio between patients with inflammatory disease versus patients with stricturing/penetrating disease phenotype (Table 5).

3.5.2. Effect of Clinical Disease Severity. There was a statistically nonsignificant trend towards decline in subcutaneous fat area (141.04 ± 77.9 cm^2 versus 95.9 ± 58.5 cm^2 versus 86.2 ± 75.5 cm^2, p = 0.10) and increase in VF/SC ratio (0.98 ± 0.4 versus 1.37 ± 0.6 versus 1.53 ± 0.9, p = 0.09) with increase in disease severity. However, there was no effect of disease severity on visceral fat area.

3.5.3. Effect of Disease Duration. Like the fat mass, the subcutaneous fat area (88.4±62.8 cm^2 versus 109.4±71.3 cm^2 versus 145.3 ± 88.2 cm^2, p = 0.15) was also lower in patients with disease duration between 1 and 5 years and disease duration > 5 years as compared to patients with disease duration less than year. There was no effect of disease duration on visceral fat area and VF/SC ratio.

3.6. Effect of Disease Duration on Body Composition in Patients of UC and CD with Disease Activity. Among 27 patients of UC with active disease, 6 had a disease duration of <1 year, 18 had a disease duration between 1 and 5 years, and 3 patients had disease duration > 5 years. Like all patients, the effect of disease duration on BMI, fat percentage, fat mass, and FFMI showed similar trends, although the difference was not significant because of small numbers (Table 6).

TABLE 6: Effect of disease duration on body composition in patients of ulcerative colitis (UC) and Crohn's disease (CD) with active disease (excluding patients in remission).

Disease duration (years)	BMI	Fat percentage	Fat mass in kg	Lean mass in kg	FFMI
Ulcerative colitis ($n = 27$)					
<1 year ($n = 6$)	20.9 ± 2.8	13.9 ± 6.7	7.6 ± 4.3	45.0 ± 6.5	17.4 ± 1.1
1–5 years ($n = 18$)	20.3 ± 3.2	12.8 ± 8.1	7.7 ± 5.7	47.6 ± 8.1	16.9 ± 1.8
>5 years ($n = 3$)	17.1 ± 2.2	6.1 ± 3.9	3.4 ± 2.7	49.5 ± 5.2	15.5 ± 1.3
p value	0.19	0.31	0.43	0.67	0.28
Crohn's disease ($n = 30$)					
<1 year ($n = 5$)	20.8 ± 5.6	11.4 ± 8.6	7.7 ± 7.6	50.7 ± 8.4	17.6 ± 2.7
1–5 years ($n = 17$)	19.4 ± 2.8	15.6 ± 9.2	7.8 ± 4.9	40.5 ± 7.0	15.7 ± 1.4
>5 years ($n = 8$)	20.2 ± 2.5	13.5 ± 8.9	7.0 ± 4.6	44.0 ± 5.6	16.8 ± 1.0
p value	0.65	0.62	0.95	0.03	0.05

Among 30 patients of CD with active disease, 5 had a disease duration of <1 year, 17 had a disease duration between 1 and 5 years, and 8 patients had disease duration > 5 years. Like all patients, the effect of disease duration on lean mass and FFMI showed similar trends ($p < 0.05$) (Table 6).

4. Discussion

The present study highlights three major findings: low lean mass and fat-free mass in patients with CD as compared to UC; progressive decline in body fat with increasing disease severity both in UC (clinical as well as endoscopic) and CD (clinical) patients; and decline in fat-free mass with increasing disease duration, again in both UC and CD patients. There was no effect on body composition of disease extent in UC, and disease behavior in CD patients. The main purpose of body composition estimation in these patients is to determine existing differences and set nutritional and therapeutic goals for patients accordingly.

Lower lean mass in CD patients reflects worse nutritional status in CD than UC patients, which could be due to pan-intestinal and transmural involvement in CD resulting in poor oral intake and malabsorption. This finding is consistent with other recent studies from Poland [7] and Hungary [9] and 2 recent systematic reviews in children and adults [24, 25]. This difference in lean mass was evident even when there was no difference in the BMI between the two groups, highlighting the fallacy of BMI in the nutritional assessment of patients with IBD. The fat mass was not different between the two groups and previous studies on this aspect have been inconsistent with some studies showing lower fat mass in CD than UC [7, 8] and others showing similar fat content between the two groups [26].

Correlation of body composition with disease severity has not been well studied, and the results have been inconsistent across literature. In a previous study done from our center, like the present study, the fat mass in patients with active CD was lower than that of patients in remission, whereas there was no difference in the fat-free mass between active CD patients and patients in remission in both the studies [10]. However, unlike the present study, the previous study also included healthy controls, and in comparison to controls, the fat mass was only lower in patients with active CD, whereas fat-free mass was lower in both active and remission groups indicating a poor recovery of lean mass in remission. Similarly, in a study of 57 patients with CD from China [11], patients with active CD had lower BMI than patients with inactive CD and in two other studies from China [11] and Brazil [8], the fat content in patients with active CD was lower than inactive CD. On the other hand, in a systematic review of 19 studies which assessed body composition in adult patients with IBD, there was no consistent association between body composition and disease activity [25]. Endoscopic severity in patients with UC also correlated negatively with fat mass in the present study, and this association was more significant than the association of clinical disease severity, thereby substantiating the association of disease severity and loss of fat mass. This correlation of endoscopic severity with fat mass is a novel concept and has not been shown in previous studies. Increasing disease activity could lead to increased utilization of lipid as a fuel substrate resulting in a reduced fat mass and a preserved fat-free mass [27].

The effect of disease duration on body composition was apparent in both UC and CD patients, but the trend was different. Among patients with UC, the effect of disease duration was seen only after 5 years, as BMI, FFMI, fat mass, and fat percentage were lower only in patients with disease duration > 5 years, whereas, among patients with CD, this effect was seen after 1 year only (lean mass, FFMI, BMI, and fat mass were lower in patients with disease duration > 1 year) indicating that malnutrition sets in early in the disease course of CD as compared to UC, and this can again be explained by the systemic nature of CD. The muscle active cytokines may stimulate protein degradation and inhibit myogenic differentiation and induce myoblast apoptosis, thereby leading to poor lean mass [28]. The corticosteroids administered to these patients may also have a negative effect on the muscle accrual as steroids are well known to enhance adiposity [29]. An inadequate and often self-restricted diet and reduced physical activity may also contribute to a reduced lean mass in these patients.

Visceral fat has been linked to pathogenesis of CD and studies have linked visceral fat with complicated disease behavior [15], postoperative complications [30, 31], and postoperative recurrence in patients with CD [12, 32]. Unlike a previous study we could not correlate visceral fat with disease behavior in our CD patients, and this could possibly be explained by difference in the patient population between the two studies. However, we could link abdominal fat with disease severity as we could demonstrate a nonsignificant negative trend of disease severity with subcutaneous fat (like the fat mass) and a positive trend with VF/SC ratio. Like the fat mass subcutaneous fat also correlated with disease duration with subcutaneous fat being lower in patients with disease duration > 1 year. We could also demonstrate a significant positive correlation between subcutaneous fat on CT and fat mass (assessed by bioimpedance), thereby indicating that in CD patients one can assess body composition with the CT. Similar results were demonstrated in a recent study from Australia where fat-free mass was correlated with skeletal muscle area on CT and fat mass was correlated with subcutaneous fat area on CT [13].

Our study has many limitations. The sample size was small and this could explain nonsignificant trend with many associations, because of type II error. Increasing the sample size could have led to more definite conclusions. We did not include healthy controls in our study, but multiple studies including a previous study from our center have already compared body composition in patients with IBD and controls, so comparison with controls would not have added to the results. Comparison of body composition in the same patients at different stages of endoscopic/clinical activity and at different time points (with respect to disease duration) would also have given better results.

To conclude, Crohn's disease patients are at a higher risk of malnutrition than ulcerative colitis patients, there is a loss of fat mass with increasing disease activity in IBD patients, and their nutritional status deteriorates with increasing disease duration (earlier in CD). Therefore, proper assessment of nutritional status along with proper measures to improve these deficiencies is very important to improve the quality of life in patients with IBD.

References

[1] V. Ahuja and R. K. Tandon, "Inflammatory bowel disease in the Asia-Pacific area: A comparison with developed countries and regional differences," *Journal of Digestive Diseases*, vol. 11, no. 3, pp. 134–147, 2010.

[2] V. Ahuja and R. K. Tandon, "Inflammatory bowel disease: The Indian augury," *Indian Journal of Gastroenterology*, vol. 31, no. 6, pp. 294–296, 2012.

[3] P. Singh, A. Ananthakrishnan, and V. Ahuja, "Pivot to Asia: Inflammatory bowel disease burden," *Intestinal Research*, vol. 15, no. 1, pp. 138–141, 2017.

[4] C. R. Fleming, "Nutrition in Patients With Crohn's Disease: Another Piece of the Puzzle," *Journal of Parenteral and Enteral Nutrition*, vol. 19, no. 2, pp. 93-94, 1995.

[5] D. Royall, G. R. Greenberg, J. P. Allard, J. P. Baker, J. E. Harrison, and K. N. Jeejeebhoy, "Critical assessment of body-composition measurements in malnourished subjects with Crohn's disease: the role of bioelectric impedance analysis," *American Journal of Clinical Nutrition*, vol. 59, no. 2, pp. 325–330, 1994.

[6] L. Tjellesen, P. K. Nielsen, and M. Staun, "Body composition by dual-energy X-ray absorptiometry in patients with Crohn's disease," *Scandinavian Journal of Gastroenterology*, vol. 33, no. 9, pp. 956–960, 1998.

[7] P. Więch, M. Binkowska-Bury, and B. Korczowski, "Body composition as an indicator of the nutritional status in children with newly diagnosed ulcerative colitis and Crohn's disease-a prospective study," *Przegląd Gastroenterologiczny*, vol. 12, no. 1, pp. 55–59, 2017.

[8] I. R. Back, S. S. Marcon, N. M. Gaino, D. S. B. Vulcano, M. S. Dorna, and L. Y. Sassaki, "Body composition in patients with Crohn's disease and ulcerative colitis," *Arq Gastroenterol*, vol. 54, no. 2, pp. 109–114, 2017.

[9] Á. A. Csontos, A. Molnár, Z. Piri, E. Pálfi, and P. Miheller, "Malnutrition risk questionnaire combined with body composition measurement in malnutrition screening in inflammatory bowel disease," *Revista Española de Enfermedades Digestivas*, vol. 109, no. 1, pp. 26–32, 2017.

[10] J. Benjamin, G. Makharia, V. Ahuja, and Y. K. Joshi, "Body composition in Indian patients with Crohn's disease during active and remission phase," *Trop Gastroenterol*, vol. 32, no. 4, pp. 285–291, 2011.

[11] T. Yan, L. Li, Q. Wu, X. Gao, P. Hu, and Q. He, "[Analysis of body composition in patients with Crohn's disease]," *Zhonghua Wei Chang Wai Ke Za Zhi*, vol. 17, no. 10, pp. 981–984, 2014.

[12] D. Q. Holt, G. T. Moore, B. J. G. Strauss, A. L. Hamilton, P. De Cruz, and M. A. Kamm, "Visceral adiposity predicts post-operative Crohn's disease recurrence," *Alimentary Pharmacology & Therapeutics*, vol. 45, no. 9, pp. 1255–1264, 2017.

[13] D. Q. Holt, B. J. G. Strauss, K. K. Lau, and G. T. Moore, "Body composition analysis using abdominal scans from routine clinical care in patients with Crohn's Disease," *Scandinavian Journal of Gastroenterology*, vol. 51, no. 7, pp. 842–847, 2016.

[14] C. Büning, C. Von Kraft, M. Hermsdorf et al., "Visceral adipose tissue in patients with Crohn's disease correlates with disease activity, inflammatory markers, and outcome," *Inflammatory Bowel Diseases*, vol. 21, no. 11, pp. 2590–2597, 2015.

[15] B. Erhayiem, R. Dhingsa, C. J. Hawkey, and V. Subramanian, "Ratio of visceral to subcutaneous fat area is a biomarker of complicated Crohn's Disease," *Clinical Gastroenterology and Hepatology*, vol. 9, no. 8, pp. 684–687.el, 2011.

[16] G. van Assche, A. Dignass, J. Panes et al., "The second European evidence-based consensus on the diagnosis and management of Crohn's disease: definitions and diagnosis," *Journal of Crohn's and Colitis*, vol. 4, no. 1, pp. 7–27, 2010.

[17] M. S. Silverberg, J. Satsangi, T. Ahmad et al., "Toward an integrated clinical, molecular and serological classification of inflammatory bowel disease: report of a Working Party of the 2005 Montreal World Congress of Gastroenterology," *Canadian Journal of Gastroenterology & Hepatology*, vol. 19, pp. 5–36, 2005.

[18] W. R. Best, J. M. Becktel, J. W. Singleton, and F. Kern Jr., "Development of a Crohn's disease activity index. National cooperative Crohn's disease study," *Gastroenterology*, vol. 70, no. 3, pp. 439–444, 1976.

[19] A. Dignass, R. Eliakim, F. Magro et al., "Second European evidence-based consensus on the diagnosis and management

of ulcerative colitis part 1: definitions and diagnosis," *Journal of Crohn's and Colitis*, vol. 6, no. 10, pp. 965–990, 2012.

[20] R. S. Walmsley, R. C. S. Ayres, R. E. Pounder, and R. N. Allan, "A simple clinical colitis activity index," *Gut*, vol. 43, no. 1, pp. 29–32, 1998.

[21] J. H. Baron, A. M. Connell, and J. E. Lennard-Jones, "Variation Between Observers in Describing Mucosal Appearances in Proctocolitis," *British Medical Journal*, vol. 1, no. 5375, pp. 89–92, 1964.

[22] R. Y. T. Sung, P. Lau, C. W. Yu, P. K. W. Lam, and E. A. S. Nelson, "Measurement of body fat using leg to leg bioimpedance," *Archives of Disease in Childhood*, vol. 85, no. 3, pp. 263–267, 2001.

[23] E. J. Boyko, W. Y. Fujimoto, D. L. Leonetti, and L. Newell-Morris, "Visceral adiposity and risk of type 2 diabetes: a prospective study among Japanese Americans," *Diabetes Care*, vol. 23, no. 4, pp. 465–471, 2000.

[24] D. Thangarajah, M. J. Hyde, V. K. S. Konteti, S. Santhakumaran, G. Frost, and J. M. E. Fell, "Systematic review: Body composition in children with inflammatory bowel disease," *Alimentary Pharmacology & Therapeutics*, vol. 42, no. 2, pp. 142–157, 2015.

[25] R. V. Bryant, M. J. Trott, F. D. Bartholomeusz, and J. M. Andrews, "Systematic review: body composition in adults with inflammatory bowel disease," *Alimentary Pharmacology & Therapeutics*, vol. 38, no. 3, pp. 213–225, 2013.

[26] R. Rocha, G. O. Santana, N. Almeida, and A. C. Lyra, "Analysis of fat and muscle mass in patients with inflammatory bowel disease during remission and active phase," *British Journal of Nutrition*, vol. 101, no. 5, pp. 676–679, 2009.

[27] G. Mingrone, A. V. Greco, G. Benedetti et al., "Increased resting lipid oxidation in Crohn's disease," *Digestive Diseases and Sciences*, vol. 41, no. 1, pp. 72–76, 1996.

[28] J. M. Burnham, J. Shults, E. Semeao et al., "Body-composition alterations consistent with cachexia in children and young adults with Crohn disease," *American Journal of Clinical Nutrition*, vol. 82, no. 2, pp. 413–420, 2005.

[29] E. Canalis, R. C. Pereira, and A. M. Delany, "Effects of glucocorticoids on the skeleton," *Journal of Pediatric Endocrinology and Metabolism*, vol. 15, no. 5, pp. 1341–1345, 2002.

[30] T. M. Connelly, R. M. Juza, W. Sangster, R. Sehgal, R. F. Tappouni, and E. Messaris, "Volumetric fat ratio and not body mass index is predictive of ileocolectomy outcomes in Crohn's disease patients," *Digestive Surgery*, vol. 31, no. 3, pp. 219–224, 2014.

[31] Z. Ding, X.-R. Wu, E. M. Remer et al., "Association between high visceral fat area and postoperative complications in patients with Crohn's disease following primary surgery," *Colorectal Disease*, vol. 18, no. 2, pp. 163–172, 2016.

[32] Y. Li, W. Zhu, J. Gong et al., "Visceral fat area is associated with a high risk for early postoperative recurrence in crohn's disease," *Colorectal Disease*, vol. 17, no. 3, pp. 225–234, 2015.

7

Thromboembolic Events Secondary to Endoscopic Cyanoacrylate Injection: Can We Foresee Any Red Flags?

Yujen Tseng,[1] Lili Ma,[2] Tiancheng Luo,[1] Xiaoqing Zeng,[1] Yichao Wei,[1] Ling Li,[3] Pengju Xu,[4] and Shiyao Chen[5]

[1]*Department of Gastroenterology, Zhongshan Hospital, Fudan University, Shanghai, China*
[2]*Department of Endoscopy Center, Zhongshan Hospital, Fudan University, Shanghai, China*
[3]*Department of Geriatrics, Zhongshan Hospital, Fudan University, Shanghai, China*
[4]*Department of Radiology, Zhongshan Hospital, Fudan University, Shanghai, China*
[5]*Department of Gastroenterology, Endoscopy Center and Evidence-Based Medicine Center, Zhongshan Hospital, Fudan University, Shanghai, China*

Correspondence should be addressed to Shiyao Chen; chen.shiyao@zs-hospital.sh.cn

Academic Editor: Fernando G. Romeiro

Background. Gastric varices (GV) are associated with high morbidity and mortality in patients with portal hypertension. Endoscopic cyanoacrylate injection is the first-line recommended therapy for GV obliteration. This study aims to explore the reason behind related adverse events and better prevent its occurrence. *Methods.* A retrospective case series study was conducted from January 1, 2013, to December 31, 2016, to identify patients who experienced severe adverse events secondary to endoscopic cyanoacrylate injection. A literature review of similar cases was performed on two medical databases, Medline and Embase. *Results.* A total of 652 patients underwent cyanoacrylate injection at our center within the study duration. Five cases of severe adverse events related to the use of tissue adhesives were identified. Detailed clinical presentation, patient treatment, and outcomes were reviewed and analyzed. Twenty-seven similar cases were identified based on the literature review providing further insight into the study. *Conclusion.* Although rare in incidence, systemic embolism associated with cyanoacrylate injection is often fatal or debilitating. This report may raise awareness in treatment protocol, including the necessity of preoperative angiographic studies, to avoid similar adverse events in clinical practice.

1. Introduction

Variceal hemorrhage is a fatal presentation of portal hypertension, commonly seen in patients with decompensated cirrhosis. Current treatment protocol for gastroesophageal varices includes primary prophylaxis, management of acute bleeding, and secondary prophylaxis [1]. According to the Baveno VI consensus, a combination of nonselective beta blockers (NSBB) and endoscopic variceal ligation (EVL) for esophageal varices and cyanoacrylate injection for gastric varices are recommended as first-line therapy [2]. Compared to esophageal varices, gastric varices are lower in prevalence but are associated with a higher risk of hemorrhage and mortality [3]. The use of *N*-butyl-2-cyanoacrylate (NB2-CYA) for gastric variceal obliteration was first reported in 1986 and is currently well recognized as first-line therapy with a high hemostasis rate [4–6]. Large cohort studies have demonstrated the safety and efficacy of cyanoacrylate injection; however others have highlighted individual adverse events [7–9]. Occurrence of systemic embolization is often associated with patient morbidity and mortality. We hereby report a series of adverse events associated with cyanoacrylate injection for the treatment of gastric varices.

2. Methods

A retrospective case series study was conducted at a tertiary hospital. The hospital database was reviewed; approval was granted by the hospital's institutional review board (IRB). All patients who underwent endoscopic procedure had

TABLE 1: Summary of patient characteristics, preoperative management, endoscopic findings, and subsequent treatment.

Patient	Cause of PH	Child-Pugh Class	Acute bleed	Preoperative drug	Endoscopic findings	Endoscopic treatment	Volume of cyanoacrylate
(1) 57 y/F	PBC	A	No	None	F0/IGV 1	NBCA	3.5 ml
(2) 74 y/M	Alcohol	A	No	None	F2/GOV2	NBCA + EIS	3 ml
(3) 50 y/M	HCV	A	No	None	F3/GOV2	NBCA + EBL	3.5 ml
(4) 51 y/M	HBV	B	Yes	Aminomethylbenzoic acid 0.4 g Etamsylate 2 g Carbazochrome 80 mg Hemocoagulase 1 IU Somatostatin 6 mg	F3/GOV2	NBCA + EBL	2.5 ml
(5) 52 y/F	PBC	B	Yes	Carbazochrome 80 mg Hemocoagulase 1 IU Somatostatin 6 mg	F3/GOV2	NBCA + EBL	1 ml

signed informed consent acknowledging the purpose and risk associated with the intervention. We included (1) patients with gastric varices with or without concurrent esophageal varices treated with injection of N-butyl-cyanoacrylate and (2) patients who experienced severe adverse events (SAE) associated with cyanoacrylate injection within 48 hours of the endoscopic procedure. SAE was defined as occurrence of death, life-threatening disability, or permanent deficit, resulting in a prolonged hospital stay.

All endoscopic procedures were commenced after an overnight fast. First, a routine endoscopy exam was performed to assess the extent of gastroesophageal varices that were classified according to Sarin's classification. Concurrent esophageal varices were graded according to the Japanese Society of Portal Hypertension [10]. Each patient received individualized therapy as deemed fit by the operator. Gastric varices were uniformly treated via the sandwich technique, which starts with an injection of lauromacrogol (Tianyu Pharmaceutical, Zhejiang, China), followed by N-butyl cyanoacrylate (Beijing Suncon Medical Adhesive, Beijing, China), and then finished with flush of lauromacrogol [11]. The number of injection sites and volume of lauromacrogol and cyanoacrylate used directly correlated with the size of the varix. Multiple injection sites were chosen in attempt to obliterate the varix or varices in one session. Volume of lauromacrogol used ranged from 2 to 10 ml, while that of cyanoacrylate ranged from 0.5 to 2 ml, per injection site. Concurrent esophageal varices were treated with either endoscopic band ligation (EBL) or endoscopic sclerotherapy injection (EIS) determined by the operator.

Patients were hospitalized for postoperative observations for 24–48 hours. Any occurrence of severe adverse events (SAE), as previously defined, was recorded. Treatment and patient response secondary to the adverse events were documented. Patient follow-ups were accomplished via telephone interviews or out-patient services to determine survival or further complications.

A literature review of case reports on adverse events related to cyanoacrylate injection was also conducted, specifically, occurrence of embolic or infarction events. Detailed search strategy of Medline (R), from 1946 to present with daily updates, and Embase, from 1974 to March 20, 2017, is provided in the Appendix.

3. Results

A thorough review of the inpatient and endoscopy database was carried out from January 1, 2013, to December 31, 2016. A total of 652 patients who underwent N-butyl-cyanoacrylate (NBCA) injection as secondary prophylaxis for gastric variceal hemorrhage were identified. Based on the a priori established inclusion criteria, the detailed hospital record and treatment protocol of 5 patients were reviewed for the purpose of this study. Three of the five patients were male, ranging from 50 to 74 years. The cause of cirrhosis was PBC in the two female patients, while the remaining were due to HBV, HCV, or alcohol, respectively. Three patients were classified as Child-Pugh Class A, while the remainder were Child-Pugh Class B. Two of the five patients were admitted to our hospital due to an episode of acute variceal hemorrhage, while others had either achieved hemodynamic stability or were admitted for a follow-up endoscopic examination. Prior to the procedure, two patients (patients (4) and (5)) received a combination of hemostatic agents and somatostatin. None of the patients had concurrent HCC or hepatic encephalopathy. Detailed patient characteristics are summarized in Table 1.

Based on the findings of the routine endoscopy, one patient had IGV Type 1, one had GOV Type 1, while three had GOV Type 2 (Figure 1). All gastric varices were treated with the sandwich technique injection of lauromacrogol and cyanoacrylate. The total volume of cyanoacrylate used ranged from 1.0 to 3.5 ml (average 2.7 ml), without exceeding 1.5 ml per injection site. Patients with concurrent esophageal varices were treated with either endoscopic band ligation (EBL) or endoscopic injection sclerotherapy (EIS).

One female patient (patient (1)) suffered from cardiac arrest during the procedure. The bedside echocardiogram revealed an enlarged right ventricle and right atrium, widened vena cava, and shrunken left ventricle. Despite aggressive measures including drug and equipment resuscitation, the patient did not survive. Patient (2) experienced fever, severe abdominal pain, and rebound tenderness after the

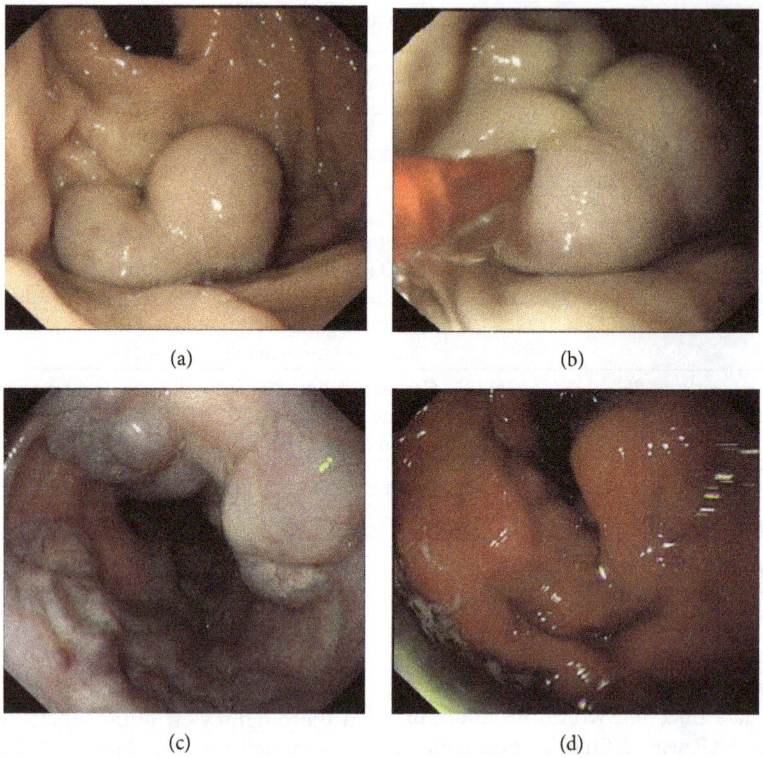

FIGURE 1: Endoscopic findings of gastroesophageal varices (IGV Type 1 and F3/GOV Type 2) with red wale sign.

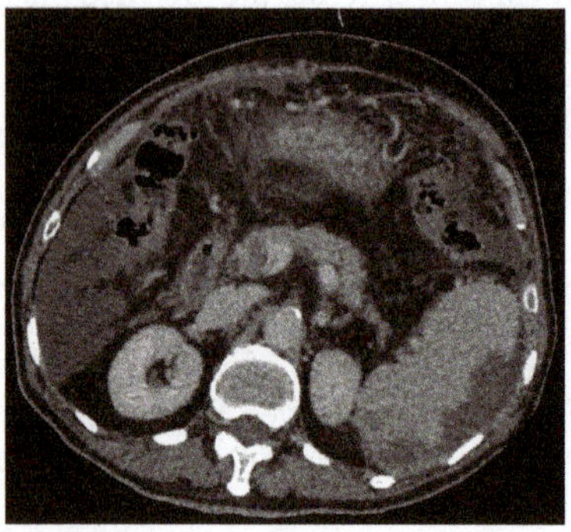

FIGURE 2: Large area splenic infarct based on CT angiography of the portal venous system.

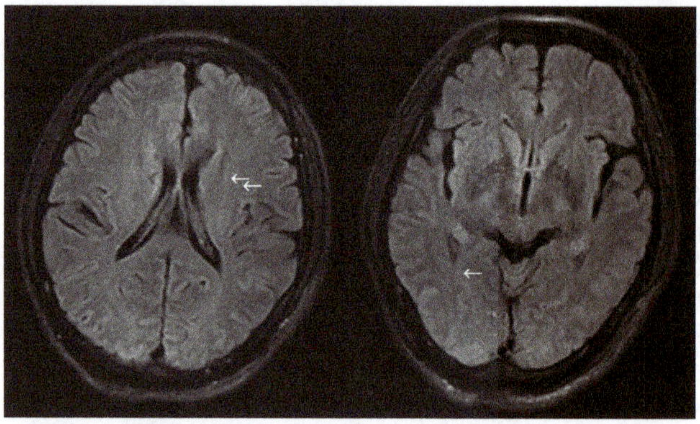

FIGURE 3: Diffuse hyperdense signals (←) on the cerebral MRI, indicative of acute cerebral infarction.

endoscopic procedure due to a large area splenic infarct (Figure 2), confirmed via CTA of the portal venous system. Two patients (patients (3) and (5)) became lethargic and confused and experienced loss of consciousness following endotherapy. Based on clinical symptoms and cerebral MRI findings, both were diagnosed with acute cerebral infarction (Figure 3). The last patient (patient (4)) experienced pain around the umbilical region with a low-grade fever (37.9°C) after the procedure. A subsequent abdominal CT and intestinal mesenteric CTA revealed intraluminal filling defects consistent with acute mesenteric ischemia (Figure 4). Detailed postoperative findings are listed in Table 2.

All patients received hemostatic medication after the endoscopic procedure as part of the standard protocol at our

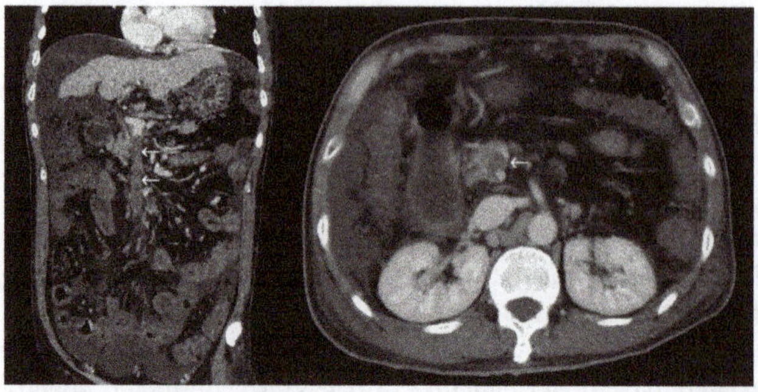

FIGURE 4: Intraluminal filling defect along the mesenteric vein and edema of the bowel wall (←).

Table 2: Postoperative events including subsequent severe adverse event (SAE), patient outcome, and probable cause.

Patient	Postoperative drug use	Adverse event	Treatment	Hospital stay	Outcome	Probable cause
(1)	None	Acute pulmonary embolism	BCLS	1 day	Death	Large spontaneous gastrorenal and splenorenal shunt
(2)	Carbazochrome 80 mg Vitamin K1 10 mg Somatostatin 6 mg	Acute splenic infarction	Dalteparin 5000 IU Antibiotics (meropenem + vancomycin)	64 days	Survival	Regurgitation of tissue adhesive through the portovenous system or probable AVM
(3)	Carbazochrome 80 mg Somatostatin 3 mg Hemocoagulase 2 U	Acute cerebral infarction	Dalteparin 5000 IU Edaravone Mannitol Dexamethasone	13 days	Survival	Spontaneous portorenal shunt
(4)	Hemocoagulase 1 IU Somatostatin 6 mg	Acute superior mesenteric infarction	LMWH 4000 IU Simethicone p.o.	9 days	Death	Regurgitation of tissue adhesive through the portovenous system or probable AVM
(5)	Hemocoagulase 1 IU Somatostatin 6 mg	Acute cerebral infarction	LMWH 4000 IU Citicoline GM-1 Dexamethasone	42 days	Survival	Spontaneous portoazygous shunt

hospital to prevent postoperative hemorrhage (Table 2). Once the patient developed signs of systemic embolization, all hemostatic agents were suspended. All patients were treated with a subcutaneous injection of low-molecular weight heparin (LMWH). Three of the four patients responded well to therapy and were subsequently discharged. Follow-up interviews confirmed survival in all three patients. However, one patient (patient (4)) developed a recurrent GI bleed, presented as melena, after 5 days of anticoagulation treatment. The patient also developed hepatic encephalopathy and deteriorated rapidly. Extraordinary life sustaining measures were refused and the patient died 9 days after the initial procedure. The overall rebleeding rate was 20% and mortality rate was 40% in the five patients who experienced SAE after cyanoacrylate injection. Of the three patients who survived (60%), only 2 received follow-up endoscopy examination. Complete variceal obliteration was observed in one patient (50%), while the other patient had recurrent gastroesophageal varices (GOV Type 2) treated with consolidation EBL plus cyanoacrylate injection.

A retrospective review of the radiological studies was conducted in attempt to identify a potential explanation for the occurrence of an embolic event. Three of the 5 patients had evident spontaneous portosystemic shunts upon review of imaging studies, including one case of portorenal shunt (patient (3), cerebral infarction), one case of portoazygous shunt (patient (5), cerebral infarction), and one case of concurrent portorenal and portosystemic shunt (patient (1), pulmonary embolism). The remaining cases of mesenteric and splenic infarction had no prominent vascular anomaly.

In order to further identify similar reports of adverse events in present literature, a detailed search of Medline (R), from 1946 to present with daily updates, and Embase, from 1974 to March 20, 2017, was conducted (the Appendix). A total of 43 and 119 reports were retrieved from each database, respectively. Forty-two duplicates were removed and a thorough review of title and abstract of 120 articles was performed. Ninety-seven reports were further eliminated due to irrelevance and finally 24 articles, along with 4 case reports identified from other sources, were included for the purpose of this literature review.

Of the 27 studies included, majority of reported adverse events were pulmonary embolism, 12/27 (44.44%), and splenic infarction, 9/27 (33.33%), while others include cases of portal vein, renal vein embolism, sclerosant extravasation, myocardial infarction, diaphragmatic embolism, cerebral infarction, right atrium emboli, esophageal variceal embolism, and subsequent septicemia or DIC. Several adverse events were attributed to cardiac abnormalities such as patent foramen ovale, prompting right-to-left shunt. Other hypotheses include volume and speed of injection or intravariceal pressure, resulting in regurgitation through the portovenous system. Interestingly, many authors presumed the presence of spontaneous portovenous shunt, such as gastrosplenorenal shunt or anomalous arteriovenous shunts, as a culprit for distant embolization. However, none of the reports provided radiological or morphological evidence of the vasculature anomaly. The results of the literature review were summarized in Table 3.

4. Discussion

Gastric varices are associated with a high morbidity and mortality rate in patients with portal hypertension. The current recommendation for first-line treatment is endoscopic injection of tissue adhesives. Obliteration can be achieved in one session, but sometimes repeat sessions are required [39]. Although cyanoacrylate injection has proven to be safe and effective, several reports on related adverse events have also

Table 3: Summary of adverse events related to cyanoacrylate injection found in current literature.

Study	Year	Country	Patient	Glue mixture (ratio), volume	Adverse event	Treatment	Outcome	Probable cause
Shim et al. [12]	1996	S. Korea	59 y/M	(0.5 : 0.8) 7 ml + 2 ml	Portal and splenic vein thrombosis	NA	NA	Large volume injection
Battaglia et al. [13]	2000	Italy	65 y/F	(1 : 1) 6 ml	Intraparenchymal subcapsular hematoma of the spleen	Splenectomy	Survival	Resin occluded branches of splenic vascularization or embolized intraparenchymal vessels and had been eliminated by macrophage action
Türler et al. [14]	2001	Germany	18 y/M	(1 : 1) 5 ml + 2 ml	Pulmonary embolism and left renal vein; recurrent left kidney abscess (5 months)	Thrombectomy and ventilation support; operative and CT-guided drainage (kidney abscess)	Survival	Spontaneous splenorenal shunt
Tan et al. [15]	2002	Malaysia	53 y/M	(0.5 : 0.7) 6 ml +1 ml	Pulmonary and splenic infarction	Supportive treatment and antibiotics	Survival	Collateral portosystemic circulation and presumable anomalous arteriovenous pulmonary shunts
Cheng et al. [16]	2004	Taiwan	65 y/F	(1 : 1) 3 ml	Sclerosant extravasation	Antibiotics and supportive treatment	Survival	High intravariceal pressure and large volume or high injection speed of tissue adhesive
Rickman et al. [17]	2004	USA	55 y/M	(1 : 1) 4 ml + 2 ml	Pulmonary emboli, splenic infarction	Oxygen support	Survival	NA
Kok et al. [18]	2004	S. Africa	24 y/F	(1 : 1) 2 ml + (1 : 2) 5 ml	Pulmonary infarction and septicemia	TIPS surgery	Death	Collateral vessels, size of varices, volume of injection, dilution of lipiodol
Upadhyay et al. [19]	2005	Oman	65 y/M	(1.5 : 2.1)	Inferior wall myocardial infarction and cortical blindness	Percutaneous occlusion of PFO followed by TIPS surgery	Survival	Patent foramen ovale
Alexander et al. [20]	2006	Australia	52 y/M	(1 : 3) 4 ml + 2 ml	Pulmonary embolism	Prednisolone and supportive treatment	Survival	Large volume injection
Liu et al. [21]	2006	Taiwan	42 y/M	(1 : 1) 2 ml	Splenic vein thrombosis	Antibiotics and supportive treatment	Survival	Volume of injection
Martins Santos et al. [22]	2007	Brazil	53 y/M	(1 : 1) 1 ml	Splenic infarction	Antibiotics and supportive treatment	Death	Arteriovenous shunt (probable)
Yu et al. [23]	2007	Taiwan	57 y/M	(1 : 0.7) 1.7 ml	Diaphragmatic embolism	Supportive treatment with narcotic analgesic and short course of terlipressin	Survival	Portophrenic shunt (probable)

Table 3: Continued.

Study	Year	Country	Patient	Glue mixture (ratio), volume	Adverse event	Treatment	Outcome	Probable cause
Chang et al. [24]	2008	Taiwan	53 y/M	(1:1) 2 ml	Pyogenic Portal venous thrombosis	Antibiotics	Death	Direct injection or regurgitation of tissue adhesive along the short gastric vein and splenic vein into the portal vein
Marion-Audibert et al. [25]	2008	France	77 y	(1:1) 1.5 ml	Pulmonary embolism	BCLS protocol	Death	Portosystemic vascular shunt (gastrosplenorenal shunt) (reconstruction with animal model)
Abdullah et al. [26]	2009	Malaysia	40 y/M	(1:1) 3 ml	Cerebral infarction	NA	Survival	Patent foramen ovale
Park et al. [27]	2010	S. Korea	34 y/M	NA	Right atrium emboli extended from inferior vena cava	NA	Survival	Gastrorenal shunt
Chen et al. [28]	2011	Taiwan	57 y/F	(1:1) 4 ml + 6 ml	Esophageal variceal embolism	Cyanoacrylate hemostasis	Survival	NA
Kazi et al. [29]	2012	Australia	44 y/F	(1:1) 4 ml	Pulmonary emboli and pulmonary infarct, resulting in DIC	Blood transfusion to correct coagulopathy	Survival	NA
Miyakoda et al. [30]	2012	Japan	76 y/F	(1:0.5) 1.5 ml + (1:0.5) 3.5 ml	Right atrium emboli	Heparin	Death	NA
Chan et al. [31]	2012	Malaysia	44 y/F	(0.5:0.8) 1.3 ml	Splenic infarction	Conservative treatment (analgesics, antihistamine, and antiemetic)	Survival	NA
Singer et al. [32]	2012	USA	75 y/M	(1:1) 3 ml	Pulmonary infarction	Empiric antibiotics and supportive care	Survival	NA
Mourin et al. [33]	2012	France	69 y/M	NA	Pulmonary infarction	Anticoagulant treatment + pneumonectomy	Death	Presumed portosystemic vascular shunts
Köksal et al. [34]	2013	Turkey	33 y/F	(1:1) 2 ml	Splenic infarction	Supportive treatment	Survival	Retrograde embolization through the splenic vein
Myung et al. [35]	2013	S. Korea	55 y/F	(1:1) 2 ml	Splenic infarction and cerebral infarction	NA	Survival	Patent foramen ovale
Nawrot et al. [36]	2014	Poland	54 y/F	(0.5:0.8) 12 ml	Pulmonary embolism with septicemia	Antibiotics	Survival	Large spontaneous splenorenal shunt
Chew et al. [37]	2014	UK	34 y/M	(1:1) 4 ml	Pulmonary emboli	Intravenous diuretics, empiric antibiotics	Survival	NA
Burke et al. [38]	2017	Australia	25 y/F	1 ml + 3 ml	Pulmonary emboli	BCLA protocol	Death	Presumed collateral circulation

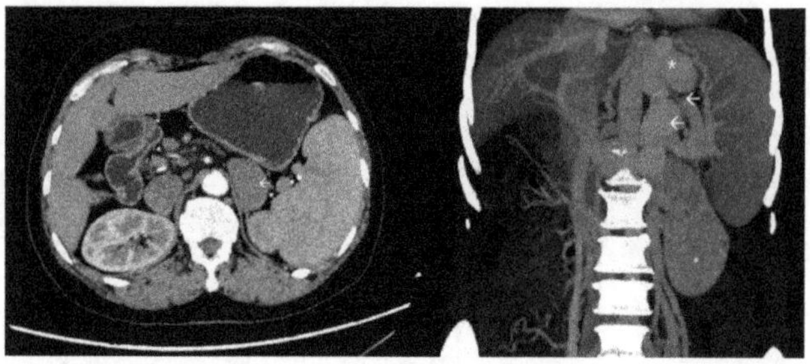

Figure 5: Spontaneous portosystemic shunt in the patient with IGV Type 1, presenting as portorenal and portosystemic shunt (←). The coronal view shows gastric varices (∗) connected to both the left renal and splenic vein through as large torturous, dilated venous shunt (←).

been documented [7]. Seewald et al. have emphasized the importance of a standardized technique, which can minimize the risk of embolization and local complications but also decrease variceal recurrence or rebleeding by effectively obliterating vessel tributaries. The recommended mixture proportion of N-butyl-2-cyanoacrylate to lipiodol is 0.5 ml : 0.8 ml, and injection of over 1 ml glue mixture may increase the risk of embolization [8, 40]. Researchers have also explored alternative treatments for gastric varices obliteration, minimizing or eliminating the use of tissue adhesives. Tan et al. conducted a randomized control trial comparing the efficacy of gastric variceal band ligation versus cyanoacrylate injection [41]. Meanwhile, Romero-Castro et al. reported fewer complications with endoscopic ultrasound-guided coil injection compared to that of traditional cyanoacrylate injection [42].

We report five cases of adverse events that occurred after the endoscopic injection of cyanoacrylate for the treatment of gastric varices. All cases involved the formation of systemic embolus, including cerebral vascular infarction, mesenteric infarction, splenic infarction, and pulmonary embolism. A retrospective review of radiological studies revealed presence of spontaneous portosystemic shunt (SPSS) in 3 patients with distant systemic emboli, including one case of portorenal shunt, one case of portoazygous shunt, and one case of concurrent portorenal and portosplenic shunt (Figure 5). Based on the clinical presentation and radiological findings, three cases can be ascertained as glue emboli, including the case of pulmonary embolism and two cases of cerebral infarction. The formation of spontaneous portosystemic shunts (SPSS) may serve as a shortcut for acute glue embolization, which calls into question the necessity of angiographic studies prior to endoscopic intervention and whether patients with diverging shunts should be tackled with a different therapeutic approach [43]. Our center has previously performed BRTO assisted cyanoacrylate injection for patients with large gastrorenal shunt or splenorenal shunt (data reported elsewhere). This procedure prevents the occurrence of systemic glue emboli for patients with evident portosystemic shunt; however, it is poorly tolerated by patients. BRTO assisted cyanoacrylate injection requires the patient to lay in a supine position with only local anesthesia and an angiography of the portosystemic system is performed via femoral access. After the portosystemic shunt is located a balloon is deployed and secured, while the endoscopist performs the subsequent cyanoacrylate injection.

The remaining cases of mesenteric infarction and splenic infarct remain controversial and cannot be ascertained as the presence of SPSS. A plausible explanation could be due to the injection of cyanoacrylate into the arterial system, which in some cases is located adjacent to the varix or is connected via an arteriovenous malformation. Glue emboli of the splenic artery may result in a large area splenic infarct as seen in patient (2). Another explanation is the regurgitation of tissue adhesives through the portovenous system, potentially due to high speed or volume injection or high intravariceal pressure. Patients with end-stage cirrhosis are also prone to clot formation, especially in the portal venous system [44]. The use of various hemostatic agents combined with a decrease in blood flow velocity, exacerbated by a stress event (endotherapy), may also be a probable explanation for an acute thrombus formation. Unlike other studies, our center employs lauromacrogol instead of lipiodol as a diluting agent for cyanoacrylate via sandwich technique [11]. Therefore, glue embolization is difficult to differentiate from a thrombus formation on imaging studies.

Antithrombotic treatment with LMWH is a fairly standard treatment protocol. However, in cases with recent interventional procedure or hemorrhagic episode, the use of LMWH can be precarious [45]. Development of a rebleed in such patients can be just as fatal as the adverse event itself. Anticoagulants are effective in the treatment of blood thrombus; however, the effect on glue emboli or improvement of patient outcome remains questionable.

The detailed literature review provided some further insights based on case reports of embolic events experienced after cyanoacrylate injection. Many authors theorized the presence of spontaneous portosystemic shunt as a probable explanation for embolization of tissue adhesives. However, no radiological or morphological evidence of vasculature malformation was provided. In our study, we meticulously reviewed the radiological imaging of all 5 patients and were able to identify the presence of spontaneous portosystemic shunt in 3/5 (60%) subjects.

Overall, the use of cyanoacrylate for gastric variceal obliteration is widely accepted with promising results. The safety of tissue adhesive injection is often guaranteed when endoscopist abides by the standardized sandwich technique [8, 40]. However, the necessity of preoperative imaging of the portovenous system should also be considered to identify patients with spontaneous portosystemic shunt (SPSS). In such cases, the risk of traditional endoscopic glue injection should be thoroughly vetted, or alternative treatment measures such as coil injection, TIPS, BRTO, or surgical therapy should be referred to. Utility of pre- and postoperative hemostatic agents should also be carefully considered to achieve a desirable hemostatic balance. Adverse events associated with tissue adhesives are often fatal and debilitating for patients; any red flags before endoscopic therapy should

Table 4

Number	Searches	Medline results	Embase results	Search type
(1)	(esophag* or esophag* gastr* or gastr* esophag* or gastr* oesophag* or gastroesophag* or gastrooesophag* or oesophag* or oesophag* gastr* or gastr*).mp. [mp = title, abstract, original title, name of substance word, subject heading word, keyword heading word, protocol supplementary concept word, rare disease supplementary concept word, unique identifier, synonyms]	169513	268529	Advanced
(2)	1 and (varic* or varix).mp.	14601	21427	Advanced
(3)	exp esophageal varices/	12569	17997	Advanced
(4)	exp gastric varices/	12569	2864	Advanced
(5)	(3) or (4)	12569	19501	Advanced
(6)	(2) or (5)	14601	22623	Advanced
(7)	(cyanoacrylate or n-butyl-2-cyanoacrylate or NBCA or NB2CYA or NB2-CYA or tissue adhesive or tissue glue or glue).mp. [mp = title, abstract, original title, name of substance word, subject heading word, keyword heading word, protocol supplementary concept word, rare disease supplementary concept word, unique identifier, synonyms]	13485	26245	Advanced
(8)	(infarct* or embol* or advers* event* or severe advers* event* or complicat*).mp. [mp = title, abstract, original title, name of substance word, subject heading word, keyword heading word, protocol supplementary concept word, rare disease supplementary concept word, unique identifier, synonyms]	1649685	3380532	Advanced
(9)	(7) and (8)	4356	10406	Advanced
(10)	(endoscop* therap* or endoscop* treat* or endoscop* inject*).mp. [mp = title, abstract, original title, name of substance word, subject heading word, keyword heading word, protocol supplementary concept word, rare disease supplementary concept word, unique identifier, synonyms]	8912	21219	Advanced
(11)	(9) and (10)	186	657	Advanced
(12)	(case or case report* or case serie* or report*).mp. [mp = title, abstract, original title, name of substance word, subject heading word, keyword heading word, protocol supplementary concept word, rare disease supplementary concept word, unique identifier, synonyms]	4746115	6342357	Advanced
(13)	(6) and (11) and (12)	43	119	Advanced

Exp, explode.

be well recognized by physicians, prompting well-rounded consideration to effectively avoid the occurrence of adverse events.

Appendix

Detailed Search Strategy

The search strategy used was Ovid Medline (R), from 1946 to present with daily updates, and Embase, from 1974 to March 20, 2017(see Table 4).

Ethical Approval

All procedures followed were in accordance with the ethical standards of the responsible committee of human experimentation (institutional and national) and with the Helsinki Declaration of 1975, as revised in 2008.

Disclosure

The abstract of this manuscript has been presented at China 17th Congress of Gastroenterology, Xi'an, China, September 14–16, 2017. This article does not contain any studies with animal subjects.

Authors' Contributions

Yujen Tseng and Lili Ma contributed equally to the manuscript and share first authorship.

Acknowledgments

This study was supported by the Innovation Fund of Shanghai Scientific Committee (no. 15411950501).

References

[1] G. Garcia-Tsao and J. Bosch, "Management of varices and variceal hemorrhage in cirrhosis," *The New England Journal of Medicine*, vol. 362, no. 9, pp. 778–832, 2010.

[2] R. de Franchis, "Expanding consensus in portal hypertension: Report of the Baveno VI Consensus Workshop: Stratifying risk and individualizing care for portal hypertension," *Journal of Hepatology*, vol. 63, no. 3, pp. 743-52, 2015.

[3] S. K. Sarin, D. Lahoti, S. P. Saxena, N. S. Murthy, and U. K. Makwana, "Prevalence, classification and natural history of gastric varices: a long-term follow-up study in 568 portal hypertension patients," *Hepatology*, vol. 16, no. 6, pp. 1343–1349, 1992.

[4] N. Soehendra, V. Nam Ch., H. Grimm, and I. Kempeneers, "Endoscopic obliteration of large esophagogastric varices with bucrylate," *Endoscopy*, vol. 18, no. 1, pp. 25-26, 1986.

[5] S. K. Sarin and S. R. Mishra, "Endoscopic Therapy for Gastric Varices," *Clinics in Liver Disease*, vol. 14, no. 2, pp. 263–279, 2010.

[6] F. Weilert and K. F. Binmoeller, "Cyanoacrylate glue for gastrointestinal bleeding," *Current Opinion in Gastroenterology* vol. 32, no. 5, pp. 358–364, 2016.

[7] K. F. Binmoeller, "Glue for gastric varices: Some sticky issues," *Gastrointestinal Endoscopy*, vol. 52, no. 2, pp. 298–301, 2000.

[8] S. Seewald, T. L. Ang, H. Imazu et al., "A standardized injection technique and regimen ensures success and safety of N-butyl-2-cyanoacrylate injection for the treatment of gastric fundal varices (with videos)," *Gastrointestinal Endoscopy*, vol. 68, no. 3, pp. 447–454, 2008.

[9] D. S. Rengstoff and K. F. Binmoeller, "A pilot study of 2-octyl cyanoacrylate injection for treatment of gastric fundal varices in humans," *Gastrointestinal Endoscopy*, vol. 59, no. 4, pp. 553–558, 2004.

[10] Y. Idezuki, "General rules for recording endoscopic findings of esophagogastric varices (1991)," *World Journal of Surgery*, vol. 19, no. 3, pp. 420–422, 1995.

[11] X. Zeng, L. Ma, Y. Tzeng et al., "Endoscopic cyanoacrylate injection with or without lauromacrogol for gastric varices: a randomized pilot study," *Journal of Gastroenterology and Hepatology*, vol. 32, no. 3, pp. 631–638, 2017.

[12] C. S. Shim, Y. D. Cho, J. O. Kim et al., "A case of portal and splenic vein thrombosis after histoacryl injection therapy in gastric varices," *Endoscopy*, vol. 28, no. 5, p. 461, 1996.

[13] G. Battaglia, T. Morbin, E. Patarnello, C. Merkel, M. C. Corona, and E. Ancona, "Visceral fistula as a complication of endoscopic treatment of esophageal and gastric varices using isobutyl-2-cyanoacrylate: Report of two cases," *Gastrointestinal Endoscopy* vol. 52, no. 2, pp. 267–270, 2000.

[14] A. Türler, M. Wolff, D. Dorlars, and A. Hirner, "Embolic and septic complications after sclerotherapy of fundic varices with cyanoacrylate," *Gastrointestinal Endoscopy*, vol. 53, no. 2, pp. 228–230, 2001.

[15] Y. M. Tan, K. L. Goh, A. Kamarulzaman et al., "Multiple systemic embolisms with septicemia after gastric variceal obliteration with cyanoacrylate," *Gastrointestinal Endoscopy*, vol. 55, no. 2, pp. 276–278, 2002.

[16] H. C. Cheng, P. N. Cheng, Y. M. Tsai, H. M. Tsai, and C. Y. Chen, "Sclerosant extravasation as a complication of sclerosing endotherapy for bleeding gastric varices," *Endoscopy*, vol. 36, no. 3, pp. 239–241, 2004.

[17] O. B. Rickman, J. P. Utz, G. L. Aughenbaugh, and C. J. Gostout, "Pulmonary embolization of 2-octyl cyanoacrylate after endoscopic injection therapy for gastric variceal bleeding," *Mayo Clinic Proceedings*, vol. 79, no. 11, pp. 1455–1458, 2004.

[18] K. Kok, R. P. Bond, I. C. Duncan et al., "Distal embolization and local vessel wall ulceration after gastric obliteration with N-butyl-2-cyanoacrylate: A case report and review of the literature," *Endoscopy*, vol. 36, no. 5, pp. 442–446, 2004.

[19] A. P. Upadhyay, R. Ananthasivan, S. Radhakrishnan, and G. Zubaidi, "Cortical blindness and acute myocardial infarction following injection of bleeding gastric varices with cyanoacrylate glue," *Endoscopy*, vol. 37, no. 10, p. 1034, 2005.

[20] S. Alexander, M. G. Korman, and W. Sievert, "Cyanoacrylate in the treatment of gastric varices complicated by multiple pulmonary emboli," *Internal Medicine Journal*, vol. 36, no. 7, pp. 462–465, 2006.

[21] C. H. Liu, F. C. Tsai, P. C. Liang, C. Z. Lee, and P. M. Yang, "Splenic vein thrombosis and Klebsiella pneumoniae septicemia after endoscopic gastric variceal obturation therapy with N-butyl-2-cyanoacrylate," *Gastrointestinal Endoscopy*, vol. 63, no. 2, pp. 336–338, 2006.

[22] M. M. Martins Santos, L. P. Correia, R. A. Rodrigues, L. H. Lenz Tolentino, A. P. Ferrari, and E. D. Libera, "Splenic artery embolization and infarction after cyanoacrylate injection for esophageal varices," *Gastrointestinal Endoscopy*, vol. 65, no. 7, pp. 1088–1090, 2007.

[23] C. F. Yu, L. W. Lin, S. W. Hung, C. T. Yeh, and C. F. Chong, "Diaphragmatic embolism after endoscopic injection sclerotherapy for gastric variceal bleeding," *The American Journal of Emergency Medicine*, vol. 25, no. 7, pp. 860–e6, 2007.

[24] C. J. Chang, Y. T. Shiau, T. L. Chen et al., "Pyogenic portal vein thrombosis as a reservoir of persistent septicemia after cyanoacrylate injection for bleeding gastric varices," *Digestion*, vol. 78, no. 2-3, pp. 139–143, 2008.

[25] A. M. Marion-Audibert, M. Schoeffler, F. Wallet et al., "Acute fatal pulmonary embolism during cyanoacrylate injection in gastric varices," *Gastroentérologie Clinique et Biologique*, vol. 32, no. 11, pp. 926–930, 2008.

[26] A. Abdullah, S. Sachithanandan, O. K. Tan et al., "Cerebral embolism following N-butyl-2-cyanoacrylate injection for esophageal postbanding ulcer bleed: A case report," *Hepatology International*, vol. 3, no. 3, pp. 504–508, 2009.

[27] J. S. Park, J. J. Park, S. K. Lim et al., "Long journey of sclerosant from the esophagus to the right atrium," *Korean Circulation Journal*, vol. 40, no. 9, pp. 468–470, 2010.

[28] P. H. Chen, M. C. Hou, H. C. Lin, and S. D. Lee, "Cyanoacrylate embolism from gastric varices may lead to esophageal variceal rupture," *Endoscopy*, vol. 43, no. 2, pp. E149–E150, 2011.

[29] S. Kazi, M. Spanger, and J. Lubel, "Gastrointestinal: Pulmonary embolism of cyanoacrylate glue following endoscopic injection of gastric varices," *Journal of Gastroenterology and Hepatology*, vol. 27, no. 12, pp. 1874-1874, 2012.

[30] K. Miyakoda, H. Takedatsu, K. Emori et al., "N-butyl-2-cyanoacrylate (histoacryl) glue in the right atrium after endoscopic injection for a ruptured duodenal varix: Complication of histoacryl injection," *Digestive Endoscopy*, vol. 24, no. 3, p. 192, 2012.

[31] R. S. Chan, A. Vijayananthan, G. Kumar, and I. N. Hilmi, "Imaging findings of extensive splenic infarction after cyanoacrylate injection for gastric varices—a case report," *Malaysian Medical Association*, pp. 424-425, 2012.

[32] A. D. Singer, G. Fananapazir, F. Maufa, S. Narra, and S. Ascher, "Pulmonary embolism following 2-octyl-cyanoacrylate/lipiodol injection for obliteration of gastric varices: An imaging perspective," *Journal of Radiology Case Reports*, vol. 6, no. 2, pp. 17–22, 2012.

[33] G. Mourin, A. Badia, A. Cazes, and B. Planquette, "An unusual cause of pulmonary artery pseudoaneurysm: Acrylate embolism," *Interactive CardioVascular and Thoracic Surgery*, vol. 15, no. 6, pp. 1082–1084, 2012.

[34] A. Ş. Köksal, E. Kayaçetin, S. Torun, V. Erkan, and R. S. Ökten, "Splenic infarction after N-butyl-2-cyanoacrylate injection for gastric varices: Why does it happen?" *Surgical Laparoscopy Endoscopy & Percutaneous Techniques*, vol. 23, no. 5, pp. e191–e193, 2013.

[35] D. S. Myung, C. Y. Chung, H. C. Park et al., "Cerebral and splenic infarctions after injection of N-butyl-2-cyanoacrylate in esophageal variceal bleeding," *World Journal of Gastroenterology*, vol. 19, no. 34, pp. 5759–5762, 2013.

[36] I. Nawrot, T. Cieciura, B. Morawski, and P. J. U. Malkowski, "Pulmonary embolism with septicemia after N-butyl-2-cyanoacrylate injection for bleeding gastric varices," *Chinese Medical Journal*, 2014.

[37] J. R. Y. Chew, A. Balan, W. Griffiths, and J. Herre, "Delayed onset pulmonary glue emboli in a ventilated patient: A rare complication following endoscopic cyanoacrylate injection for gastric variceal haemorrhage," *BMJ Case Reports*, vol. 2014, Article ID 206461, 2014.

[38] M. P. Burke, C. O'Donnell, and Y. Baber, "Death from pulmonary embolism of cyanoacrylate glue following gastric varix endoscopic injection," *Forensic Science, Medicine and Pathology*, vol. 13, no. 1, pp. 82–85, 2017.

[39] S. K. Sarin and A. Kumar, "Endoscopic Treatment of Gastric Varices," *Clinics in Liver Disease*, vol. 18, no. 4, pp. 809–827, 2014.

[40] S. Seewald, P. V. J. Sriram, M. Naga et al., "Cyanoacrylate glue in gastric variceal bleeding," *Endoscopy*, vol. 34, no. 11, pp. 926–932, 2002.

[41] P. C. Tan, M. C. Hou, H. C. Lin et al., "A randomized trial of endoscopic treatment of acute gastric variceal hemorrhage: N-butyl-2-cyanoacrylate injection versus band ligation," *Hepatology*, vol. 43, no. 4, pp. 690–697, 2006.

[42] R. Romero-Castro, M. Ellrichmann, C. Ortiz-Moyano et al., "EUS-guided coil versus cyanoacrylate therapy for the treatment of gastric varices: A multicenter study (with videos)," *Gastrointestinal Endoscopy*, vol. 78, no. 5, pp. 711–721, 2013.

[43] M. Takashi, M. Igarashi, S. Hino et al., "Portal hemodynamics in chronic portal-systemic encephalopathy - Angiographic study in seven cases," *Journal of Hepatology*, vol. 1, no. 5, pp. 467–476, 1985.

[44] F. Nery, S. Chevret, B. Condat et al., "Causes and consequences of portal vein thrombosis in 1,243 patients with cirrhosis: results of a longitudinal study," *Hepatology*, vol. 61, no. 2, pp. 660–667, 2015.

[45] A. Andriulli, A. Tripodi, P. Angeli et al., "Hemostatic balance in patients with liver cirrhosis: report of a consensus conference," *Digestive and Liver Disease*, vol. 48, no. 5, pp. 455–467, 2016.

8

Low Total Dose of Anti-Human T-Lymphocyte Globulin (ATG) Guarantees a Good Glomerular Filtration Rate after Liver Transplant in Recipients with Pretransplant Renal Dysfunction

Cristina Dopazo,[1] Ramón Charco,[1] Mireia Caralt,[1] Elizabeth Pando,[1] José Luis Lázaro,[1] Concepción Gómez-Gavara,[1] Lluis Castells,[2] and Itxarone Bilbao[1]

[1] *Department of HPB Surgery and Transplants, Hospital Universitario Vall d'Hebron, Universidad Autónoma de Barcelona, Barcelona, Spain*
[2] *Hepatology Unit, Department of Internal Medicine, Hospital Vall d'Hebron, CIBERehd, Universidad Autónoma de Barcelona, Barcelona, Spain*

Correspondence should be addressed to Cristina Dopazo; cdopazo@vhebron.net

Academic Editor: Stefano Gitto

We aimed to evaluate the safety and efficacy of low doses of anti-T-lymphocyte globulin (ATG)-based immunosuppression in preserving renal function and preventing liver rejection in liver transplant (LT) recipients with pretransplant renal dysfunction. We designed a prospective single-center cohort study analyzing patients with pre-LT renal dysfunction defined as eGFR<60 mL/min/1.73m^2, who underwent induction therapy with ATG (*ATG group, n=20)*. This group was compared with a similar retrospective cohort treated with basiliximab (*BAS group, n=20*). An economic analysis between both induction therapies was also undertaken. In the *ATG group,* 45% and 50% of patients had recovered their renal function without acute cellular rejection (ACR) episodes at day 7 and 1 month after LT, respectively, versus 40% and 55% of patients in *the BAS group* (p=1). Renal function improved in both groups over time and no differences between groups were observed regarding one-year eGRF and one-year probability of ACR. Cost per patient of the ATG course was 403€ (r: 126-756) versus 2,524€ of the basiliximab course (p=0.001). In conclusion, induction with low dose of ATG or basiliximab in patients with pretransplant renal dysfunction is a good strategy for preserving posttransplant renal function; however the use of low-dose ATG resulted in a substantial reduction in drug costs. This trail is registered with *ClinicalTrials.gov number:* NCT01453218.

1. Introduction

Renal dysfunction in liver transplantation (LT) is one of the major concerns hindering posttransplant patient management and determining worse prognosis [1–3].

Renal dysfunction in cirrhotic patients is of multiple well-known causes [3–5]. According to published data, approximately 30% of cirrhotic patients on the waiting list for LT have some degree of renal impairment [6]. After LT, impaired renal function tends to recover partially or completely unless advanced parenchymatous lesions are significantly involved as a major cause of the dysfunction [7–12].

In this scenario, the feasibility of delaying the introduction of calcineurin inhibitors (CNI) in patients with a high risk of immediate posttransplant renal dysfunction, as in critically ill patients with severe ascites, hepatorenal syndrome, or pre-LT renal dysfunction in whom it would be desirable to allow their renal function to return to normal before the introduction of nephrotoxic CNI as part of a maintenance immunosuppressive regimen has already been demonstrated [13–20]. This practice is usually accompanied by induction immunosuppression therapy consisting of a chimeric monoclonal interleukin-2-receptor (CD25 antigen) antibody administered on day 0 and day 4 after LT.

Anti-human T-lymphocyte globulin (ATG) is an alternative to interleukin-2-receptor antagonistic induction therapy, with greater immunosuppressive power but higher hematologic and infectious adverse event rates widely reported in renal transplantation [20–25]. For this reason, induction therapies using polyclonal anti-thymocyte globulins in LT are not universally used since the liver is assumed to be less immunogenic than kidney grafts.

Considering the lower immunogenicity of the liver, we designed a study to evaluate the safety and efficacy of an immunosuppressor regimen plus induction therapy with low-dose ATG in preserving renal function and preventing liver rejection in LT recipients with pretransplant renal dysfunction.

2. Methods

2.1. Study Design. A prospective single-center cohort study of adult LT recipients with a pretransplant renal dysfunction (*ATG group*) was designed to evaluate the efficacy and safety of induction therapy with ATG plus steroids and tacrolimus (TAC). Pre-LT renal dysfunction was defined as an estimated glomerular filtration rate (eGFR) < 60 mL/min/1.73m^2 under the MDRD4 formula on the day of LT.

Inclusion Criteria. Adult patients on the waiting list for LT from brain-dead donors with pre-LT renal dysfunction were included. In cases of cirrhosis due to hepatitis C virus (HCV) infection, negative HCV-RNA was required.

Exclusion Criteria. Exclusion criteria included retransplantation, multiorgan transplantation, acute liver failure, severe leucopenia (<1.2x10E9/L), and/or thrombocytopenia (<50x10E9/L).

Patients in the ATG study group were compared with a historical cohort of patients with pretransplant renal dysfunction (eGFR < 60 mL/min/1.73m^2 under the MDRD4 formula on the day of LT), who underwent LT and received monoclonal interleukin-2-receptor (basiliximab) as induction therapy (*BAS group*). For every ATG patient, we retrospectively selected 1 age (+/-10 years), sex, diagnosis, and MELD score matched patients for comparison (1:1 matching).

The study was conducted in compliance with the provisions of the Declaration of Helsinki and Good Clinical Practice guidelines. This study was approved by the Hospital Vall d'Hebron Institutional Review Board (Barcelona, Spain). All patients provided their written informed consent form prior to initiation of the study and were allowed to withdraw at any time. The trial was registered with ClinicalTrials.gov number NCT01453218.

2.2. Immunosuppression with ATG Induction. Patients in the *ATG group* received induction therapy with anti-human T-lymphocyte globulin (Grafalon; Neovii Biotech GMBH; Germany). ATG was intravenously (i.v.) administered on Intensive Care Unit (ICU) admission at a dose of 1mg/kg/bodyweight. All patients were premedicated with methylprednisolone 250mg i.v., dexchlorpheniramine 5mg i.v., and paracetamol 1g. Following doses were given on days 2 and 4 with dose adjustment according to CD2/CD3 levels (>20cel/μL). The third dose of ATG on day 4 was omitted if CD2/CD3 levels were below 20 cel/μL and platelet counts < 50,000cells/mm^3 on the day after the second dose. CD2/CD3 levels were also measured on days 7 and 14 after LT.

TAC initiation was delayed until at least the second day depending on urine output of more than 50ml/h and if improvement in eGFR was observed (≥ 30 mL/min/1.73m^2). TAC was introduced at a low dose (0.05mg/Kg twice daily) and dosage adjustments were made to achieve a 12-hour trough level of 5 to 8 ng/dL during the first 3 months and less than 5 ng/dL thereafter if no rejection occurred.

Methylprednisolone was started at ICU admission coinciding with ATG premedication at doses of 250mg i.v., followed by 200mg i.v. per day, tapered to 20mg orally per day over 6 days. During follow-up, methylprednisolone was reduced to 16mg orally per day at the 4th week, tapered to minimum doses for the following three months, and discontinued in all patients with normal liver function, except those with autoimmune disease.

Mycophenolate mofetil (MMF) at a dose of 1g twice a day was introduced on day 7 if TAC trough level failed to reach an adequate level and platelet count was > 50x10E9/L.

2.3. Immunosuppression with Basiliximab Induction. Patients in the *BAS group* received induction therapy with basiliximab (Simulect; Novartis, Basel, Switzerland) 20mg intravenously on day 0 intraoperatively after allograft reperfusion and on day 4 after LT.

The initiation of low TAC doses followed the same criteria as in the *ATG group.* Methylprednisolone 500 mg i.v. was administered intraoperatively, followed by 200mg i.v. per day, decreasing to 20mg orally per day over 6 days. During follow-up, methylprednisolone was reduced according to the same protocol as in the ATG group.

MMF at doses of 1g twice a day was started from day 1 if the platelet count was > 50x10E9/L.

2.4. Cytomegalovirus (CMV) and Pneumocystis Carinii Prophylaxis. All patients with a high risk for cytomegalovirus (CMV) infection (donor-positive, recipient-negative) received at least 3 months' prophylaxis with valganciclovir. CMV viral load was monitored weekly by PCR during the first month after transplant and monthly thereafter.

Additionally, pneumocystis carinii prophylaxis with trimethoprim and sulfamethoxazole or pentamidine was mandatory for all patients for at least 6 months.

2.5. Acute Cellular Rejection (ACR) Treatment. All suspected ACR episodes were proven by biopsy (BPAR) and stratified according to BANFF criteria [26]: indeterminate (portal inflammatory infiltrate that failed to meet the criteria for the diagnosis of ACR), mild (rejection infiltrate in a minority of triads that is generally mild and confined within the portal spaces), moderate (rejection infiltrate expanding most or all of the triads), and severe (moderate plus spillover into periportal areas and moderate to severe perivenular inflammation that extends into the hepatic parenchyma and is associated with perivenular hepatocyte necrosis). Treatment included 3 boluses of methylprednisolone (500 mg i.v.) if episodes were moderate or severe or increased doses of TAC if mild.

2.6. Endpoints. The primary efficacy endpoint was the combination of absence of ACR episodes and eGFR ≥ 60 mL/min/1.73m^2 at day 7 and 1 month after transplantation. Secondary endpoints were one-year patient and graft survival, incidence of infections including CMV (PCR>1000 copies/ μL), and the incidence of adverse events directly associated with ATG focused mainly on hematologic events (leucopenia and thrombocytopenia).

Demographic and baseline data of the recipients, donors, and surgical procedure were prospectively recorded in a database. During post-LT follow-up, documentation of clinical signs and laboratory data were obtained at baseline, days 7 and 14, and months 1, 3, 6, 9, and 12.

Follow-up was one year.

2.7. Cost Study. A financial analysis was also made to compare the impact of ATG induction therapy with that of our standard treatment with basiliximab. The analysis was based on the cost of the number of doses administered.

2.8. Statistical Analysis. This was an exploratory study and sample size determination was not based on statistical power. A preanalysis was conducted with 40 subjects (20 in each arm) and the behavior of this group was considered the population estimate.

Categorical variables were summarized as counts and percentages and continuous variables as medians with range. Group comparisons were made by the Mann–Whitney test for continuous data and chi-square test with Fisher's correction for categorical data. The Friedman test was used to detect differences among different values of one variable. Time to reach ACR was calculated with the Kaplan Meier method using the log-rank test for treatment comparisons.

In order to increase statistical power, a primary combined endpoint was used as a single dichotomous outcome. The composite endpoint was considered when BPAR was absent and eGFR ≥ 60 mL/min/1.73m^2 was present.

Differences were considered statistically significant when $p < 0.05$. Statistical analysis was performed using IBM SPSS Statistics 23.0 software.

3. Results

From January 2012 to December 2016, twenty patients received ATG as immunosuppression induction therapy. They were compared with 20 matched patients who received basiliximab immunosuppression induction therapy from January 2005 to December 2011. No differences were found between groups regarding age, sex, primary liver disease, comorbidities, and MELD; however, significant differences were observed regarding pre-LT eGFR between groups. No patients were on hemodialysis at the time of LT *(see Table 1).*

3.1. ATG Dosage. Median first ATG dose was 74±10mg. Thirteen (65%) patients received a second dose, mean 79±7mg, and four patients (20%) received a third dose, mean of 78±16mg.

CD2/CD3 levels dropped to a median of 70 cel/ μL (r: 10-297) after the first ATG dose and to 28 cel/ μL (r: 0-240) after the second. Fourteen days after LT, CD2/CD3 levels had returned to normal range [median 330 cel/ μL (49-1350)].

Table 1: Patient characteristics and surgical data.

	ATG Group (n=20)	BAS group (n=20)	p-value
Age (years)	60(±6)	57 (±7)	0.143
Male, n (%)	18 (90%)	17 (85%)	1
Primary liver disease			0.215
Alcoholic	11 (55%)	11(55%)	
Hepatitis C	4 (20%)	8 (40%)	
HCC	3 (15%)	1 (5%)	
Hepatitis B	1 (5%)	-	
NASH	1 (5%)	-	
Pre-LT Arterial Hypertension, n (%)	6 (30%)	5 (25%)	0.723
Pre-LT Diabetes Mellitus, n (%)	10 (50%)	4 (20%)	0.096
Pre-LT Cardiologic Disease, n(%)	4 (20%)	-	0.106
Median pre-eGFR (mL/min/1.73m^2)	49±9	34±12	0.001
MELD score	20 (±7)	26 (±9)	0.065
Cold ischemia time (min)	325±85	370±96	0.070
Warm ischemia time (min)	45±19	39±10	0.254
Intraoperative transfusion			
Red blood cells (Unit)	5 (0-26)	6 (4-11)	0.060
Fresh Frozen Plasma (Unit)	2 (0-18)	8 (0-16)	0.003
Platelets (Unit)	0 (0-10)	2 (0-20)	0.068
Piggy-back with portacaval shunt	11 (55%)	17 (85%)	0.082
Hospital Stay (days)	20 (11-90)	15 (10-114)	0.242

NASH, nonalcoholic steatohepatitis; eGFR, estimated glomerular filtration rate, and MELD; model for end-stage liver disease.

3.2. Basiliximab Dosage. All patients in the *BAS group* received the two doses of 20 mg i.v. of basiliximab at day 0 and day 4 after LT.

3.3. CNI Administration. The introduction of TAC was delayed a mean of 5±2 days in the *ATG group* compared to a mean of 2±0.5 days in the *BAS group* (p=0.001). No differences were found in mean TAC levels between groups at day 7 after LT [3 ng/dL (r: 1-8) in the *ATG group* versus 5 ng/dL (r: 1-9) in the *BAS group*, p=0.29], not even at one, 3, 6, and 12-months after transplant. See *Figure 1.*

3.4. Endpoints

3.4.1. Primary Combined Endpoint. Efficacy of primary combined endpoints had been achieved in 45% and 50% of patients at day 7 and 1 month after LT, respectively, in the *ATG group* versus 40% and 55% of patients at day 7 and 1 month after LT, respectively, in *the BAS group* (p=1).

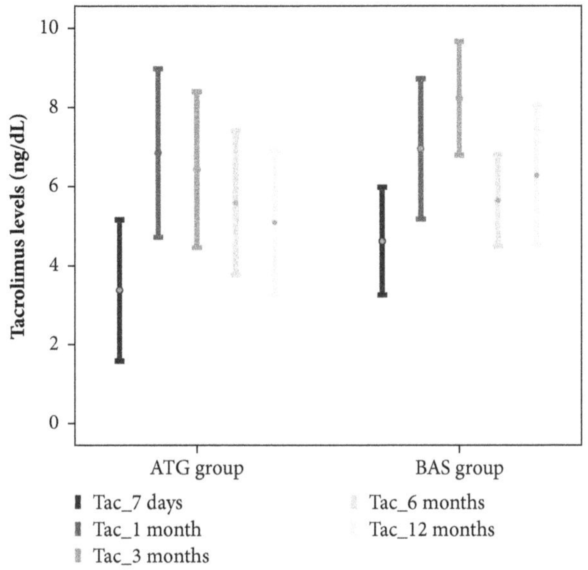

Figure 1: Tacrolimus levels after liver transplantation.

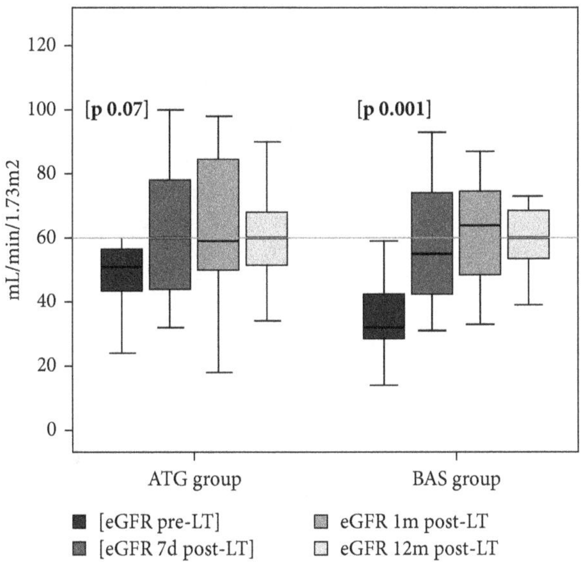

Figure 2: Glomerular filtration rate between groups at one year.

3.4.2. Renal Function. Ten of 20 patients (50%) had recovered their renal function (eGFR ≥60 mL/min/1.73m^2) at day 7 after LT, continuing with the same percentage 1 month after LT in the ATG group. Eight of 20 patients (40%) and 11 of 20 patients (55%) had recovered their renal function (eGFR ≥60 mL/min/1.73m^2) at day 7 and 1 month after LT, respectively, in the BAS group; these differences were not significant between groups.

Evolution of eGFR is shown in *Figure 2*. An improvement in renal function was observed over time in both groups, being only significant at 7 days after LT compared to before LT in BAS group.

No differences were observed during follow-up and renal function at one year after LT was 58±16 mL/min/1.73m^2 in the *ATG group* versus 62±16 mL/min/1.73m^2 in the *BAS group* (p=0.31).

Table 2: Results of secondary endpoints.

	ATG Group (n=20)	BAS group (n=20)	p-value
One-year patient and graft survival	95%	95%	1
Infection	6 (30%)	7 (35%)	0.510
(i) Cholangitis (gram-negative bacteria)	3	1	
(ii) Diarrheas (Clostridium difficile)	3	-	
(iii) Pneumonia (Klebsiella pneumoniae)	-	2	
(iv) Urinary tract infection (E. coli)	-	2	
(v) MRSA infection (central vein catheter)	-	1	
(vi) Oral Candidiasis	-	1	
CMV infection	9 (45%)	7 (35%)	0.519
Adverse events related to ATG			
Thrombocytopenia	3 (15%)		
Thrombocytopenia + Leukopenia	1 (5%)		

MRSA, methicillin-resistant Staphylococcus aureus.

3.4.3. ACR Episodes. ACR had occurred in 2 patients (10%) in the ATG group and none in the BAS group at day 7 after LT (p= 0.48). No more ACR episodes were observed in either group up to the end of the first month after LT.

Although the probability of BPAR was 2-fold higher in the *ATG group* compared with the BAS group, these differences were not significant (Figure 3). Eight patients (40%) in the *ATG group* presented some ACR episode during follow-up: 4 were moderate and 4 mild. ACR was reported in four patients (20%) in the *BAS group:* 2 were moderate and 2 mild. All cases in both groups were successfully treated with boluses of methylprednisolone and/or increased doses of TAC. There were no episodes of severe ACR.

3.4.4. Secondary Endpoints. Regarding mortality only two patients died during follow-up, one in each group. One in the *ATG group* was due to biliary complications related to hepatic artery thrombosis and further sepsis 2 months after LT. The other was a 69-year-old patient who died from decompensated cirrhosis due to chronic rejection 11 months after LT. TAC had to be withdrawn at day 28 owing to severe neurologic symptoms; however ductopenia appeared in the liver biopsy over 6 months later and the patient was treated with methylprednisolone, mTOR, and reintroduction of TAC. No clinical and pathologic response occurred.

No patients underwent retransplantation during follow-up, leading to 1-year graft and patient survival of 95% (*Table 2*).

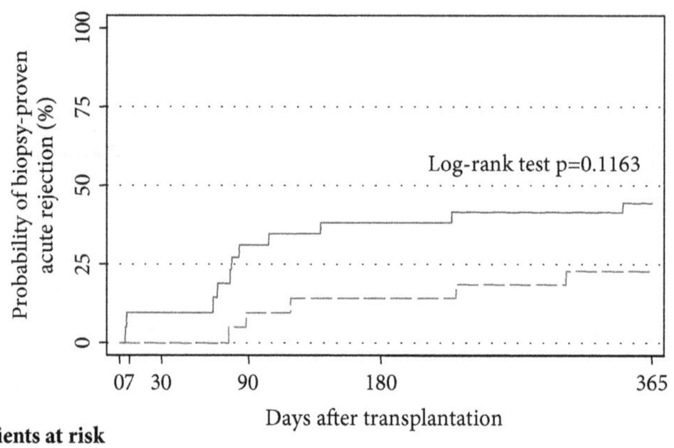

Patients at risk

ATG group	(0) 20	(5)	19	(2)	19	(2)	19
BAS group	(0) 20	(2)	20	(1)	20	(2)	19

——— ATG
– – – BAS

Figure 3: Cumulative probability of biopsy-proven rejection after transplantation.

No differences in the infection rate were observed between groups. Results of secondary endpoints at the end of follow-up are shown in *Table 2*.

3.5. Costs. The use of low-dose ATG resulted in a substantial reduction in drug costs compared to basiliximab. The *ATG group* received a median dose of 1.96 mg/kg (r: 0.65-4.16) and a median total dose of 160 mg (r: 50-300). Using a wholesale acquisition cost for a 100-mg vial of ATG (Grafalon; Neovii Biotech GMBH; Germany) (252€) at our facility, the median drug cost for a course/patient of ATG induction was 403€ (r:126-756) versus 2,524 € per patient in the *BAS group* (p=0.001).

4. Discussion

This study demonstrated that induction therapy based on low-dose ATG preserves renal function in cirrhotic patients undergoing LT with pretransplant renal dysfunction.

ATG induction has been widely used in kidney transplantation. Results in this setting revealed fewer ACR episodes and less delayed graft function. Studies are divided into those that use a standard course (1.5mg/Kg for five to six doses) [21–24] and those that use a short course (1.5g/Kg for three to five doses) [27, 28] showing the same benefits and less degree of leucopenia and thrombocytopenia.

The use of any antibody therapy for induction in liver transplantation remains controversial [29–31]. The liver is considered an immunologically privileged organ and the use of antibodies to prevent rejection has been perceived as unnecessary and may increase the risk of overimmunosuppression. In a five-year randomized prospective study published by Boillot et al. [31] in the pre-MELD era, ATG induction in LT failed to exert any beneficial effect on rejection prevention and patient and graft survival.

However, the role of ATG induction in LT has been revisited in recent years and seems to provide the same benefits using a short-course therapy, permitting delayed CNI introduction at low doses to avoid CNI-induced renal impairment [17, 18].

Previous studies in LT reported a low ACR rate and renal function recovery in the early posttransplant period in patients at high risk of acute renal failure using variable doses of ATG induction therapy, around 1mg/kg - 2mg/kg per day over 3 days [15–19]. More recently, Yoo et al. [20] published their experience in the largest series including 500 patients who underwent a steroid-free protocol with ATG induction given at 3mg/Kg divided into two doses of 1.5mg/kg. They obtained excellent results with an ACR rate of 23% in five-year follow-up, good outcomes, low complication rates, and good renal function preservation. Moreover, Montenovo et al. [25] retrospectively compared, for the first time, the clinical effects of ATG versus basiliximab as induction therapies in LT in a population with normal pretransplant renal function. The ATG was administered at 1.5mg/kg/day over 3 days with delayed TAC introduction. Their results showed a significantly lower ACR rate in favor of ATG (18% versus 27%) and decreased creatinine levels in both groups in a median follow-up of 5 years; however, no data on eGFR were reported.

In concordance with these results, our study showed delayed introduction of reduced-dose TAC under the protection of induction therapy based on low doses of ATG in patients with pretransplant renal dysfunction to be associated with a low ACR rate in the first month after LT and renal function recovery with no increase in the infection rate. The fact that the use of polyclonal antibodies did not increase the risk of infections in our series may be related to the low total median ATG dose used (1.96 mg/kg), lower than reported by other authors [17–19].

The most significant finding in our study was that approximately half of the patients treated with either of the induction therapies already had normal renal function with no rejection episodes at one week after LT. Results one month later were similar. The main causes of renal function recovery were good function of the new liver and the delay in CNI initiation. Thus, rationale for using ATG or basiliximab is to increase the immunosuppressive effect meanwhile to prevent ACR until renal function improves, and not because they have a direct effect. It is important to point out that although the number of patients who achieved normal renal function was the same in both groups at one week after LT, TAC was introduced significantly later in the ATG group. The reason was that the authors assumed the more immunosuppressive effect to be associated with the polyclonal antibodies, and thus overimmunosuppression by TAC addition was avoided. However, rejection occurred in 10% of patients in the ATG group during the first month after LT, a rate similar to that reported in other studies [20–25]. Improvement in renal function was observed in both groups over time, with no significant differences at one year after LT.

The disappointing result in our series was that the probability of rejection was double in the ATG group at the end of the study compared with the BAS group. These differences were not significant, probably due to the small number of patients in each group. We cannot rule out the possibility that a higher total ATG dose might improve these results; however, we should point out that the ACR rate remained low during the first month after transplant. Nevertheless, all ACR episodes were mild or moderate and none were corticoid-resistant.

Regarding the safety of ATG administration, it was well tolerated and only 4 patients presented thrombocytopenia or leucopenia which was easily managed by dose reduction or interruption, with platelets and leucocytes being in normal range at one month after transplant, similar to report by other studies [18–20]. Moreover, excellent one-year patient and graft survival were reported in both groups and neither of the two deaths during follow-up could be attributed to the induction therapy.

The greatest benefit of the use of low-dose ATG as induction therapy was the significant financial saving due to the direct cost of the drug compared to basiliximab. The average saving was more than 2,000€ per LT patient. The literature reported two economic analyses in the kidney transplant setting. Marfo et al. [28] compared the clinical and economic impact of using short-course versus standard-course ATG, with no significant differences in acute rejection episodes and a significant cost reduction using the short course. Recently, Cremashi et al. [32] compared quality-adjusted life years (QALYs) between ATG and basiliximab, with a modest increase in QALYs and lower long-term costs in the ATG cohort. However, no data on liver transplantation were reported.

The major limitations of this study were the low number of patients owing to the exploratory nature of the trial and bias in inclusion criteria. Patients with severe thrombocytopenia or leucopenia were not included in the ATG group, which probably selected patients with less portal hypertension and who were less critically ill compared with the BAS group. This became evident as shown by the higher pretransplant eGFR and lower MELD score in the ATG group. Despite that, not differences in outcomes were observed between groups.

In summary, induction therapy with low doses of ATG or anti-IL2 antagonists in cirrhotic patients with pretransplant renal dysfunction are good strategies for preserving posttransplant renal function, with the cost of ATG being much lower. Owing to a direct effect of ATG on platelets and leucocytes, induction with these antibodies should not be recommended in patients with severe thrombocytopenia or leucopenia, findings that are more frequent in very advanced cirrhosis with severe portal hypertension. Nevertheless, it should be taken into account that our study included a small number of patients, and thus, prospective, randomized, control studies are required to confirm these results.

Abbreviations

ACR: Acute cellular rejection
ATG: Anti-human T-lymphocyte globulin
BPAR: Biopsy-proven acute rejection
CMV: Cytomegalovirus
CNI: Calcineurin inhibitors
eGFR: Estimated glomerular filtration rate
HCV: Hepatitis C virus
ICU: Intensive care unit
i.v.: Intravenously
LT: Liver transplantation
MELD: Model for end-stage liver disease
MMF: Mycophenolate mofetil
PCR: Polymerase chain reaction
TAC: Tacrolimus.

Acknowledgments

The authors thank Christine O'Hara for English language edition, Santiago Pérez-Hoyos for statistical analysis, and Esther Delgado for secretarial work.

References

[1] A. Pawarode, D. M. Fine, and P. J. Thuluvath, "Independent risk factors and natural history of renal dysfunction in liver transplant recipients," *Liver Transplantation*, vol. 9, no. 7, pp. 741–747, 2003.

[2] J. B. Cabezuelo, P. Ramirez, F. Acosta et al., "Prognostic factors of early acute renal failure in liver transplantation," *Transplantation Proceedings*, vol. 34, no. 1, pp. 254-255, 2002.

[3] J. M. Moreno, V. Cuervas-Mons, and E. Rubio, "Chronic renal dysfunction after liver transplantation in adult patients: prevalence, risk factors, and impact on mortality," *Transplantation Proceedings*, vol. 35, no. 5, pp. 1907-1908, 2003.

[4] T. A. Gonwa, M. L. Mai, L. B. Melton et al., "End-stage renal disease (ESRD) after orthotopic liver transplantation (OLTX)

using calcineurin-based immunotherapy: risk of development and treatment," *Transplantation*, vol. 72, no. 12, pp. 1934–1939, 2001.

[5] N. C. Fisher, P. G. Nightingale, B. K. Gunson, G. W. Lipkin, and J. M. Neuberger, "Chronic renal failure following liver transplantation: A retrospective analysis," *Transplantation*, vol. 66, no. 1, pp. 59–66, 1998.

[6] A. O. Ojo, P. J. Held, F. K. Port et al., "Chronic renal failure after transplantation of a nonrenal organ," *The New England Journal of Medicine*, vol. 349, no. 10, pp. 931–940, 2003.

[7] A. S. Paramesh, S. Roayaie, Y. Doan et al., "Post-liver transplant acute renal failure: Factors predicting development of end-stage renal disease," *Clinical Transplantation*, vol. 18, no. 1, pp. 94–99, 2004.

[8] M. S. Campbell, D. S. Kotlyar, C. M. Brensinger et al., "Renal function after orthotopic liver transplantation is predicted by duration of pretransplantation creatinine elevation," *Liver Transplantation*, vol. 11, no. 9, pp. 1048–1055, 2005.

[9] I. Bilbao, R. Charco, J. Balsells et al., "Risk factors for acute renal failure requiring dialysis after liver transplantation," *Clinical Transplantation*, vol. 12, no. 2, pp. 123–129, 1998.

[10] M. L. Gallardo, M. E. Herrera Gutierrez, G. S. Pérez, E. C. Balsera, J. F. Fernández Ortega, and G. Q. García, "Risk factors for renal dysfunction in the postoperative course of liver transplant," *Liver Transplantation*, vol. 10, no. 11, pp. 1379–1385, 2004.

[11] C. Duvoux and G. P. Pageaux, "Immunosuppression in liver transplant recipients with renal impairment," *Journal of Hepatology*, vol. 54, no. 5, pp. 1041–1054, 2011.

[12] L. Castells, C. Balsells, and I. Bilbao, "Early detection, prevention and management of renal failure in liver transplantation," *Gastroenterol Hepatol*, vol. 37, 2014.

[13] J. D. Eason, G. E. Loss, J. Blazek, S. Nair, and A. L. Mason, "Steroid-free liver transplantation using rabbit antithymocyte globulin induction: Results of a prospective randomized trial," *Liver Transplantation*, vol. 7, no. 8, pp. 693–697, 2001.

[14] J. D. Eason, S. Nair, A. J. Cohen, J. L. Blazek, and G. E. Loss Jr., "Steroid-free liver transplantation using rabbit antithymocyte globulin and early tacrolimus monotherapy," *Transplantation*, vol. 75, no. 8, pp. 1396–1399, 2003.

[15] J. I. Tchervenkov, G. N. Tzimas, M. Cantarovich, J. S. Barkun, and P. Metrakos, "The impact of thymoglobulin on renal function and calcineurin inhibitor initiation in recipients of orthotopic liver transplant: A retrospective analysis of 298 consecutive patients," *Transplantation Proceedings*, vol. 36, no. 6, pp. 1747–1752, 2004.

[16] A. J. Tector, J. A. Fridell, R. S. Mangus et al., "Promising early results with immunosuppression using rabbit anti-thymocyte globulin and steroids with delayed introduction of tacrolimus in adult liver transplant recipients," *Liver Transplantation*, vol. 10, no. 3, pp. 404–407, 2004.

[17] T. Soliman, H. Hetz, C. Burghuber et al., "Short-term induction therapy with anti-thymocyte globulin and delayed use of calcineurin inhibitors in orthotopic liver transplantation," *Liver Transplantation*, vol. 13, no. 7, pp. 1039–1044, 2007.

[18] I. Bajjoka, L. Hsaiky, K. Brown, and M. Abouljoud, "Preserving renal function in liver transplant recipients with rabbit anti-thymocyte globulin and delayed initiation of calcineurin inhibitors," *Liver Transplantation*, vol. 14, no. 1, pp. 66–72, 2008.

[19] R. S. Mangus, J. A. Fridell, R. M. Vianna, P. Y. Kwo, J. Chen, and A. J. Tector, "Immunosuppression induction with rabbit anti-thymocyte globulin with or without rituximab in 1000 liver transplant patients with long-term follow-up," *Liver Transplantation*, vol. 18, no. 7, pp. 786–795, 2012.

[20] M. C. Yoo, J. M. Vanatta, K. A. Modanlou et al., "Steroid-free liver transplantation using rabbit antithymocyte globulin induction in 500 consecutive patients," *Transplantation*, vol. 99, no. 6, pp. 1231–1235, 2015.

[21] D. C. Brennan, J. A. Daller, K. D. Lake, D. Cibrik, and D. Del Castillo, "Rabbit antithymocyte globulin versus basiliximab in renal transplantation," *The New England Journal of Medicine*, vol. 355, no. 19, pp. 1967–1977, 2006.

[22] O. Thomusch, M. Wiesener, M. Opgenoorth et al., "Rabbit-ATG or basiliximab induction for rapid steroid withdrawal after renal transplantation (Harmony): an open-label, multicentre, randomised controlled trial," *The Lancet*, vol. 388, no. 10063, pp. 3006–3016, 2016.

[23] L. Penninga, A. Wettergren, C. H. Wilson et al., *Antibody inductions versus placebo, no induction or another type of antibody induction for liver transplant recipients*, 2014.

[24] P. Hill, N. B. Cross, A. N. Barnett, S. C. Palmer, and A. C. Webster, "Polyclonal and monoclonal antibodies for induction therapy in kidney transplant recipients," *Cochrane Database of Systematic Reviews*.

[25] M. I. Montenovo, F. G. Jalikis, M. Li et al., "Superior patient and graft survival in adult liver transplant with rabbit antithymocyte globulin induction: Experience with 595 patients," *Experimental and Clinical Transplantation*, vol. 15, no. 4, pp. 425–431, 2017.

[26] A. J. Demetris, K. P. Batts, A. P. Dhillon et al., "Banff schema for grading liver allograft rejection: an international consensus document," *Hepatology*, vol. 25, no. 3, pp. 658–663, 1997.

[27] M. Grafals, B. Smith, N. Murakami et al., "Immunophenotyping and efficacy of low dose ATG in non-sensitized kidney recipients undergoing early steroid withdrawal: a randomized pilot study," *PLoS ONE*, vol. 9, no. 8, Article ID e104408, 2014.

[28] K. Marfo, E. Akalin, C. Wang, and A. Lu, "Clinical and economic analysis of short-course versus standard-course antithymocyte globulin (rabbit) induction therapy in deceased-donor renal transplant recipients," *American Journal of Health-System Pharmacy*, vol. 68, no. 23, pp. 2276–2282, 2011.

[29] J. M. Langrehr, M. Glanemann, O. Guckelberger et al., "A randomized, placebo-controlled trial with anti-interleukin-2 receptor antibody for immunosuppressive induction therapy after liver transplantation," *Clinical Transplantation*, vol. 12, no. 4, pp. 303–312, 1998.

[30] E. Benedetti, D. Bogetti, H. N. Sankary, G. Chejfec, S. Cotler, and G. Testa, "Can thymoglobulin (TG) induction protects liver allografts from ischemia/reperfusion injury (IRI)?" *Transplantation*, vol. 78, p. 118, 2004.

[31] O. Boillot, B. Seket, J. Dumortier et al., "Thymoglobulin induction in liver transplant recipients with a tacrolimus, mycophenolate mofetil, and steroid immunosuppressive regimen: A five-year randomized prospective study," *Liver Transplantation*, vol. 15, no. 11, pp. 1426–1434, 2009.

[32] L. Cremaschi, R. von Versen, T. Benzing et al., "Induction therapy with rabbit antithymocyte globulin versus basiliximab after kidney transplantation: a health economic analysis from a German perspective," *Transplant International*, vol. 30, no. 10, pp. 1011–1019, 2017.

9

Efficacy and Safety of Immunosuppressive Therapy for PBC–AIH Overlap Syndrome Accompanied by Decompensated Cirrhosis

Xiaoli Fan,[1] Yongjun Zhu,[1] Ruoting Men,[1] Maoyao Wen,[1] Yi Shen,[1] Changli Lu,[2] and Li Yang[1]

[1]*Department of Gastroenterology & Hepatology, West China Hospital, Sichuan University, Chengdu, Sichuan 610041, China*
[2]*Department of Pathology, West China Hospital, Sichuan University, Chengdu, Sichuan 610041, China*

Correspondence should be addressed to Li Yang; yangli_hx@scu.edu.cn

Academic Editor: Kusum Kharbanda

Aim. To explore the efficacy and safety of immunosuppressive therapy for the treatment of primary biliary cirrhosis-autoimmune hepatitis (PBC-AIH) overlap syndrome accompanied by decompensated cirrhosis. *Methods.* A cohort study was performed to evaluate the usefulness of immunosuppressive therapy in this unique group. This cohort study was performed between October 2013 and June 2017 and included 28 biopsy-proven patients diagnosed according to the Paris criteria. The therapies included ursodeoxycholic acid (UDCA) alone (N=14) or in combination with immunosuppression (IS) therapy (N=14). The primary endpoints were biochemical remission, liver-related adverse events, transplant-free survival, and drug side-effects. *Results.* The frequency of biochemical remission for the AIH features was significantly higher in the UDCA+IS group than in the UDCA-only group (60.0 versus 9.1%, P=0.024) after 12 months of therapy but not after 3 and 6 months (28.6 versus 0%, P=0.165; 35.7 versus 7.1%, P=0.098). The rates of liver-related adverse events were lower in the combined group (2/14 versus 9/14, P=0.018). The Kaplan-Meier estimate showed that the transplant-free survival was distinct between the two groups (P=0.019). In the UDCA+IS group, mild and transient leukopenia occurred in two patients receiving azathioprine (AZA), and an infection was observed in one patient receiving mycophenolate mofetil (MMF). *Conclusions.* PBC-AIH patients with decompensated cirrhosis receiving a combination of UDCA and immunosuppressors presented with higher biochemical remission rates and experienced fewer liver-related adverse events, implying that the combined treatment might be a better therapeutic option for strictly defined decompensated PBC-AIH overlap syndrome.

1. Introduction

Autoimmune liver disease (AILD) comprises a group of immune-mediated liver diseases that include autoimmune hepatitis (AIH), primary biliary cirrhosis (PBC), and primary sclerosing cholangitis (PSC) [1]. The occurrence of overlapping syndromes at different disease stages (so-called overlap syndromes) is not rare, with PBC-AIH overlap syndrome being the most common [2]. The prevalence of PBC-AIH overlap syndrome is approximately 8–10% in adult patients with either PBC or AIH [3, 4], and this low incidence contributes to imprecise diagnostic criteria; furthermore, no standard therapy is currently available. According to the most recent guidelines based on the results of small studies, a combination of ursodeoxycholic acid (UDCA) and immunosuppressants is often recommended for PBC-AIH in clinical practice [5–7].

Risk stratification was recently performed by a panel of experts on the topic of cirrhosis [8]. The survival rates of compensated and decompensated cirrhosis are strikingly different, and the median survival time of the latter may be less than 2 years [9, 10]. PBC-AIH patients presenting with already advanced cirrhosis may die in the early phase of treatment because of complications related to immunosuppression; however, there are no data supporting this finding [11]. Hence, the present study was undertaken to analyse a single-centre cohort of PBC-AIH patients with decompensated cirrhosis. The present study was initiated to determine whether immunosuppressive therapy could be used in a cohort of decompensated PBC-AIH patients to obtain a biochemical response and to control the disease progression and the cost in terms of adverse reactions.

2. Materials and Methods

2.1. Inclusion Criteria. West China Hospital is a 4300-bed tertiary teaching hospital affiliated with Sichuan University. The hospital has a liver transplant unit (Liver Transplantation Centre, West China Hospital) and is the leading hospital in the western areas of China.

Cases were prospectively recruited between October 2013 and June 2017 using an electronic database of AILD, which was established in October 2013. Twenty-eight consecutive patients with PBC-AIH with decompensated cirrhosis strictly according to the Paris criteria were incorporated. The study was approved by the Ethics Committee of West China Hospital.

As recommended by the Paris criteria, the patients were diagnosed with PBC when they met 2 or more of the following diagnostic criteria: (1) the presence of anti-mitochondrial antibodies (AMA), (2) an alkaline phosphatase (ALP) level at least 2-fold the upper normal limit (UNL) or a gamma-glutamyl transpeptidase (GGT) level at least 5-fold the UNL, and (3) a liver biopsy specimen exhibiting florid bile duct lesions. Patients were diagnosed with AIH when they met 2 or more of the following criteria: (1) an alanine aminotransferase (ALT) level at least 5-fold the UNL, (2) serum IgG at least 2-fold the UNL or a positive test for smooth muscle antibodies (SMA), and (3) a liver biopsy exhibiting moderate or severe periportal or periseptal lymphocytic piecemeal necrosis. In our setting, only simultaneous forms of PBC-AIH overlap syndrome were enrolled, because fewer patients had the consecutive forms, which might have raised different diagnostic and therapeutic issues [12, 13]. Patients with viral hepatitis, nonalcoholic steatohepatitis, drug-induced liver disease, Wilson's disease, or other causes of liver damage were excluded through a careful history analysis and evaluation. Overlap with suspected PSC and acute severe AIH, as defined according to the proposed criteria, was also excluded [14].

Cirrhosis was diagnosed according to the histological analysis, unequivocal imaging, or endoscopic examination [15]. Decompensation was diagnosed by the presence of clinical complications, including ascites, variceal hemorrhage, and hepatic encephalopathy (HE) [8].

2.2. Clinical and Laboratory Analyses. The biochemical, serological, radiological, and histological data, treatment strategies, and outcomes were recorded for the patients with PBC-AIH with decompensated cirrhosis. The laboratory measurements included total bilirubin (TBIL), ALT, aspartate aminotransferase (AST), ALP, GGT, albumin (ALB), globulin (GLB), IgG, IgM, antinuclear antibody (ANA), liver-kidney microsomal antibody (LKM), soluble liver antigen (SLA), antibody against liver cytosol type 1 antigen (LC-1), routine blood measurements, and noninvasive hepatic fibrosis parameters. Child-Pugh scores were collected at baseline. All parameters were examined in the Department of Laboratory Medicine of West China Hospital, which was certified by the College of American Pathologists (CAP).

The imaging tests included ultrasonography (US), computed tomography (CT), and/or magnetic resonance imaging (MRI).

All patients underwent follow-up, including clinical and laboratory evaluations, every 1–3 months.

2.3. Treatment. A total of 28 consecutive decompensated PBC-AIH patients were enrolled in this open, real-world, observational study. Because the optimal type of treatment was not known, the managing physician was free to decide whether he would treat the patients with UDCA alone or combined with immunosuppressants. The patients treated with UDCA alone received a 13–15 mg/kg/d dose. In the UDCA+IS group (N=14), the patients were given an initial dose of 12-40 mg/d of methylprednisolone, simultaneously. Induction therapy was response-guided and individualized for the 14 patients and was gradually reduced. Azathioprine (AZA) (50-100 mg/d) was combined with UDCA and steroids for 12 patients in the UDCA+IS group, whereas mycophenolate mofetil (MMF) was combined with UDCA and steroids for one patient when the total bilirubin level was above 100 μmol/L and the other one was merely given UDCA and steroids. Proton pump inhibitors (PPIs) were used to prevent peptic ulcers or bleeding during corticosteroid reduction, and vitamin D and calcium were introduced to prevent osteoporosis and fractures.

Prior to the initiation of corticosteroid therapy, an absence of infection was confirmed by negative cultures of blood samples, ascites fluids, and urine specimens and chest X-ray or CT. Common complications were prevented and treated according to accepted clinical management guidelines.

2.4. Pathological Examination. Liver samples were acquired by ultrasound-guided percutaneous needle biopsy of the liver. The tissues were fixed in 10% formaldehyde (Kelong, China), embedded in paraffin, and used for haematoxylin and eosin (H&E) staining, Masson trichrome staining, special staining, and immunohistochemical staining to examine the histological characteristics. Finally, two pathologists (Changli Lu and Jianping Liu) from the Pathology Department of West China Hospital (certified by CAP) interpreted the samples. Diagnostic pathological changes in AIH were recorded, including interface hepatitis, lymphoplasmacytic infiltrate, hepatocyte resetting, and emperipolesis. Pathological changes used for the diagnosis of PBC included florid duct lesion, bile duct damage, ductular proliferation, and cholestasis. The activity grade (G0–4) and fibrosis stage (S0–4) were assessed, according to the Scheuer system [16–19].

2.5. Outcomes Assessment. The primary effectiveness assessment was biochemical remission of AIH features (normalization of transaminases and IgG after starting therapy, as determined using existing guidelines). Liver-related adverse events

TABLE 1: Demographic and clinical features, laboratory parameters, prognostic scores, and decompensation characteristics between the two groups.

Variables	UDCA-only group (N=14)	UDCA+IS group (N=14)	*P* value
Age at entry (years)	60.0 (51.3, 61.3)	48.0 (42.5, 53.5)	0.024
Gender (F/M)	13/1	12/2	>0.999
TBIL, μmol/L	29.0 (23.2, 41.1)	38.9 (35.2, 127.1)	0.035
ALT, IU/L	66.5 (44.8, 127.0)	112.0 (45.7, 174.5)	0.401
AST, IU/L	103.5 (78.5, 129.8)	170.0 (91.0, 212.5)	0.401
ALP, IU/L	349.5 (257.8, 519.0)	294.0 (196.5, 430.5)	0.285
GGT, IU/L	268.5 (157.0, 656.3)	229.5 (51.8, 293.5)	0.285
ALB, g/L	37.6 (31.8, 39.9)	32.3 (29.9, 35.5)	0.031
GLB, g/L	43.4 (37.4, 47.1)	45.4 (35.3, 50.2)	0.511
INR	1.1 (1.0, 1.2)	1.1 (1.0, 1.2)	0.734
Cr, μmol/L	57.3 (51.8, 66.3)	53.5 (43.3, 61.3)	0.137
ANA positive, N (%)	13/14	12/14	>0.999
AMA positive, N (%)	9/14	9/14	>0.999
LKM positive, N (%)	0	0	-
LC-1 positive, N (%)	0	0	-
SLA positive, N (%)	0	0	-
Concurrent autoimmune diseases, N (%)	4/14	6 /14	0.695
IgG (g/L)	22.8 (20.2, 25.7)	28.6 (19.7, 32.4)	0.125
IgM (g/L)	2.2 (1.3, 5.7)	2.7 (2.4, 3.0)	0.306
APRI score	3.9 (2.2, 5.3)	6.4 (3.9, 7.2)	0.051
FIB-4 index	6.6 (4.9, 8.7)	11.7 (6.7, 18.9)	0.075
Complications			
Ascites	12/14	10/14	0.648
Variceal bleeding	2/14	4/14	0.648
Prognostic scores			
Child-Pugh score	6.5 (6.0, 7.0)	8.0 (6.0, 8.0)	0.265

Note. UDCA, ursodeoxycholic acid; IS, immunosuppressants; TBIL, total bilirubin; ALT, alanine aminotransferase; AST, aspartate aminotransferase; ALP, alkaline phosphatase; GGT, gamma-glutamyl transpeptidase; ALB, albumin; GLB, globulin; ANA, antinuclear antibody; AMA, anti-mitochondrial antibody; LKM, liver–kidney microsomal antibody; LC-1, antibody against liver cytosol type 1 antigen; SLA, soluble liver antigen/liver pancreas antibody; APRI, aspartate aminotransferase to platelet ratio index; FIB-4, fibrosis 4 index.

were determined if the patients experienced the following: (1) worsening of existing hepatic decompensation, (2) a new decompensation event other than the event present at the initiation of therapy, (3) liver failure, or (4) transplantation or death attributable to decompensation events. The transplant-free survival was compared additionally. The evaluation of drug side-effects included diarrhoea, steroid-specific side effects (i.e., osteoporosis, fractures, moon face, or acne), infection, and myelosuppression. All safety assessments were performed for the total patient cohort. Patients were followed until May 2018.

2.6. Statistical Analysis. Continuous data are presented as medians and quartiles, and categorical data are expressed as percentages. The Mann–Whitney U test was used for comparisons of continuous variables. The Chi-square test or Fisher's exact test was used to analyse differences in categorical variables between two independent groups where appropriate. A P-value <0.05 was considered significant. Data processing was performed with the SPSS software package (SPSS version 24.0 for Windows, IBM Corp., Armonk, NY, USA).

3. Results

3.1. Basic Information. A total of 28 patients diagnosed with PBC-AIH accompanied by decompensated cirrhosis were enrolled in the cohort study (Figure 1). Table 1 presents the clinical and biochemical characteristics of the two groups. For the UDCA alone group, the median age at treatment initiation was 60.0 (51.3, 61.3) years, and the female-to-male ratio was 13:1. For the UDCA+IS group, the median age was 48.0 (42.5, 53.5) years, and the female-to-male ratio was 12:2. AMA was positive in 64.2% of patients (9 of 14) in the both the UDCA alone group and UDCA+IS group (P>0.999). SLA, LC-1, and LKM were negative in the enrolled patients. At the time of study inclusion, the patients who did not receive immunosuppressants had lower total bilirubin (TBIL) levels (29.0 versus 38.9 IU/L, P=0.035) and higher albumin (ALB) levels (37.6 versus 32.3 IU/L, P=0.031) than the combined

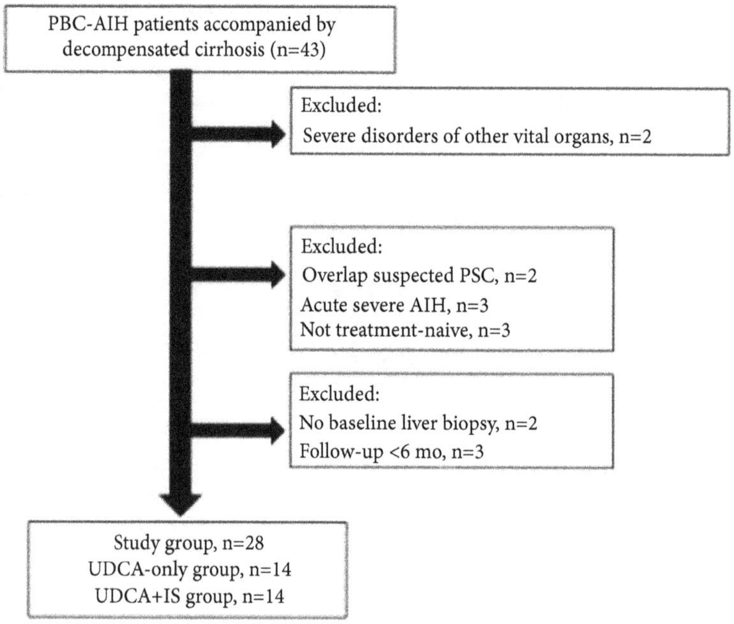

FIGURE 1: Study flowchart for patient inclusion.

TABLE 2: Comparison of symptoms between the two groups at baseline.

Symptoms	**UDCA-only group (N=14)**	**UDCA+IS group (N=14)**	***P* value**
Jaundice	3 (21.4%)	6(42.9%)	0.420
Ventosity	5(35.7%)	3(21.4%)	0.678
Fatigue	4(28.6%)	3(21.4%)	>0.999
Lower limb swelling	3(21.4%)	4(28.6%)	>0.999
Anorexia	2(14.3%)	3(21.4%)	>0.999
Arthralgia	2(14.3%)	4(28.6%)	0.648
Yellow urine	2(14.3%)	3(21.4%)	>0.999
Abdominal pain	3(21.4%)	2(14.3%)	>0.999
Weight loss	2(14.3%)	1(7.2%)	>0.999
Nausea	1(7.2%)	1(7.2%)	-
None	1(7.2%)	1(7.2%)	>0.999

group. All patients were diagnosed with decompensated cirrhosis prior to treatment (Table 1).

The common clinical symptoms are shown in Table 2. Jaundice and ventosity were the two most common symptoms in all patients. The symptoms at presentation were similar in the two groups.

3.2. Histological Features in the Study Cohort. All 28 patients had biopsy specimens available at diagnosis and presented with a typical picture of AIH features, with moderate to severe interface hepatitis and lymphocytic infiltrates, as well as PBC features. Severe interface hepatitis was only observed in 2 patients in the combined group. Hepatocellular rosette formation was noted in 8 and 10 patients in the two groups, respectively. Lymphoplasmacytic infiltrate was found in most patients, whereas emperipolesis was not observed. Bile duct damage was found in 13 and 10 patients in the two groups, whereas ductopenia was observed in 9 and 6 patients, respectively. Ductular proliferation, which was revealed by staining for cytokeratin 7, was observed in 11 and 9 patients in the two groups, respectively (Table 3). Figure 2 presents the features of a biopsy specimen from a patient who received UDCA plus immunosuppressant treatment.

3.3. Treatment Response. Table 4 shows the treatment response rates for both patient groups. At the end of the study, 42.9% (12/28) of the patients reached complete biochemical remission. Overall, the response rates after 3, 6, and 12 months of therapy were 14.2% (4/28), 21.4% (6/28), and 33.3% (7/28), respectively. The remission rate after 12 months was significantly higher in the combined group than in the UDCA-only group (60.0 versus 9.1%, P=0.024). Although not statistically significant, the biochemical remission rates seem to be higher in the combined group after 3 and 6 months of therapy (28.6 versus 0%, P=0.098 and 35.7 versus 7.1%, P=0.165).

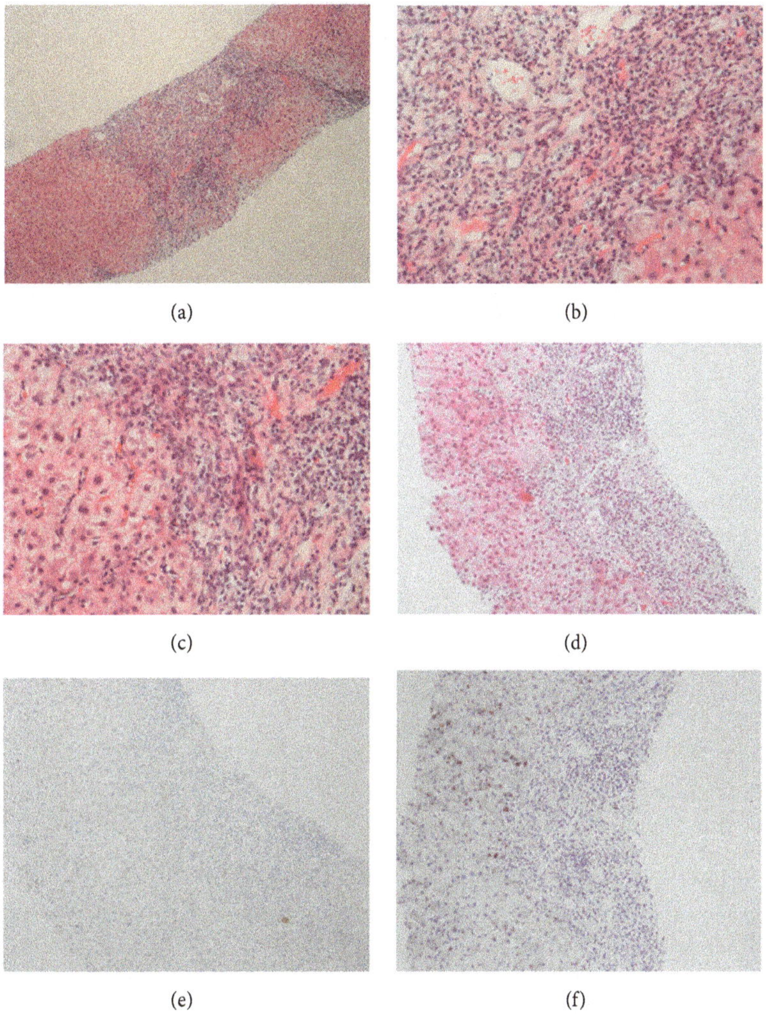

FIGURE 2: Histological features of decompensated PBC-AIH patients. (a) Bridging necrosis and moderate to severe interface hepatitis (×100, HE staining); (b) prominent interface hepatitis with numerous plasma cells (×400, HE staining); (c) typical rosetting of hepatocytes in the area of interface hepatitis (×400, HE staining); (d), (e), (f) interlobular bile duct loss without a significant ductular reaction (×200, HE staining, CK7 staining, and copper staining in sequence).

TABLE 3: Histological features of the decompensated PBC-AIH patients.

Variables	UDCA-only group (N=14)	UDCA+IS group (N=14)	*P* value
Number of portal areas	10	9	0.541
Severe interface hepatitis	0/14	2/14	0.481
Moderate interface hepatitis	14/14	12/14	0.481
Hepatocyte rosette formation	8/14	10/14	0.695
Lymphoplasmacytic infiltrate	13/14	13/14	>0.999
Emperipolesis	0/14	0/14	-
Bile duct damage	13/14	10/14	0.326
Ductopenia	9/14	6/14	0.449
Bile duct proliferation	11/14	9/14	0.678
Cholestasis	7/14	6/14	>0.999
G0/1/2/3/4 (N)	0/0/2/12/0	0/1/2/7/4	0.374
S0/1/2/3/4 (N)	0/3/4/5/2	0/0/3/8/3	0.117

Note. UDCA, ursodeoxycholic acid; IS, immunosuppressants.

TABLE 4: Response to treatment in AIH features after 3, 6, and 12 months of therapy.

Variables	Overall (n=28, %)	UDCA-only group (n=14), %	UDCA+IS group (n=14), %	*P* value
3-month remission	4(14.2%)	0(0%)	4(28.6%)	0.098
6-month remission	6(21.4%)	1(7.1%)	5(35.7%)	0.165
12-month remission*	7(33.3%)#	1(9.1%)##	6(60.0%)	0.024

*Twenty-one patients were treated for more than 12 months in total.
#Eleven patients were treated for more than 12 months in the UDCA-only group.
##Ten patients were treated for more than 12 months in the UDCA+IS group.

TABLE 5: Liver-related adverse events in the two groups.

Variables	UDCA-only group (N=14)	UDCA+IS group (N=14)	*P* value
Adverse events	9/14(64.3%)	2/14(14.3%)	0.018
Severe ascites	4(28.6%)	1(7.1%)	0.326
Variceal bleeding	1(7.1%)	0	>0.999
Liver failure	4(28.6%)	1(7.1%)	0.596
Transplantation/liver-related death	4/14(28.6%)	1/14(7.1%)	0.326

Note. UDCA, ursodeoxycholic acid; IS, immunosuppressants.

The symptoms of 12/14 (85.7%) of patients in the combined group have improved significantly, while the rate of symptom improvement was 71.4% (P=0.353).

3.4. Liver-Related Adverse Events and Transplant Free Survival Period. Table 5 shows the clinical outcomes at the end of the study. During the study period, the rates of liver-related adverse events were 64.3% (9 of 14) and 14.3% (2 of 14) in the UDCA alone group and the combination group, respectively (*P*=0.018). Thus, a total of 11 patients experienced liver-related adverse events during the follow-up. The median follow-up time was 18.0 (13.3, 20.8) months and was similar for patients in the UDCA-only group and the combined group [20.0 (13.5, 26.8) months, respectively (P=0.427]. To date, relapses during maintenance therapy have not been observed, and immunosuppression has not been withdrawn.

Liver transplantations were more commonly observed in the UDCA-only group and the combined group (4/14 vs 1/14, P=0.326). No patient died till the end of follow-up. The reasons for liver transplantation were cholestasis (N=3), esophagogastric hemorrhage (N=1), and refractory ascites (N=1). In the 5 patients who received liver transplantations in the two groups, none died posttransplantation. The Kaplan-Meier estimate showed that the transplant-free survival was distinct between the two groups (P=0.019) (Figure 3).

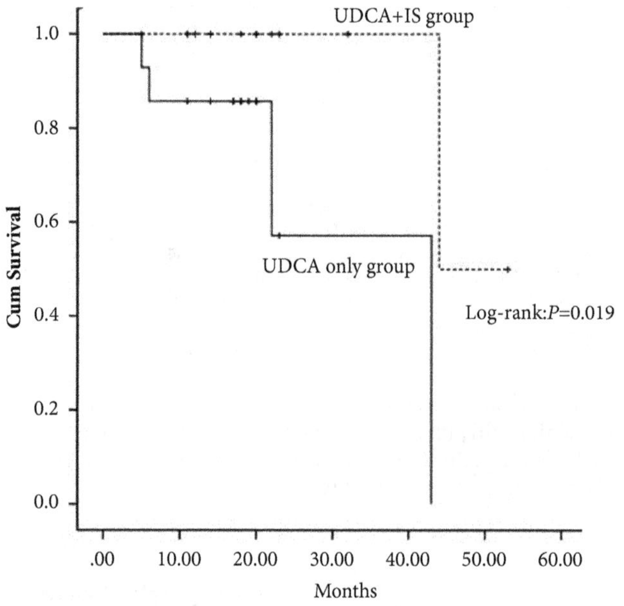

FIGURE 3: Transplant-free survival between the two groups (log-rank, P = 0.019).

3.5. Drug Side-Effects. Seven patients experienced transient diarrhoea after UDCA treatment. Corticosteroid-related side effects were noted in 35.7% (5 of 14) of the patients in the combined group. Most of these effects were mild, steroid-specific side effects, such as acne and moon face, and most resolved after dose reduction. Two patients in the UDCA+IS group experienced mild leukopenia (white blood count values of 3.0×10^9/L and 2.49×10^9/L) during the first 60 days of AZA treatment. AZA was not discontinued, because the white blood counts increased gradually and thereafter remained stable. A mild urinary tract infection occurred in one patient who received MMF during the first 60 days of AZA treatment.

4. Discussion

This cohort study was the first to assess the real-world effectiveness and safety of immunosuppressors in decompensated PBC-AIH patients. Six patients (60%) receiving UDCA plus immunosuppressors achieved biochemical remission, whereas only one patient (9.1%) achieved biochemical remission 12 months after beginning therapy. Patients treated with a combination of UDCA and immunosuppressors experienced fewer liver-related adverse events and obtained longer transplant-free survival, implying that the natural history and progression of decompensated PBC-AIH may also be haltered and averted.

Biochemical remission is a predictor of histologic outcome in PBC-AIH and may postpone the progression of cirrhosis [20]. In the present study, biochemical remission occurred in 60.0% of patients treated with a combination of UDCA and immunosuppression. Our data were consistent with the results from other studies, although these studies did not investigate advanced cirrhosis. A multicentre retrospective study with 88 patients with PBC-AIH found that the combination of UDCA and immunosuppression was effective in 73% of patients who were not previously treated or did not respond to UDCA alone [20]. Chazouilleres et al. found that fibrosis progression occurred more frequently in noncirrhotic patients under UDCA monotherapy (4/8) than under combined therapy (0/6) (P=0.04) [21]. Similar results were obtained in a recent meta-analysis, which found that combination therapy with UDCA and corticosteroids was more effective than UDCA alone [6]. In our study, most of the biochemical and immune parameters improved dramatically in both groups after treatment, whereas the immune variable IgG, which is a hallmark of liver inflammation and the treatment response [5], did not decrease in the UDCA group. However, the TBIL values, which were used as one element to evaluate AIH remission [22], did not significantly differ before and after treatment in either group (data not shown). Early studies have suggested that UDCA alone can help achieve biochemical and histological improvements in PBC-AIH patients, but the patient groups of the studies being compared did not focus on PBC–AIH overlap syndrome accompanied by decompensated cirrhosis [23, 24]. Hence, our data, similar to data from other studies, emphasize that the administration of immunosuppressors aids the hepatic immune response in this group of patients.

The median survival time for decompensated cirrhosis may be less than 2 years [9, 10]. Recent EASL guidelines proposed that treatment was probably no longer indicated in AIH patients with decompensated cirrhosis unless they had a high inflammatory score on the liver biopsy. However, limited studies have offered real-world data for the responses, outcomes, and side effects in AIH or PBC-AIH patients with decompensated cirrhosis [5, 25]. In the present study, the data showed a benefit on the progression of advanced cirrhosis in the UDCA+IS group during the observation period (median, 15.0 months). This result was in line with another study. Wang et al. found that immunosuppression treatment helped 62.5% of AIH patients with decompensated cirrhosis revert to compensated cirrhosis and that the rate of transplant-free survival was significantly greater in patients who received corticosteroids compared to those who did not [25]. Although the relationship between PBC-AIH overlap syndrome and AIH alone is complex, their results implied that immunosuppressive treatment could interrupt the progression of autoimmune-mediated advanced cirrhosis by controlling the hepatic immune response. In our study, all the patients were diagnosed according to Paris criteria; that is, PBC patients were diagnosed with AIH when they met 2 or more of the criteria, which meant that our patients were with histological features of active liver inflammation, rather than quiet or burnt-out cirrhosis. In that situation, more emphasis would be needed on the treat complications to prolong the transplant-free survival. Hence, individualized protocols are needed for different clinical situations. However, further prospective studies with more patients and long-term follow-ups may provide more robust evidence.

Prior to starting therapy, the risks and benefits of immunosuppressive treatment must be weighed. In our study, 12 patients (85.7%) received an initial methylprednisolone dose of 24 mg/d that was rapidly tapered according to the treatment response. The methylprednisolone doses for the other two patients were 12 mg/d and 48 mg/d. No serious side-effects of methylprednisolone were observed in our study, which was mostly attributed to our positive strategies used for tapering, preventive medications, and monitoring. In the 12 patients who received AZA as an adjuvant drug, transient leukopenia occurred in 2 patients (14.2%). Our data were not consistent with Heneghan et al. [26], who found that advanced fibrosis but not the thiopurine methyltransferase (TPMT) genotype or activity predicted azathioprine toxicity in AIH patients. In our patients, *NUDT15* (i.e., rs116855232) and *TPMT* (i.e., rs1142345) SNPs were genotyped using a real-time PCR method. No TPMT genetic variants were genotyped in these 12 patients, but heterozygous *NUDT15* R139C genotypes were found in the 2 patients who experienced leukopenia (data not shown). Hence, adjusting the azathioprine dosage may be considered according to the rs116855232 genotype rather than advanced fibrosis or cirrhosis. Hence, the rate of leukopenia was relatively low and acceptable. However, whether the *TPMT* and *NUDT* genotypes were associated with leukopenia in these PBC-AIH patients is unknown. Also, the infection rate was 7.1%, which was in line with Wang et al. (10.9%) [25].

The present study has some limitations. First, this investigation was a single-centre cohort study. Given this experimental approach, avoiding confounding factors was relatively difficult, and some data were not available. Second, because decompensated cirrhosis is an uncommon and advanced presentation of this disease, obtaining larger sample sizes is difficult in real-word studies. The current lack of controlled trials makes the results of small studies on rare diseases helpful and informative. Furthermore, because the mortality rate is as high as 85% over 5 years in patients with decompensation who do not receive a liver transplant, conducting a prospective study with extended follow-up can be very difficult. Third, no histological evaluations were performed after therapy to confirm the histological validity of this study.

In conclusion, we found that PBC-AIH patients with decompensated cirrhosis receiving a combination of UDCA and immunosuppressors presented higher biochemical remission rates, fewer liver-related adverse events, and longer transplant-free survival, implying that combined treatment might be a better therapeutic option for strictly defined PBC-AIH overlap syndrome accompanied by decompensated cirrhosis.

Authors' Contributions

Xiaoli Fan and Yongjun Zhu contributed equally to this work.

Acknowledgments

This work was supported by grants from the National Natural Science Foundation of China [no. 81770568 to Li Yang] and Fundamental Research Funds for the Central Universities [no. 2012017yjsy198 to Xiaoli Fan].

References

[1] A. J. Czaja, "Frequency and nature of the variant syndromes of autoimmune liver disease," *Hepatology*, vol. 28, no. 2, pp. 360–365, 1998.

[2] C. Rust and U. H. Beuers, "Overlap syndromes among autoimmune liver diseases," *World Journal of Gastroenterology*, vol. 14, no. 21, pp. 3368–3373, 2008.

[3] O. Chazouillères, D. Wendum, L. Serfaty, S. Montembault, O. Rosmorduc, and R. Poupon, "Primary biliary cirrhosis-autoimmune hepatitis overlap syndrome: clinical features and response to therapy," *Hepatology*, vol. 28, no. 2, pp. 296–301, 1998.

[4] A. Heurgué, F. Vitry, M.-D. Diebold et al., "Overlap syndrome of primary biliary cirrhosis and autoimmune hepatitis: A retrospective study of 115 cases of autoimmune liver disease," *Gastroentérologie Clinique et Biologique*, vol. 31, no. 1, pp. 17–25, 2007.

[5] "Corrigendum to "EASL Clinical Practice Guidelines: Autoimmune hepatitis" [J Hepatol 2015;63:971–1004]," *Journal of Hepatology*, vol. 63, no. 6, pp. 1543-1544, 2015.

[6] H. Zhang, S. Li, J. Yang et al., "A meta-analysis of ursodeoxycholic acid therapy versus combination therapy with corticosteroids for PBC-AIH-overlap syndrome: Evidence from 97 monotherapy and 117 combinations," *Przegląd Gastroenterologiczny*, vol. 10, no. 3, pp. 148–155, 2015.

[7] G. M. Hirschfield, U. Beuers, C. Corpechot et al., "EASL Clinical Practice Guidelines: The diagnosis and management of patients with primary biliary cholangitis," *Journal of Hepatology*, vol. 67, no. 1, pp. 145–172, 2017.

[8] G. Garcia-Tsao, J. G. Abraldes, A. Berzigotti, and J. Bosch, "Portal hypertensive bleeding in cirrhosis: risk stratification, diagnosis, and management: 2016 practice guidance by the American Association for the study of liver diseases," *Hepatology*, vol. 65, no. 1, pp. G310–G335, 2017.

[9] A. Zipprich, G. Garcia-Tsao, S. Rogowski, W. E. Fleig, T. Seufferlein, and M. M. Dollinger, "Prognostic indicators of survival in patients with compensated and decompensated cirrhosis," *Liver International*, vol. 32, no. 9, pp. 1407–1414, 2012.

[10] G. D'Amico, L. Pasta, A. Morabito et al., "Competing risks and prognostic stages of cirrhosis: A 25-year inception cohort study of 494 patients," *Alimentary Pharmacology & Therapeutics*, vol. 39, no. 10, pp. 1180–1193, 2014.

[11] A. W. Lohse and G. Mieli-Vergani, "Autoimmune hepatitis," *Journal of Hepatology*, vol. 55, no. 1, pp. 171–182, 2011.

[12] K. M. Boberg, R. W. Chapman, G. M. Hirschfield, A. W. Lohse, M. P. Manns, and E. Schrumpf, "Overlap syndromes: the International Autoimmune Hepatitis Group (IAIHG) position statement on a controversial issue," *Journal of Hepatology*, vol. 54, no. 2, pp. 374–385, 2011.

[13] P. J. Trivedi and G. M. Hirschfield, "Review article: Overlap syndromes and autoimmune liver disease," *Alimentary Pharmacology & Therapeutics*, vol. 36, no. 6, pp. 517–533, 2012.

[14] R. T. Stravitz, J. H. Lefkowitch, R. J. Fontana et al., "Autoimmune acute liver failure: proposed clinical and histological criteria," *Hepatology*, vol. 53, no. 2, pp. 517–526, 2011.

[15] D. Schuppan and N. H. Afdhal, "Liver cirrhosis," *The Lancet*, vol. 371, no. 9615, pp. 838–851, 2008.

[16] P. J. Scheuer, "Classification of chronic viral hepatitis: a need for reassessment," *Journal of Hepatology*, vol. 13, no. 3, pp. 372–374, 1991.

[17] C. Sempoux and J. Rahier, "Histological scoring of chronic hepatitis," *Acta Gastro-Enterologica Belgica*, vol. 67, no. 3, pp. 290–293, 2004.

[18] A. W. H. Chan, R. C. K. Chan, G. L. H. Wong et al., "Evaluation of histological staging systems for primary biliary cirrhosis: Correlation with clinical and biochemical factors and significance of pathological parameters in prognostication," *Histopathology*, vol. 65, no. 2, pp. 174–186, 2014.

[19] T. Namisaki, K. Moriya, M. Kitade et al., "Clinical significance of the Scheuer histological staging system for primary biliary cholangitis in Japanese patients," *European Journal of Gastroenterology & Hepatology*, vol. 29, no. 1, pp. 23–30, 2017.

[20] E. Ozaslan, C. Efe, A. Heurgué-Berlot et al., "Factors associated with response to therapy and outcome of patients with primary biliary cirrhosis with features of autoimmune hepatitis," *Clinical Gastroenterology and Hepatology*, vol. 12, no. 5, pp. 863–869, 2014.

[21] O. Chazouillères, D. Wendum, L. Serfaty, O. Rosmorduc, and R. Poupon, "Long term outcome and response to therapy of primary biliary cirrhosis - Autoimmune hepatitis overlap syndrome," *Journal of Hepatology*, vol. 44, no. 2, pp. 400–406, 2006.

[22] M. P. Manns, A. J. Czaja, J. D. Gorham et al., "Diagnosis and management of autoimmune hepatitis," *Hepatology*, vol. 51, no. 6, pp. 2193–2213, 2010.

[23] E. J. Heathcote, K. Cauch-Dudek, S. Joshi et al., "Primary biliary cirrhosis with additional features of autoimmune hepatitis: Response to therapy with ursodeoxycholic acid," *Hepatology*, vol. 35, no. 2, pp. 409–413, 2002.

[24] F. Günsar, U. S. Akarca, G. Ersöz, Z. Karasu, G. Yüce, and Y. Batur, "Clinical and biochemical features and therapy responses in primary biliary cirrhosis and primary biliary cirrhosis-autoimmune hepatitis overlap syndrome," *Hepato-Gastroenterology*, vol. 49, no. 47, pp. 1195–1200, 2002.

[25] Z. Wang, L. Sheng, and Y. Yang, "he Management of Autoimmune Hepatitis Patients with Decompensated Cirrhosis: Real-World Experience and a Comprehensive Review," *Clinical reviews in allergy & immunology*, vol. 52, no. 3, pp. 424–435, 2016.

[26] M. A. Heneghan, M. L. Allan, J. D. Bornstein, A. J. Muir, and D. A. Tendler, "Utility of thiopurine methyltransferase genotyping and phenotyping, and measurement of azathioprine metabolites in the management of patients with autoimmune hepatitis," *Journal of Hepatology*, vol. 45, no. 4, pp. 584–591, 2006.

10

A Systematic Review of the Efficacy and Safety of Fecal Microbiota Transplant for *Clostridium difficile* Infection in Immunocompromised Patients

Oluwaseun Shogbesan,[1] Dilli Ram Poudel,[2] Samjeris Victor,[3] Asad Jehangir,[2] Opeyemi Fadahunsi,[4] Gbenga Shogbesan,[5] and Anthony Donato[1]

[1]*Department of Medicine, Tower Health System, Sixth Avenue and Spruce Street, West Reading, PA 19611, USA*
[2]*Hospitalist Services, Tower Health System, Sixth Avenue and Spruce Street, West Reading, PA 19611, USA*
[3]*Department of Biochemistry & Molecular Biology, Pennsylvania State University, State College, PA 16801, USA*
[4]*Division of Cardiology, Dalhousie University, Halifax, NS B3H 4RS, Canada*
[5]*Department of Internal Medicine, Piedmont Athens Regional Medical Center, Athens, GA 30606, USA*

Correspondence should be addressed to Oluwaseun Shogbesan; oluwaseun.shogbesan@readinghealth.org

Academic Editor: Salvatore Oliva

Background. Fecal microbiota transplantation (FMT) has been shown to be effective in recurrent *Clostridium difficile* (CD) infection, with resolution in 80% to 90% of patients. However, immunosuppressed patients were often excluded from FMT trials, so safety and efficacy in this population are unknown. *Methods.* We searched MEDLINE and EMBASE for English language articles published on FMT for treatment of CD infection in immunocompromised patients (including patients on immunosuppressant medications, patients with human immunodeficiency virus (HIV), inherited or primary immunodeficiency syndromes, cancer undergoing chemotherapy, or organ transplant, including-bone marrow transplant) of all ages. We excluded inflammatory bowel disease patients that were not on immunosuppressant medications. Resolution and adverse event rates (including secondary infection, rehospitalization, and death) were calculated. *Results.* Forty-four studies were included, none of which were randomized designs. A total of 303 immunocompromised patients were studied. Mean patient age was 57.3 years. Immunosuppressant medication use was the reason for the immunocompromised state in the majority (77.2%), and 19.2% had greater than one immunocompromising condition. Seventy-six percent were given FMT via colonoscopy. Of the 234 patients with reported follow-up outcomes, 207/234 (87%) reported resolution after first treatment, with 93% noting success after multiple treatments. There were 2 reported deaths, 2 colectomies, 5 treatment-related infections, and 10 subsequent hospitalizations. *Conclusion.* We found evidence that supports the use of FMT for treatment of CD infection in immunocompromised patients, with similar rates of serious adverse events to immunocompetent patients.

1. Introduction

Clostridium difficile (CD) infection is the leading cause of healthcare-associated diarrheal illness in the United States, affecting nearly 500,000 patients annually [1, 2]. Both incidence and severity of CD infection have increased over the past two decades, and CD infection is now responsible for 29,000 deaths/year within 30 days of diagnosis [1]. Immunocompromised patients, including those receiving immunosuppressant medications or patients with human immunodeficiency virus (HIV) and transplants, seem to be at increased risk of hospitalization and recurrence of CD infection as the immune system is an important defense for both protection and recovery from infection [3–6].

Antibiotics have long been the mainstay of treatment for CD infection. However, 25% of patients suffer recurrence of CD infection within 60 days of antibiotic therapy [7, 8]. FMT has emerged as an effective alternative for the relapsed and refractory CD infection patients with reported success rates of 80-90% in clinical trials [9, 10]. Due to safety concerns related to introducing bacterial therapy in immunocompromised patients, those with immunocompromised states have been excluded from most trials, and guidelines currently recommend caution in these patient populations due to the absence of safety and efficacy data [11, 12].

The aim of our study is to conduct a systematic review of the existing literature to collate the evidence for efficacy and safety of FMT in immunocompromised population.

2. Methods

We searched PubMed, EMBASE, and Google Scholar for English language articles published on FMT for treatment of CD infection from inception through May 2017.

These databases were searched using the search terms under 2 broad search themes of "*Clostridium difficile*" and "fecal microbiota transplantation" and were combined using a Boolean operator AND (see supplementary file 1). For the term "*Clostridium difficile*", we used a combination of MeSH entry term words *Clostridium difficile* and *C. difficile*. For the MeSH term "fecal microbiota transplantation", we used synonyms for fecal microbiota transplantation, intestinal microbiota transfer, donor feces infusion, and stool transplant. We made the decision not to include the term "immunocompromised" due to concerns that our search would not capture the patients broadly enough. We instead reviewed all individual articles for descriptions of treated patients who matched our definition of immunocompromised.

We defined a patient as immunocompromised if that patient was receiving immunosuppressive agents (including but not limited to mTOR inhibitors, calcineurin inhibitors, anti-TNF agents, other biologic agents, high dose steroids > 20 mg/day or ≥ 1 mg/kg for > 14 days), patients with human immunodeficiency virus (HIV) infection (regardless of CD4 count), acquired immune deficiency syndrome (AIDS), inherited or primary immunodeficiency syndromes, hematologic malignancy or solid tumor (active with treatment in past 3 months or in remission for less than 5 years), solid organ transplant, and/or bone marrow transplant. We excluded inflammatory bowel disease (IBD) patients that were not receiving immunosuppressant medications. We also excluded patient with chronic medical conditions such as chronic liver disease, chronic kidney disease, and autoimmune conditions not on immunosuppressant. We included patients of all age groups.

Our outcomes of interest were clinical resolution of diarrhea, bacteriologic resolution, treatment failure, adverse events, and mortality. Clinical or bacteriologic resolution was defined as absence of diarrhea or need for further CDI treatment after FMT within the study or follow-up period clinically or with C. difficile toxin testing, respectively. Treatment failure was defined as nonresponse or recurrence of diarrhea with or without positive C. difficile toxin. We defined post-FMT death as any death within 30 days of FMT.

We reviewed all study types with original data published in English language. The reference lists of included articles and chosen articles were manually hand-searched for additional articles. Our eligibility criteria for inclusion were as follows: (1) studies of any type on human subjects with a full published manuscript who met at least one of our definitions for immunocompromised, (2) received fecal transplant via any method for a laboratory-confirmed, symptomatic CD infection, and (3) any of the outcomes of interest was reported in the manuscript. We included patients who received FMT in inpatient, outpatient, or home setting. We excluded studies that evaluated FMT for non-CD illness. We excluded conference abstracts to avoid duplication of our study population with a subsequent full publication. We excluded studies that did not report on any of our outcomes or had mixed population of immunocompromised and immunocompetent patients that did not report outcomes of immunocompromised population separately.

Three reviewers (YF, SV, and OS) independently screened titles and abstracts and excluded irrelevant studies. Full manuscript review was conducted by three investigators (YF, SV, and OS) to determine inclusion eligibility. Disagreement on inclusion was adjudicated by a third investigator (AD). Data extraction was performed by 3 investigators (GS, AJ, and SV) and reviewed for accuracy by a third investigator (OS).

We extracted data on patient's characteristics including age, gender, number of CD infections prior to FMT, interventions prior to FMT, time from index CD infection diagnosis to FMT, method of diagnosis of index CD infection, and reasons for immune compromise. We collected study characteristics including study type, location, clinical setting, and duration of study including length of follow-up period. We also extracted FMT treatment data, including delivery method (upper GI infusion, capsule ingestion, colonoscopic infusion, or enema), number of treatments, whether fresh or frozen stool was administered, treatment dose infused, stool donor relationship (related or unrelated), pretransplant bowel preparation, and pretransplant use of antibiotics. Outcome data collected included resolution of clinical symptoms, treatment failure after single FMT, all-cause mortality within 30 days, number of relapses, and need for additional FMT prior to resolution. We also categorized adverse events including colectomy, CD/FMT-related deaths, new hospitalizations, life-threatening events, need for surgery, infection complications, IBD flares, and time from infection to adverse event. A CD/FMT-related adverse event was defined as any complication or new event occurring within 30 days of first FMT. Duplicate patient entries were identified and removed. Authors were contacted for clarification on data where necessary.

We assessed study quality using questions from the NIH quality assessment tool for case series studies. We conducted quality assessment only on studies with at least five patients in original study population (Supplementary file 2) [57].

We did pooled studies and calculated resolution and adverse event rates with 95% confidence interval using STATA version 13 (College Station, TX). We set statistical significance at $p \leq 0.05$. Some studies reported adverse events but had missing data for efficacy. Given the importance of adverse event outcomes in immunocompromised patients, we conducted separate efficacy and safety analyses.

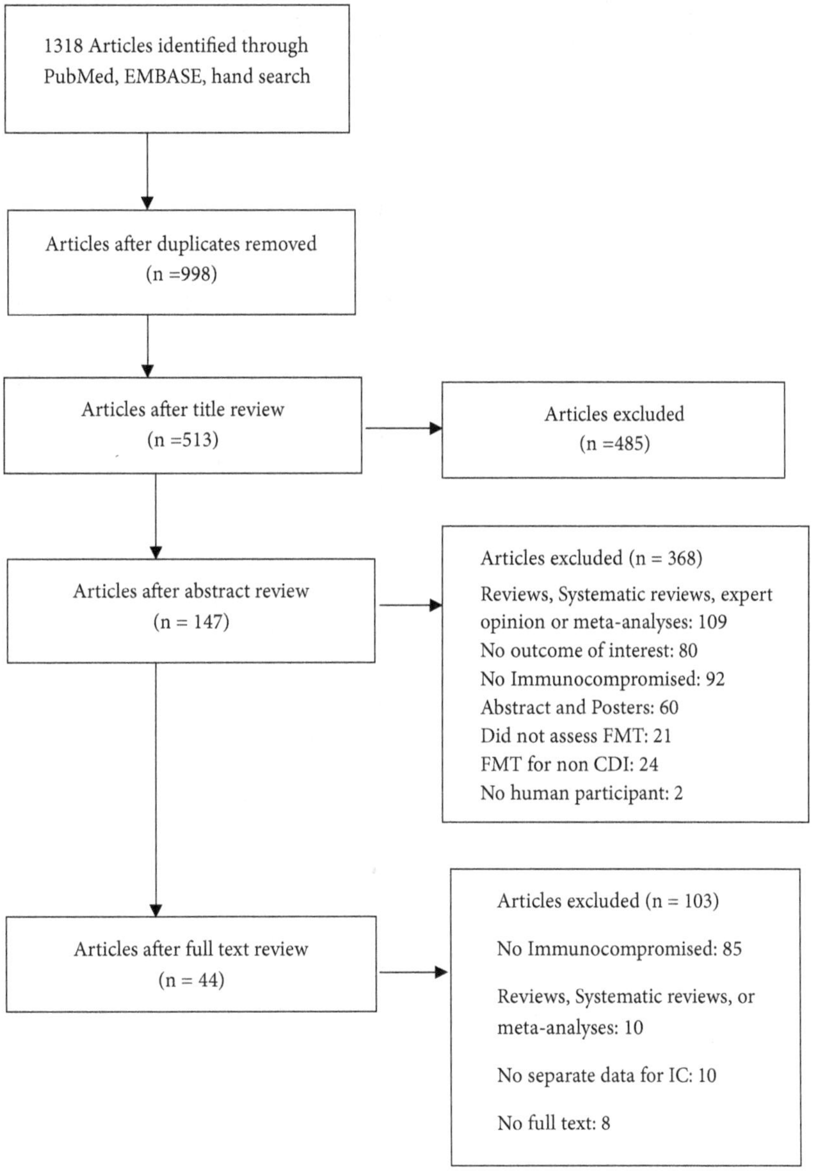

FIGURE 1: Flowchart for study selection.

There were no randomized controlled trials and study heterogeneity between the nonrandomized trials precluded performing a meta-analysis on our included studies.

3. Results

We identified 44 studies which met inclusion criteria describing 303 patients (Figure 1) [13–56]. Forty-three were single cases or case series and one was a retrospective cohort study, and no randomized designs were identified (Table 1). Of those studies reporting gender, 62% were females and 38% were males. The mean age was 57.3 years (range: 2-88 years). The most common reason for the immunocompromised state was use of immunosuppressant medication (77.2%). Other reasons for being immunocompromised included solid organ transplant (18.2%), active malignancy including lymphoma or leukemia (16.2%), hematopoietic stem cell transplant (2.5%), and HIV/AIDS (2.1%). There was more than one immunocompromising condition in 19.9% of patients.

Patient averaged about 2.5 episodes of CD prior to first FMT. Most patients (73.7%) had received other treatments for CD infection, mainly antibiotics, before FMT, with many (48.6%) receiving 2 or more CD infection treatments prior to FMT. Treatments other than antibiotics prior to FMT included probiotics, intravenous immunoglobulin, and surgery. For patients that received antibiotics prior to FMT, antibiotics were stopped on average about 1.5 days (range: 0-3, SD: 0.55 days) prior to FMT procedure.

Colonoscopy was the route of delivery of FMT in 76% of patients, while 21% had stool transplanted via ingestion of capsules or other upper gastrointestinal route (nasal tubes or endoscopy). Retention enema was performed in 7.6 % of patients. Most patients (95%) received fresh stool, while

Table 1: Summary of included articles.

Author, Year	Article type	N patients included	Immunocompromised	FMT delivery	N transplant	Stool (g or volume (mL per transplant	Donor relationship	AE
Aas, 2003 [13]	Case series	1	Leukemia	NG Tube	1	30 g/25 ml	NR	No
Aratari, 2015 [14]	Case report	1	IBD on IS	Colonoscopy	1	150 g	UR	No
Bilal, 2015 [15]	Case report	1	Liver and kidney transplant on tacrolimus	Colonoscopy	1	180 ml	R	No
Blackburn, 2015 [16]	Case report	1	Leukemia	Colonoscopy	1	NR	NR	No
de Castro, 2015 [17]	Case Report	1	ALL s/p HSCT	Upper Endoscopy	1	NR	NR	No
Duplessis, 2012 [18]	Case report	1	CD on IS	UG Upper Endoscopy	1	75 g/200 ml	R	No
Ehlermann, 2014 [19]	Case report	1	Heart transplant	Upper Endoscopy	1	100 ml	R	No
Elopre, 2013 [20]	Case series	2	AIDS, DM + AIDS	Upper Endoscopy	1	30 g/25 ml	R	No
Fischer, 2016 [21]	Cohort	101	Multiple defined	Colonoscopy	1	NR	NR	NR
Friedman-Moraco, 2014 [22]	Case series	2	SOT	Upper Endoscopy and Colonoscopy	2	30 g/80-325 ml	R	Yes
Garborg, 2010 [23]	Case series	1	AML	Upper Endoscopy	1	50-100 g/200 ml	R	No
Gathe, 2016 [24]	Case report	1	HIV	Colonoscopy, Enema and Nasogastric tube	4	NR	R	No
Guiterrez-Delgado, 2016 [25]	Case series	1	Acute leukemia	Colonoscopy	2	NR	UR	No
Gweon, 2015 [26]	Case report	1	Thyroid cancer	Colonoscopy and Upper Endoscopy	1	75 g	UR	No
Hirsch, 2015 [27]	Case series	5	Lymphoma, AML, Renal cell CA, IS	Oral (ingested	1-4	2.3 g (6-22 capsules)	UR	Yes
Hourigan, 2015 [28]	Case series	3	IBD on IS	Colonoscopy	1	92 g	R	No
Kelly, 2014 [29]	Case series	46*	IS, SOT, Severe/end stage chronic disease, Cancer, HIV	Colonoscopy#	1-2	NR	NR	Yes
Khoruts, 2016 [30]	Case series	38	SOT, IS	Colonoscopy	1	NR	NR	NR
Kronman, 2014 [31]	Case series	3	IBD on IS	NG Tube	1	30-60 ml	R	No
Laszlo, 2016 [32]	Case series	1	UC on IS	Colonoscopy	1	150 ml	R	Yes
Lee, 2014 [33]	Case report	1	Liver transplant	Upper Endoscopy	2	NR	R	Yes
Lee CH, 2014 [34]	Case series	3	Renal transplant	Enema	1-4	100 ml	UR	No
Loke, 2016 [35]	Case report	1	Specific Antibody Deficiency (SAD	Colonoscopy	1	50 g/500 ml	R	NR

Table 1: Continued.

Author, Year	Article type	N patients included	Immunocompromised	FMT delivery	N transplant	Stool (g or volume (mL per transplant	Donor relationship	AE
Mandalia, 2016 [36]	Case series	37	HIV, AIDS, malignancy, IS	NR	1-3	NR	NR	Yes
Mattila, 2012 [37]	Case series	3	Lung transplant	Colonoscopy	1-2	100 ml	R and UR	No
Mittal, 2015 [38]	Case report	1	Diffuse large B cell non-Hodgkin's lymphoma +UC	Enema	2	NR	NR	Yes
Neemann, 2015 [39]	Case report	1	ALL s/p HSCT	Upper Endoscopy	1	30 ml	R	NR
Ott, 2017 [40]	Case series	3	Kidney transplant, HIV, Colon Cancer	Upper Endoscopy	1	NR	R and UR	No
Pathak, 2014 [41]	Case series	3	Adenocarcinoma left colon, Renal transplant, Cancer	Colonoscopy	1	6-8 teaspoons, 40-500ml	R	No
Pierog, 2014 [42]	Case series	2	IBD on IS	Colonoscopy	1	60 ml	R	Yes
Porter, 2014 [43]	Case report	1	B cell CLL	Upper Endoscopy	6	50 g	UR	NR
Quera, 2013 [44]	Case report	1	CD on IS	Colonoscopy	1	NR	NR	Yes
Ramay, 2015 [45]	Case report	1	Heart transplant	Colonoscopy	2	250 ml	UR	No
Ray, 2014 [46]	Case series	2	Multiple	Colonoscopy	1	60 ml	R	No
Rubin, 2012 [47]	Case series	15	Malignant disease	Upper Endoscopy	1	30 g/25 ml	R	No
Russell, 2014 [48]	Case series	1	UC on IS	Colonoscopy	1	30-40 g/250 ml	R	Yes
Schunemann, 2013 [49]	Case report	1	AIDS	Colonoscopy and Upper Endoscopy	2	NR	R	No
Silverman, 2010 [50]	Case series	3	Lymphoma, liver transplant	Enema	1	50 ml	R	Yes
Stripling, 2015 [51]	Case report	1	Cardiac, kidney transplant on IS	Upper Endoscopy	1	NR	R	No
Trubiano, 2014 [52]	Case report	1	Diffuse large B cell lymphoma	Upper Endoscopy	2	260 ml	R	No
Webb, 2016 [53]	Case series	5	HSCT	NJ tube	1	25-100 g	NR	Yes
Weingarden, 2013 [54]	Case series	1	Metastatic Ovarian cancer	Colonoscopy	1	NR	UR	Yes
Yoon, 2010 [55]	Case series	2	Colon cancer, Breast cancer	Colonoscopy	1	NR	R	No
Zainah, 2012 [56]	Case report	1	UC on IS	Colonoscopy	1	300 ml	R	No

AE= adverse events; ALL= acute lymphocytic leukemia; AML= acute myeloid leukemia; CA= cancer; CD=Crohn's disease; CLL= chronic lymphocytic leukemia; E= enema; HIV= human immunodeficiency virus: IBD= inflammatory bowel disease: IS= immunosuppressant; HSCT= hematopoietic stem cell transplant; LTE= letter to editor; NG= nasogastric tube; NR= not reported or no separate patient level data on immunocompromised patients; R= related (genetically or household; SOT= solid organ transplant; UC= ulcerative colitis; UG= upper gastrointestinal endoscopy; and UR= unrelated

*= more IC patients but only including those with separate data that we could match to IC status, outcome, and AE

#= article reports where most centers used colonoscopy; possibly some included patients had other route of delivery.

5% utilized commercially prepared products. Among those reporting source of stool, a related donor was employed in 75% of patients.

A total of 234 patients had data on outcome and were included in the efficacy analysis. Of these, 206 (87.7%) had clinical resolution of CD infection after first FMT treatment, while 93% had resolution after 2 or more FMT attempts. Comparing rate of resolution by delivery method, colonoscopy delivered FMT had an 84% success rate, while upper gastrointestinal delivery (via endoscopy, capsule, and nasogastric or nasojejunal tubes) resulted in 92% success rate ($p = 0.202$). In terms of number of immunocompromising conditions, patients with one condition had a success rate of 93%, while those with two or more immunocompromising conditions were resolved 78% of the time (Odds ratio (OR) 0.24, 95% CI: 0.11- 0.51, $p<0.0001$).

All 303 patients were included in the safety analysis. There were 2 reported deaths. Both deaths were in patients with solid organ transplants. One patient died 13 days after successful FMT, with death due to progressive pneumonia, while the second patient died 1 day after FMT following aspiration pneumonitis during sedation for colonoscopy. Other reported adverse events include 2 colectomies, 5 episodes of bacteremia or infection, 10 subsequent hospitalizations, 7 otherwise unspecified life-threatening complications, and 7 flares of inflammatory bowel disease. Twenty-eight patients had other complications including abdominal pain, irritable bowel syndrome, nausea, fever, and diverticulitis post-FMT procedure. Mean time to adverse event was 26.6 days (range: 0-56, SD: 34.3 days) from FMT (Table 2).

Twenty of the included 43 case reports/studies had at least 5 patients in the original study population. Only 10 studies showed adequate reporting in all of six essential domains of study quality (study objective, case definition, outcome measure definition, FMT procedure, adequacy of follow-up, and donor characteristics), with others missing 1 to 3 of these elements (Supplementary file 2).

4. Discussion

Our review identified an 88% success rate after a single FMT and 93% after multiple FMTs in our immunocompromised population, which parallels the 80-90% success rates reported in the general population [9, 10]. Patients with a single immunocompromising factor had a higher rate of treatment success when compared to patients with multiple immunocompromising factors ($p<0.001$). In comparison, a retrospective series by Kelly et al. looking at 80 immunocompromised patients with CD infection treated with FMT reported a 78% cure rate following a single FMT and 89% cure rate with multiple FMT [28]. Of these 80 patients, 38 met our inclusion criteria and were included in our analyses. A recent systematic review and meta-analysis by Ianiro et al. found a similar cure rate of 93% after multiple FMT with a 76% cure rate after a single FMT [58]. While Ianiro et al. excluded case reports and case series with less than 10 patients who received FMT for CDI with a minimum of 8 weeks follow-up, our study focused on only immunocompromised patients regardless of the study size given our already limited study population.

Safety concerns were the rationale for excluding immunocompromised patients from clinical trials and expression of caution in guidelines for FMT. We identified just 2 deaths among out 303 patients with 30 days of FMT. Both deaths were reported in a retrospective review by Kelly et al. but we could not directly ascertain whether those deaths were directly related to FMT, to the CD infection or the patient's underlying immunocompromised states. Other deaths in our included studies were either not related to FMT (post-colectomy complications) or occurred beyond 30 days after FMT [23, 37]. Of those reporting rehospitalization following FMT, 8.3% reported this. While fecal transplant has been associated with reactivation of existing immune-mediated disorders or new disorders such as immune thrombocytopenia, rheumatoid arthritis in immunocompetent patients following treatment, this side effect was not identified in our study [59]. It is possible that the underlying immunosuppressed states of our study population may have suppressed any adverse immunologic responses observed in immunocompetent patients.

Our study has the following strengths. It addresses a very specific population with CD infection that has a higher incidence of CD infection with higher risk of recurrence and would ideally benefit from FMT. In addition, we included only patients who met a standard, predetermined definition of immunosuppression. However, our study has some limitations. We reviewed case reports and series, as there were no RCTs that were identified for inclusion. Inclusion of case reports with possibility of publication bias towards positive results might account for the high success rate after a single FMT. Missing data on demographics, method of stool transplantation, volume and amount of stool, and relationships of donor and recipients were common in our review and were also noted in a similar review by Bafeta et al. [60]. One clinical trial had immunocompromised patients that met inclusion criteria but had a mixed population of patients that included immunocompetent patients and did not provide separate data on the included immunocompromised population and therefore could not be included in our study [61]. Our efforts at contacting authors to provide data on immunocompromised patients were unsuccessful. In the absence of clinical trials, overall studies were too heterogeneous precluding a meta-analysis.

5. Conclusion

In conclusion, FMT in immunocompromised appears to have comparable efficacy and safety data to those on patients with intact immunity. However, due to heterogeneity of immunosuppression subtype, no solid conclusion can be made about any single specific immunocompromised states or a combination regarding response to FMT. Further randomized trials including these patient populations would be appropriate.

Disclosure

An abstract of the manuscript was presented at the American College of Gastroenterology (ACG) Annual Scientific Meeting in October 2016 as a poster presentation.

TABLE 2: Adverse events (AE) in immunocompromised patients with recurrent CD infection treated with FMT.

Author, Year	Patients with events (N)	Type of AE
Friedman-Moraco, 2014 [22]	1	Life threatening event: ischemic stroke
Hirsch, 2015 [27]	1	New Hospitalization
	1	Life threatening event
	1	Abdominal pain
Kelly, 2014 [29]	1	Colectomy
	1	Death
	1	Death
	5	New Hospitalization
	1	Life threatening event
	3	Infection: pneumonia, Influenza, Pertussis
	4	IBD flare
	11	Others:
		Hip pain
		Nausea
		Bloating
		Fever
		Diarrhea
		Abdominal pain
		Catheter infection
		Self-limited diarrhea
		Minor mucosal tear during colonoscopy
Laszlo, 2016 [32]	1	Others: Mild abdominal pain
Lee, 2014 [34]	1	New Hospitalization/Life threatening event
Mandalia, 2016 [36]	3	IBD flare
	1	Diverticulitis
Mittal, 2015 [38]	1	New Hospitalization
Pierog, 2014 [42]	1	Life-threatening event/New Hospitalizations/Surgery
Quera, 2013 [44]	1	Life threatening event
		Infection: Pan-sensitive *E. coli*
Russell, 2014 [48]	1	Colectomy/New Hospitalization/Life threatening events/Surgery
Silverman, 2010 [50]	3	IBS
Webb, 2016 [53]	5	Abdominal pain
Weingarden, 2013 [54]	1	Colectomy

AE= adverse event; IBS= irritable bowel syndrome.

Authors' Contributions

Oluwaseun Shogbesan contributed to conceptualizing, search, data abstraction, and manuscript writing. Samjeris Victor contributed to search, data abstraction, and manuscript writing. Dilli Ram Poudel contributed to data analysis, conceptualizing, and manuscript writing. Opeyemi Fadahunsi contributed to search. Asad Jehangir contributed to data abstraction. Gbenga Shogbesan contributed to data abstraction and conceptualizing. Anthony Donato contributed to conceptualizing and manuscript writing

Acknowledgments

The authors would like to thank Alex Short for her contribution to the search strategy. An abstract of the manuscript was presented at the American College of Gastroenterology (ACG) Annual Scientific Meeting in October 2016 as a poster presentation.

References

[1] F. C. Lessa, L. G. Winston, and L. C. McDonald, "Emerging infections program C. difficile surveillance team. Burden of Clostridium difficile infection in the United States," *The New England Journal of Medicine*, vol. 372, pp. 2369-2370, 2015.

[2] E. M. Drozd, T. J. Inocencio, S. Braithwaite et al., "Mortality, hospital costs, payments, and readmissions associated with clostridium difficile infection among medicare beneficiaries," *Infectious Diseases in Clinical Practice*, vol. 23, no. 6, pp. 318–323, 2015.

[3] M. Kamboj, C. Son, S. Cantu et al., "Hospital-onset clostridium difficile infection rates in persons with cancer or Hematopoietic stem cell transplant: A C3IC network report," *Infection Control and Hospital Epidemiology*, vol. 33, no. 11, pp. 1162–1164, 2012.

[4] C. D. Alonso and M. Kamboj, "Clostridium difficile infection (CDI) in solid organ and hematopoietic stem cell transplant recipients," *Current Infectious Disease Reports*, vol. 16, p. 414, 2014.

[5] S. Raza, M. A. Baig, H. Russell, Y. Gourdet, and B. J. Berger, "*Clostridium difficile* infection following chemotherapy," *Recent Patents on Anti-Infective Drug Discovery*, vol. 5, no. 1, pp. 1–9, 2010.

[6] S. Schneeweiss, J. Korzenik, D. H. Solomon, C. Canning, J. Lee, and B. Bressler, "Infliximab and other immunomodulating drugs in patients with inflammatory bowel disease and the risk of serious bacterial infections," *Alimentary Pharmacology & Therapeutics*, vol. 30, no. 3, pp. 253–264, 2009.

[7] C. P. Kelly and J. T. LaMont, "Clostridium difficile—more difficult than ever," *The New England Journal of Medicine*, vol. 359, no. 18, pp. 1932–1940, 2008.

[8] L. V. McFarland, G. W. Elmer, and C. M. Surawicz, "Breaking the cycle: Treatment strategies for 163 cases of recurrent Clostridium difficile disease," *American Journal of Gastroenterology*, vol. 97, no. 7, pp. 1769–1775, 2002.

[9] E. van Nood, A. Vrieze, and M. Nieuwdorp, "Duodenal infusion of donor feces for recurrent clostridium difficile," *The New England Journal of Medicine*, vol. 368, no. 5, pp. 407–415, 2013.

[10] G. Cammarota, L. Masucci, G. Ianiro et al., " Randomised clinical trial: faecal microbiota transplantation by colonoscopy vs. vancomycin for the treatment of recurrent ," *Alimentary Pharmacology & Therapeutics*, vol. 41, no. 9, pp. 835–843, 2015.

[11] J. S. Bakken, T. Borody, L. J. Brandt et al., "Treating clostridium difficile infection with fecal microbiota transplantation," *Clinical Gastroenterology and Hepatology*, vol. 9, no. 12, pp. 1044–1049, 2011.

[12] H. Sokol, T. Galperine, N. Kapel et al., "Faecal microbiota transplantation in recurrent Clostridium difficile infection: Recommendations from the French Group of faecal microbiota transplantation," *Digestive and Liver Disease*, vol. 48, pp. 242–247, 2016.

[13] J. Aas, C. E. Gessert, and J. S. Bakken, "Recurrent Clostridium difficile colitis: Case series involving 18 patients treated with donor stool administered via a nasogastric tube," *Clinical Infectious Diseases*, vol. 36, no. 5, pp. 580–585, 2003.

[14] A. Aratari, G. Cammarota, and C. Papi, "Fecal microbiota transplantation for recurrent C. difficile infection in a patient with chronic refractory ulcerative colitis," *Journal of Crohn's and Colitis*, vol. 9, no. 4, p. 367, 2015.

[15] M. Bilal, R. Khehra, C. Strahotin, and R. Mitre, "Long-term follow-up of fecal microbiota transplantation for treatment of recurrent clostridium difficile infection in a dual solid organ transplant recipient," *Case Reports in Gastroenterology*, vol. 9, pp. 156–159, 2015.

[16] L. M. Blackburn, A. Bales, M. Caldwell, L. Cordell, S. Hamilton, and H. Kreider, "Fecal microbiota transplantation in patients with cancer undergoing treatment," *Clinical Journal of Oncology Nursing*, vol. 19, no. 1, pp. 111–114, 2015.

[17] C. G. de Castro, A. J. Ganc, R. L. Ganc, M. S. Petrolli, and N. Hamerschlack, "Fecal microbiota transplant after hematopoietic SCT: Report of a successful case," *Bone Marrow Transplantation*, vol. 50, no. 1, p. 145, 2015.

[18] C. A. Duplessis, D. You, M. Johnson, and A. Speziale, "Efficacious outcome employing fecal bacteriotherapy in severe Crohn's colitis complicated by refractory Clostridium difficile infection," *Infection*, vol. 40, no. 4, pp. 469–472, 2012.

[19] P. Ehlermann, A. O. Dösch, and H. A. Katus, "Donor fecal transfer for recurrent Clostridium difficile-associated diarrhea in heart transplantation," *The Journal of Heart and Lung Transplantation*, vol. 33, no. 5, pp. 551–553, 2014.

[20] L. Elopre and M. Rodriguez, "Fecal microbiota therapy for recurrent Clostridium difficile infection in HIV-infected persons," *Annals of Internal Medicine*, vol. 158, no. 10, pp. 779–780, 2013.

[21] M. Fischer, D. Kao, C. Kelly et al., "Fecal Microbiota Transplantation is Safe and Efficacious for Recurrent or Refractory Clostridium difficile Infection in Patients with Inflammatory Bowel Disease," *Inflammatory Bowel Diseases*, vol. 22, no. 10, pp. 2402–2409, 2016.

[22] R. J. Friedman-Moraco, A. K. Mehta, G. M. Lyon, and C. S. Kraft, "Fecal microbiota transplantation for refractory Clostridium difficile colitis in solid organ transplant recipients," *American Journal of Transplantation*, vol. 14, no. 2, pp. 477–480, 2014.

[23] K. Garborg, B. Waagsbø, A. Stallemo, J. Matre, and A. Sundøy, "Results of faecal donor instillation therapy for recurrent Clostridium difficile-associated diarrhoea," *Infectious Diseases*, vol. 42, no. 11-12, pp. 857–861, 2010.

[24] J. C. Gathe, E. M. Diejomaoh, C. C. Mayberry, and J. B. Clemmons, "Fecal Transplantation for Clostridium Difficile - "all Stool May Not Be Created Equal"," *Journal of the International Association of Providers of AIDS Care*, vol. 15, no. 2, pp. 107-108, 2016.

[25] E. M. Gutiérrez-Delgado, E. Garza-González, M. A. Martínez-Vázquez et al., "Fecal transplant for Clostridium difficile infection relapses using "pooled" frozen feces from non-related donors," *Acta Gastro-Enterologica Belgica*, vol. 79, no. 2, pp. 268–270, 2016.

[26] T.-G. Gweon, K. J. Lee, D. Kang et al., "A case of toxic megacolon caused by *Clostridium difficile* infection and treated with fecal microbiota transplantation," *Gut and Liver*, vol. 9, no. 2, pp. 247–250, 2015.

[27] B. E. Hirsch, N. Saraiya, K. Poeth, R. M. Schwartz, M. E. Epstein, and G. Honig, "Effectiveness of fecal-derived microbiota transfer using orally administered capsules for recurrent Clostridium difficile infection," *BMC Infectious Diseases*, vol. 15, p. 191, 2015.

[28] S. K. Hourigan, L. A. Chen, Z. Grigoryan et al., "Microbiome changes associated with sustained eradication of *Clostridium difficile* after single faecal microbiota transplantation in children with and without inflammatory bowel disease," *Alimentary Pharmacology & Therapeutics*, vol. 42, no. 6, pp. 741–752, 2015.

[29] C. R. Kelly, C. Ihunnah, M. Fischer et al., "Fecal microbiota transplant for treatment of *Clostridium difficile* infection in

immunocompromised patients," *American Journal of Gastroenterology*, vol. 109, no. 7, pp. 1065–1071, 2014.

[30] A. Khoruts, K. M. Rank, K. M. Newman et al., "Inflammatory Bowel Disease Affects the Outcome of Fecal Microbiota Transplantation for Recurrent Clostridium difficile Infection," *Clinical Gastroenterology and Hepatology*, vol. 14, no. 10, pp. 1433–1438, 2016.

[31] M. P. Kronman, H. J. Nielson, A. L. Adler et al., "Fecal microbiota transplantation via nasogastric tube for recurrent clostridium difficile infection in pediatric patients," *Journal of Pediatric Gastroenterology and Nutrition*, vol. 60, no. 1, pp. 23–26, 2015.

[32] M. Laszlo, L. Ciobanu, V. Andreica, and O. Pascu, "Fecal transplantation indications in ulcerative colitis. preliminary study," *Clujul Medical*, vol. 89, no. 2, pp. 224–228, 2016.

[33] C. H. Lee, J. E. Belanger, Z. Kassam et al., "The outcome and long-term follow-up of 94 patients with recurrent and refractory Clostridium difficile infection using single to multiple fecal microbiota transplantation via retention enema," *European Journal of Clinical Microbiology & Infectious Diseases*, vol. 33, no. 8, pp. 1425–1428, 2014.

[34] T. J. Lee and C. M. Jones, "A report of fecal transplantation for refractory clostridium difficile colitis in an orthotopic liver transplant recipient," *Journal of Gastroenterology and Hepatology Research*, vol. 3, no. 11, pp. 1357–1359, 2014.

[35] P. Loke, R. G. Heine, V. McWilliam, D. J. S. Cameron, M. L. K. Tang, and K. J. Allen, "Fecal microbial transplantation in a pediatric case of recurrent Clostridium difficile infection and specific antibody deficiency," *Pediatric Allergy and Immunology*, vol. 27, no. 8, pp. 872–874, 2016.

[36] A. Mandalia, A. Ward, W. Tauxe, C. S. Kraft, and T. Dhere, "Fecal transplant is as effective and safe in immunocompromised as non-immunocompromised patients for Clostridium difficile," *International Journal of Colorectal Disease*, vol. 31, no. 5, pp. 1059-1060, 2016.

[37] E. Mattila, R. Uusitalo-Seppälä, M. Wuorela et al., "Fecal transplantation, through colonoscopy, is effective therapy for recurrent *Clostridium difficile* infection," *Gastroenterology*, vol. 142, no. 3, pp. 490–496, 2012.

[38] C. Mittal, N. Miller, A. Meighani, B. R. Hart, A. John, and M. Ramesh, "Fecal microbiota transplant for recurrent Clostridium difficile infection after peripheral autologous stem cell transplant for diffuse large B-cell lymphoma," *Bone Marrow Transplantation*, vol. 50, no. 7, p. 1010, 2015.

[39] K. Neemann, D. D. Eichele, P. P. W. Smith, R. Bociek, M. Akhtari, and A. Freifeld, "Fecal microbiota transplantation for fulminant *Clostridium difficile* infection in an allogeneic stem cell transplant patient," *Transplant Infectious Disease*, vol. 14, no. 6, pp. E161–E165, 2012.

[40] S. J. Ott, G. H. Waetzig, A. Rehman et al., "Efficacy of Sterile Fecal Filtrate Transfer for Treating Patients With Clostridium difficile Infection," *Gastroenterology*, vol. 152, no. 4, pp. 799–811, 2017.

[41] R. Pathak, H. A. Enuh, A. Patel, and P. Wickremesinghe, "Treatment of relapsing clostridium difficile infection using fecal microbiota transplantation," *Clinical and Experimental Gastroenterology*, vol. 7, pp. 1–6, 2013.

[42] A. Pierog, A. Mencin, and N. R. Reilly, "Fecal microbiota transplantation in children with recurrent clostridium difficile infection," *The Pediatric Infectious Disease Journal*, vol. 33, no. 11, pp. 1198–1200, 2014.

[43] R. J. Porter, "Pulsed faecal microbiota transplantation for recalcitrant recurrent Clostridium difficile infection," *Clinical Microbiology and Infection*, vol. 21, no. 3, pp. e23–e24, 2015.

[44] R. Quera, R. Espinoza, C. Estay, and D. Rivera, "Bacteremia as an adverse event of fecal microbiota transplantation in a patient with Crohn's disease and recurrent Clostridium difficile infection," *Journal of Crohn's and Colitis*, vol. 8, no. 3, pp. 252-253, 2014.

[45] F. H. Ramay, A. Amoroso, E. C. Von Rosenvinge, and K. Saharia, "Fecal microbiota transplantation for treatment of severe, recurrent, and refractory clostridium difficile infection in a severely immunocompromised patient," *Infectious Diseases in Clinical Practice*, vol. 24, no. 4, pp. 237–240, 2016.

[46] A. Ray, R. Smith, and J. Breaux, "Fecal microbiota transplantation for clostridium difficile infection: The ochsner experience," *The Ochsner Journal*, vol. 14, no. 4, pp. 538–544, 2014.

[47] T. A. Rubin, C. E. Gessert, J. Aas, and J. S. Bakken, "Fecal microbiome transplantation for recurrent Clostridium difficile infection: Report on a case series," *Anaerobe*, vol. 19, no. 1, pp. 22–26, 2013.

[48] G. H. Russell, J. L. Kaplan, I. Youngster et al., "Fecal transplant for recurrent clostridium difficile infection in children with and without inflammatory bowel disease," *Journal of Pediatric Gastroenterology and Nutrition*, vol. 58, no. 5, pp. 588–592, 2014.

[49] M. Schünemann and M. Oette, "Fecal microbiota transplantation for Clostridium difficile-associated colitis in a severely immunocompromized critically ill AIDS patient: A case report," *AIDS*, vol. 28, no. 5, pp. 798-799, 2014.

[50] M. S. Silverman, I. Davis, and D. R. Pillai, "Success of Self-Administered Home Fecal Transplantation for Chronic Clostridium difficile Infection," *Clinical Gastroenterology and Hepatology*, vol. 8, no. 5, pp. 471–473, 2010.

[51] J. Stripling, R. Kumar, J. W. Baddley et al., "Loss of vancomycin-resistant enterococcus fecal dominance in an organ transplant patient with clostridium difficile colitis after fecal microbiota transplant," *Open Forum Infectious Diseases*, vol. 2, no. 2, 2015.

[52] J. A. Trubiano, A. George, J. Barnett et al., "A different kind of "allogeneic transplant": Successful fecal microbiota transplant for recurrent and refractory Clostridium difficile infection in a patient with relapsed aggressive B-cell lymphoma," *Leukemia & Lymphoma*, vol. 56, no. 2, pp. 512–514, 2015.

[53] B. J. Webb, A. Brunner, C. D. Ford, M. A. Gazdik, F. B. Petersen, and D. Hoda, "Fecal microbiota transplantation for recurrent Clostridium difficile infection in hematopoietic stem cell transplant recipients," *Transplant Infectious Disease*, vol. 18, no. 4, pp. 628–633, 2016.

[54] A. R. Weingarden, M. J. Hamilton, M. J. Sadowsky, and A. Khoruts, "Resolution of severe clostridium difficile infection following sequential fecal microbiota transplantation," *Journal of Clinical Gastroenterology*, vol. 47, no. 8, pp. 735–737, 2013.

[55] S. S. Yoon and L. J. Brandt, "Treatment of refractory/recurrent C. difficile-associated disease by donated stool transplanted via colonoscopy: A case series of 12 patients," *Journal of Clinical Gastroenterology*, vol. 44, no. 8, pp. 562–566, 2010.

[56] H. Zainah and A. Silverman, "Fecal bacteriotherapy: A case report in an immunosuppressed patient with ulcerative colitis and recurrent," *Case Reports in Infectious Diseases*, vol. 2012, Article ID 810943, 2 pages, 2012.

[57] "Study Quality Assessment tools," in *Quality Assessment Tool for Case series Studies*, National Heart, Lung, and Blood institute, https://www.nhlbi.nih.gov/health-topics/study-quality-assessment-tools.

[58] G. Ianiro, M. Maida, J. Burisch et al., "Efficiacy of different faecal microbiota transplantation protocols for *Clostridium difficile* infection: A systematic review and meta-analysis," *United European Gastroenterology Journal*, pp. 1–13, 2018.

[59] L. J. Brandt, O. C. Aroniadis, M. Mellow et al., "Long-term follow-up of colonoscopic fecal microbiota transplant for recurrent *Clostridium difficile* infection," *American Journal of Gastroenterology*, vol. 107, no. 7, pp. 1079–1087, 2012.

[60] A. Bafeta, A. Yavchitz, C. Riveros, R. Batista, and P. Ravaud, "Methods and reporting studies assessing fecal microbiota transplantation: A systematic review," *Annals of Internal Medicine*, vol. 167, no. 1, pp. 34–39, 2017.

[61] C. H. Lee, T. Steiner, E. O. Petrof et al., "Frozen vs fresh fecal microbiota transplantation and clinical resolution of diarrhea in patients with recurrent clostridium difficile infection a randomized clinical trial," *Journal of the American Medical Association*, vol. 315, no. 2, pp. 142–149, 2016.

11

Choice of Allograft in Patients Requiring Intestinal Transplantation

Genevieve Huard,[1,2,3] Thomas Schiano,[1,2] Jang Moon,[1] and Kishore Iyer[1]

[1] *Intestinal Rehabilitation and Transplantation Program, Recanati/Miller Transplantation Institute, Mount Sinai Medical Center, New York, NY, USA*
[2] *Division of Liver Diseases, Mount Sinai Medical Center, New York, NY, USA*
[3] *Division of Liver Diseases, Centre Hospitalier de l'Université de Montréal, Montréal, QC, Canada*

Correspondence should be addressed to Genevieve Huard; genevieve.huard@umontreal.ca

Academic Editor: Michael Beyak

Intestinal transplantation (ITx) is indicated in patients with irreversible intestinal failure (IF) and life-threatening complications related to total parenteral nutrition (TPN). ITx can be classified into three main types. Isolated intestinal transplantation (IITx), that is, transplantation of the jejunoileum, is indicated in patients with preserved liver function. Combined liver-intestine transplantation (L-ITx), that is, transplantation of the liver and the jejunoileum, is indicated in patients with liver failure related to TPN. Thus, patients with cirrhosis or advanced fibrosis should receive a combined allograft, while patients with lower grades of liver fibrosis can usually safely undergo ITx. Reflecting their degree of sickness, the waitlist mortality rate and the early posttransplant outcomes of patients receiving L-ITx are worse than IITx. However, L-ITx is associated with better long-term graft and patient survival. Multivisceral transplantation (MVTx), that is, transplantation of the organs dependent on the celiac axis and superior mesenteric artery, can be classified into full MVTx if it includes the liver and modified MVTx if it does not. The most common indications for MVTx are extensive portomesenteric thrombosis and diffuse gastrointestinal pathology such as motility disorders and polyposis syndrome. Every patient with IF should undergo a multidisciplinary evaluation by an experienced ITx team.

1. Introduction

Intestinal failure (IF) is defined as a critical reduction of the functional gut mass leading to the inability to maintain fluid, electrolyte, and protein-energy balance such that intravenous supplementation becomes necessary [1–3]. The development of successful intestinal and multivisceral transplantation is one of the most recent milestones in the field of intestinal rehabilitation and solid organ transplantation [4]. Currently, intestinal transplantation (ITx) is offered to patients with irreversible IF and total parenteral nutrition (TPN) failure in which survival on TPN is compromised [2, 5, 6]. TPN-related complications recognized as indications for ITx by the Center for Medicare and Medicaid Services are the following: impending or overt liver failure related to TPN (parenteral nutrition associated liver disease (PNALD)), impending loss of vascular access for TPN administration, multiple episodes of catheter-related sepsis, a single episode of life-threatening catheter-related sepsis, or frequent episodes of significant dehydration despite supplemental fluid administration (Table 1) [2, 7–9].

In the past decade, the outcomes of ITx have greatly improved. As shown in the most recent report from the Intestinal Transplant Registry (ITR) (worldwide data), the current 1-, 5-, and 10-year patient survival rates after ITx are 77%, 58%, and 47%, respectively [10, 11]. Moreover, the current 1-, 5-, and 10-year graft survival rates are 71%, 50%, and 41%, respectively [10, 11].

The jejunoileum is the defining component of any ITx. Depending on the inclusion of other organs along with the jejunoileum, ITx can be classified into three main categories: isolated intestinal transplantation (IITx) with or without colon, combined liver-intestine transplantation (L-ITx), and multivisceral transplantation (MVTx) [12] (Figure 1). While

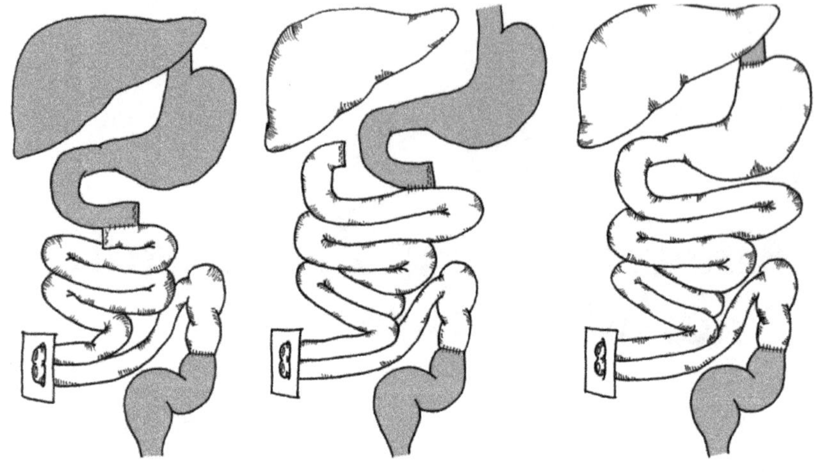

FIGURE 1: Types of allograft in intestinal transplantation. (a) Isolated intestine transplantation (IITx), (b) combined liver-intestine transplantation (L-ITx), and (c) multivisceral transplantation (MVTx). *Note.* Organs in grey represent native organs and dashed organs represent transplanted organs.

controversy persists regarding nomenclature, MVTx may be defined as the replacement of organs depending on the celiac trunk and superior mesenteric artery (SMA), that is, the stomach, liver, pancreas, duodenum, jejunum, and ileum [12]. MVTx can be "full" if it includes the liver or "modified" (MMVTx) if it does not include the liver [12]. According to the most recent report from the ITR, from 2001 to 2011, 46.6% of ITx were IITx, 26.6% were combined L-ITx, 21.3% were MVTx, and 5.5% were MMVTx [10, 11]. More recently, the proportion of ITx including the liver as part of the allograft is greatly decreased. Forty-eight percent of the allografts included the liver between 2001 and 2011 as compared to 61.8% and 53.2% between 1985–1995 and 1995–2001, respectively [10, 11].

The choice of intestinal allograft depends on many factors including the underlying pathology leading to irreversible IF, the absence or presence of simultaneous organ dysfunction (e.g., chronic renal failure, diabetes, and liver failure), age and size of the patient (there are donor-recipient match size issues in smaller patients), anatomy of the recipient, organ availability in the different organ procurement organizations, and transplant center expertise or preferences [12]. Currently, there is no published consensus regarding the choice of allograft in patients requiring ITx. Herein, we critically review the current literature regarding the complex decision-making process deciding on the type of allograft needed in patients requiring ITx.

2. Intestinal Failure and Intestinal Rehabilitation

Soon after an extensive intestinal resection, several physiological adaptation mechanisms such as increased villous height and crypt depth as well as intestinal dilatation are initiated and continue over the first two years in order to restore nutritional autonomy [1, 13, 14]. Usually, these adaptation mechanisms are sufficient to enhance the absorptive surface area of the residual small bowel (SB) and intravenous nutritional support is therefore temporary in the majority of the cases [1]. In cases in which these adaptive mechanisms are insufficient, nutritional dependency becomes irreversible and long-term TPN is the standard therapy [15, 16]. In such circumstances, intestinal rehabilitation should be attempted in order to safely reduce the need for TPN and therefore avoid the complications related to long-term TPN. Intestinal transplantation should only be considered after failure of dedicated attempts at intestinal rehabilitation and after the development of life-threatening complications related to TPN [2, 5, 7].

Given the complexity of the management of patients with IF, such patients should be referred to and followed by a multidisciplinary program with expertise in IF and intestinal rehabilitation [17]. Early referral to such a program is associated with better outcomes, reduced morbidity, and reduced mortality in patients with IF [7, 18].

TABLE 1: TPN-related complications warranting intestinal transplantation (Medicare and Medicare Services).

Impending or overt liver failure related to PNALD
≥2 episodes per year of catheter-related sepsis requiring hospitalization
≥1 episode of life-threatening infection (fungemia, septic shock, ARDS)
Impending loss of vascular access for TPN administration (thrombosis of ≥2 central veins)
Repeated episodes of significant dehydration despite IV fluids administration in supplement to TPN

Note. PNALD: parenteral nutrition associated liver disease; ARDS: adult respiratory distress syndrome; TPN: total parenteral nutrition.

The first step of intestinal rehabilitation is usually proper dietary management and adjunctive medications [20, 21]. In general, such patients benefit from hyperphagia to compensate for their malabsorptive state. Moreover, they should be encouraged to have small and frequent meals to improve absorption [15]. Patients with colon in continuity with SB usually benefit from a diet rich in complex carbohydrates and low in fat [15, 22]. Finally, these patients should be encouraged to limit their fluid intakes and to consume isoosmotic fluids such as the oral rehydration solution in order to optimize water and sodium absorption [15, 21, 23].

In addition to dietary modifications, several medications are recommended in patients with IF in order to avoid dehydration associated with high stoma outputs. Proton pump inhibitors are usually recommended in the first few months following an extensive intestinal resection in order to compensate for the hypergastrinemia state and the consequent gastric acid hypersecretion [24, 25]. The use of antidiarrhoeal medications such as loperamide is standard in patients with IF in order to increase intestinal transit time and therefore improve absorption and reduce stoma output [15]. When clinically appropriate, enterocyte growth factors should be considered to promote the physiological adaptation mechanisms [14]. Recently, recombinant human glucagon-like peptide- (GLP-) 2 analog (teduglutide) has been shown to reduce the volume and the number of days of TPN support [26–28]. The underlying mechanism of action of teduglutide probably involves mucosal growth by promoting intestinal crypt cell proliferation and inhibiting apoptosis [29]. Moreover, GLP-2 analogs have been shown to increase intestinal transit time and decrease gastric emptying and gastric acid secretion [30].

Finally, several surgical techniques are now available for patients with irreversible IF. Whenever possible, the continuity between the SB and the colon should be restored in order to improve fluid and energy balance [15]. When clinically appropriate, surgical lengthening procedures (i.e., STEP procedure nad Bianchi procedure) should be considered before referral for intestinal transplantation [31, 32].

Given all these recent improvements in the management of patients with IF, intestinal transplantation should therefore only be considered in the minority of patients who failed dedicated attempts at intestinal rehabilitation.

3. Isolated Intestine Transplantation

IITx is indicated for patients with irreversible IF and preserved liver function [12, 33]. Currently, the most common indications for IITx in patients with irreversible IF are impending vascular access loss for TPN administration and repeated or life-threatening line sepsis [2]. IITx should only be considered in patients who failed dedicated attempts at intestinal rehabilitation.

The venous drainage of the allograft may be achieved through orthotopic portal drainage but is more usually achieved systemically through direct anastomosis to the inferior vena cava (IVC). The initial attempts to drain isolated intestinal allografts systemically came in patients receiving IITx in the presence of moderate degrees of liver fibrosis, where systemic venous drainage was considered safer by avoiding venous anastomosis against higher vascular resistance. In the published Miami and Pittsburgh experiences, systemic compared to portal drainage was not associated with increased risk of patient or graft loss [34, 35]. However, in the Miami series, systemic drainage was associated with an increased risk of Gram-negative bacteremia and pneumonia, possibly reflecting the important role of the liver in the clearance of translocated intestinal bacteria [34]. Interestingly, systemic drainage was not associated with increased risk of hepatic encephalopathy [34], although at our center we have had 3 (unreported) cases of episodic hyperammonemia and concomitant mental status changes in patients whose isolated intestinal allografts were drained systemically. The Pittsburgh experience also revealed that systemic drainage was not associated with an increased risk of rejection [35]. Thus, the technically easier systemic venous drainage does not appear to be associated with significant adverse outcomes [34, 35].

In patients suffering concomitantly from pancreatic insufficiency, such as in patients with type 1 diabetes or cystic fibrosis, the pancreas can also be included in the allograft, either as a composite graft or simultaneous implantation of the intestine and pancreas from the same donor [12]. The indications for combined intestinal and kidney transplant are not as well defined in the current literature. Clearly, patients on long-term hemodialysis at the time of evaluation for IITx should be evaluated for concurrent kidney transplant [36]. Also, given that the incidence of chronic renal failure is greater than 20% five years after ITx, patients with abnormal renal function going into transplant should be evaluated for possible concurrent kidney transplantation [37, 38]. Avoidance of early renal insufficiency is of major importance given that it will have a significant impact on immunosuppression and fluid management in the posttransplant setting. Moreover, as shown in the published experience from Los Angeles, renal dysfunction (GFR < 75% of normal) at day 7, 1 month, and 1 year after ITx was associated with an increased risk of death (HR: 1.5, 1.2, and 6.0, resp.) [39].

In some centers, the right hemicolon (vascularized by the SMA) and the ileocecal valve are now routinely included in the allograft of patients undergoing IITx [12, 40]. In an early report of 71 ITx, including 29 colon-containing allografts, inclusion of the colon appeared to be significantly associated with decreased graft and patient survival [41]. However, these early findings were not subsequently confirmed and the practice of colon inclusion has resumed in some centers since the publication of the Paris and the Miami experiences [40, 42]. In the Paris series, 23/36 children received an allograft including the colon (17 were L-ITx) and colonic inclusion had no impact on patient or graft survival [42]. Kato et al. reported on 93 ITx that included the colon out of a total of 245 ITx [40]. Inclusion of the colon was not associated with decreased graft or patient survival [40]. Moreover, colonic inclusion was associated with a higher frequency of formed stools after stoma closure (67% in patients with colon inclusion versus 48.5% in patients who did not receive a colon as part of the allograft) [40]. Since the publication of those two recent series, it is now believed that colonic inclusion has no unfavorable impact on the posttransplant outcomes of ITx. According to the most recent ITR report, in 2012, 30% of the intestinal allografts included the colon in comparison to 4% in 2000 [10]. Colonic inclusion may improve quality of life after transplantation, being associated with less diarrhea after stoma reversal. Moreover, as demonstrated in the ITR report, colonic inclusion increased the likelihood of being free from TPN and intravenous fluid supplementation by 5% in comparison to those who did not receive a colonic segment, reflecting the important role of the colon in fluid and free fatty acid absorption [10]. In this same report, colonic inclusion did not increase the risk of rejection after transplantation [10]. Of note, the inclusion of colon in the allograft does not allow the performance of ITx without a temporary ileostomy. The presence of a temporary ileostomy is essential for easy access to the allograft for endoscopic monitoring after transplantation. The inclusion of the ileocecal valve may increase the difficulty in endoscopically accessing the ileal component of the graft after ITx and, thus, a temporary ileostomy remains essential [40]. In the Miami series, there were no cases of acute cellular rejection (ACR) restricted to the colonic segment of the allograft [40].

The intestinal allograft is highly immunogenic and chimeric, containing a large amount of lymphoid tissue (gut-associated lymphoid tissue) with the genotype of the epithelial cells remaining mainly that of the donor [2, 35, 43]. The outcomes of IITx are thus marked by high rates of ACR [35]. Also, the rates of ACR after IITx are higher than those seen after L-ITx or MVTx, that is, after transplantation of a liver-containing allograft [35, 44–47]. It is thought that the transplantation of the liver in association with the intestine promotes tolerance towards the bowel graft by inducing the production of regulatory T-cells and the deletion of alloreactive T-cells [19, 35, 48]. A multivisceral allograft might confer even more protection against severe ACR of the intestinal allograft in comparison to L-ITx [46]. MMVTx, that is, allograft not including the liver, may also confer protection against ACR in comparison to ITx [44]. One theory to explain this finding is that the risk of ACR might be related to the relative proportion of donor lymphoid tissue transplanted with the allograft compared to the remaining recipient lymphoid tissue [44]. MVTx and MMVTx come by default with a larger amount of lymphoid tissue and may thus be more capable of inducing tolerance towards the intestinal allograft [44]. In the preinduction era, ACR of the intestinal allograft in the first 30 days after transplantation was reported to be as high as 88% [49]. Currently, according to the most recent report from the Scientific Registry of Transplant Recipients (SRTR), the cumulative incidence of ACR after ITx is 39% at 12 months and 44% at 24 months [19].

4. Combined Liver-Intestine Transplantation

L-ITx is indicated for patients with irreversible IF despite intestinal rehabilitation and impending or overt liver failure related to TPN (PNALD) [2, 12, 33, 50–52]. Usually, the liver is transplanted en bloc along with the pancreas and small bowel in order to avoid hilar dissection and decrease the risk of vascular and biliary complications after transplantation [6, 53, 54].

Historically, ITx was most commonly performed in combination with a liver allograft, since most patients listed for ITx also had advanced PNALD. As per the 2005 United Network for Organ Sharing (UNOS) data, 74% of the patients listed for ITx also required listing for a liver transplant, either before (10%), simultaneously (52%), or after (12%) an ITx [52]. Since 2008, proportionally less L-ITx are performed compared to IITx [19]. According to the last SRTR report, in 2012, only 42% of ITx included a liver allograft [19]. This recent reduction in the number of L-ITX performed annually is most likely a reflection of the advances in the understanding of the physiopathological mechanisms of PNALD and of the improved care of patients on long-term TPN. In addition to TPN composition optimization and lipid restriction, fish oil emulsions (Omegaven) are now available in many countries [55, 56]. Replacement of the soy-based lipid emulsions by omega-3 rich lipid emulsions is associated with rapid improvement of cholestasis in the majority of the cases [56–58]. However, whether this biochemical cholestasis reversal is associated with hepatic fibrosis regression remains highly controversial [55, 56, 58–61].

Currently, there is no clear consensus defining when a liver should be included in the allograft [50]. Patients on TPN who develop cirrhosis have essentially a 100% mortality rate at 5 years without transplantation [52, 62]. Chan and coworkers reported 6 individuals with end-stage liver disease (ESLD) related to TPN with universal mortality, occurring at a median of 10.8 months following the first elevation of bilirubin [63]. Another study showed a 1-year and 2-year survival rates of only 30% and 22%, respectively, in patients listed for L-ITx who did not undergo ITx [64]. Given these results, it is generally accepted that individuals with cirrhosis secondary to TPN and those with advanced stages of fibrosis should be considered for concurrent liver transplantation [12, 33, 50–52]. As a general rule, patients with biopsy-proven advanced fibrosis (F3-F4) and those with clinical signs of cirrhosis (portal hypertension, coagulopathy) should not receive an IITx. In the cases of lesser grades of fibrosis, PNALD may regress or resolve after a successful IITx allowing for weaning and eventual withdrawal of TPN [12, 50, 51]. In one series, four patients having liver fibrosis stage 2 or 3 underwent IITx. Nine months after transplant, all patients showed regression of liver fibrosis with an improvement of at least one stage on posttransplant liver biopsy [65]. Moreover, early cirrhosis reversal 17 months after a successful IITx and TPN weaning has been demonstrated [66]. Since evaluation of the extent of PNALD may be challenging, a liver biopsy should be performed prior to ITx in patients with persistent elevation of the total bilirubin and/or low platelet counts in order to guide the choice of allograft. When possible, a transjugular liver biopsy should be chosen over a percutaneous liver biopsy, since this procedure also allows for measurement of the portal pressure gradient, recognizing that, in the patient with short bowel, wedge pressure measurements may grossly underestimate actual portal venous pressures.

Massive resection of the small bowel and thus decreased portal venous return to the liver can mask the presence of advanced fibrosis with clinical portal hypertension not occurring. Hence, patients with extreme short bowel syndrome may not manifest the usual stigmata of ESLD in the form of ascites or esophageal varices, and synthetic dysfunction is a very late and poor prognostic sign. In these patients, presence of hepatosplenomegaly, thrombocytopenia, and engorged superficial abdominal veins may be the only signs of ESLD with portal hypertension and constitute absolute indications for liver replacement in addition to the intestine.

An important consideration in the choice of allograft is the higher mortality on the waiting list in patients waiting for L-ITx compared to those listed for IITx [19, 50, 52, 62, 67–69]. Since the creation of the waiting list for ITx in 1994, the mortality in candidates listed for L-ITx has greatly exceeded that of all other solid organ transplant candidates [50, 67]. The worse short-term prognosis of patients listed for L-ITx was not appropriately taken into account in the previous organ allocation systems and these patients were thus disadvantaged compared to other liver transplant (LT) candidates [62, 68, 69]. Prior to 2002, it was estimated that 86% of all deaths occurring in patients listed for ITx were in those waiting for L-ITx [62]. Also, children seemed to be disproportionately affected given that 83% of all deaths were in pediatric candidates [62]. In February 2002, the MELD and PELD scores were implemented to better prioritize patients at higher risk of short-term mortality on the waiting list [69, 70]. Despite the fact that MELD and PELD scores are based on objective criteria, candidates listed for L-ITx were unfortunately still at higher risk of death and less likely to be transplanted compared to their counterparts listed for LT or IITx [71, 72]. To account for the higher mortality risk in patients with IF and PNALD listed for L-ITx, modifications to the MELD and PELD scoring systems were implemented in 2005 and 2007 [69]. Currently, when an adult's MELD score does not adequately reflect the severity of his condition, an appeal for extra MELD points can be filed with the Regional Review Board (UNOS policy 3.6.4.1 Adult Candidate Status). For children below 12 years and adolescents aged between 12 and 17 years listed for L-ITx, extra 23 points are currently added to their natural PELD score to account for their higher mortality risk on the waiting list [69]. Moreover, in 2005, a status IB was created for pediatric candidates waiting for L-ITx [69]. Following these modifications to the MELD and PELD scores, Kaplan et al. assessed the impact of these modifications on the waiting list mortality of L-ITx candidates [69]. According to their analysis of UNOS data from 1999 to 2009, the policy modifications were highly effective in eliminating the mortality disparities on the waiting list for adults with a MELD score over 15 points [69]. However, adult patients listed for L-ITx with MELD score under 15 points were still disproportionately at higher risk of mortality compared to their LT counterparts [69]. This same study revealed an improvement in the waiting list mortality for pediatric candidates but the policy revisions were not sufficient to completely eliminate the mortality disparities between L-ITx and isolated LT pediatric candidates [69]. According to the most recent SRTR report, 11.6% (6.7 deaths/100 waitlist years in 2010–2012 versus 51.0/100 waitlist year in 1998-1999) of ITx candidates died on the waiting list in 2012 [19]. Despite the recent improvement in the waitlist mortality for L-ITx, in 2012, the waiting list mortality rate was still almost 10 times higher for L-ITx candidates (14.2 deaths/100 waitlist years) versus IITx candidates (1.5 deaths/100 waitlist years) (Figure 2) [19]. Regional disparities in PELD/MELD scores at the time of transplantation and waitlist mortality continue to be significant, forcing a need to search for alternative strategies to tackle this issue [50, 52, 73].

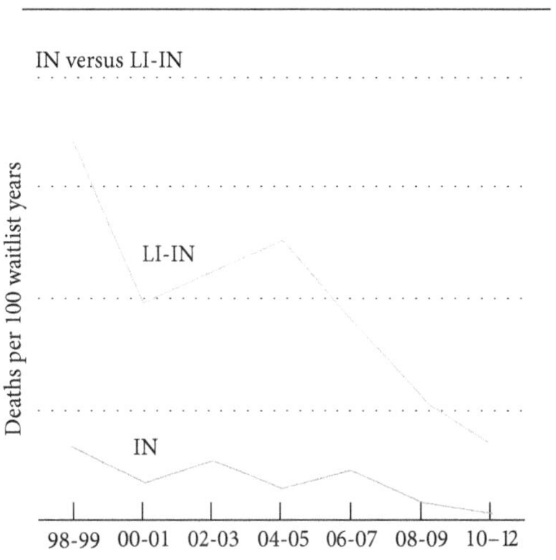

FIGURE 2: Waitlist mortality among patients listed for isolated intestinal transplantation and combined liver-intestine transplantation. *Notes.* (1) From SRTR report 2012 [19]. (2) LI-IN: combined liver-intestine transplantation; IN: isolated intestinal transplantation.

IITx can sometimes be performed if the chances of survival while waiting for a L-ITx are estimated to be lower than the chances of survival after IITx and if there is an expectation that the native liver will recover after successful intestinal engraftment. Such an approach is associated with a potential risk of liver decompensation and encephalopathy after IITx. If the posttransplant course is uncomplicated and the TPN can be weaned, it appears that liver function can be preserved without liver replacement. While it is unclear whether biochemical improvement in liver function is paralleled by histological improvement, we have reported downstaging of fibrosis in a small number of patients after IITx and even reversal of TPN-related cirrhosis 17 months after IITx [65, 66].

L-ITx carries a higher early postoperative mortality rate but a better long-term graft and patient survival rates compared to IITx [52]. The higher initial mortality rate seen in L-ITx recipients is thought to be, in part, secondary to their poorer clinical status going into transplant compared to their IITx counterparts [48, 52, 62]. Moreover, when life-threatening complications such as infections or PTLD occur after transplant, the intestinal allograft can be removed and all immunosuppression ceased in the IITx recipients with TPN being reinstituted [62, 68, 74]. This life-saving option is not possible in the L-ITx recipients, making them less easily

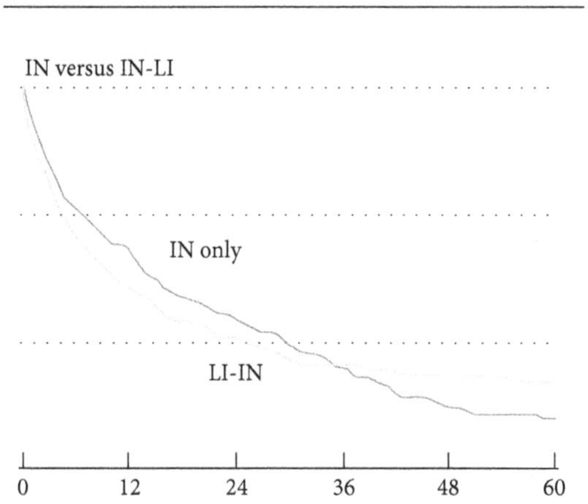

Figure 3: Graft survival after isolated intestinal transplantation versus combined liver-intestine transplantation. *Notes.* (1) From SRTR report 2012 [19]. (2) LI-IN: combined liver-intestine transplantation; IN: isolated intestinal transplantation.

salvageable when similar complications occur after transplant [62, 68, 74]. However, as shown in the last SRTR report, 3 years after transplantation, L-ITx recipients demonstrate better long-term outcomes compared to their IITx counterparts [19] (Figure 3). These better long-term outcomes may be related to the liver-induced tolerance towards the allograft, with decreased risk of ACR and chronic rejection [35, 48].

5. Multivisceral and Modified Multivisceral Transplantation

In many centers, the term MVTx is used to refer to allografts including the stomach and the duodenum in continuity with the jejunoileum [2, 12]. MVTx can also refer to the transplantation of all organs dependent on the celiac artery axis and the SMA (stomach, liver, pancreas, duodenum, and jejunoileum) [12, 50, 75–77]. This definition distinguishes MVT from L-ITx, only by the inclusion of the stomach in the former. An alternative definition that has not been widely accepted distinguishes MVTx only by the need for upper abdominal exenteration and not by the inclusion or exclusion of the stomach. Moreover, a multivisceral allograft can be "full" (MVTx) if it includes the liver and "modified" (MMVTx) if it does not [12, 50, 75–77].

The number and the type of organs included in a multiorgan allograft depend largely on the underlying pathology leading to transplant [12, 33]. Currently, the most frequent indication for MVTx is extensive portomesenteric thrombosis with hepatic decompensation and/or life-threatening bleeding complications related to portal hypertension [2, 12, 33, 50–52]. In this particular situation, the extensive vascular thrombosis surgically precludes an isolated LT [2, 12, 33, 50–52]. Furthermore, the alternate approach of isolated LT with cavoportal hemitransposition is associated with poor patient and graft survival and usually does not provide adequate decompression of the thrombosed portomesenteric and splenic systems [78]. As a result, patients can still experience complications related to portal hypertension [78]. Other common indications for MVTx are familial polyposis syndromes (familial adenomatous polyposis, Peutz-Jeghers syndrome), massive abdominal desmoid tumors, and locally aggressive benign tumors requiring total exenteration [12, 33]. Traumatic loss of abdominal viscera, such as can be seen after major motor vehicle accidents, is also an indication for MVTx [12, 33]. Diffuse gastrointestinal motility disorders, such as chronic intestinal pseudoobstruction (CIPO), scleroderma, and hollow visceral myopathy syndrome, can also warrant a MVTx [12, 33]. Of note, whenever the native liver function is preserved and it is surgically feasible, the allograft should not include the liver.

Some indications for MVTx warrant further clarifications. In the case of diffuse portomesenteric thrombosis in association with cirrhosis, the extent of the venous thrombosis usually surgically contraindicates the transplantation of an isolated liver for technical reasons and inability to provide portal venous inflow. In this situation, a full MVTx should be performed and is usually associated with excellent outcomes [79]. In the case of diffuse portomesenteric and splenic thrombosis in a noncirrhotic patient who develops life-threatening bleeding from portal hypertension, the decision to perform a MVTx should be reserved only after the patient has failed attempts at TIPS and/or surgical shunts [35, 80]. In patients having familial adenomatous polyposis, some centers advocate for MVTx given the increased risk of malignancy in the pancreaticoduodenal complex [75]. Duodenal adenomatosis, a premalignant condition, may warrant duodenectomy and pancreatectomy as an attempt to prevent malignant transformation after transplantation [75]. This surgical approach with subsequent MVTx should be considered in patients with FAP, mostly in the presence of advanced dysplastic changes, rapidly growing adenomas, and a family history of duodenal cancer [75]. For CIPO, there is no current consensus on the number and the type of organs that should be included in the allograft. Given the diffuse nature of the motility disorder, some centers advocate for the inclusion of the stomach as part of the allograft, while others perform ITx with or without hemigastrectomy and gastrojejunostomy to favor gastric emptying [81, 82].

A last point to consider in the decision to perform a MVTx is that posttransplantation outcomes are marked by increased risks of infections compared to IITx [35, 46, 83]. Moreover, it appears that the risks of CMV and PTLD are higher after MVTx, contributing to the less favorable outcomes of MVTx [83]. A recent series also reported a mildly increased risk of graft versus host disease (GVHD) compared to other types of ITx: 14% for MVTx, 10% for MMVTx, 8% for L-ITx, and 6% for ITx [35].

6. Isolated Liver Transplantation

Some centers have advocated isolated LT for children who develop ESLD secondary to TPN before full expected intestinal adaptation occurs. Such an approach can be justified in certain children who demonstrate a reasonable tolerance to enteral feeding, usually defined as greater than 50% of the total caloric needs, and continuous signs of progressive intestinal adaptation [84–87]. In children, the length of small bowel cannot be used to predict the likelihood of nutritional independency. However, isolated LT should not be performed when the remaining length of functioning small bowel is less than 25 cm [84, 85].

The rationale justifying the performance of an isolated LT in these children is that ESLD and portal hypertension can blunt further intestinal adaptation and can also preclude the performance of surgical lengthening procedures that could allow for TPN weaning [84–86]. Moreover, the outcomes of ITx and, more specifically, L-ITx are still not as good as those for LT and can justify proceeding to an isolated LT in particular cases [84–86]. In some very sick children, the availability of a living liver donor may also justify the decision to perform an isolated LT. Also, such an adult liver allograft might confer a greater resistance against the development of PNALD and allow more time for maximal intestinal adaptation [84–86].

The largest series published to date on isolated LT in children with IF and advanced PNALD is the experience from Omaha [84, 85]. In this series, 23 children who were estimated to have a good prognosis for nutritional independence following maximal gut adaptation received an isolated LT between 1995 and 2004. Of these 23 patients, 17 had long-term survival, with 1-year and 5-year patient survival rates of 82% and 72%, respectively, and 1-year and 5-year graft survival rates of 75% and 60%, respectively. Of those 17 patients, 14 were weaned from TPN after a median of 3 months. Of note, the majority of the patients weaned from TPN (8/14) required long-term supplemental enteral feeds to maintain adequate growth. Among the three patients who could not be completely weaned from TPN, one patient developed recurrent PNALD and required listing for L-ITx. Among the six children who died after isolated LT for PNALD, one patient died because of recurrent PNALD and four died of infectious complications. The recurrence of PNALD after isolated LT is not well defined in the literature. In one small series, three children underwent isolated LT for PNALD, none of whom were definitively weaned from TPN. Among those three patients, recurrence of PNALD after LT was seen in one patient, who ultimately died [86].

7. Summary

With recent improvements in immunosuppression, induction protocols, and posttransplantation management, ITx is now associated with improved patient and graft survival. The jejunoileum is the central component of every ITx. The choice of allograft is complex and every patient should undergo a multidisciplinary evaluation. ITx in patients with short gut syndrome should only be considered in those who failed dedicated intestinal rehabilitation attempts and after the development of life-threatening complications related to TPN. Inclusion of the right hemicolon should be performed in patients without full native colon in order to improve quality of life after ileostomy reversal and to optimize fluid reabsorption. In patients with PNALD, a transjugular liver biopsy should be performed and L-ITx should be considered in patients with advanced fibrosis. In patients requiring ITx for extensive portomesenteric thrombosis, this procedure should only be considered after all the other therapeutic options have failed. In the case of diffuse gastrointestinal pathology such as polyposis syndrome and motility disorders, MVTx should be considered on a case by case basis. Finally, an isolated LT can be considered in children demonstrating progressive intestinal adaptation and ESLD related to the TPN. However, when such an approach is chosen, the undefined risk of PNALD recurrence should be considered.

Abbreviations

ITx:	Intestinal transplantation
IF:	Intestinal failure
TPN:	Total parenteral nutrition
PNALD:	Parenteral nutrition associated liver disease
ITR:	Intestinal transplant registry
SB:	Small bowel
IITx:	Isolated intestinal transplantation
L-ITx:	Combined liver-intestine transplantation
MVTx:	Multivisceral transplantation
SMA:	Superior mesenteric artery
MMVTx:	Modified multivisceral transplantation
GLP:	Glucagon-like peptide
IVC:	Inferior vena cava
ACR:	Acute cellular rejection
SRTR:	Scientific registry of transplant recipients
UNOS:	United network for organ sharing
ESLD:	End-stage liver disease
LT:	Liver transplantation
CIPO:	Chronic intestinal pseudoobstruction
GVHD:	Graft versus host disease.

References

[1] A. Walther, A. Coots, J. Nathan, S. Kocoshis, and G. Tiao, "Physiology of the small intestine after resection and transplant," *Current Opinion in Gastroenterology*, vol. 29, no. 2, pp. 153–158, 2013.

[2] T. M. Fishbein, "Intestinal transplantation," *The New England Journal of Medicine*, vol. 361, no. 10, pp. 998–1008, 2009.

[3] S. Lal, A. Teubner, and J. L. Shaffer, "Review article: intestinal failure," *Alimentary Pharmacology and Therapeutics*, vol. 24, no. 1, pp. 19–31, 2006.

[4] K. M. Abu-Elmagd, G. Costa, G. J. Bond et al., "Five hundred intestinal and multivisceral transplantations at a single center: major advances with new challenges," *Annals of Surgery*, vol. 250, no. 4, pp. 567–581, 2009.

[5] L. Pironi, F. Joly, A. Forbes et al., "Long-term follow-up of patients on home parenteral nutrition in Europe: implications for intestinal transplantation," *Gut*, vol. 60, no. 1, pp. 17–25, 2011.

[6] D. Sudan, "The current state of intestine transplantation: indications, techniques, outcomes and challenges," *American Journal of Transplantation and the American Society of Transplant Surgeons*, vol. 14, no. 9, pp. 1976–1984, 2014.

[7] L. Pironi, O. Goulet, A. Buchman et al., "Outcome on home parenteral nutrition for benign intestinal failure: a review of the literature and benchmarking with the european prospective survey of espen," *Clinical Nutrition*, vol. 31, no. 6, pp. 831–845, 2012.

[8] S. S. Kaufman, J. B. Atkinson, A. Bianchi et al., "Indications for pediatric intestinal transplantation: a position paper of the American Society of Transplantation. Pediatric transplantation," *Pediatric Transplantation*, vol. 5, no. 2, pp. 80–87, 2001.

[9] M. Medicare, "Department of Health and Human Services. centers for the medicare and medicaid services. program memorandum intermediaries/carriers," *Intestinal and Multi-Visceral Transplantation*, Article ID AB-02-040, pp. 02–040, 2002.

[10] ITR, "Bi-annual report," in *Intestinal Transplant Registry*, D. Grant, Ed., Toronto, Canada, 2014.

[11] D. Grant, K. Abu-Elmagd, G. Mazariegos et al., "Intestinal transplant registry report: global activity and trends," *The American Society of Transplantation and the American Society of Transplant Surgeons*, vol. 15, no. 1, pp. 210–219, 2015.

[12] A. Nickkholgh, P. Contin, K. Abu-Elmagd et al., "Intestinal transplantation: review of operative techniques," *Clinical Transplantation*, vol. 27, supplement 25, pp. 56–65, 2013.

[13] K. A. Tappenden, "Intestinal adaptation following resection," *Journal of Parenteral and Enteral Nutrition*, vol. 38, supplement 1, pp. 23–31, 2014.

[14] K. Abu-Elmagd, "The concept of gut rehabilitation and the future of visceral transplantation," *Nature Reviews Gastroenterology and Hepatology*, vol. 12, no. 2, pp. 108–120, 2015.

[15] L. Pironi, J. Arends, F. Bozzetti et al., "ESPEN guidelines on chronic intestinal failure in adults," *Clinical Nutrition*, vol. 35, no. 2, pp. 247–307, 2016.

[16] P. W. Wales, N. Allen, P. Worthington, D. George, C. Compher, and D. Teitelbaum, "Clinical Guidelines: support of pediatric patients with intestinal failure at risk of parenteral nutrition-associated liver disease," *Journal of Parenteral and Enteral Nutrition*, vol. 38, no. 5, pp. 538–557, 2014.

[17] T. M. Fishbein, T. Schiano, N. LeLeiko, and wtal, "An integrated approach to intestinal failure: results of a new program with total parenteral nutrition, bowel rehabilitation, and transplantation," *Journal of Gastrointestinal Surgery*, vol. 6, no. 4, pp. 554–562, 2002.

[18] J. D. Stanger, C. Oliveira, C. Blackmore, Y. Avitzur, and P. W. Wales, "The impact of multi-disciplinary intestinal rehabilitation programs on the outcome of pediatric patients with intestinal failure: a systematic review and meta-analysis," *Journal of Pediatric Surgery*, vol. 48, no. 5, pp. 983–992, 2013.

[19] J. M. Smith, M. A. Skeans, S. P. Horslen et al., "Annual data report: intestine. american journal of transplantation," *Journal of the American Society of Transplantation and the American Society of Transplant Surgeons*, vol. 14, supplement 1, pp. 97–111, 2014.

[20] P. B. Jeppesen, "Pharmacologic options for intestinal rehabilitation in patients with short bowel syndrome," *Journal of Parenteral and Enteral Nutrition*, vol. 38, supplement 1, pp. 45s–52s, 2014.

[21] L. E. Matarese, "Nutrition and fluid optimization for patients with short bowel syndrome," *Journal of Parenteral and Enteral Nutrition*, vol. 37, no. 2, pp. 161–170, 2013.

[22] I. Nordgaard, B. S. Hansen, and P. B. Mortensen, "Importance of colonic support for energy absorption as small-bowel failure proceeds," *American Journal of Clinical Nutrition*, vol. 64, no. 2, pp. 222–231, 1996.

[23] J. M. D. Nightingale, J. E. Lennard-Jones, E. R. Walker, and M. J. G. Farthing, "Oral salt supplements to compensate for jejunostomy losses: comparison of sodium chloride capsules, glucose electrolyte solution, and glucose polymer electrolyte solution," *Gut*, vol. 33, no. 6, pp. 759–761, 1992.

[24] N. S. Williams, P. Evans, and R. F. G. J. King, "Gastric acid secretion and gastrin production in the short bowel syndrome," *Gut*, vol. 26, no. 9, pp. 914–919, 1985.

[25] P. B. Jeppesen, M. Staun, L. Tjellesen, and P. B. Mortensen, "Effect of intravenous ranitidine and omeprazole on intestinal absorption of water, sodium, and macronutrients in patients with intestinal resection," *Gut*, vol. 43, no. 6, pp. 763–769, 1998.

[26] S. J. D. O'Keefe, P. B. Jeppesen, R. Gilroy, M. Pertkiewicz, J. P. Allard, and B. Messing, "Safety and efficacy of teduglutide after 52 weeks of treatment in patients with short bowel intestinal failure," *Clinical Gastroenterology and Hepatology*, vol. 11, no. 7, pp. 815–823, 2013.

[27] P. B. Jeppesen, M. Pertkiewicz, B. Messing et al., "Teduglutide reduces need for parenteral support among patients with short bowel syndrome with intestinal failure," *Gastroenterology*, vol. 143, no. 6, pp. 1473.e3–1481.e3, 2012.

[28] P. B. Jeppesen, R. Gilroy, M. Pertkiewicz, J. P. Allard, B. Messing, and S. J. O'Keefe, "Randomised placebo-controlled trial of teduglutide in reducing parenteral nutrition and/or intravenous fluid requirements in patients with short bowel syndrome," *Gut*, vol. 60, no. 7, pp. 902–914, 2011.

[29] P. Arda-Pirincci and S. Bolkent, "The role of glucagon-like peptide-2 on apoptosis, cell proliferation, and oxidant-antioxidant system at a mouse model of intestinal injury induced by tumor necrosis factor-alpha/actinomycin D," *Molecular and Cellular Biochemistry*, vol. 350, no. 1-2, pp. 13–27, 2011.

[30] J. J. Meier, M. A. Nauck, A. Pott et al., "Glucagon-like peptide 2 stimulates glucagon secretion, enhances lipid absorption, and inhibits gastric acid secretion in humans," *Gastroenterology*, vol. 130, no. 1, pp. 44–54, 2006.

[31] H. B. Kim, D. Fauza, J. Garza, J.-T. Oh, S. Nurko, and T. Jaksic, "Serial transverse enteroplasty (STEP): a novel bowel lengthening procedure," *Journal of Pediatric Surgery*, vol. 38, no. 3, pp. 425–429, 2003.

[32] A. Bianchi, "Intestinal loop lengthening—A technique for increasing small intestinal length," *Journal of Pediatric Surgery*, vol. 15, no. 2, pp. 145–151, 1980.

[33] L. E. Matarese, G. Costa, G. Bond et al., "Therapeutic efficacy of intestinal and multivisceral transplantation: survival and nutrition outcome," *Nutrition in Clinical Practice*, vol. 22, no. 5, pp. 474–481, 2007.

[34] T. Berney, T. Kato, S. Nishida et al., "Portal versus systemic drainage of small bowel allografts: comparative assessment of survival, function, rejection, and bacterial translocation," *Journal of the American College of Surgeons*, vol. 195, no. 6, pp. 804–813, 2002.

[35] K. M. Abu-Elmagd, G. Costa, G. J. Bond et al., "Five hundred intestinal and multivisceral transplantations at a single center: major advances with new challenges," *Annals of Surgery*, vol. 250, no. 4, pp. 567–581, 2009.

[36] L. J. Ceulemans, Y. Nijs, F. Nuytens et al., "Combined kidney and intestinal transplantation in patients with enteric hyperoxaluria

secondary to short bowel syndrome," *American Journal of Transplantation*, vol. 13, no. 7, pp. 1910–1914, 2013.

[37] A. O. Ojo, P. J. Held, F. K. Port et al., "Chronic renal failure after transplantation of a nonrenal organ," *The New England Journal of Medicine*, vol. 349, no. 10, pp. 931–940, 2003.

[38] R. L. Ruebner, P. P. Reese, M. R. Denburg, P. L. Abt, and S. L. Furth, "End-stage kidney disease after pediatric nonrenal solid organ transplantation," *Pediatrics*, vol. 132, no. 5, pp. e1319–e1326, 2013.

[39] M. J. Watson, R. S. Venick, F. Kaldas et al., "Renal function impacts outcomes after intestinal transplantation," *Transplantation*, vol. 86, no. 1, pp. 117–122, 2008.

[40] T. Kato, G. Selvaggi, J. J. Gaynor et al., "Inclusion of donor colon and ileocecal valve in intestinal transplantation," *Transplantation*, vol. 86, no. 2, pp. 293–297, 2008.

[41] S. Todo, J. Reyes, H. Furukawa et al., "Outcome analysis of 71 clinical intestinal transplantations," *Annals of Surgery*, vol. 222, no. 3, pp. 270–282, 1995.

[42] O. Goulet, F. Auber, L. Fourcade et al., "Intestinal transplantation including the colon in children," *Transplantation Proceedings*, vol. 34, no. 5, pp. 1885–1886, 2002.

[43] H. Remotti, S. Subramanian, M. Martinez, T. Kato, and M. S. Magid, "Small-bowel allograft biopsies in the management of small-intestinal and multivisceral transplant recipients: histopathologic review and clinical correlations," *Archives of Pathology & Laboratory Medicine*, vol. 136, pp. 761–71, 2012.

[44] G. Selvaggi, J. J. Gaynor, J. Moon et al., "Analysis of acute cellular rejection episodes in recipients of primary intestinal transplantation: A single center, 11-year experience," *American Journal of Transplantation*, vol. 7, no. 5, pp. 1249–1257, 2007.

[45] H. Takahashi, G. Selvaggi, S. Nishida et al., "Organ-specific differences in acute rejection intensity in a multivisceral transplant," *Transplantation*, vol. 81, no. 2, pp. 297–299, 2006.

[46] A. G. Tzakis, T. Kato, S. Nishida et al., "The Miami experience with almost 100 multivisceral transplants," *Transplantation Proceedings*, vol. 38, no. 6, pp. 1681–1682, 2006.

[47] K. Abu-Elmagd, J. Reyes, G. Bond et al., "Clinical intestinal transplantation: a decade of experience at a single center," *Annals of Surgery*, vol. 234, no. 3, pp. 404–417, 2001.

[48] O. Goulet, D. Damotte, and S. Sarnacki, "Liver-induced immune tolerance in recipients of combined liver-intestine transplants," *Transplantation Proceedings*, vol. 37, no. 4, pp. 1689–1690, 2005.

[49] J. Reyes, J. Bueno, S. Kocoshis et al., "Current status of intestinal transplantation in children," *Journal of Pediatric Surgery*, vol. 33, no. 2, pp. 243–254, 1998.

[50] J. P. Fryer, "The current status of intestinal transplantation," *Current Opinion in Organ Transplantation*, vol. 13, no. 3, pp. 266–272, 2008.

[51] D. N. Gotthardt, A. Gauss, U. Zech et al., "Indications for intestinal transplantation: recognizing the scope and limits of total parenteral nutrition," *Clinical Transplantation*, vol. 27, no. 25, pp. 49–55, 2013.

[52] A. L. Buchman, K. Iyer, and J. Fryer, "Parenteral nutrition-associated liver disease and the role for isolated intestine and intestine/liver transplantation," *Hepatology*, vol. 43, no. 1, pp. 9–19, 2006.

[53] D. L. Sudan, K. R. Iyer, A. Deroover et al., "A new technique for combined liver/small intestinal transplantation," *Transplantation*, vol. 72, no. 11, pp. 1846–1848, 2001.

[54] A. N. Langnas, B. W. Shaw Jr., D. L. Antonson et al., "Preliminary experience with intestinal transplantation in infants and children," *Pediatrics*, vol. 97, no. 4, pp. 443–448, 1996.

[55] D. F. Mercer, B. D. Hobson, R. T. Fischer et al., "Hepatic fibrosis persists and progresses despite biochemical improvement in children treated with intravenous fish oil emulsion," *Journal of Pediatric Gastroenterology and Nutrition*, vol. 56, no. 4, pp. 364–369, 2013.

[56] V. E. de Meijer, K. M. Gura, H. D. Le, J. A. Meisel, and M. Puder, "Fish oil-based lipid emulsions prevent and reverse parenteral nutrition-associated liver disease: the Boston experience," *Journal of Parenteral and Enteral Nutrition*, vol. 33, no. 5, pp. 541–547, 2009.

[57] E. Venecourt-Jackson, S. J. Hill, and R. S. Walmsley, "Successful treatment of parenteral nutrition-associated liver disease in an adult by use of a fish oil-based lipid source," *Nutrition*, vol. 29, no. 1, pp. 356–358, 2013.

[58] Z. Xu, Y. Li, J. Wang, B. Wu, and J. Li, "Effect of omega-3 polyunsaturated fatty acids to reverse biopsy-proven parenteral nutrition-associated liver disease in adults," *Clinical Nutrition*, vol. 31, no. 2, pp. 217–223, 2012.

[59] C. S. Matsumoto, S. S. Kaufman, E. R. Island et al., "Hepatic explant pathology of pediatric intestinal transplant recipients previously treated with omega-3 fatty acid lipid emulsion," *Journal of Pediatrics*, vol. 165, no. 1, pp. 59–64, 2014.

[60] J. S. Soden, M. A. Lovell, K. Brown, D. A. Partrick, and R. J. Sokol, "Failure of resolution of portal fibrosis during omega-3 fatty acid lipid emulsion therapy in two patients with irreversible intestinal failure," *Journal of Pediatrics*, vol. 156, no. 2, pp. 327–331, 2010.

[61] D. L. Burns and B. M. Gill, "Reversal of parenteral nutrition-associated liver disease with a fish oil-based lipid emulsion (Omegaven) in an adult dependent on home parenteral nutrition," *Journal of Parenteral and Enteral Nutrition*, vol. 37, no. 2, pp. 274–280, 2013.

[62] J. Fryer, S. Pellar, D. Ormond, A. Koffron, and M. Abecassis, "Mortality in candidates waiting for combined liver-intestine transplants exceeds that for other candidates waiting for liver transplants," *Liver Transplantation*, vol. 9, no. 7, pp. 748–753, 2003.

[63] S. Chan, K. C. McCowen, B. R. Bistrian et al., "Incidence, prognosis, and etiology of end-stage liver disease in patients receiving home total parenteral nutrition," *Surgery*, vol. 126, no. 1, pp. 28–34, 1999.

[64] J. Bueno, S. Ohwada, S. Kocoshis et al., "Factors impacting the survival of children with intestinal failure referred for intestinal transplantation," *Journal of Pediatric Surgery*, vol. 34, no. 1, pp. 27–33, 1999.

[65] M. I. Fiel, B. Sauter, H.-S. Wu et al., "Regression of hepatic fibrosis after intestinal transplantation in total parenteral nutrition liver disease," *Clinical Gastroenterology and Hepatology*, vol. 6, no. 8, pp. 926–933, 2008.

[66] M. I. Fiel, H.-S. Wu, K. Iyer, G. Rodriguez-Laiz, and T. D. Schiano, "Rapid reversal of parenteral-nutrition-associated cirrhosis following isolated intestinal transplantation," *Journal of Gastrointestinal Surgery*, vol. 13, no. 9, pp. 1717–1723, 2009.

[67] J. P. Roberts, R. S. Brown Jr., E. B. Edwards et al., "Liver and intestine transplantation," *Journal of the American Society of Transplantation and the American Society of Transplant Surgeons*, vol. 3, Supplement 4, pp. 78–90, 2003.

[68] J. P. Fryer and K. Iyer, "Innovative approaches to improving organ availability for small bowel transplant candidates," *Gastroenterology*, vol. 130, no. 2, supplement 1, pp. S152–S157, 2006.

[69] J. Kaplan, L. Han, W. Halgrimson, E. Wang, and J. Fryer, "The impact of MELD/PELD revisions on the mortality of liver-intestine transplantation candidates," *American Journal of Transplantation*, vol. 11, no. 9, pp. 1896–1904, 2011.

[70] R. Wiesner, E. Edwards, R. Freeman et al., "Model for end-stage liver disease (MELD) and allocation of donor livers," *Gastroenterology*, vol. 124, no. 1, pp. 91–96, 2003.

[71] G. V. Mazariegos, D. E. Steffick, S. Horslen et al., "Intestine transplantation in the United States, 1999–2008," *American Society of Transplantation and the American Society of Transplant Surgeons*, vol. 10, no. 4, pp. 1020–1034, 2010.

[72] N. Chungfat, I. Dixler, V. Cohran, A. Buchman, M. Abecassis, and J. Fryer, "Impact of parenteral nutrition-associated liver disease on intestinal transplant waitlist dynamics," *Journal of the American College of Surgeons*, vol. 205, no. 6, pp. 755–761, 2007.

[73] S. E. Gentry, A. B. Massie, S. W. Cheek et al., "Addressing geographic disparities in liver transplantation through redistricting," *American Journal of Transplantation*, vol. 13, no. 8, pp. 2052–2058, 2013.

[74] T. Fishbein, S. Florman, G. Gondolesi, and R. Decker, "Noncomposite simultaneous liver and intestinal transplantation," *Transplantation*, vol. 75, no. 4, pp. 564–565, 2003.

[75] R. J. Cruz Jr., G. Costa, G. J. Bond et al., "Modified multivisceral transplantation with spleen-preserving pancreaticoduodenectomy for patients with familial adenomatous polyposis 'gardner's syndrome'," *Transplantation*, vol. 91, no. 12, pp. 1417–1423, 2011.

[76] R. J. Cruz Jr., G. Costa, G. Bond et al., "Modified "liver-sparing" multivisceral transplant with preserved native spleen, pancreas, and duodenum: technique and long-term outcome," *Journal of Gastrointestinal Surgery*, vol. 14, no. 11, pp. 1709–1721, 2010.

[77] J. P. Fryer, "Intestinal transplantation: current status," *Gastroenterology Clinics of North America*, vol. 36, no. 1, pp. 145–159, 2007.

[78] A. G. Tzakis, P. Kirkegaard, A. D. Pinna et al., "Liver transplantation with cavoportal hemitransposition in the presence of diffuse portal vein thrombosis," *Transplantation*, vol. 65, no. 5, pp. 619–624, 1998.

[79] R. M. Vianna, R. S. Mangus, C. Kubal, J. A. Fridell, T. Beduschi, and A. Joseph Tector, "Multivisceral transplantation for diffuse portomesenteric thrombosis," *Annals of Surgery*, vol. 255, no. 6, pp. 1144–1150, 2012.

[80] G. Costa, R. J. Cruz, and K. M. Abu-Elmagd, "Surgical shunt versus TIPS for treatment of variceal hemorrhage in the current era of liver and multivisceral transplantation," *Surgical Clinics of North America*, vol. 90, no. 4, pp. 891–905, 2010.

[81] L. Sigurdsson, J. Reyes, S. A. Kocoshis et al., "Intestinal transplantation in children with chronic intestinal pseudo- obstruction," *Gut*, vol. 45, no. 4, pp. 570–574, 1999.

[82] M. Masetti, F. Di Benedetto, N. Cautero et al., "Intestinal transplantation for chronic intestinal pseudo-obstruction in adult patients," *American Journal of Transplantation*, vol. 4, no. 5, pp. 826–829, 2004.

[83] M. E. De Vera, J. Reyes, J. Demetris et al., "Isolated intestinal versus composite visceral allografts: causes of graft failure," *Transplantation Proceedings*, vol. 32, no. 6, pp. 1221–1222, 2000.

[84] J. F. Botha, W. J. Grant, C. Torres et al., "Isolated liver transplantation in infants with end-stage liver disease due to short bowel syndrome," *Liver Transplantation : Official Publication of the American Association for the Study of Liver Diseases and the International Liver Transplantation Society*, vol. 12, pp. 1062–1066.

[85] S. P. Horslen, D. L. Sudan, K. R. Iyer et al., "Isolated liver transplantation in infants with end-stage liver disease associated with short bowel syndrome," *Annals of Surgery*, vol. 235, no. 3, pp. 435–439, 2002.

[86] I. R. Diamond, P. W. Wales, D. R. Grant, and A. Fecteau, "Isolated liver transplantation in pediatric short bowel syndrome: is there a role?" *Journal of Pediatric Surgery*, vol. 41, no. 5, pp. 955–959, 2006.

[87] N. R. Barshes, B. A. Carter, S. J. Karpen, C. A. O'Mahony, and J. A. Goss, "Isolated orthotopic liver transplantation for parenteral nutrition-associated liver injury," *Journal of Parenteral and Enteral Nutrition*, vol. 30, no. 6, pp. 526–529, 2006.

12

Transcriptome Analysis of Porcine PBMCs Reveals the Immune Cascade Response and Gene Ontology Terms Related to Cell Death and Fibrosis in the Progression of Liver Failure

YiMin Zhang,[1] Li Shao,[1] Ning Zhou,[1] JianZhou Li,[1] Yu Chen,[2] Juan Lu,[1] Jie Wang,[1] ErMei Chen,[1] ZhongYang Xie,[1] and LanJuan Li[1]

[1] *State Key Laboratory for Diagnosis and Treatment of Infectious Diseases, Collaborative Innovation Center for Diagnosis and Treatment of Infectious Diseases, The First Affiliated Hospital, College of Medicine, Zhejiang University, Hangzhou, Zhejiang Province, China*
[2] *Department of Experimental Animals, Zhejiang Academy of Traditional Chinese Medicine, Hangzhou, Zhejiang Province, China*

Correspondence should be addressed to LanJuan Li; ljli@zju.edu.cn

Academic Editor: En-Qiang Chen

Background. The key gene sets involved in the progression of acute liver failure (ALF), which has a high mortality rate, remain unclear. This study aims to gain a deeper understanding of the transcriptional response of peripheral blood mononuclear cells (PBMCs) following ALF. *Methods.* ALF was induced by D-galactosamine (D-gal) in a porcine model. PBMCs were separated at time zero (baseline group), 36 h (failure group), and 60 h (dying group) after D-gal injection. Transcriptional profiling was performed using RNA sequencing and analysed using DAVID bioinformatics resources. *Results.* Compared with the baseline group, 816 and 1,845 differentially expressed genes (DEGs) were identified in the failure and dying groups, respectively. A total of five and two gene ontology (GO) term clusters were enriched in 107 GO terms in the failure group and 154 GO terms in the dying group. These GO clusters were primarily immune-related, including genes regulating the inflammasome complex and toll-like receptor signalling pathways. Specifically, GO terms related to cell death, including apoptosis, pyroptosis, and autophagy, and those related to fibrosis, coagulation dysfunction, and hepatic encephalopathy were enriched. Seven Kyoto Encyclopedia of Genes and Genomes (KEGG) pathways, cytokine-cytokine receptor interaction, hematopoietic cell lineage, lysosome, rheumatoid arthritis, malaria, and phagosome and pertussis pathways were mapped for DEGs in the failure group. All of these seven KEGG pathways were involved in the 19 KEGG pathways mapped in the dying group. *Conclusion.* We found that the dramatic PBMC transcriptome changes triggered by ALF progression was predominantly related to immune responses. The enriched GO terms related to cell death, fibrosis, and so on, as indicated by PBMC transcriptome analysis, seem to be useful in elucidating potential key gene sets in the progression of ALF. A better understanding of these gene sets might be of preventive or therapeutic interest.

1. Introduction

Acute liver failure (ALF) is a severe syndrome characterised by hepatic encephalopathy and coagulation dysfunction, which can lead to multiorgan failure and death [1–3]. High morbidity and mortality following ALF are major problems worldwide [2, 3]. Thus, a thorough understanding of key genes or gene sets that regulate the progression of ALF is required.

The development of second-generation sequencing, particularly RNA-sequencing (RNA-Seq), has made it possible to perform global analysis of changes in gene expression during the course of a disease [4–6].

Taking biopsy samples during an ALF flare places the patient at high risk for lethal bleeding. More importantly, biopsy would influence the progression of ALF.

Analysis of the transcriptome of peripheral blood mononuclear cells (PBMCs) has successfully elucidated the mechanisms of numerous complex diseases and vaccination models [7–10]. These studies showed that analysing the PBMC transcriptome is helpful in identifying key genes and gene sets that control disease progression.

Here, we performed a comparative analysis of PBMC transcriptome in a porcine model of D-galactosamine- (D-gal-) induced ALF to identify candidate genes and gene sets that play important roles in the progression of ALF.

2. Materials and Methods

2.1. Porcine Model of D-gal-Induced ALF. A D-gal-induced ALF porcine model was used as previously described by our group [11]. Briefly, male Bama experimental miniature pigs were used and 1.3 g/kg body weight D-gal (Hanhong Chemical, Shanghai, China) was intravenously injected to induce ALF. Blood samples were collected at baseline (time zero) and 36 and 60 h after D-gal injection. Pigs were sacrificed after blood sample collection at 60 h. The general medical condition of the experimental pigs was monitored throughout the experiment.

All animal experiments were conducted in the Department of Experimental Animals, Zhejiang Academy of Traditional Chinese Medicine, China, and approved by the Animal Care Ethics Committee of the Academy. All experimental animals were treated humanely.

2.2. Clinical Parameters following D-gal-Induced Porcine ALF. At 0, 36, and 60 h, parameters to quantify the severity of liver failure were collected including the international normalization ratio (INR), and alanine aminotransferase, aspartate aminotransferase, alkaline phosphatase, γ-glutamyl transpeptidase, total bilirubin, and creatinine levels.

Blood ammonia was measured using an ammonia test kit (ARKRAY, Tokyo, Japan) with a detection range between 10 and 400 μg/dL. INR was quantified using STA-R (Diagnostic Stago, Asnieres, France) in the emergency laboratory at the First Affiliated Hospital, College of Medicine, Zhejiang University. Serum alanine aminotransferase, aspartate aminotransferase, alkaline phosphatase, γ-glutamyl transpeptidase, total bilirubin, and creatinine levels were measured using an automated biochemical analyser (Abbott Aeroset; Abbott Laboratories, Chicago, IL, USA) in the same laboratory.

2.3. PBMC Isolation and RNA Extraction. PBMCs were isolated using Ficoll-Histopaque (Sigma Aldrich, St. Louis, MO, USA) immediately after blood sample collection. Subsequently, total RNA was extracted using RNeasy Mini kits (QIAGEN, Hilden, Germany) according to the manufacturer's instructions. All RNA samples were stored at −80°C for future analysis.

2.4. mRNA Library Construction, RNA-Sequencing, and Data Analysis. Total RNA (1 μg) was thawed to create a library using TruSeq Stranded RNA LT Guide (Illumina, San Diego, CA, USA) according to the manufacturer's instructions. An Agilent 2100 bioanalyser (Santa Clara, CA, USA) was used to evaluate the concentration and size distribution of complementary DNA (cDNA) in the library before sequencing with the Illumina HiSequation 2500 system. The high-throughput sequencing was performed according to the manufacturer's instructions (Illumina HiSequation 2500 User Guide).

The raw data were filtered by FASTX (ver. 0.0.13) before mapping to the genome using TopHat (ver. 2.0.9). Gene fragments were counted using HTSeq followed by trimmed mean of M values (TMM) normalization. Significantly differentially expressed genes (DEGs) were identified using Cufflinks (ver. 2.2.1) [12]. DEGs were then submitted to Visualisation and Integrated Discovery analysis (DAVID; ver. 6.8) [13] for gene ontology (GO) term enrichment and clustering and Kyoto Encyclopedia of Genes and Genomes (KEGG) pathway mapping using default parameters, except for an EASE score setting of 0.05.

2.5. Validation of RNA-Seq Data by qRT-PCR. Quantitative RT-PCR was performed on selected genes to validate the data obtained from mRNA sequencing. Briefly, total RNA was reverse-transcribed into cDNA using the Fast Quant RT kit (Tiangen, Beijing, China). All qRT-PCR was conducted using SYBR Green SuperReal PreMix Plus (FP205; Tiangen) on an ABI 7900HT (Applied Biosystems, Foster City, CA, USA). Experimental conditions included a 3-min cycle at 94°C followed by 40 cycles of 20 s at 94°C, 20 s at 58°C, and 20 s at 72°C.

Each qRT-PCR run was performed in triplicate with two biological replicates. Beta-2-microglobulin (B2M) was used as the reference gene for data normalization, as previously described. A correlation analysis of the fold change of selected genes between qRT-PCR and RNA-Seq was performed.

2.6. Statistical Analysis. RNA-seq data analyses were described previously in Section 2.4. Other statistical analyses were performed by Graphpad Prism (Version 5.0, GraphPad Software, San Diego, United States). Biochemical parameters in the progress of ALF were compared using Student's t-test. Linear regression was performed in validation of RNA-Seq data by qRT-PCR. A p value less than 0.05 was considered significant.

3. Results

3.1. Clinical Features and Biochemical Parameters of D-gal-Induced ALF in Pigs. All animals enrolled in this experiment were healthy, with a good appetite and response to the D-gal injection at time zero (baseline). The ALF model was successfully established in all the animals at 36 h (failure) after D-gal injection. The pigs stopped eating and became obviously restless, with yellow urine. At 60 h post-injection (dying), the pigs showed ataxia and symptoms of hepatic encephalopathy, with no reaction to painful stimuli.

The biochemical parameters as ALF progressed are listed in Table 1. Liver failure was identified by the progressive increase in liver enzymes, bilirubin, blood ammonia, and the international normalization ratio in both the failure and dying groups as compared to the baseline group. A deviation of bilirubin and liver enzymes, or elevated total bilirubin with decreased liver enzymes, was observed in the dying group but not in the failure group.

Table 1: Biochemical parameters in a porcine model of ALF.

Parameters	Baseline	Failure	Dying
International normalization ratio	0.9 ± 0.05	2.7 ± 0.2**	4.8 ± 0.8**
Ammonia (μg/dl)	22.3 ± 3.1	76.5 ± 8.7**	225.5 ± 47.4**
Alanine aminotransferase (U/L)	56.3 ± 8.0	311.5 ± 65.0*	230.3 ± 46.5*
Aspartate aminotransferase (U/L)	36.0 ± 3.3	5023.8 ± 1034.6*	1788.5 ± 263.6**
Alkaline phosphatase (U/L)	72.8 ± 16.9	232.8 ± 53.4*	564.0 ± 82.6**
γ-Glutamyl transpeptidase (U/L)	64.5 ± 9.6	77.0 ± 5.1	96.3 ± 5.0*
Total bilirubin (μmol/L)	2.3 ± 0.3	40.8 ± 5.7**	70.8 ± 7.6**
Creatinine (mmol/L)	58.0 ± 2.1	59.3 ± 6.4	49.5 ± 3.3

Data are means ± SEM. $^{*}p < 0.05$, $^{**}p < 0.01$ versus baseline.

Table 2: Qualitative analysis of PBMC RNA-Seq data in a porcine model of ALF.

Sample name	Raw reads	Q20 value	Clean reads	Mapped reads	Genic reads	Percentage of genic reads	Expressed gene number
Baseline-1	80,876,352	94.80%	77,508,054	63,736,589	51,530,237	80.80%	15,249
Baseline-2	122,478,648	95.40%	117,994,584	64,288,782	47,627,719	74.10%	14,990
Baseline-3	97,633,918	95.10%	93,252,338	76,290,007	48,400,655	63.40%	15,470
Baseline-4	91,203,498	95.30%	87,519,976	70,759,871	54,612,207	77.20%	15,642
Dying-1	106,182,528	95.20%	101,728,266	83,553,821	57,816,273	69.20%	15,563
Dying-2	93,997,436	95.20%	90,503,598	74,471,193	60,365,900	81.10%	15,101
Dying-3	118,901,914	94.90%	91,408,790	73,952,809	57,686,330	78.00%	15,712
Dying-4	84,848,674	95.30%	81,623,206	67,004,468	55,869,637	83.40%	15,343
Failure-1	80,262,120	95.20%	76,885,638	63,014,127	49,808,658	79.00%	15,297
Failure-2	100,438,952	95.30%	100,291,397	82,963,827	68,021,072	82.00%	15,812
Failure-3	86,394,661	94.90%	66,295,638	54,080,154	38,129,055	70.50%	15,228
Failure-4	99,697,480	94.80%	95,927,678	79,312,204	60,637,999	76.50%	15,404

3.2. Statistical Analysis of PBMC Transcriptome Data. RNA-Seq was performed in a total of 12 samples, with 4 samples in each group (baseline, failure, and dying). More than 9 Gb sequence data was the yield in each sample. Overall, 80.3–122.5 million raw reads per sample were generated with the quality of over 94.8% Q20, in which 66.3–118.0 million were clean reads.

A total of 54.1–83.5 million reads were mapped to the porcine genome, in which 63.4–83.4% fell in genic regions while the remaining were in intergenic regions. 14,990 to 15,812 expressed genes were identified (fragments per kilobase of exon per million mapped reads [FPKM] > 0) in each sample, respectively. Detailed information is presented in Table 2.

3.3. Differential Expression of Genes Associated with the Progression of D-gal-Induced ALF. DEGs during progression of D-gal-induced ALF were identified using Cufflinks (ver. 2.2.1). Genes were identified as significantly different with a false discovery rate (FDR) when the adjusted p value was (<0.05) and a greater than twofold log change was evident. Compared to the baseline group, 816 DEGs (Supplementary Table 1) were identified in the failure group and 1,845 DEGs (Supplementary Table 2) were identified in the dying group. A total of 590 identified genes overlapped between the two groups. Details are presented in Figure 1.

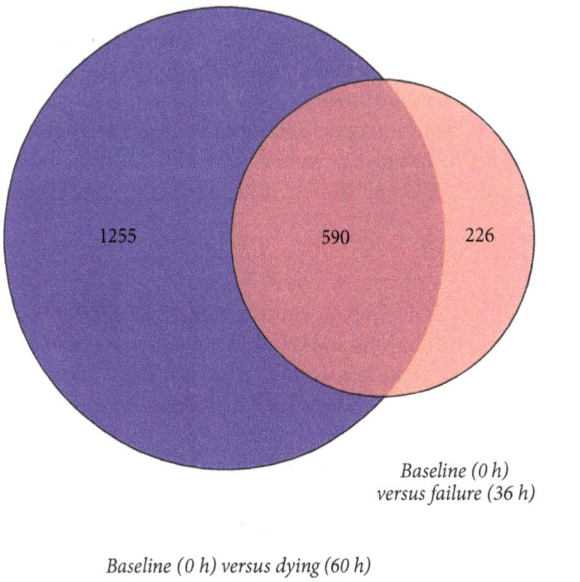

Figure 1: Differential expression of genes involved in the progression of acute liver failure (ALF).

3.4. Progression of D-gal-Induced ALF: GO Analysis. GO enrichment analysis and term clustering were performed to identify DEGs in the failure and dying groups as compared to the baseline group. In total, 107 GO terms were enriched for DEGs identified in the failure group, of which 76 were within the biological process (BP) category, 15 were within the cellular component (CC) category, and 16 were within the molecular function (MF) category. Among these GO terms, 26 were grouped into five independent clusters. The GO terms in the five clusters were related to positive regulation of the inflammatory response, the inflammasome complex, the toll-like receptor (TLR) signalling pathway, cell chemotaxis, and semaphorin receptor activity. With the exception of predominantly innate immune-related terms, important GO terms related to cell death were also enriched for processes such as apoptosis and pyroptosis. GO terms related to autophagy, another type of programmed cell death, were also identified. These terms are the regulation of autophagy, phagocytic vesicles, and lysosomes. Terms related to the process of liver fibrosis included gene sets important in the negative regulation of the fibroblast growth factor receptor signalling pathway and semaphorin receptor activity, and so on. Moreover, GO terms related to coagulation dysfunction and hepatic encephalopathy were also enriched, such as blood coagulation, astrocyte development, and the semaphorin-plexin signalling pathway involved in axon guidance, branchiomotor neuron axon guidance, and so on.

In total, 154 GO terms were enriched for the DEGs identified in the dying group, which included 104 BP terms, 25 CC terms, and 25 MF terms. Overall, 20 out of 154 GO terms were included in two clusters. The representative GO terms in these clusters were related to regulation of the inflammatory response and the inflammasome complex. Most enriched GO terms were predominantly immune-related. Other important GO terms were related to cell death, including apoptotic processes, apoptotic-signalling pathways, negative regulation of apoptotic processes, pyroptosis, autophagy, lysosomal membrane, and lysosomal lumen. Fibrosis-related terms such as collagen catabolic processes and collagen binding were also enriched; hepatic encephalopathy-related GO term, astrocyte development, was also enriched.

Details of GO enrichment and clustering are presented in Figure 2.

3.5. KEGG Pathways Involved in the Progression of D-gal-Induced ALF. KEGG pathway mapping was used to study the molecular interactions and relation networks of the identified DEGs participating in metabolism, cellular processes and so on following D-gal-induced ALF. A total of seven KEGG pathways were mapped from DEGs identified in the failure group, all of which overlapped with the 19 identified KEGG pathways in the dying group. The seven KEGG pathways that were common to both included cytokine-cytokine receptor interaction, hematopoietic cell lineage, lysosome, rheumatoid arthritis, malaria, phagosome, and pertussis pathways. The remaining 12 KEGG pathways identified in the dying group were predominantly immune-related pathways, such as the NF-kappa B signalling pathway, the tumour necrosis factor (TNF) signalling pathway, and the complement and coagulation cascade pathways. KEGG pathways of diseases characterised by impaired liver function, such as Chagas disease (American trypanosomiasis), *Salmonella* infection, and Legionellosis, were also mapped using KEGG pathway mapping. Details are presented in Table 3.

3.6. Validation of RNA-Seq Data by qRT-PCR Analysis. To validate the RNA-Seq data, qRT-PCR of 12 selected genes was performed. The forward and reverse pairs of qRT-PCR primers for each gene are listed in Supplementary Table 3. Linear correlation analysis was conducted between the RNA-Seq and qRT-PCR results, which showed that the fold changes were significantly concordant between RNA-Seq and qRT-PCR data ($r = 0.95$, $p < 0.0001$). Results are shown in Figure 3 and Supplementary Table 4.

4. Discussion

ALF is a syndrome characterised by severe coagulopathy due to liver dysfunction and altered consciousness as a result of hepatic encephalopathy [3]. These features of ALF can be revealed at the PBMC level by transcriptome analysis, with the enriched GO term of blood coagulation and the mapped KEGG pathway of complement and coagulation cascades. Vemuganti et al. reported that, in association with hepatic encephalopathy, axon guidance micro-RNA levels changed in the cerebral cortex of a rat model of ALF [14]. In this study, three GO terms—branchiomotor neuron axon guidance, the semaphorin-plexin signalling pathway involved in axon guidance, and the cortical cytoskeleton—were identified. KEGG mapping analysis also identified disease-related KEGG pathways characterised by liver dysfunction, such as malaria, Chagas disease (American trypanosomiasis), *Salmonella* infection, and Legionellosis. The ability of PBMCs to migrate in a transendothelial manner and establish a dialogue between cells in solid organs has been reported previously [15–17]. These findings may explain the transcriptome changes observed in PBMCs that parallel the changes observed in solid organs, such as the liver and brain.

Previous studies have revealed extensive differential gene expression detected in the liver during the progression of ALF [18]. In this study, compared to the baseline group, the number of DEGs identified in the dying group was more extensive than in the failure group (1845 and 816 genes, resp.), which suggests that the cascades identified by PBMC transcriptome analysis change as ALF progresses. In addition, seven common KEGG pathways were identified for DEGs in both the failure and dying groups, which showed that the key pathways triggered by ALF result in further cascades at the transcriptome level.

Systemic inflammatory responses play an important role in the progression of ALF. Several key innate and adaptive immune mechanisms of ALF have been described previously, including acquired neutrophil dysfunction [19, 20], TLR function [21–23], and the important actions of chemokine and cytokine storms [24, 25]. All of these immune-related changes were identified in our GO enrichment and KEGG pathway mapping studies, which included genes involved in neutrophil chemotaxis, the TLR signalling pathway, and the TNF signalling pathway, among others.

Cell death plays an important role in ALF [26, 27]. Apoptosis is a form of hepatocyte death that contributes to

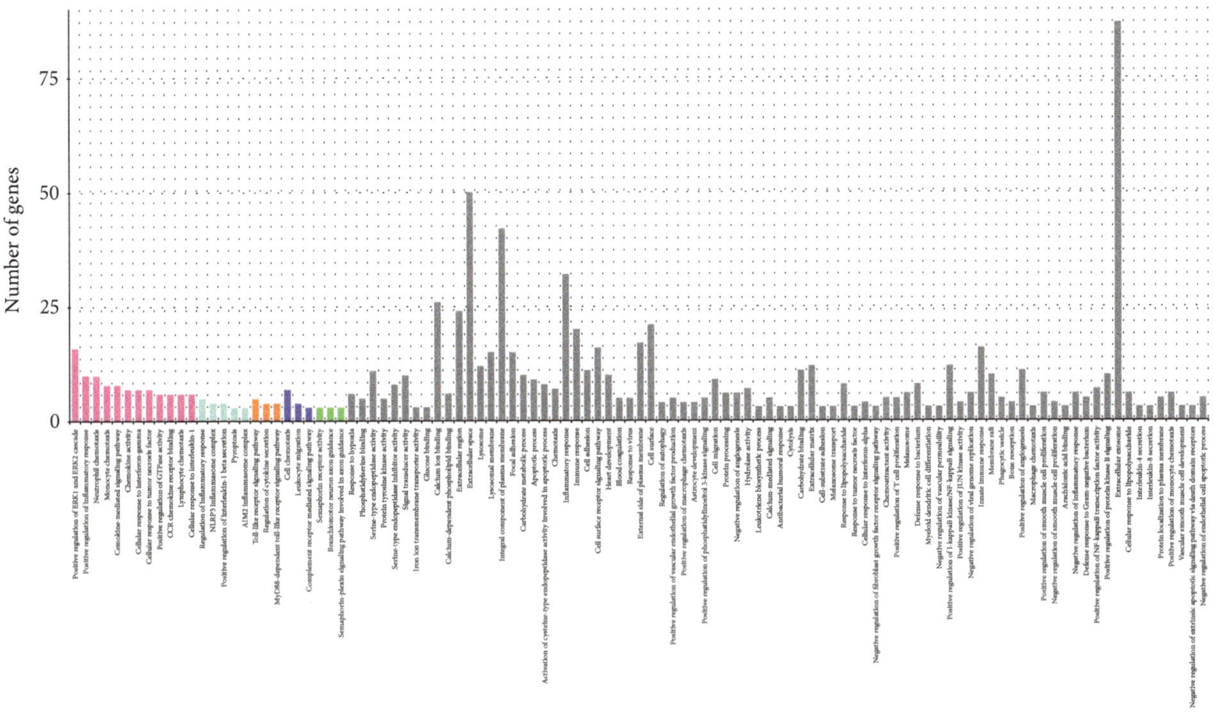

(a)

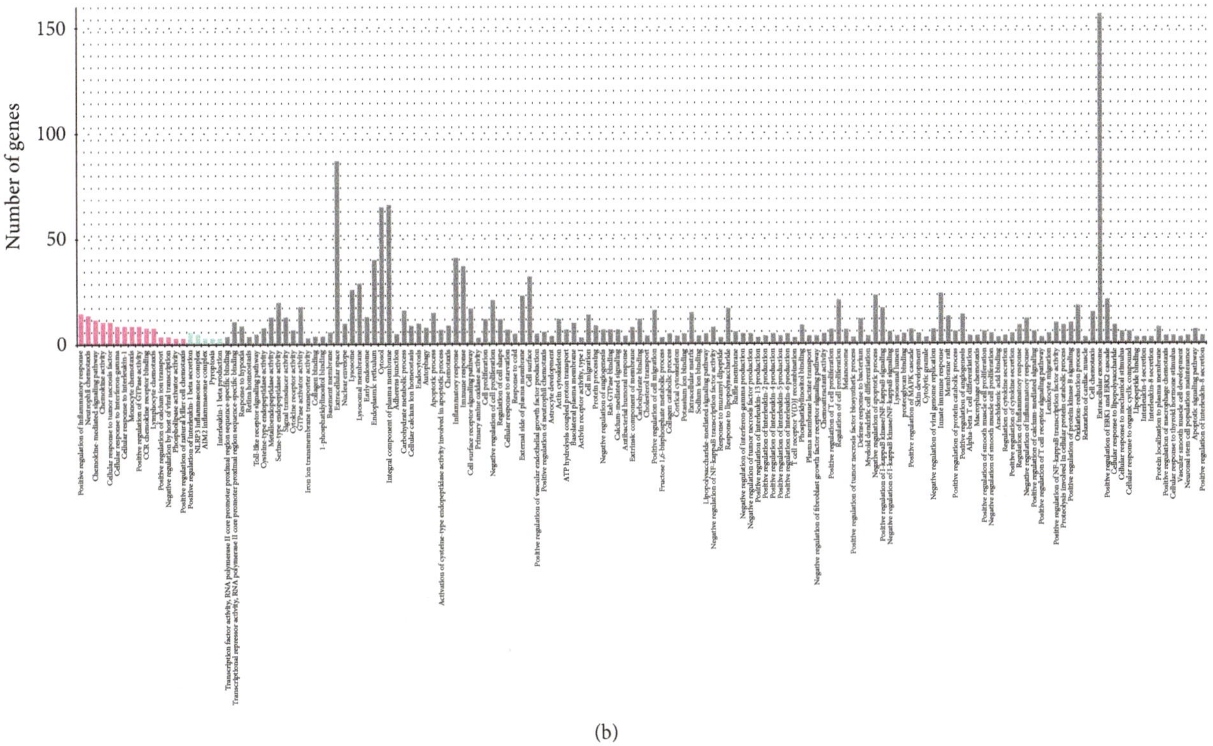

(b)

FIGURE 2: (a) Gene ontology (GO) terms of differentially expressed genes (DEGs) in the failure versus baseline group. (b) GO terms of DEGs in the dying versus baseline group.

ALF [28, 29]. Evidence of apoptotic pathways was identified in our transcriptome analysis. Two GO terms, the apoptotic process and apoptotic-signalling pathways, were enriched. Apart from apoptosis, recent research has focused on a new form of proinflammatory cell death known as pyroptosis [30]. Until now, studies on pyroptosis in ALF have been limited [31, 32]. Furthermore, to the best of our knowledge, a role for pyroptosis in drug-induced ALF has not been reported previously. The enrichment of pyroptosis GO terms following D-gal-induced ALF suggests that pyroptosis is an important

TABLE 3: KEGG pathways involved in the progression of ALF.

Name	Failure versus baseline			Dying versus baseline		
	Mapped genes	Fold enrichment	FDR adjusted p	Mapped genes	Fold enrichment	FDR adjusted p
Cytokine-cytokine receptor interaction	25	3.0	$4.3E-04$	38	2.5	$3.0E-05$
Hematopoietic cell lineage	13	4.4	$3.8E-03$	15	2.7	$2.1E-02$
Lysosome	14	3.2	$2.1E-02$	34	4.2	$2.9E-10$
Rheumatoid arthritis	12	3.7	$2.3E-02$	21	3.5	$7.0E-05$
Malaria	9	4.6	$2.6E-02$	14	3.9	$1.4E-03$
Phagosome	15	2.7	$3.9E-02$	26	2.5	$1.1E-03$
Pertussis	10	3.7	$4.4E-02$	20	3.9	$4.0E-05$
NF-kappa B signaling pathway				19	3.1	$1.3E-03$
Transcriptional misregulation in cancer				26	2.4	$1.6E-03$
Chagas disease (American trypanosomiasis)				20	2.7	$3.3E-03$
Leishmaniasis				14	3.3	$6.6E-03$
TNF signaling pathway				19	2.5	$8.5E-03$
Salmonella infection				16	2.8	$8.8E-03$
Complement and coagulation cascades				14	2.8	$2.1E-02$
Mineral absorption				10	3.4	$3.1E-02$
Osteoclast differentiation				20	2.2	$3.2E-02$
Legionellosis				12	2.8	$4.4E-02$
Pentose phosphate pathway				7	4.6	$4.6E-02$
Histidine metabolism				7	4.6	$4.6E-02$

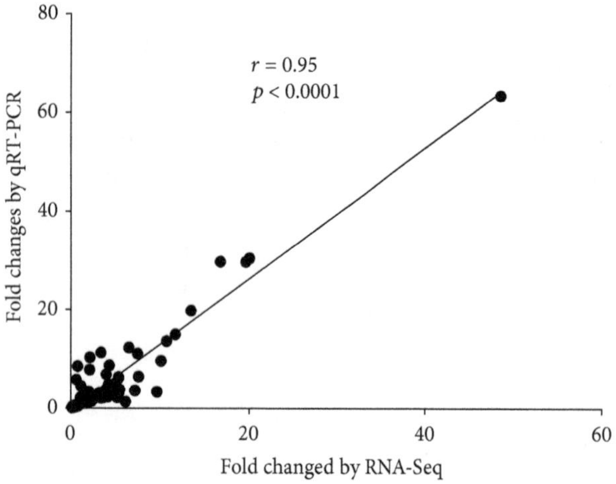

FIGURE 3: Correlation of gene fold changes between RNA-sequencing (RNA-Seq) and qRT-PCR analysis.

route to cell death in a model of drug-induced ALF and therefore merits further study. In addition to pyroptosis, necrapoptosis, also known as aponecrosis or apoptotic necrosis, is an important proinflammatory cell death pattern that shared common features and pathways with both apoptosis and necrosis [33, 34]. Also, this cell death pattern was found in liver injury [35, 36]. The necrapoptosis GO term or KEGG pathway was not enriched or mapped in this study. The possible reason might be that this cell demise pattern has not been annotated in databases of GO (http://geneontology.org/) and KEGG (http://www.kegg.jp/), for we cannot retrieve it in either of two databases so far. However, GO term, the adenosine triphosphate (ATP) hydrolysis coupled proton transport, was enriched in this study. ATP has been proved as a key factor to determine the way out of necrapoptosis [34]. This might verify from another aspect in transcriptome level that necrapoptosis is an important cell death pattern involved in the progression of ALF.

Autophagy is a lysosomal pathway tasked with the process of self-degradation of cellular components by the sequestration of these components in double-membrane autophagosomes [37]. It has been widely reported that autophagy plays an important role in cancer and other chronic diseases of the organs [38–42]. Autophagy is an important current research topic in models of liver disease [43–45]. However, currently there are limited data on the role of autophagy in the progression of ALF [46, 47]. In this study, GO terms such as autophagy, regulation of autophagy, and phagocytic-vehicle were all enriched. Two KEGG pathways of lysosomal and phagosome regulation were mapped. These results provide another potential avenue of transcriptome-level research on the influence of autophagy on the progression of ALF.

The role of fibrosis in the progression of chronic liver disease has been widely studied. Although fibrosis is observed in ALF [48], an understanding of the underlying mechanisms remains limited. GO terms related to the collagen-related component of liver fibrosis, such as collagen catabolic processes and collagen binding, were also enriched in this study. Semaphorin families are regulators of the progression of fibrosis in chronic liver diseases [49, 50]. However, the role of semaphorin families in ALF remains unknown. Semaphorin receptor activity GO terms were also found in this study, which constitutes another interesting avenue for research.

In conclusion, this study identified dramatic changes in the PBMC transcriptome predominantly related to immune responses in ALF. Enriched GO terms related to coagulation dysfunction, hepatic encephalopathy, and mapped KEGG pathways of diseases characterised by liver injury demonstrated that the PBMC transcriptome reflects the features of ALF. The enrichment of GO terms related to cell death and fibrosis indicates that PBMC transcriptome analysis is a useful method to elucidate potential key gene sets involved in ALF progression. Thus, a better understanding of the gene sets identified in this study may contribute to ALF prevention or treatment.

Authors' Contributions

YiMin Zhang and Li Shao contributed equally to this paper; LanJuan Li and YiMin Zhang designed the study; YiMin Zhang, Ning Zhou, JianZhou Li, Yu Chen, and Juan Lu performed experiments; Li Shao, ErMei Chen, Jie Wang, and ZhongYang Xie collected the data. YiMin Zhang and Li Shao analysed the data and wrote the paper.

Acknowledgments

This work was supported by China National Science and Technology Major Project, no. 2017ZX10202202; National Natural Science Foundation of China, no. 81600497; and Zhejiang CTM Science and Technology Project, no. 2011ZB061.

References

[1] J. Polson and W. M. Lee, "AASLD position paper: The management of acute liver failure," *Hepatology*, vol. 41, no. 5, pp. 1179–1197, 2005.

[2] S. L. Flamm, Y.-X. Yang, S. Singh et al., "American Gastroenterological Association Institute Guidelines for the Diagnosis and Management of Acute Liver Failure," *Gastroenterology*, vol. 152, no. 3, pp. 644–647, 2017.

[3] J. Wendon, J. Cordoba, A. Dhawan et al., "EASL clinical practical guidelines on the management of acute (fulminant) liver failure," *Journal of Hepatology*, vol. 66, no. 5, pp. 1047–1081, 2017.

[4] T. A. Skvortsov, D. V. Ignatov, K. B. Majorov, A. S. Apt, and T. L. Azhikina, "Mycobacterium tuberculosis transcriptome profiling in mice with genetically different susceptibility to tuberculosis," *Acta Naturae*, vol. 5, no. 17, pp. 62–69, 2013.

[5] H. Kalam, M. F. Fontana, and D. Kumar, "Alternate splicing of transcripts shape macrophage response to Mycobacterium tuberculosis infection," *PLoS Pathogens*, vol. 13, no. 3, Article ID e1006236, 2017.

[6] C. Rippe, B. Zhu, K. K. Krawczyk et al., "Hypertension reduces soluble guanylyl cyclase expression in the mouse aorta via the Notch signaling pathway," *Scientific Reports*, vol. 7, no. 1, article no. 1334, 2017.

[7] J. Chesne, R. Danger, K. Botturi et al., "Systematic analysis of blood cell transcriptome in EndStage chronic respiratory diseases," *PLoS ONE*, vol. 9, no. 10, Article ID e109291, 2014.

[8] S. Tattermusch, J. A. Skinner, D. Chaussabel et al., "Systems biology approaches reveal a specific interferon-inducible signature in HTLV-1 associated myelopathy," *PLoS Pathogens*, vol. 8, no. 1, Article ID e1002480, 2012.

[9] T. D. Querec, R. S. Akondy, E. K. Lee et al., "Systems biology approach predicts immunogenicity of the yellow fever vaccine in humans," *Nature Immunology*, vol. 10, no. 1, pp. 116–125, 2009.

[10] J. S. Tsang, P. L. Schwartzberg, Y. Kotliarov et al., "Global analyses of human immune variation reveal baseline predictors of postvaccination responses," *Cell*, vol. 157, no. 2, pp. 499–513, 2014.

[11] N. Zhou, J. Li, Y. Zhang et al., "Efficacy of coupled low-volume plasma exchange with plasma filtration adsorption in treating pigs with acute liver failure: a randomised study," *Journal of Hepatology*, vol. 63, no. 2, pp. 378–387, 2015.

[12] C. Trapnell, A. Roberts, L. Goff et al., "Differential gene and transcript expression analysis of RNA-seq experiments with TopHat and Cufflinks," *Nature Protocols*, vol. 7, no. 3, pp. 562–578, 2012.

[13] D. W. Huang, B. T. Sherman, and R. A. Lempicki, "Systematic and integrative analysis of large gene lists using DAVID bioinformatics resources," *Nature Protocols*, vol. 4, no. 1, pp. 44–57, 2009.

[14] R. Vemuganti, V. R. Silva, S. L. Mehta, and A. S. Hazell, "Acute liver failure-induced hepatic encephalopathy is associated with changes in microRNA expression profiles in cerebral cortex of the rat," *Metabolic Brain Disease*, vol. 29, no. 4, pp. 891–899, 2014.

[15] R. B. Meeker, D. C. Bragg, W. Poulton, and L. Hudson, "Transmigration of macrophages across the choroid plexus epithelium in response to the feline immunodeficiency virus," *Cell and Tissue Research*, vol. 347, no. 2, pp. 443–455, 2012.

[16] Y. Huang, X.-Y. Zhu, M.-R. Du, and D.-J. Li, "Human trophoblasts recruited T lymphocytes and monocytes into decidua by secretion of chemokine CXCL16 and interaction with CXCR6 in the first-trimester pregnancy," *The Journal of Immunology*, vol. 180, no. 4, pp. 2367–2375, 2008.

[17] T. Zhang, L. Tian, G. Hu, K. Teng, and X. Mu, "Microvascular endothelial cells play potential immunoregulatory roles in the immune response to foot-and-mouth disease vaccines," *Cell Biochemistry & Function*, vol. 29, no. 5, pp. 394–399, 2011.

[18] F. Chen, H.-H. Zhu, L.-F. Zhou et al., "Genes related to the very early stage of ConA-induced fulminant hepatitis: A gene-chip-based study in a mouse model," *BMC Genomics*, vol. 11, no. 1, article no. 240, 2010.

[19] N. J. Taylor, A. Nishtala, G. K. Manakkat Vijay et al., "Circulating neutrophil dysfunction in acute liver failure," *Hepatology*, vol. 57, no. 3, pp. 1142–1152, 2013.

[20] P. E. Marques, S. S. Amaral, D. A. Pires et al., "Chemokines and mitochondrial products activate neutrophils to amplify organ injury during mouse acute liver failure," *Hepatology*, vol. 56, no. 5, pp. 1971–1982, 2012.

[21] S. Zhang, N. Yang, S. Ni et al., "Pretreatment of lipopolysaccharide (LPS) ameliorates D-GalN/LPS induced acute liver failure through TLR4 signaling pathway," *International Journal of Clinical and Experimental Pathology*, vol. 7, no. 10, pp. 6626–6634, 2014.

[22] N. Shah, M. Montes De Oca, M. Jover-Cobos et al., "Role of toll-like receptor 4 in mediating multiorgan dysfunction in mice with acetaminophen induced acute liver failure," *Liver Transplantation*, vol. 19, no. 7, pp. 751–761, 2013.

[23] R. Sehgal, S. Patra, P. David et al., "Impaired monocyte-macrophage functions and defective toll-like receptor signaling in hepatitis E virus-infected pregnant women with acute liver failure," *Hepatology*, vol. 62, no. 6, pp. 1683–1696, 2015.

[24] L. Collin, P. Moulin, M. Jungers, and A. P. Geubel, "Epstein-Barr virus (EBV)-induced liver failure in the absence of extensive liver-cell necrosis: A case for cytokine-induced liver dysfunction?" *Journal of Hepatology*, vol. 41, no. 1, pp. 174-175, 2004.

[25] J. Li, X. Zhu, F. Liu et al., "Cytokine and autoantibody patterns in acute liver failure," *Journal of Immunotoxicology*, vol. 7, no. 3, pp. 157–164, 2010.

[26] Z. Cao, F. Li, X. Xiang et al., "Circulating cell death biomarker: Good candidates of prognostic indicator for patients with hepatitis B virus related acute-on-chronic liver failure," *Scientific Reports*, vol. 5, Article ID 14240, 2015.

[27] H. Bantel and K. Schulze-Osthoff, "Mechanisms of cell death in acute liver failure," *Frontiers in Physiology*, vol. 3, article no. 79, 2012.

[28] J. An, C. Harms, G. Lättig-Tünnemann et al., "TAT-apoptosis repressor with caspase recruitment domain protein transduction rescues mice from fulminant liver failure," *Hepatology*, vol. 56, no. 2, pp. 715–726, 2012.

[29] P. Zhang, M. Zhang, M. Wan et al., "Tamoxifen Attenuates Lipopolysaccharide/Galactosamine-induced acute liver failure by antagonizing hepatic inflammation and apoptosis," *Immunological Investigations*, vol. 46, no. 3, pp. 284–294, 2017.

[30] K. R. Bortoluci and R. Medzhitov, "Control of infection by pyroptosis and autophagy: Role of TLR and NLR," *Cellular and Molecular Life Sciences*, vol. 67, no. 10, pp. 1643–1651, 2010.

[31] Y. Geng, Q. Ma, Y.-N. Liu et al., "Heatstroke induces liver injury via IL-1β and HMGB1-induced pyroptosis," *Journal of Hepatology*, vol. 63, no. 3, article no. 5648, pp. 622–633, 2015.

[32] Y. L. Chen, G. Xu, X. Liang et al., "Inhibition of hepatic cells pyroptosis attenuates CLP-induced acute liver injury," *American journal of translational research*, vol. 8, no. 12, pp. 5685-95, 2016.

[33] L. Formigli, L. Papucci, A. Tani et al., "Aponecrosis: morphological and biochemical exploration of a syncretic process of cell death sharing apoptosis and necrosis," *Journal of Cellular Physiology*, vol. 182, no. 1, pp. 41–49, 2000.

[34] J. J. Lemasters, T. Qian, L. He et al., "Role of mitochondrial inner membrane permeabilization in necrotic cell death, apoptosis, and autophagy," *Antioxidants & Redox Signaling*, vol. 4, no. 5, pp. 769–781, 2002.

[35] A. M. El-Gibaly, C. Scheuer, M. D. Menger, and B. Vollmar, "Improvement of rat liver graft quality by pifithrin-α-mediated inhibition of hepatocyte necrapoptosis," *Hepatology*, vol. 39, no. 6, pp. 1553–1562, 2004.

[36] H. Jaeschke and J. J. Lemasters, "Apoptosis versus oncotic necrosis in hepatic ischemia/reperfusion injury," *Gastroenterology*, vol. 125, no. 4, pp. 1246–1257, 2003.

[37] C. He and D. J. Klionsky, "Regulation mechanisms and signaling pathways of autophagy," *Annual Review of Genetics*, vol. 43, pp. 67–93, 2009.

[38] Z. Zhong, E. Sanchez-Lopez, and M. Karin, "Autophagy, inflammation, and immunity: a troika governing cancer and its treatment," *Cell*, vol. 166, no. 2, pp. 288–298, 2016.

[39] J. Moscat and M. T. Diaz-Meco, "p62 at the crossroads of autophagy, apoptosis, and cancer," *Cell*, vol. 137, no. 6, pp. 1001–1004, 2009.

[40] Z. V. Wang, B. A. Rothermel, and J. A. Hill, "Autophagy in hypertensive heart disease," *The Journal of Biological Chemistry*, vol. 285, no. 12, pp. 8509–8514, 2010.

[41] T. Kimura, Y. Isaka, and T. Yoshimori, "Autophagy and kidney inflammation," *Autophagy*, vol. 13, no. 6, pp. 997–1003, 2017.

[42] K. Mizumura, S. Cloonan, and M. E. Choi, "Autophagy: Friend or Foe in Lung Disease?" *Annals of the American Thoracic Society*, vol. 13, 1, pp. S40–S47, 2016.

[43] X.-M. Yin, W.-X. Ding, and W. Gao, "Autophagy in the liver," *Hepatology*, vol. 47, no. 5, pp. 1773–1785, 2008.

[44] C. Zhang and A. M. Cuervo, "Restoration of chaperone-mediated autophagy in aging liver improves cellular maintenance and hepatic function," *Nature Medicine*, vol. 14, no. 9, pp. 959–965, 2008.

[45] P.-E. Rautou, A. Mansouri, D. Lebrec, F. Durand, D. Valla, and R. Moreau, "Autophagy in liver diseases," *Journal of Hepatology*, vol. 53, no. 6, pp. 1123–1134, 2010.

[46] F. Ren, L. Zhang, X. Zhang et al., "Inhibition of glycogen synthase kinase 3beta promotes autophagy to protect mice from acute liver failure mediated by peroxisome proliferator-activated receptor alpha," *Cell death & disease*, vol. 7, article e2151, 2016.

[47] L. Jin, H. Gao, J. Wang et al., "Role and regulation of autophagy and apoptosis by nitric oxide in hepatic stellate cells during acute liver failure," *Liver International*, vol. 37, no. 11, pp. 1651–1659, 2017.

[48] Y. He, L. Jin, J. Wang, Z. Yan, T. Chen, and Y. Zhao, "Mechanisms of fibrosis in acute liver failure," *Liver International*, vol. 35, no. 7, pp. 1877–1885, 2015.

[49] T. Yagai, A. Miyajima, and M. Tanaka, "Semaphorin 3E secreted by damaged hepatocytes regulates the sinusoidal regeneration and liver fibrosis during liver regeneration," *The American Journal of Pathology*, vol. 184, no. 8, pp. 2250–2259, 2014.

[50] S. De Minicis, C. Rychlicki, L. Agostinelli et al., "Semaphorin 7A contributes to TGF-β-mediated liver fibrogenesis," *The American Journal of Pathology*, vol. 183, no. 3, pp. 820–830, 2013.

13

Choosing an Animal Model for the Study of Functional Dyspepsia

Yang Ye,[1,2] Xue-Rui Wang,[1] Yang Zheng,[1] Jing-Wen Yang,[1] Na-Na Yang,[1,2] Guang-Xia Shi,[1] and Cun-Zhi Liu[1]

[1] *Acupuncture and Moxibustion Department, Beijing Hospital of Traditional Chinese Medicine Affiliated to Capital Medical University, Beijing Key Laboratory of Acupuncture Neuromodulation, Beijing, China*
[2] *Beijing University of Chinese Medicine, Beijing, China*

Correspondence should be addressed to Cun-Zhi Liu; lcz623780@126.com

Academic Editor: Yousuke Nakai

Functional dyspepsia (FD) is a common functional gastrointestinal disorder with pain or discomfort in the upper abdomen as the main characteristic. The prevalence of FD worldwide varies between 5% and 11%. This condition adversely affects attendance and productivity in the workplace. Emerging evidence is beginning to unravel the pathophysiologies of FD, and new data on treatment are helping to guide evidence-based practice. In order to better understand the pathophysiologies of FD and explore better treatment options, various kinds of animal models of FD have been developed. However, it is unclear which of these models most closely mimic the human disease. This review provides a comprehensive overview of the currently available animal models of FD in relationship to the clinical features of the disease. The rationales, methods, merits, and disadvantages for modelling specific symptoms of FD are discussed in detail.

1. Introduction

Functional dyspepsia (FD) is a highly prevalent gastrointestinal disorder that is clinically characterized by diverse symptomatology including a sensation of pain or burning in the epigastrium, postprandial fullness, early satiety, bloating, and nausea [1]. The global prevalence of uninvestigated dyspepsia in adults is 20.8%, but this figure varies depending on the geographical location and the definition of disease [2]. Although the pathological mechanisms underlying FD have not yet been fully elucidated, existing research indicates that the etiology of FD is multifactorial. Delayed gastric emptying, impaired gastric fundus accommodation, visceral hypersensitivity, and various psychosocial factors are considered to be the major pathophysiologic disturbances of FD [3].

Animal models have been extensively used to determine pathological mechanisms and to develop new therapies for human diseases including FD. Many attempts have been performed to model various aspects of FD. Results from these animal studies have benefited our understanding of the pathophysiology of this disease and helped to identify potential therapies [4]. Despite developments in our understanding of FD, scientists around the world have not yet developed a specific treatment or preventive drug for this disorder [5]. Therefore, FD animal models will continue to have a critical role in drug screening and therapy development, which could eventually lead to potential therapeutic strategies for FD patients. Various types of FD animal models are employed in the current preclinical studies [4]. A common question about the FD animal models is which of these models most closely simulate the clinical and pathologic features of the human disease?

In this review article, we will summarize progress that has been made in modelling FD in experimental animals from the perspective of the pathophysiological features and clinical symptoms. The animals used for in vivo FD studies have included rats, mice, and dogs. But here, we will primarily focus on rat models because rats are the most commonly used animals for modelling FD (Table 1). Understanding the fundamental methodology, strengths, and weaknesses of the various kinds of modelling methods will help in the choice of the most suitable model for a particular purpose and question of interest. Furthermore, we will propose developmental directions of FD animal model for future studies.

2. Pathophysiological Features of FD

2.1. Delayed Gastric Emptying. Delayed gastric emptying is considered to be a pathophysiological feature of FD that is closely related to dyspepsia symptoms [41]. A study showed that the prevalence of delayed emptying in FD patients ranges between 20 and 35% [42]. When food moves to the small intestine FD symptoms including fullness, bloating, and belching develop [43]. Many prokinetic agents have been used in the treatment of FD, such as cisapride, domperidone, and itopride [44].

2.2. Impaired Gastric Fundic Accommodation. Gastric accommodation is mediated by the activation of noncholinergic nerves in the gastric wall that result in the production and diffusion of nitric oxide to gastric smooth muscles [45]. Impaired gastric fundic accommodation, a vagal reflex, refers to slow gastric emptying and the failure of the gastric fundus to reflex after a meal [46]. Impaired accommodation is a frequently encountered pathophysiological abnormality in FD [47]. Research has shown that 40% of dyspeptic patients have impaired accommodation, and this is associated with early satiety and weight loss [48].

2.3. Visceral Hypersensitivity. Visceral hypersensitivity has been considered to play an important role in the generation of FD symptoms [49]. Data show that 30% of patients with functional dyspepsia have evidence of hypersensitivity to gastric distention [50]. In addition, the duodenum is recognized as a site involved in symptom generation in FD through increased sensitivity to acid and lipids [51]. Visceral hypersensitivity may result from alterations in the peripheral or central nervous system and the etiology is complex [52]. Stimuli including hollow organ distension, inflammation, traction on the mesentery, and ischemia may lead to visceral hypersensitivity under the pathological circumstances [53]. Visceral hypersensitivity to distention in FD is associated with symptoms of early satiety, abdominal pain, postprandial pain, excessive belching, nausea, and unexplained weight loss [54].

2.4. Psychological Distress. Psychological distress including anxiety and depression is related to FD and may precede the onset of FD in some people [55]. The relationship of FD with anxiety and depression is complex and may be associated with processing of negative stimulus in the central nervous system and brain-gut axis [56]. The detection rates of depression and anxiety symptoms in patients with functional dyspepsia are 34.36% and 25.55%, respectively [57]. Because of the potential role of psychological distress in FD, antidepressants have been recommended as a therapy [3].

3. Drug Administration Animal Models

3.1. Clonidine Injection

Rationale. Sympathetic and parasympathetic control of gastric motility is a classic example of norepinephrine and acetylcholine triggering opposing actions [58, 59]. It is well known that both norepinephrine and acetylcholine are important regulators of gastrointestinal motility, and inhibition to acetylcholine degradation has been reported to enhance gastric motility [6]. As an α_2-adrenoceptor agonist, clonidine is used to suppress the release of acetylcholine from cholinergic neurons. This could ultimately lead to hypomotility, delayed gastric emptying, and intestinal transit [60, 61].

Methods. In the clonidine-induced motility dysfunction model, clonidine is subcutaneously administered to animals [7].

Features. Clonidine injection mainly leads to motility dysfunction including hypomotility and delayed gastric emptying by inhibiting acetylcholine activity [6–8]. There are no reports to suggest that this model could be used to induce other pathological features of FD, such as impaired fundic accommodation or visceral hypersensitivity. In addition, the motility dysfunction caused by clonidine is temporary in animals, so gastrointestinal motility should be evaluated shortly after the clonidine administration. Therefore, this is a transitory FD animal model which specifically focuses on the gastrointestinal motility dysfunction.

3.2. Atropine Injection

Rationale. The effects of acetylcholine on gastrointestinal contractility are mainly regulated by muscarinic acetylcholine receptors [62]. So the activity of muscarinic acetylcholine receptors is directly tied to the gastrointestinal motility [63]. Atropine, a muscarinic acetylcholine receptor antagonist, could be used to induce delay in gastrointestinal transit [10].

Methods. Different methods exist to establish an atropine-induced FD animal model. Atropine can be injected subcutaneously or intraperitoneally to make a delayed gastrointestinal transit model [10, 11].

Features. This is another motility dysfunction model that exerts its effect by directly acting on the cholinergic system. It also persists for a short time and only induces delayed gastrointestinal transit.

3.3. Dopamine Injection

Rationale. Dopamine inhibits acetylcholine release and gastric motility and it has been proposed as a possible neurotransmitter in gastric relaxation [64, 65]. The effect of dopamine has been thought to be mediated through the dopamine-2 receptor and dopamine-3 receptor [65]. Therefore, dopamine could be used to induce delayed gastric emptying in FD animal studies.

Table 1: Animal models of functional dyspepsia.

Approach	Species	Mechanism	Pharmacologic action	T/C	Year	Reference
Drug administration animal models						
Clonidine injection	SD rats, ICR mice, Beagle dogs	α2-Adrenoceptor agonists	Delays gastric emptying and intestinal transit	T	2011, 2012, 2015, 2016	[2, 6–9]
Atropine injection	SD rats, ICR mice	Muscarinic acetylcholine receptor antagonists	Delays gastrointestinal transit	T	2008, 2012	[10, 11]
Dopamine injection	ICR mice	Dopamine agonists	Delays gastric emptying	T	2012, 2016	[9, 10]
Apomorphine injection	SD rats, ICR mice	Dopamine receptor agonists	Delays gastric emptying	T	2008, 2010, 2011, 2015	[2, 11–13]
5-HT injection	ICR mice	5-HT agonists	Delays gastric emptying and reduces small intestinal motility	T	2012	[10]
5-HT_3 receptor agonist injection	ICR mice	5-HT receptor agonists	Delays gastric emptying and reduces small intestinal motility	T	2012	[10]
CRF injection	SD rats	Stress hormone	Delays gastric emptying	T	2012	[14]
Cisplatin injection	SD rats, Swiss mice	Gastrointestinal side effects	Delays gastric emptying	T	2008, 2012	[11, 15]
Soybean oil administration	SD rats	Gastric motility	Delays gastric emptying	T	2012	[14]
Neonatal intervention animal models						
Neonatal gastric irritation	SD rats	Mild gastritis in early life	Delays gastric emptying, induces gastric hypersensitivity, impairs accommodation, increases depressive and anxious behaviors	C	2008, 2011, 2014, 2017,	[16–21]
Neonatal colon inflammation	SD rats	Colitis in early life	Delays gastric emptying, induces gastric hypersensitivity, increases depressive behaviors	C	2013, 2016, 2017	[21–24]
Neonatal maternal separation	Wistar rats	Childhood trauma	Delays gastric emptying	C	2015, 2016	[25, 26]
Stress stimulation animal models						
Restraint stress	Wistar rats, ICR mice,	Chronic stresses	Delays gastric emptying	C	2008, 2015	[2, 26–28]
Water-immersion restraint stress	SD rats, Wistar rats	Acute stresses	Delays gastric emptying	T	2013, 2016	[25, 29]
Tail clamping	SD rats, Wistar rats	Chronic stresses	Delays gastric emptying, increases anxious behaviors	C	2011, 2016	[30–32]
CMUS	SD rats	Chronic stresses	Increases depressive behaviors	C	2017	[33]
Other intervention animal models						
Gastric distension	Wistar rats	Abdominal muscle	Induces visceral hyperalgesia	C	2011	[34]
Laparotomy	SD rats	Local inflammation	Delays gastrointestinal transit	C	2008, 2015	[11, 35]
Duodenal acidification	SD rats	Duodenum	Induces gastric hypersensitivity	T	2014	[36]
Chronic high-fat feeding	SD rats	Gastric motility	Delays gastric emptying	C	2015	[37]

Table 1: Continued.

Approach	Species	Mechanism	Pharmacologic action	T/C	Year	Reference
Special species animal models						
FSL rats	FSL rats	Genetic depression	Delays gastric emptying, impairs accommodation, increases depressive behaviors	C	2005	[38]
WKY rats	WKY rats	Genetic anxiety	Impairs accommodation, increases anxious behaviors	C	2007	[39]
BB-DP rats	BB-DP rats	Genetic impaired accommodation	Impairs gastric accommodation	C	2014	[40]
Compound factors animal models						
Neonatal colon inflammation followed by adult gastric irritation	SD rats	Colitis in early life and gastritis	Delays gastric emptying, induces gastric hypersensitivity, increases depressive behaviors	C	2017	[21]
Neonatal maternal separation followed by adult restraint stress	Wistar rats	Childhood trauma and chronic stresses	Delays gastric emptying	C	2015, 2016	[25, 26]

T, temporary; C, continuous; SD, Sprague-Dawley; ICR, Institute of Cancer Research; 5-HT, 5-Hydroxytryptamine; CRF, corticotropin-releasing factor; CMUS, chronic mild unpredictable stimulation; FSL, Flinders Sensitive Line; WKY, Wistar Kyoto; BB-DP, BioBreeding diabetes-prone.

Methods. In this model, dopamine is intraperitoneally administered to animals [9, 10].

Features. This is also a transient delayed gastric emptying FD model. As dopamine is degraded, the delayed gastric emptying will return to normal again.

3.4. Apomorphine Injection

Rationale. Dopamine delays gastric emptying, and inhibiting the effect of dopamine is achieved by activating dopamine receptors [65]. As a dopamine receptor agonist, apomorphine inhibits gastrointestinal motor function [12, 66].

Methods. Animals are subcutaneously injected with apomorphine to induce delayed gastric emptying [12, 13].

Features. This model is similar to the dopamine-induced delayed gastric emptying model. It could be used as a FD model when gastric motility needs to be evaluated.

3.5. 5-Hydroxytryptamine Injection

Rationale. 5-Hydroxytryptamine (5-HT) plays an important role in the regulation of gastrointestinal motility [67]. Gastrointestinal contraction amplitude is increased by 5-HT primarily via a cholinergic pathway. Furthermore, $5HT_3$ receptors and $5HT_1$-like and/or $5HT_{2C}$ receptors are responsible for 5HT-induced gastrointestinal contractions [67].

Methods. In this model, 5-HT is intraperitoneally injected into animals [10].

Features. 5-HT is used to induce reductions in gastric emptying and small intestinal motility. It is a short-term FD model which only concentrates on impaired gastrointestinal motility.

3.6. 5-HT3 Receptor Agonist Injection

Rationale. One of the most well-established physiological roles of the $5\text{-}HT_3$ receptor is to regulate gastrointestinal motility [68]. 5HT-induced inhibition of gastrointestinal dynamics might be partially achieved via $5HT_3$ receptors [67]. $5\text{-}HT_3$ receptor agonists suppress gastric emptying and gastrointestinal motility [10].

Methods. A $5\text{-}HT_3$ receptor agonist is intraperitoneally injected into animals to induce a reduction in gastric emptying and small intestinal motility [10].

Features. This model is similar to the 5-HT-induced delayed gastric emptying model. The motility of the small intestine is reduced by $5\text{-}HT_3$ receptor agonist injection [10]. In another study, m-chlorophenylbiguanide (m-CPBG) was employed to induce a FD animal model as a selective $5\text{-}HT_3$ receptor agonist [9].

3.7. Corticotropin-Releasing Factor Injection

Rationale. Acute stress induces a delay in gastric emptying through a peripheral sympathetic pathway [69]. Corticotropin-releasing factor (CRF), a pituitary hormone secreted in response to stress, is closely related to stress-induced abnormal colonic responses such as stimulation of motility, transit, defecation, and occurrence of diarrhea [70].

Methods. CRF is intravenously injected into animals in this model [14].

Features. Delayed gastric emptying is induced by CRF injection and this effect is temporary. CRF has been reported to be involved in visceral hypersensitivity, but this role of CRF has not been investigated in FD animal studies [70].

3.8. Cisplatin Injection

Rationale. Cisplatin, an effective chemotherapeutic agent that has been widely used in the treatment of various cancers, causes severe side effects on gastrointestinal function such as a delay in gastric emptying as well as nausea and vomiting [11]. Delayed gastrointestinal transit induced by cisplatin could be used to mimic the impaired gastric motility of FD.

Methods. Cisplatin is intraperitoneally injected to animals to induce inhibition of gastric emptying [11, 15].

Features. Cisplatin injection induces delayed gastric emptying, which could be used to mimic the gastrointestinal motility dysfunction of FD, but cisplatin also causes many other serious side effects such as kidney and liver damage, which is a drawback of this method [71, 72].

3.9. Soybean Oil Administration

Rationale. Soybean oil, a common dietary fat, is mostly used for frying and baking. In biomedical science, soybean oil is commonly used to investigate biological reactions to dietary fat [73]. It is known that fat can delay gastric emptying [74, 75]. Soybean oil has been used to induce delayed gastric emptying model [14, 76].

Methods. After the deprivation of food and water, soybean oil is orally administrated to animals [14].

Features. This model uses soybean oil to inhibit gastric emptying in a dose-dependent manner [14].

4. Neonatal Intervention Animal Models

4.1. Neonatal Gastric Irritation

Rationale. This FD model refers to the neonatal administration of a mild irritant, which results in transient superficial sloughing of the gastric epithelium [16]. Iodoacetamide has been reported to cause mild gastritis, along with impairments of gastric sensory and motor function [77, 78]. The neonatal period is a time of known neuronal vulnerability to long-term plasticity [79, 80]. Therefore, gastric irritation with iodoacetamide in the neonatal period leads to gastric hypersensitivity and motor dysfunction that persist into adulthood without significant morphologic and histologic changes in the stomach [16–19].

Methods. In this model, animal pups are given 0.1% iodoacetamide in a sucrose solution by oral gavage daily for six consecutive days. After the gastric irritation, animals are then fed normally until adulthood [16].

Features. Neonatal iodoacetamide treatment early in life induces gastric hypersensitivity, motor dysfunction, and impaired accommodation in adulthood. In addition, gastric irritation in the neonatal period also leads to a long-lasting increase in depression-like and anxiety-like behaviors [20]. Overall, neonatal gastric irritation is a classical and comprehensive method to induce a FD animal model. A clear understanding of the mechanisms responsible for the pathophysiology of this model need to be elucidated in future studies.

4.2. Neonatal Colon Inflammation

Rationale. Trinitrobenzene sulfonic acid (TNBS) induces chronic colonic inflammation in rodent animals [81]. In this pathological process, prostanoid concentrations are increased causing macroscopic and microscopic gastrointestinal lesions [82, 83]. In addition, intraluminal administration of TNBS also induces FD-like gastric hypersensitivity and anxiety behaviors [22, 23]. Early life inflammation leads to a high risk for the development of FD in adulthood [84, 85].

Methods. Animal pups receive TNBS acid in 10% ethanol in saline through a catheter inserted 2 cm into the distal colon on postnatal day 10 without anesthesia. The animals are kept in a head-down position for about 2 minutes during the administration of TNBS and the anus is held closed for 1 minute to prevent leakage of the TNBS solution. Six to eight weeks later, the now-adult animals are used as an FD model [21, 22].

Features. TNBS-induced colon inflammation is a classical method to induce a colitis animal model. This model presents multiple pathological characteristics of FD including gastric hypersensitivity, delayed gastric emptying, and depression-like behaviors [21–24]. Therefore, it is another comprehensive model of FD. Due to the toxicity of TNBS, the mortality rate of neonatal colon inflammation was 4.1% [22].

4.3. Neonatal Maternal Separation

Rationale. Adverse physiological or psychological experiences in early life are associated with the development of FD symptoms [84, 86]. Childhood trauma might lead to a more sensitive response of the hypothalamus-pituitary-adrenal (HPA) axis, motor dysfunction of the gastrointestinal tract, and dyspeptic symptoms in adult FD patients [25]. Neonatal maternal separation is a well-established experimental model of early life stress which has been used in many studies [87, 88].

Methods. Animal pups are removed from their mother's cage and placed in an individual cage for three consecutive hours daily. This process lasts for 12 or 19 days [25, 26]. The pups are returned to their mother cage after maternal separation. On postnatal day 22, all pups are weaned. These animals are used in FD models when they reach adulthood. To avoid hormonal cycle-induced variations, only male pups are used.

Features. Exposure of animals to neonatal maternal separation leads to structural changes in gastric enteric glial cells and a delay in gastric emptying. The effect of inducing FD is limited when neonatal maternal separation is used independently. Therefore, it is better to combine neonatal maternal separation with another method to establish a good FD animal model [25, 26].

5. Stress Stimulation Animal Models

5.1. Restraint Stress

Rationale. Psychological and physiological stresses such as restraint stress have been shown to inhibit antral motility and gastric emptying in animals [89–91]. Delayed gastric emptying is related to the stress-induced sympathetic activation, which is accompanied by increased stress hormones and active ghrelin [26]. Furthermore, stress hormones and active ghrelin play key roles in mediating gastric motility [26, 92].

Methods. Animals are restrained in cylindrical, well-ventilated, and stainless steel tubes for 60 or 90 min once a day for seven days [26–28].

Features. In this model, physiologic and psychological stresses are used to induce feeding inhibition and delayed gastric emptying. Chronic stress is established in this animal model because the stress status lasts for seven days.

5.2. Water-Immersion Restraint Stress

Rationale. Mental and physical stress exert an inhibitory effect on the gastrointestinal tract via various mediators including catecholamine, CRF, and ghrelin [93, 94]. Acute stressors may have profound effects on intestinal epithelial physiology, stimulating ion secretion, and reducing barrier function [95]. The model of water-immersion restraint stress produces both physical and psychological stresses [29].

Methods. The total body of the animal from head to lower hind limbs is tightly placed in cages, and the entire body except the head is immersed vertically to the level of the xiphoid process in a water bath for several hours. The stress session is performed only once [25, 29].

Features. This stress model is reported to increase plasma adrenocorticotrophic hormone (ACTH) and cortisol levels [29]. It also induces delay in gastric emptying [25]. However, this is an acute stress model instead of a chronic stress model, which may differ from human pathophysiology.

5.3. Tail Clamping

Rationale. Stress is found to contribute to gastrointestinal motility disorders [96]. Tail clamping angers animals and causes fighting, which may lead to anxiety-like behaviors and delayed gastric emptying.

Methods. Animals' tails are clamped with sponge forceps distally to anger them and cause fighting. This is performed for 30 minutes at a time, but without injury. This procedure is repeated four times daily for seven continuous days [30–32].

Features. Animals appear dispirited, irritable, nervous, and anxious and lose their appetite after tail clamping. The gastric myoelectrical main frequency, power, and the percentage of slow wave duality of the animals decrease significantly. Tail clamping also induces delay in gastric emptying and an increase in serum nitric oxide [32]. It is another chronic stress model which combines mental and physical stresses.

5.4. Chronic Mild Unpredictable Stimulation

Rationale. Chronic mild unpredictable stimulation (CMUS) is a classical method to induce depression in animals [97]. Patients with FD have been reported to score highly for anxiety and depressive symptoms [57]. The depression-like behaviors due to CMUS are similar to symptoms of some FD patients.

Methods. FD is established through CMUS, which included bondage, swim-induced fatigue, electrical stimulation, fasting, and concussion. The stimulation is performed every day for three continuous weeks [33].

Features. CMUS is a common experimental depression model. This model could be used to focus on depression in FD patients. After CMUS, the weight of animals decreases and the numbers of crossings, cleanings, and stand-up times decrease.

6. Other Intervention Animal Models

6.1. Gastric Distension

Rationale. Visceral hyperalgesia plays an important role in the pathophysiology of FD and may partially result from sensitization of primary afferent fibers innervating the gastrointestinal tract [98]. The visceromotor response to gastric distension could be used to study visceral hyperalgesia in conscious animals. Abdominal muscle contractions in response to balloon gastric distention are regarded as an indicator of visceral pain.

Methods. A flexible latex balloon catheter is surgically placed into the stomach though a small incision. A force transducer is then sutured to the abdominal external oblique muscle to measure the number of abdominal contractions as an indicator of visceral pain sensation [34].

Features. Gastric distension-induced visceromotor response is a special FD model which replicates visceral hyperalgesia for FD. The limitation of this model is that it does not reproduce other aspects of FD, such as delayed gastric emptying, impaired gastric fundic accommodation, and depression-like behaviors.

6.2. Laparotomy

Rationale. Laparotomy followed by intestinal manipulation has been used as a classical method to induce postoperative ileus animal model [99]. After laparotomy and intestinal manipulation, spinal afferents and the motor nucleus of the vagus nerve are activated. They activate many inhibitory pathways involving adrenergic neurons and nitrergic and vipergic neurons, which then reduce the motility of gastrointestinal tract. After the early neurogenic phase, local inflammation becomes the leading cause of continuous gastrointestinal hypomotility [100].

Methods. After a rat is anesthetized, a laparotomy is performed using a three-centimeter midline incision. The small intestine and caecum are gently pulled out of the abdominal cavity and the small intestine is gently manipulated with the fingers for ten minutes. After manipulation, the small intestine and caecum are replaced and the surgical wound is sutured [35].

Features. Laparotomy can be used to establish animal model of delayed gastrointestinal transit. It is easy to perform and the results are reliable. However, this model only mimics impaired gastrointestinal motility of FD.

6.3. Duodenal Acidification

Rationale. Hypersensitivity in gastric perception is considered to be one cause of FD [3]. Clinical studies have shown the involvement of duodenal acidification-induced gastric hypersensitivity in the pathogenesis of FD [101, 102].

Methods. 0.01 mol/L hydrochloric acid (HCl) is infused into the proximal duodenum at a rate of 0.1 ml/min [36].

Features. Duodenal infusion of HCl enhances the gastric nociceptive response in conscious animals. This model is able to accurately mimic the clinical findings of gastric hypersensitivity induced by duodenal acidification.

6.4. Chronic High-Fat Feeding

Rationale. High-fat feeding is relevant to FD and bile acids affect gastrointestinal motility [103, 104]. Increased levels of circulating bile acids induced by chronic high-fat feeding upregulate neuronal nitric oxide synthase (nNOS) and bile acid receptor 1 (TGR5) expression in the gastric myenteric plexus, resulting in enhanced noncholinergic relaxation and delayed gastric emptying [37].

Methods. Animals are fed a high-fat diet for two consecutive weeks. The high-fat diet includes 58% kcal fat [37].

Features. High-fat feeding for two weeks leads to delay in gastric emptying. This model mimics the clinical situation of FD from a dietary perspective. It is a useful tool to investigate effective treatments for FD induced by chronic high-fat feeding.

7. Special Species Animal Models

7.1. Flinders Sensitive Line Rats

Rationale. Flinders Sensitive Line (FSL) rats, selectively bred for hypersensitivity to cholinergic stimuli, were originally proposed as a genetic animal model of depression [105]. Like some depressed humans, FSL rats show hypersensitivity to cholinergic agonists, are less active, exhibit higher rapid eye movement sleep, and respond to antidepressants [106, 107]. Anxiety and depression are associated with FD and may precede the onset of the disorder in some people [55]. As the FSL rats show some behavioral similarities to FD patients, this species could be used in FD models.

Features. FSL rats have disturbed gastric motility, reflected as both an increased gastric accommodation rate and gastric volume during gastric distension, which then leads to a delay in gastric emptying [38]. Although FSL rats show some features similar to some FD patients, the increase in gastric accommodation in FSL rats is contrary to the reduced accommodation often seen in FD patients. FSL rats may be useful to study certain aspects of FD, such as depression and delayed gastric emptying.

7.2. Wistar Kyoto Rats

Rationale. Wistar Kyoto (WKY) rats, a high-anxiety strain considered to be hyperresponsive to stress, are also a recognized animal model of impaired gastric accommodation [108, 109]. The WKY rats exhibit some of the pathophysiological characteristics of some FD patients, such as impaired gastric accommodation and anxiety.

Features. During gastric distension, WKY rats have a lower intragastric volume, indicating impaired gastric accommodation. The impaired gastric accommodation seen in WKY is associated with an increased cholinergic activity of the gastric vagal nerves [109]. In WKY rats, impaired accommodation of smooth muscles might not be a widespread phenomenon along the gastrointestinal tract but rather a local disturbance [39]. WKY rats may be useful to study certain FD patients who have both impaired gastric accommodation and anxiety.

7.3. BioBreeding Diabetes-Prone Rats

Rationale. Normoglycemic BioBreeding diabetes-prone (BB-DP) rats display both altered fundic motor control and impaired gastric accommodation, which is at least partially caused by a loss in nitrergic nervous function. Normoglycemic BB-DP rats provide a spontaneous model for inflammation-induced impaired gastric accommodation [40].

Features. This impaired accommodation is associated with low-grade inflammation and loss of neuronal isoform of nitric oxide synthase proteins which develop over time in this model [40]. The normoglycemic BB-DP rats may help us to understand the pathophysiological mechanisms in FD patients with inflammation-induced impaired gastric accommodation and develop new medications for these people.

8. Animal Models Multiple Features

8.1. Neonatal Colon Inflammation Followed by Adult Gastric Irritation

Rationale. Neonatal colon inflammation is combined with adult gastric irritation to establish a FD animal model. TNBS-induced colonic inflammation in animal pups leads to gastric hypersensitivity, delayed gastric emptying, and depression-like behaviors. Gastric irritation via iodoacetamide causes impaired gastric sensory and motor dysfunction.

Methods. Neonatal animals are treated with TNBS followed by treatment with 0.1% iodoacetamide for seven days at 6–8 weeks of age [21].

Features. This model concentrates the advantages of two kinds of methods and presents typical pathophysiological characteristics of FD, such as early satiety, delayed gastric emptying, gastric hypersensitivity, and depression-like behaviors. But it does not worsen the symptoms of FD compared to neonatal colon inflammation alone [21].

8.2. Neonatal Maternal Separation Followed by Adult Restraint Stress

Rationale. Neonatal maternal separation leads to delayed gastric emptying in adulthood. Restraint stress also suppresses antral motility and delays gastric emptying. The gastric motility may be even worse when the two models are combined together.

Methods. Animal pups are separated from their parents and placed in individual cages in another room for three hours daily. Restraint stress was performed for one week when the animals reached adulthood [25, 26].

Features. Neonatal maternal separation followed by adult restraint stress induces a more severe delay in gastric emptying compared with neonatal maternal separation or restraint

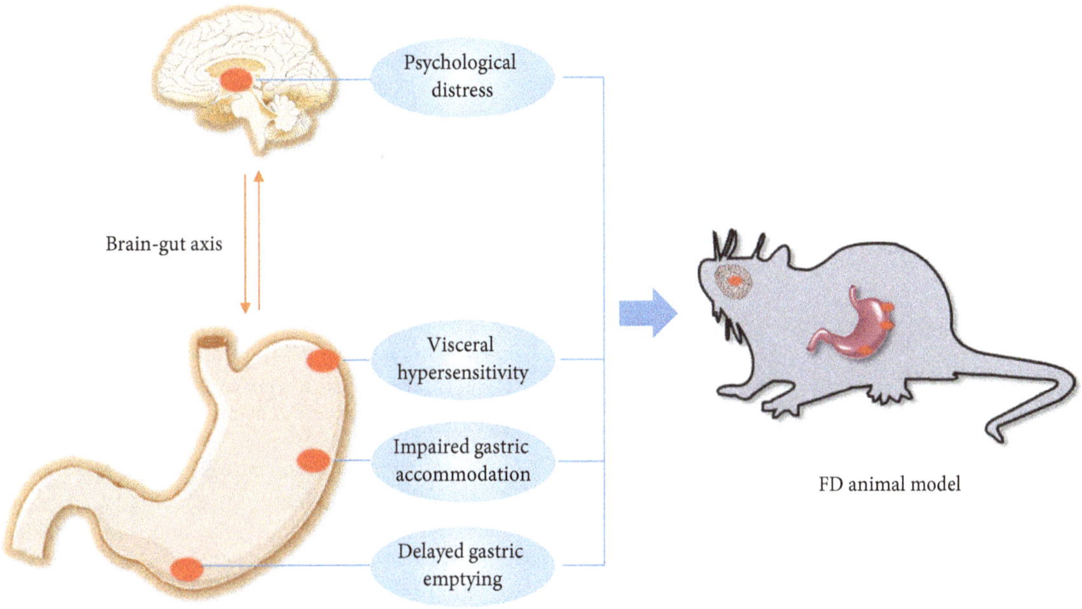

FIGURE 1: Delayed gastric emptying, impaired gastric accommodation, visceral hypersensitivity, and psychological distress are the major pathophysiologic disturbances of FD. These points are also targets of FD animal model.

stress alone. This compound model causes a relatively serious delay of gastric motility.

9. Which Animal Model Is Most Suited to Study FD?

An ideal animal model should mimic the disease conditions and outcomes as close as possible to the human condition. The ideal model may offer an opportunity to understand molecular mechanisms that lead to disease development and help to develop new drugs. All the above animal models of FD were established on the basis of the following features: delayed gastric emptying, impaired gastric accommodation, visceral hypersensitivity, and psychological distresses (Figure 1). Different FD animal models have different merits. For example, clonidine injection has been used mainly to induce delay in gastric emptying and BB-DP rats are used mainly for impaired gastric accommodation. Among these models, neonatal gastric irritation is the best model because it presents the main pathophysiological characteristics of FD.

It is unrealistic to expect any animal model to mimic every facet of the complex disturbances typical for FD. The decision about which particular model should be chosen to study FD will depend on the study aims and questions of interest. Compound animal model that include two or more factors that contribute to FD development may be preferable. To date few studies have used compound animal model in preclinical studies of FD. These complex models might be more promising in future studies because they can reproduce the pathogenic lesions that underlie the disease in humans from different aspects. Additionally, genetic approaches might also be used to generate animal models of FD.

10. Conclusion

FD adversely affects attendance and productivity in the workplace and causes enormous expense for patients and society [110]. Although a cure for this disease is still far in the future, some progress in terms of the development and characterization of FD animal models has been made. Various kinds of methods have been employed to establish FD models from different pathological perspectives. Delayed gastric emptying, impaired gastric accommodation, visceral hypersensitivity, and psychological distresses are the main targets for establishing FD models. Different animal models are better suited for modelling certain aspects of FD. The most appropriate model according to the reasons for the experiment. Although great challenges remain, the development of FD animal models that offer pathophysiological characteristics similar to FD patients should be encouraged. Good models will help us better understand the mechanisms of FD and give us a better chance to develop effective therapies.

Abbreviations

FD:	Functional dyspepsia
5-HT:	5-Hydroxytryptamine
m-CPBG:	m-Chlorophenylbiguanide
CRF:	Corticotropin-releasing factor
TNBS:	Trinitrobenzene sulfonic acid

HPA: Hypothalamus-pituitary-adrenal
ACTH: Adrenocorticotrophic hormone
CMUS: Chronic mild unpredictable stimulation
HCI: Hydrochloric acid
TGR5: Bile acid receptor 1
nNOS: Neuronal nitric oxide synthase
FSL: Flinders Sensitive Line
WKY: Wistar Kyoto
BB-DP: BioBreeding diabetes-prone.

Acknowledgments

This research was supported by the Capital Characteristic Key Program of Beijing Science and Technology Commission (Grant no. Z161100000516007).

References

[1] N. J. Talley, G. R. Locke III, and B. D. Lahr, "Functional dyspepsia, delayed gastric emptying, and impaired quality of life," *Gut*, vol. 55, no. 7, pp. 933–939, 2006.

[2] A. C. Ford, A. Marwaha, R. Sood, and P. Moayyedi, "Global prevalence of, and risk factors for, uninvestigated dyspepsia: a meta-analysis," *Gut*, vol. 64, pp. 1049–1057, 2015.

[3] N. J. Talley and A. C. Ford, "Functional dyspepsia," *The New England Journal of Medicine*, vol. 373, no. 19, pp. 1853–1863, 2015.

[4] M. Camilleri, L. Bueno, and V. Andresen, "Pharmacological, pharmacokinetic, and pharmacogenomic aspects of functional gastrointestinal disorders," *Gastroenterology*, 2016.

[5] G. F. Longstreth, "Functional dyspepsia - managing the conundrum," *The New England Journal of Medicine*, vol. 354, no. 8, pp. 791–793, 2006.

[6] Y. Matsunaga, T. Tanaka, K. Yoshinaga et al., "Acotiamide hydrochloride (Z-338), a new selective acetylcholinesterase inhibitor, enhances gastric motility without prolonging QT interval in dogs: comparison with cisapride, itopride, and mosapride," *The Journal of Pharmacology and Experimental Therapeutics*, vol. 336, no. 3, pp. 791–800, 2011.

[7] M. Kawachi, Y. Matsunaga, T. Tanaka et al., "Acotiamide hydrochloride (Z-338) enhances gastric motility and emptying by inhibiting acetylcholinesterase activity in rats," *European Journal of Pharmacology*, vol. 666, no. 1-3, pp. 218–225, 2011.

[8] K. Nagahama, Y. Matsunaga, M. Kawachi et al., "Acotiamide, a new orally active acetylcholinesterase inhibitor, stimulates gastrointestinal motor activity in conscious dogs," *Neurogastroenterology & Motility*, vol. 24, no. 6, pp. 566–e256, 2012.

[9] T. Asano, S. Aida, S. Suemasu, and T. Mizushima, "Anethole restores delayed gastric emptying and impaired gastric accommodation in rodents," *Biochemical and Biophysical Research Communications*, vol. 472, no. 1, pp. 125–130, 2016.

[10] Y. Kimura and M. Sumiyoshi, "Effects of an Atractylodes lancea rhizome extract and a volatile component β-eudesmol on gastrointestinal motility in mice," *Journal of Ethnopharmacology*, vol. 141, no. 1, pp. 530–536, 2012.

[11] T. H. Lee, J. J. Choi, D. H. Kim et al., "Gastroprokinetic effects of DA-9701, a new prokinetic agent formulated with Pharbitis Semen and Corydalis Tuber," *Phytomedicine*, vol. 15, no. 10, pp. 836–843, 2008.

[12] T. H. Lee, M. Son, and S. Y. Kim, "Effects of corydaline from corydalis tuber on gastric motor function in an animal model," *Biological & Pharmaceutical Bulletin*, vol. 33, no. 6, pp. 958–962, 2010.

[13] T. H. Lee, K. H. Kim, S. O. Lee, K. R. Lee, M. Son, and M. Jin, "Tetrahydroberberine, an isoquinoline alkaloid isolated from corydalis tuber, enhances gastrointestinal motor function," *The Journal of Pharmacology and Experimental Therapeutics*, vol. 338, no. 3, pp. 917–924, 2011.

[14] T. Hirata, Y. Keto, M. Yamano, T. Yokoyama, T. Sengoku, and N. Seki, "Inhibitory effect of ramosetron on corticotropin releasing factor- and soybean oil-induced delays in gastric emptying in rats," *Journal of Gastroenterology and Hepatology*, vol. 27, no. 9, pp. 1505–1511, 2012.

[15] F. Borrelli, B. Romano, I. Fasolino et al., "Prokinetic effect of a standardized yarrow (Achillea millefolium) extract and its constituent choline: Studies in the mouse and human stomach," *Neurogastroenterology & Motility*, vol. 24, no. 2, pp. 164–e90, 2012.

[16] L.-S. Liu, J. H. Winston, M. M. Shenoy, G.-Q. Song, J. D. Z. Chen, and P. J. Pasricha, "A rat model of chronic gastric sensorimotor dysfunction resulting from transient neonatal gastric irritation," *Gastroenterology*, vol. 134, no. 7, pp. 2070–2079, 2008.

[17] S. Li and J. D. Z. Chen, "Down-regulation of a-type potassium channel in gastric-specific DRG neurons in a rat model of functional dyspepsia," *Neurogastroenterology & Motility*, vol. 26, no. 7, pp. 962–970, 2014.

[18] J. Zhou, S. Li, Y. Wang et al., "Effects and mechanisms of auricular electroacupuncture on gastric hypersensitivity in a rodent model of functional dyspepsia," *PLoS ONE*, vol. 12, no. 3, Article ID e0174568, 2017.

[19] L. S. Liu, M. Shenoy, and P. J. Pasricha, "The analgesic effects of the GABAB receptor agonist, baclofen, in a rodent model of functional dyspepsia," *Neurogastroenterology & Motility*, vol. 23, no. 4, p. 356, 2011.

[20] L. Liu, Q. Li, R. Sapolsky et al., "Transient gastric irritation in the neonatal rats leads to changes in hypothalamic CRF expression, depression- and anxiety-like behavior as adults," *PLoS ONE*, vol. 6, no. 5, Article ID e19498, 2011.

[21] J. H. Winston, J. E. Aguirre, X.-Z. Shi, and S. K. Sarna, "Impaired Interoception in a Preclinical Model of Functional Dyspepsia," *Digestive Diseases and Sciences*, pp. 1–11, 2017.

[22] J. H. Winston and S. K. Sarna, "Developmental origins of functional dyspepsia-like gastric hypersensitivity in rats," *Gastroenterology*, vol. 144, no. 3, pp. 570–e3, 2013.

[23] J. H. Winston and S. K. Sarna, "Enhanced sympathetic nerve activity induced by neonatal colon inflammation induces gastric hypersensitivity and anxiety-like behavior in adult rats," *American Journal of Physiology-Gastrointestinal and Liver Physiology*, vol. 311, no. 1, pp. G32–G39, 2016.

[24] Q. Li, J. H. Winston, and S. K. Sarna, "Noninflammatory upregulation of nerve growth factor underlies gastric hypersensitivity induced by neonatal colon inflammation," *American Journal of Physiology-Regulatory, Integrative and Comparative Physiology*, vol. 310, no. 3, pp. R235–R242, 2016.

[25] K. Tominaga, Y. Fujikawa, F. Tanaka et al., "Structural changes in gastric glial cells and delayed gastric emptying as responses to

early life stress and acute adulthood stress in rats," *Life Sciences*, vol. 148, pp. 254–259, 2016.

[26] H. Abdel-Aziz, W. Wadie, H. F. Zaki et al., "Novel sequential stress model for functional dyspepsia: efficacy of the herbal preparation STW5," *Phytomedicine*, vol. 22, no. 5, pp. 588–595, 2015.

[27] K. Seto, T. Sasaki, K. Katsunuma, N. Kobayashi, K. Tanaka, and J. Tack, "Acotiamide hydrochloride (Z-338), a novel prokinetic agent, restores delayed gastric emptying and feeding inhibition induced by restraint stress in rats," *Neurogastroenterology & Motility*, vol. 20, no. 9, pp. 1051–1059, 2008.

[28] H. Zhang, T. Han, L.-N. Sun et al., "Regulative effects of essential oil from Atractylodes lancea on delayed gastric emptying in stress-induced rats," *Phytomedicine*, vol. 15, no. 8, pp. 602–611, 2008.

[29] H. S. Lee, D.-K. Kim, Y. B. Kim, and K. J. Lee, "Effect of acute stress on immune cell counts and the expression of tight junction proteins in the duodenal mucosa of rats," *Gut and Liver*, vol. 7, no. 2, pp. 190–196, 2013.

[30] G. Zhang, S. Xie, W. Hu et al., "Effects of electroacupuncture on interstitial cells of cajal (ICC) ultrastructure and connexin 43 protein expression in the gastrointestinal tract of functional dyspepsia (FD) rats," *Medical Science Monitor*, vol. 22, pp. 2021–2027, 2016.

[31] W. Wei, X. Li, J. Hao et al., "Proteomic analysis of functional dyspepsia in stressed rats treated with traditional Chinese medicine 'Wei Kangning'," *Journal of Gastroenterology and Hepatology*, vol. 26, no. 9, pp. 1425–1433, 2011.

[32] X.-J. Wang, J.-S. Guo, Y. Xu et al., "Effect of Shuwei Decoction on rats with functional dyspepsia," *Chinese Journal of Integrative Medicine*, pp. 1–6, 2016.

[33] J.-J. Qiu, Z. Liu, P. Zhao et al., "Gut microbial diversity analysis using Illumina sequencing for functional dyspepsia with liver depression-spleen deficiency syndrome and the interventional Xiaoyaosan in a rat model," *World Journal of Gastroenterology*, vol. 23, no. 5, pp. 810–816, 2017.

[34] Y. Seto, N. Yoshida, and H. Kaneko, "Effects of mosapride citrate, a 5-HT4-receptor agonist, on gastric distension-induced visceromotor response in conscious rats," *Journal of Pharmacological Sciences*, vol. 116, no. 1, pp. 47–53, 2011.

[35] B. K. Poudel, J. Y. Yu, Y. S. Kwon et al., "The pharmacological effects of benachio-F® on rat gastrointestinal functions," *Biomolecules & Therapeutics*, vol. 23, no. 4, pp. 350–356, 2015.

[36] M. Nakata-Fukuda, T. Hirata, Y. Keto, M. Yamano, T. Yokoyama, and Y. Uchiyama, "Inhibitory effect of the selective serotonin 5-HT3 receptor antagonist ramosetron on duodenal acidification-induced gastric hypersensitivity in rats," *European Journal of Pharmacology*, vol. 731, no. 1, pp. 88–92, 2014.

[37] H. Zhou, S. Zhou, J. Gao, G. Zhang, Y. Lu, and C. Owyang, "Upregulation of bile acid receptor TGR5 and nNOS in gastric myenteric plexus is responsible for delayed gastric emptying after chronic high-fat feeding in rats," *American Journal of Physiology-Gastrointestinal and Liver Physiology*, vol. 308, no. 10, pp. G863–G873, 2015.

[38] H. Mattsson, Z. Arani, M. Astin, A. Bayati, D. H. Overstreet, and A. Lehmann, "Altered neuroendocrine response and gastric dysmotility in the flinders sensitive line rat," *Neurogastroenterology & Motility*, vol. 17, no. 2, pp. 166–174, 2005.

[39] V. Martínez, M. Ryttinger, M. Kjerling, and M. Astin-Nielsen, "Characterisation of colonic accommodation in Wistar Kyoto rats with impaired gastric accommodation," *Naunyn-Schmiedeberg's Archives of Pharmacology*, vol. 376, no. 3, pp. 205–216, 2007.

[40] C. Vanormelingen, T. Vanuytsel, T. Masaoka et al., "The normoglycaemic biobreeding rat: a spontaneous model for impaired gastric accommodation," *Gut*, vol. 65, no. 1, pp. 73–81, 2016.

[41] H. Asano, T. Tomita, K. Nakamura et al., "Prevalence of gastric motility disorders in patients with functional dyspepsia," *Journal of Neurogastroenterology and Motility*, vol. 23, no. 3, pp. 392–399, 2017.

[42] G. Sarnelli, P. Caenepeel, B. Geypens, J. Janssens, and J. Tack, "Symptoms associated with impaired gastric emptying of solids and liquids in functional dyspepsia," *American Journal of Gastroenterology*, vol. 98, no. 4, pp. 783–788, 2003.

[43] M. M. Walker and N. J. Talley, "The role of duodenal inflammation in functional dyspepsia," *Journal of Clinical Gastroenterology*, vol. 51, no. 1, pp. 12–18, 2017.

[44] P. Moayyedi, S. Soo, J. Deeks, B. Delaney, M. Innes, and D. Forman, "Pharmacological interventions for non-ulcer dyspepsia," *Cochrane Database of Systematic Reviews*, no. 4, Article ID CD001960, 2004.

[45] S. Kindt and J. Tack, "Impaired gastric accommodation and its role in dyspepsia," *Gut*, vol. 55, no. 12, pp. 1685–1691, 2006.

[46] F. Carbone and J. Tack, "Gastroduodenal mechanisms underlying functional gastric disorders," *Digestive Diseases*, vol. 32, no. 3, pp. 222–229, 2014.

[47] H. Piessevaux, J. Tack, S. Walrand, S. Pauwels, and A. Geubel, "Intragastric distribution of a standardized meal in health and functional dyspepsia: Correlation with specific symptoms," *Neurogastroenterology & Motility*, vol. 15, no. 5, pp. 447–455, 2003.

[48] J. Tack, H. Piessevaux, B. Coulie, P. Caenepeel, and J. Janssens, "Role of impaired gastric accommodation to a meal in functional dyspepsia," *Gastroenterology*, vol. 115, no. 6, pp. 1346–1352, 1998.

[49] O. S. Van Boxel, J. J. M. Ter Linde, P. D. Siersema, and A. J. P. M. Smout, "Role of chemical stimulation of the duodenum in dyspeptic symptom generation," *American Journal of Gastroenterology*, vol. 105, no. 4, pp. 803–811, 2010.

[50] M. Camilleri and V. Stanghellini, "Current management strategies and emerging treatments for functional dyspepsia," *Nature Reviews Gastroenterology & Hepatology*, vol. 10, no. 3, pp. 187–194, 2013.

[51] K. J. Lee and J. Tack, "Duodenal implications in the pathophysiology of functional dyspepsia," *Journal of Neurogastroenterology and Motility*, vol. 16, no. 3, pp. 251–257, 2010.

[52] B. Feng, J. H. La, E. S. Schwartz, and G. F. Gebhart, "Neural and neuro-immune mechanisms of visceral hypersensitivity in irritable bowel syndrome," *American Journal of Physiology-Gastrointestinal and Liver Physiology*, vol. 302, no. 10, pp. G1085–G1098, 2012.

[53] J. M. Rosen, "Visceral hypersensitivity and electromechanical dysfunction as therapeutic targets in pediatric functional dyspepsia," *World Journal of Gastrointestinal Pharmacology and Therapeutics*, vol. 5, no. 3, p. 122, 2014.

[54] J. Tack, P. Caenepeel, B. Fischler, H. Piessevaux, and J. Janssens, "Symptoms associated with hypersensitivity to gastric distention in functional dyspepsia," *Gastroenterology*, vol. 121, no. 3, pp. 526–535, 2001.

[55] P. Aro, N. J. Talley, S. Johansson, L. Agréus, and J. Ronkainen, "Anxiety is linked to new-onset dyspepsia in the Swedish

population: a 10-Year Follow-up Study," *Gastroenterology*, vol. 148, no. 5, pp. 928–937, 2015.

[56] I.-S. Lee, H. Wang, Y. Chae, H. Preissl, and P. Enck, "Functional neuroimaging studies in functional dyspepsia patients: a systematic review," *Neurogastroenterology & Motility*, vol. 28, no. 6, pp. 793–805, 2016.

[57] A.-Z. Zhang, Q.-C. Wang, K.-M. Huang et al., "Prevalence of depression and anxiety in patients with chronic digestive system diseases: A multicenter epidemiological study," *World Journal of Gastroenterology*, vol. 22, no. 42, pp. 9437–9444, 2016.

[58] V. M. Smirnov and A. E. Lychkova, "Synergism of sympathetic and parasympathetic systems in the regulation of gastric motility," *Bulletin of Experimental Biology and Medicine*, vol. 134, no. 1, pp. 12–14, 2002.

[59] T. J. Ridolfi, W.-D. Tong, T. Takahashi, L. Kosinski, and K. A. Ludwig, "Sympathetic and parasympathetic regulation of rectal motility in rats," *Journal of Gastrointestinal Surgery*, vol. 13, no. 11, pp. 2027–2033, 2009.

[60] T. Asai, W. W. Mapleson, and I. Power, "Differential effects of clonidine and dexmedetomidine on gastric emptying and gastrointestinal transit in the rat," *British Journal of Anaesthesia*, vol. 78, no. 3, pp. 301–307, 1997.

[61] T. Asano, S. Aida, S. Suemasu, K. Tahara, K.-I. Tanaka, and T. Mizushima, "Aldioxa improves delayed gastric emptying and impaired gastric compliance, pathophysiologic mechanisms of functional dyspepsia," *Scientific Reports*, vol. 5, Article ID 17519, 2015.

[62] A. E. Bharucha, K. Ravi, and A. R. Zinsmeister, "Comparison of selective M3 and nonselective muscarinic receptor antagonists on gastrointestinal transit and bowel habits in humans," *American Journal of Physiology-Gastrointestinal and Liver Physiology*, vol. 299, no. 1, pp. G215–G219, 2010.

[63] X. Gao, Y. Zhao, Y. Su et al., "β1/2 or M2/3 receptors are required for different gastrointestinal motility responses induced by acupuncture at heterotopic or homotopic acupoints," *PLoS ONE*, vol. 11, no. 12, Article ID e0168200, 2016.

[64] N. G. Levein, S. E. Thörn, and M. Wattwil, "Dopamine delays gastric emptying and prolongs orocaecal transit time in volunteers," *European Journal of Anaesthesiology*, vol. 16, no. 4, pp. 246–250, 1999.

[65] P. Kashyap, M.-A. Micci, S. Pasricha, and P. J. Pasricha, "The D2/D3 agonist PD128907 (R-(+)-trans-3,4a,10b-tetrahydro-4-Propyl-2H,5H- [1]benzopyrano[4,3-b]-1,4-oxazin-9-ol) inhibits stimulated pyloric relaxation and spontaneous gastric emptying," *Digestive Diseases and Sciences*, vol. 54, no. 1, pp. 57–62, 2009.

[66] J. P. Blancquaert, R. A. Lefebvre, and J. L. Willems, "Gastric relaxation by intravenous and intracerebroventricular administration of apomorphine, morphine and fentanyl in the conscious dog," *Arch Int Pharmacodyn Ther*, vol. 256, no. 1, pp. 153-154, 1982.

[67] M. Nakajima, Y. Shiihara, Y. Shiba et al., "Effect of 5-hydroxytryptamine on gastrointestinal motility in conscious guinea-pigs," *Neurogastroenterology & Motility*, vol. 9, no. 4, pp. 205–214, 1997.

[68] T. K. MacHu, "Therapeutics of 5-HT_3 receptor antagonists: current uses and future directions," *Pharmacology & Therapeutics*, vol. 130, no. 3, pp. 338–347, 2011.

[69] Y.-S. Jung, M.-Y. Kim, H. S. Lee, S. L. Park, and K. J. Lee, "Effect of DA-9701, a novel prokinetic agent, on stress-induced delayed gastric emptying and hormonal changes in rats," *Neurogastroenterology & Motility*, vol. 25, no. 3, pp. 254–e166, 2013.

[70] Y. Taché, V. Martinez, L. Wang, and M. Million, "CRF 1 receptor signaling pathways are involved in stress-related alterations of colonic function and viscerosensitivity: Implications for irritable bowel syndrome," *British Journal of Pharmacology*, vol. 141, no. 8, pp. 1321–1330, 2004.

[71] B. Deng, Y. Lin, S. Ma et al., "The leukotriene B4-leukotriene B4 receptor axis promotes cisplatin-induced acute kidney injury by modulating neutrophil recruitment," *Kidney International*, 2016.

[72] N. A. El-Shitany and B. Eid, "Proanthocyanidin protects against cisplatin-induced oxidative liver damage through inhibition of inflammation and NF-$\kappa\beta$/TLR-4 pathway," *Environmental Toxicology*, vol. 32, no. 7, pp. 1952–1963, 2017.

[73] D. M. Savastano and M. Covasa, "Intestinal nutrients elicit satiation through concomitant activation of CCK1 and 5-HT3 receptors," *Physiology & Behavior*, vol. 92, no. 3, pp. 434–442, 2007.

[74] G. Stacher, H. Bergmann, G. Gaupmann et al., "Fat preload delays gastric emptying: reversal by cisapride.," *British Journal of Clinical Pharmacology*, vol. 30, no. 6, pp. 839–845, 1990.

[75] G. Stacher, H. Bergmann, C. Schneider et al., "Effects of the 5-HT3 receptor antagonist ICS 205-930 on fat-delayed gastric emptying and antral motor activity.," *British Journal of Clinical Pharmacology*, vol. 30, no. 1, pp. 41–48, 1990.

[76] K. Tachiyashiki and K. Imaizumi, "Effects of vegetable oils and C18-unsaturated fatty acids on plasma ethanol levels and gastric emptying in ethanol-administered rats," *Journal of Nutritional Science and Vitaminology*, vol. 39, no. 2, pp. 163–176, 1993.

[77] H. Nishio, Y. Hayashi, S. Terashima, and K. Takeuchi, "Role of endogenous nitric oxide in mucosal defense of inflamed rat stomach following iodoacetamide treatment," *Life Sciences*, vol. 79, no. 16, pp. 1523–1530, 2006.

[78] K. Bielefeldt, N. Ozaki, and G. F. Gebhart, "Mild gastritis alters voltage-sensitive sodium currents in gastric sensory neurons in rats," *Gastroenterology*, vol. 122, no. 3, pp. 752–761, 2002.

[79] Z. D. Jiang, X. M. Shao, and A. R. Wilkinson, "Changes in BAER amplitudes after perinatal asphyxia during the neonatal period in term infants," *Brain & Development*, vol. 28, no. 9, pp. 554–559, 2006.

[80] Z. D. Jiang, D. M. Brosi, X. M. Shao, and A. R. Wilkinson, "Sustained depression of brainstem auditory electrophysiology during the first months in term infants after perinatal asphyxia," *Clinical Neurophysiology*, vol. 119, no. 7, pp. 1496–1505, 2008.

[81] A. Sarkate and S. S. Dhaneshwar, "Investigation of mitigating effect of colon-specific prodrugs of boswellic acid on 2,4,6-trinitrobenzene sulfonic acidinduced colitis in Wistar rats: Design, kinetics and biological evaluation," *World Journal of Gastroenterology*, vol. 23, no. 7, pp. 1147–1162, 2017.

[82] H. Hoshino, S. Sugiyama, A. Ohara, H. Goto, Y. Tsukamoto, and T. Ozawa, "Mechanism and prevention of chronic colonic inflammation with trinitrobenzene sulfonic acid in rats," *Clinical and Experimental Pharmacology and Physiology*, vol. 19, no. 10, pp. 717–722, 1992.

[83] T. Karaca, Y. H. Uz, S. Demirtas, I. Karaboga, and G. Can, "Protective effect of royal jelly in 2,4,6 trinitrobenzene sulfonic acid-induced colitis in rats," *Iranian Journal of Basic Medical Sciences*, vol. 18, no. 4, pp. 370–379, 2015.

[84] B. Geeraerts, L. Van Oudenhove, B. Fischler et al., "Influence of abuse history on gastric sensorimotor function in functional dyspepsia," *Neurogastroenterology & Motility*, vol. 21, no. 1, pp. 33–41, 2009.

[85] D. K. Chitkara, M. A. L. van Tilburg, N. Blois-Martin, and W. E. Whitehead, "Early life risk factors that contribute to irritable bowel syndrome in adults: a systematic review," *American Journal of Gastroenterology*, vol. 103, no. 3, pp. 765–774, 2008.

[86] L. Van Oudenhove, J. Vandenberghe, R. Vos, B. Fischler, K. Demyttenaere, and J. Tack, "Abuse history, depression, and somatization are associated with gastric sensitivity and gastric emptying in functional dyspepsia," *Psychosomatic Medicine*, vol. 73, no. 8, pp. 648–655, 2011.

[87] Y. Yang, Z. Cheng, H. Tang et al., "Neonatal maternal separation impairs prefrontal cortical myelination and cognitive functions in rats through activation of wnt signaling," *Cerebral Cortex*, vol. 27, no. 5, pp. 2871–2884, 2017.

[88] S. Y. Shin, S. H. Han, R.-S. Woo, S. H. Jang, and S. S. Min, "Adolescent mice show anxiety- and aggressive-like behavior and the reduction of long-term potentiation in mossy fiber-CA3 synapses after neonatal maternal separation," *Neuroscience*, vol. 316, pp. 221–231, 2016.

[89] G. A. Carrasco and L. D. Van De Kar, "Neuroendocrine pharmacology of stress," *European Journal of Pharmacology*, vol. 463, no. 1-3, pp. 235–272, 2003.

[90] V. Martinez, L. Wang, M. Million, J. Rivier, and Y. Taché, "Urocortins and the regulation of gastrointestinal motor function and visceral pain," *Peptides*, vol. 25, no. 10, pp. 1733–1744, 2004.

[91] Y. Nakade, D. Tsuchida, H. Fukuda, M. Iwa, T. N. Pappas, and T. Takahashi, "Restraint stress delays solid gastric emptying via a central CRF and peripheral sympathetic neuron in rats," *American Journal of Physiology-Regulatory, Integrative and Comparative Physiology*, vol. 288, no. 2, pp. R427–R432, 2005.

[92] H. Taniguchi, H. Ariga, J. Zheng et al., "Endogenous ghrelin and 5-HT regulate interdigestive gastrointestinal contractions in conscious rats," *American Journal of Physiology-Gastrointestinal and Liver Physiology*, vol. 295, no. 2, pp. G403–G411, 2008.

[93] T. Nozu, S. Kumei, K. Takakusaki, and T. Okumura, "Water-avoidance stress enhances gastric contractions in freely moving conscious rats: Role of peripheral CRF receptors," *Journal of Gastroenterology*, vol. 49, no. 5, pp. 799–805, 2014.

[94] J. Zheng, A. Dobner, R. Babygirija, K. Ludwig, and T. Takahashi, "Effects of repeated restraint stress on gastric motility in rats," *American Journal of Physiology-Regulatory, Integrative and Comparative Physiology*, vol. 296, no. 5, pp. R1358–R1365, 2009.

[95] P. R. Saunders, U. Kosecka, D. M. McKay, and M. H. Perdue, "Acute stressors stimulate ion secretion and increase epithelial permeability in rat intestine," *American Journal of Physiology*, vol. 267, no. 5, pp. G794–G799, 1994.

[96] J. E. Kellow, P. M. Langeluddecke, G. M. Eckersley, M. P. Jones, and C. C. Tennant, "Effects of acute psychologic stress on small-intestinal motility in health and the irritable bowel syndrome," *Scandinavian Journal of Gastroenterology*, vol. 27, no. 1, pp. 53–58, 1992.

[97] J. Li, Y. Li, B. Zhang, X. Shen, and H. Zhao, "Why depression and pain often coexist and mutually reinforce: Role of the lateral habenula," *Experimental Neurology*, vol. 284, pp. 106–113, 2016.

[98] J. Vandenberghe, R. Vos, P. Persoons, K. Demyttenaere, J. Janssens, and J. Tack, "Dyspeptic patients with visceral hypersensitivity: sensitisation of pain specific or multimodal pathways?" *Gut*, vol. 54, no. 7, pp. 914–919, 2005.

[99] F. O. The, G. E. Boeckxstaens, S. A. Snoek et al., "Activation of the cholinergic anti-inflammatory pathway ameliorates postoperative ileus in mice," *Gastroenterology*, vol. 133, no. 4, pp. 1219–1228, 2007.

[100] G. E. Boeckxstaens and W. J. de Jonge, "Neuroimmune mechanisms in postoperative ileus," *Gut*, vol. 58, no. 9, pp. 1300–1311, 2009.

[101] M. Ishii, H. Kusunoki, N. Manabe et al., "Evaluation of duodenal hypersensitivity induced by duodenal acidification using transnasal endoscopy," *Journal of Gastroenterology and Hepatology*, vol. 25, no. 5, pp. 913–918, 2010.

[102] K. Lee, "Influence of duodenal acidification on the sensorimotor function of the proximal stomach in humans," *The American Journal of Physiology - Gastrointestinal and Liver Physiology*, vol. 286, no. 2, pp. 278G–284, 2004.

[103] A. N. Pilichiewicz, K. L. Feltrin, M. Horowitz et al., "Functional dyspepsia is associated with a greater symptomatic response to fat but not carbohydrate, increased fasting and postprandial CCK, and diminished PYY," *American Journal of Gastroenterology*, vol. 103, no. 10, pp. 2613–2623, 2008.

[104] N. A. M. Van Ooteghem, M. Samsom, K. J. Van Erpecum, and G. P. Van Berge-Henegouwen, "Effects of ileal bile salts on fasting small intestinal and gallbladder motility," *Neurogastroenterology & Motility*, vol. 14, no. 5, pp. 527–533, 2002.

[105] D. H. Overstreet, "The flinders sensitive line rats: a genetic animal model of depression," *Neuroscience & Biobehavioral Reviews*, vol. 17, no. 1, pp. 51–68, 1993.

[106] D. H. Overstreet, O. Pucilowski, A. H. Rezvani, and D. S. Janowsky, "Administration of antidepressants, diazepam and psychomotor stimulants further confirms the utility of Flinders Sensitive Line rats as an animal model of depression," *Psychopharmacology*, vol. 121, no. 1, pp. 27–37, 1995.

[107] D. H. Overstreet, "Behavioral characteristics of rat lines selected for differential hypothermic responses to cholinergic or serotonergic agonists," *Behavior Genetics*, vol. 32, no. 5, pp. 335–348, 2002.

[108] W. P. Paré, "The performance of WKY rats on three tests of emotional behavior," *Physiology & Behavior*, vol. 51, no. 5, pp. 1051–1056, 1992.

[109] M. Astin Nielsen, A. Bayati, and H. Mattsson, "Wistar Kyoto rats have impaired gastric accommodation compared to sprague dawley rats due to increased gastric vagal cholinergic tone," *Scandinavian Journal of Gastroenterology*, vol. 41, no. 7, pp. 773–781, 2006.

[110] B. E. Lacy, K. T. Weiser, A. T. Kennedy, M. D. Crowell, and N. J. Talley, "Functional dyspepsia: the economic impact to patients," *Alimentary Pharmacology & Therapeutics*, vol. 38, no. 2, pp. 170–177, 2013.

14

Alpha-Fetoprotein as a Predictive Marker for Patients with Hepatitis B-Related Acute-on-Chronic Liver Failure

Xiaoping Wang,[1,2] Caifei Shen,[1] Jianjiang Yang,[1] Xianjun Yang,[3] Sen Qin,[1,2] Haijun Zeng,[1] Xiaoling Wu,[1] Shanhong Tang ,[1,2] and Weizheng Zeng [1]

[1] *Department of Gastroenterology, Chengdu Military General Hospital, Chengdu, Sichuan, China*
[2] *College of Medicine, Southwest Jiaotong University, Chengdu, Sichuan, China*
[3] *Chengdu Military Command Disease Prevention and Control Center, Chengdu, Sichuan, China*

Correspondence should be addressed to Shanhong Tang; 15928956390@163.com and Weizheng Zeng; zengweizheng@163.com

Academic Editor: Yu-Chen Fan

Background and Aims. The value of alpha-fetoprotein (AFP) in hepatitis B-related acute-on-chronic liver failure (HBACLF) is not fully understood. The present study aimed to evaluate the prognostic effect of AFP on the prediction of HBACLF outcomes. *Methods.* We investigated a cohort of patients with HBACLF admitted from January 2013 to May 2017. The endpoint of followup was 180 days, death, or liver transplantation. AFP concentrations were estimated on admission. To make statistical comparisons, we used chi-squared test, receiver operating characteristic (ROC) curve analysis, survivorship curve analysis, and Cox proportional-hazards model. *Results.* A total of 92 patients (81.5% male, median age of 46 years) were included. Overall survival rate within 180 days was 43.48%, and the value of $\log_{10}{}^{AFP} \geq 2.04$ indicated a better prognosis with 76.9% specificity and 62.5% sensitivity for patients with HBACLF. Age (HR 1.041), total bilirubin (HR 1.004), $\log_{10}{}^{AFP}$ (HR 2.155), and INR (HR 1.446) were found to be risk factors of survival. *Conclusion.* AFP could be a useful marker to predict outcomes of acute-on-chronic liver failure.

1. Introduction

Acute-on-chronic liver failure (ACLF) is defined by a rapid progression in hepatic dysfunction induced by certain precipitating events due to previous liver diseases, resulting in multisystem organ failure and high short-term mortality [1]. There is no specific treatment for ACLF, and the most effective therapy is liver transplantation. However, the shortage of liver donations has largely hindered its wide implementation. Supporting the regeneration of hepatocytes and preventing the complications tend to decrease the mortality of ACLF, and artificial liver support is a useful method to manage ACLF [2]. The aetiologies of ACLF vary between territories. Viral infections are more common in Asia, while there is a wide prevalence of alcoholic cirrhosis and nonalcoholic fatty liver in American and European countries [3–6]. With a carrier rate of hepatitis B virus (HBV) surface antigen at approximately 8% in adults, China exhibits a high morbidity of hepatitis B, which is the most common aetiological factor of ACLF [7].

Some scoring systems efficiently assess the severity and mortality of ACLF, such as SOFA score [8], MELD [9], and King's College Criteria [10]. Other parameters including bilirubin and international normalized ratio (INR) are treated as prognostic markers in clinical practice as well. Those methods primarily focus on the impaired hepatic function, while seldom did researchers concentrate on parameters of hepatocyte regeneration and evaluate their prognostic value for ACLF. Typically, AFP is the most abundant plasma protein in foetuses, and serum AFP remains elevated in infant livers until several weeks after birth. High serum AFP expression in adults generally indicates a high possibility of hepatocellular carcinoma in patients with chronic hepatitis or cirrhosis [11]. Meanwhile, AFP is considered a biomarker of proliferating liver stem cells in liver injury conditions as well, and the recruitment of liver progenitor cells is associated with a better outcome for liver failure [12, 13].

The discovery of AFP dates back to 1960s. Since then, AFP has been investigated in the field of liver diseases. Previous

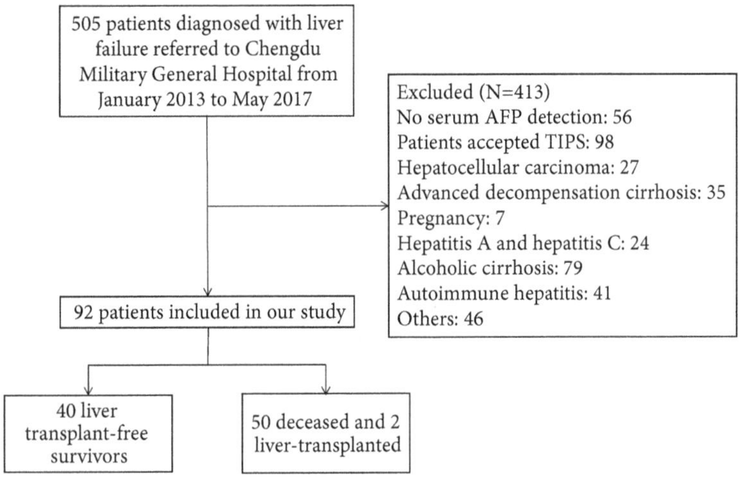

FIGURE 1: Inclusion and exclusion criteria for the study.

studies demonstrated that AFP was a vital prognostic marker for outcomes in patients with acute liver failure [14–16]. However, few studies evaluated the outcomes of ACLF from the perspective of hepatocyte regeneration. As we know, ACLF exhibits a small window during which liver dysfunction may be reversed, and the repair of liver tissues is tightly correlated with hepatocyte regeneration, which presents as increased AFP levels. Therefore, we performed a retrospective study to identify whether AFP was a valid predictive indicator of outcomes in ACLF patients.

2. Materials and Methods

2.1. Study Population. We concentrated on a cohort of patients with hepatitis B-related acute-on-chronic liver failure (HBACLF). A total of 505 patients with suspected ACLF were enrolled in our study from January 2013 to May 2017 at Chengdu Military General Hospital, Sichuan, China. Researchers who undertook the work of selecting cases as the main subjects were blind to the serum AFP concentrations of those patients. ACLF is diagnosed according to the criteria of Asian Pacific Association for the Study of the Liver (APASL): serum bilirubin $\geq 85\,\mu$mol/L, INR ≥ 1.5 or prothrombin activity $\leq 40\%$, any degree of encephalopathy and/or clinical ascites within 4 weeks, and an evidence of ongoing chronic liver diseases [3]. Patients who were diagnosed with ACLF and aged 18 to 75 years were included. A total of 413 patients in our database were excluded for the following reasons: (1) lack of serum AFP concentrations; (2) manifestation of decompensated liver cirrhosis prior to ACLF diagnosis, such as ascites and variceal haemorrhage; (3) patients with portal hypertension who received a transjugular intrahepatic portosystemic shunt (TIPS); (4) patients pathologically diagnosed with or clinically suspected for hepatocellular carcinoma; (5) other malignancies such as gastric cancer; (6) pregnancy; (7) HIV or hepatotropic virus infection other than HBV; and (8) other preexisting chronic liver diseases, such as fatty liver, autoimmune hepatitis, and alcoholic cirrhosis (Figure 1). The final cohort contained 92 patients with a median age of 46 years (range, 18–75 years), and all patients received antiviral therapy by orally taking tenofovir or entecavir. Besides, reduced glutathione was given to protect the liver from subsequent damage.

2.2. Clinical and Biological Parameters. The clinical parameters included ascites and hepatic encephalopathy (HE). The biological parameters included AFP, INR, and total bilirubin. The serum AFP levels were measured on admission.

2.3. Followup. The end point of observation was 180 days, death, or liver transplantation. Forty of the 92 patients survived spontaneously, 50 patients died, and 2 patients received liver transplantation.

2.4. Statistical Analysis. Results are presented as means and standard deviations (SDs) and median and range appropriately. The chi-squared test was used to compare rates between groups. Receiver operating characteristic (ROC) curve analysis was performed. Survival was estimated by Kaplan-Meier method, and differences were evaluated with log-rank test. Cox proportional-hazards model was adopted to estimate the risk factors of survival. Data were analyzed using SPSS version 16.0 software (IBM Corporation, Somers, NY, USA). Differences were considered to be of statistical significance when the P value ≤ 0.05.

3. Results

3.1. Baseline Characteristics. Ninety-two patients were incorporated in our study, including 17 women (18.5%). The population was divided into two groups based on the prognosis of ACLF. In total, there were 40 liver transplant-free survivors, 50 deceased patients, and 2 liver-transplanted patients. Table 1 depicts the demographic and biochemical characters of the two groups. Age, total bilirubin, AFP, and INR differed significantly between transplant-free survivors and those who deceased or got liver-transplanted.

3.2. AFP as a Predictor for Prognosis of HBACLF. The recruitment of functional hepatocytes is the key to the recovery

Table 1: Characteristic comparisons between subgroups.

Variables	Transplant-free survival group ($n = 40$)	Deceased and transplanted group ($n = 52$)	P value
Age*, y	41.83 (12.37)	50.31 (13.10)	0.002
Male n, %	33 (82.50%)	42 (80.77%)	0.832
Total bilirubin#, μmol/L	261.89 (86.98–496.59)	386.55 (137.45–723.22)	<0.001
AFP#, ng/ml	148.80 (8.50–2375.30)	43.21 (1.10–1495.80)	<0.001
INR#	1.83 (1.50–4.31)	2.21 (1.51–5.70)	0.001

AFP, alpha-fetoprotein; INR, international normalized ratio; *normally distributed continuous variable; #not normally distributed continuous variable.

Table 2: Univariate and multivariate Cox regression analysis for survival.

Parameter	Univariate Cox regression ($n = 92$)				Multivariate Cox regression ($n = 92$)			
	P	HR	CI		P	HR	CI	
Age*	0.003	1.033	1.011	1.056	<0.001	1.041	1.019	1.063
Total bilirubin*	<0.001	1.004	1.002	1.006	<0.001	1.004	1.002	1.006
INR*	0.001	1.564	1.200	2.039	0.015	1.446	1.074	1.948
$\log_{10}^{AFP}$#	<0.001	2.908	1.603	5.274	0.018	2.155	1.139	4.076
Ascites#	0.407							
HE#	0.163							

AFP, alpha-fetoprotein; INR, international normalized ratio; HE, hepatic encephalopathy; HR, hazard ratio; and CI, confidence interval; *continuous variables and #categorical variables ($\log_{10}^{AFP}$ was sorted into subgroups: $\log_{10}^{AFP} \geq 2$ and $\log_{10}^{AFP} < 2$. No statistical significance was attained between patients with or without ascites and HE).

of the impaired liver function. To estimate the outcome of ACLF from the perspective of hepatocyte regeneration, we evaluated the predictive value of AFP by creating an equation, namely, $\log_{10}^{AFP}$, to assess the prognosis of HBACLF. A receiver operating characteristic curve was created for this parameter to predict the outcome of ACLF patients. The area under the curve was 0.725. A cut-off point of $\log_{10}^{AFP} \geq 2.04$ was suggested to indicate a better outcome with 76.9% specificity and 62.5% sensitivity (Figure 2).

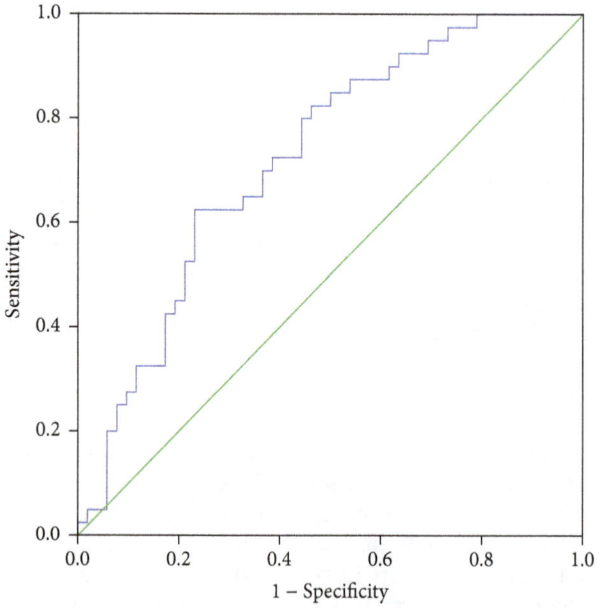

Figure 2: ROC curve for $\log_{10}^{AFP}$ in predicting the outcome of HBACLF ($n = 92$).

3.3. $\log_{10}^{AFP}$ *Is a Risk Factor of Survival for HBACLF.* Patients with chronic hepatitis B-related ACLF exhibited an incredibly high mortality within 180 days in our observation. The transplant-free survival rate at 30 days was 72.83%, and it gradually declined to 43.48% at 180 days of followup (Figure 3(a)). Given that patients would probably have a better outcome when $\log_{10}^{AFP}$ was approximately higher than 2, we then chose $\log_{10}^{AFP}$ as a categorical variable to assess the survival of HBACLF. In addition, we also adopt demographic parameters and serum biochemical parameters which were considered as representatives of the hepatic function. By using Cox proportional-hazards model, $\log_{10}^{AFP}$ was found to be an independent factor of survival as a categorical variable, as with continuous variables including age, INR, and levels of total bilirubin (Table 2). There were 41 patients whose $\log_{10}^{AFP} \geq 2$, and this group of patients was more likely to exhibit a longer survival time. The transplant-free survival rates at 30, 90, and 180 days were 58.82% versus 90.24% ($P = 0.001$), 39.22% versus 83.93% ($P < 0.001$), and 29.41% versus 58.54% ($P = 0.005$), respectively, in groups of patients with $\log_{10}^{AFP} < 2$ and ≥ 2 (Figure 3(b)).

4. Discussion

The idea of ACLF was first proposed to describe the acute liver damage of an ongoing chronic liver disease in 1995 [17]. There

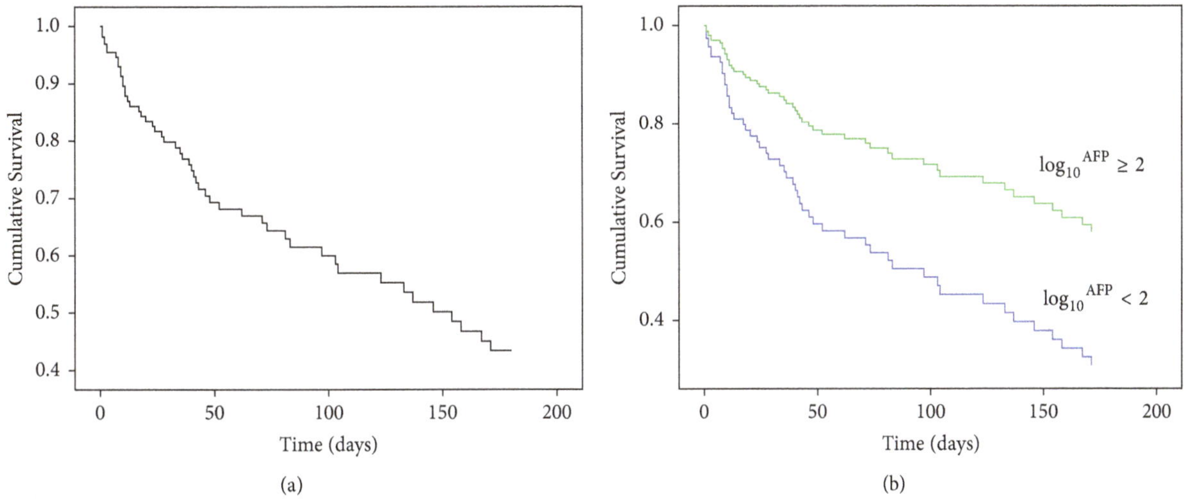

FIGURE 3: (a) Graph of multivariate Cox regression survival curve of the total population ($n = 92$). (b) Graph of multivariate Cox regression survival curve for patients with $\log_{10}{}^{AFP} \geq 2$ ($n = 41$) and $\log_{10}{}^{AFP} < 2$ ($n = 51$).

are more than 13 different definitions of ACLF worldwide, which vary from the West to the East. An acute insult may lead to rapid and progressive liver failure in patients with chronic liver diseases and result in high short-term mortality of approximately 50–90% because of the limited functional reserve of the liver [1, 18].

China exhibits a high morbidity of hepatitis B and HBACLF. There are studies estimating the severity and outcomes of HBACLF by establishing prognostic scoring models. Previous studies illustrated that the liver volume [19], lymphocyte-monocyte ratio [20], albumin-bilirubin score [21], logistic regression model [22], macrophage inflammatory protein 3α [23], and other methods [24–26] could be simple and sensitive models to evaluate the severity and prognosis of ACLF, which would be practically useful in clinic. Those methods mainly concentrated on the severity of liver injury, and the parameters in those models were generally to reflect the condition of liver function. It is known to us that the prognosis of ACLF depends on the extent of liver injury, the capability of hepatocyte regeneration, and the prevention of multiple organ failure. There are a number of studies evaluating the prognosis of ACLF from the perspective of liver function; however, limited researches have assessed the outcome of ACLF by adopting parameters reflecting hepatocyte regeneration. AFP is a biomarker of liver renovation; thus, we investigated the prognostic value of AFP in ACLF for that the magnitude of in the increased AFP levels is closely related to hepatocyte regeneration after acute or superimposed hepatic injury. Previous studies demonstrated that AFP was a prognostic marker in patients with acute liver failure [27, 28]. However, limited studies demonstrated a correlation between AFP levels and the outcomes of patients with ACLF, especially patients with acute hepatic failure based on chronic HBV infection.

AFP is not detected in normal adult serum. In 1963, Abelev et al. [29] found that a type of murine embryonal α-globulin, which was originally called AFP, could be detected in normal or malignant hepatocyte proliferation in adult rats. Then, AFP was considered a marker of hepatocyte regeneration, and the capacity of hepatocyte regeneration is key to the reversal of liver injury. The present study assessed the predictive value of AFP in the prognosis of hepatitis B-related acute-on-chronic liver failure because these patients always exhibited bad progress, and the short-term mortality is dramatically high. Valid predictive models and intensive care are necessary in the management of ACLF because some individuals regain their health following liver injury recovery and hepatocyte regeneration. Our study demonstrated that the parameter $\log_{10}{}^{AFP}$ was a helpful marker to predict the outcomes of ACLF. A higher AFP concentration could predict a better outcome of HBACLF, and $\log_{10}{}^{AFP} \geq 2$ could indicate a longer short-term survival time for patients with ACLF. Therefore, we speculated that the concentration of AFP may be positively related to the capacity for liver regeneration in the condition of acute liver injury on the basis of chronic liver diseases, apart from malignancies such as hepatocellular carcinoma and gastric cancer.

Consistent with Katoonizadeh's research [18], our study indicated that the difference of age was of statistical significance between survivors and those who deceased or got liver transplanted. Elderly patients exhibit a weakened condition of body function, which may result in multiple organ failure when there was a hypohepatia already. And we suspected that the number of functional hepatocytes may be lower in the elderly than young adults. In addition, total bilirubin and INR were found to be risk factors of survival as well. Previous studies demonstrated that a higher level of bilirubin was associated with a poor outcome in patients with liver failure because the dysfunctional liver exhibited deficient bilirubin metabolism, which demonstrates that the extent of damage to hepatocytes was extremely serious [8, 30]. Impeded hepatic synthetic function reduces the production of prothrombin and other proteins in the liver, which accounts for the higher level of INR, and a higher degree of INR indicates an unfavourable prognosis [31].

One limitation of our study was the lack of dynamic observations of AFP levels. A persistently low AFP may be interpreted as regenerative failure in protracted cases but ultimately leads to death. Some patients with low AFP concentrations on admission ultimately survived because liver tissue repair occurred followed with a serially intensive care. Other parameters, such as HBeAg, creatinine, albumin, and some scoring systems, could also help assess the outcome of ACLF. Therefore, further studies of multifactor-correlated prognostic models are needed.

5. Conclusion

In summary, AFP is an indicator of the prognosis of hepatitis B-related acute-on-chronic liver failure. Higher levels of AFP concentrations could predict a better outcome of HBACLF, and $\log_{10}^{\text{AFP}} \geq 2$ would indicate a longer survival time.

Authors' Contributions

Shanhong Tang designed the study and carried it out. Sen Qin and Haijun Zeng joined in data collection. Xianjun Yang and Jianjiang Yang conducted data analysis. Xiaoping Wang and Caifei Shen drafted the manuscript. Xiaoling Wu and Weizheng Zeng helped to finalize the manuscript. All of the authors read and approved the manuscript. Xiaoping Wang and Caifei Shen equally contributed to this work.

Acknowledgments

This work was supported by the grant from the National Natural Science Foundations of China 81401993 (to Shanhong Tang).

References

[1] S. K. Sarin and A. Choudhury, "Acute-on-chronic liver failure: Terminology, mechanisms and management," *Nature Reviews Gastroenterology & Hepatology*, vol. 13, no. 3, pp. 131–149, 2016.

[2] L. L. Kjaergard, J. Liu, B. Als-Nielsen, and C. Gluud, "Artificial and bioartificial support systems for acute and acute-on-chronic liver failure: A systematic review," *Journal of the American Medical Association*, vol. 289, no. 2, pp. 217–222, 2003.

[3] S. K. Sarin, C. K. Kedarisetty, Z. Abbas et al., "Acute-on-chronic liver failure: consensus recommendations of the Asian Pacific Association for the Study of the Liver (APASL) 2014," *Hepatology International*, vol. 8, no. 4, pp. 453–471, 2014.

[4] J. Wendon, J. Cordoba, A. Dhawan et al., "EASL clinical practical guidelines on the management of acute (fulminant) liver failure," *Journal of Hepatology*, vol. 66, no. 5, pp. 1047–1081, 2017.

[5] J. Polson and W. M. Lee, "AAFOL Disease, AASLD position paper: the management of acute liver failure: update 2011," *National Guideline Clearinghouse*, vol. 65, no. 1, pp. 1433–1441, 2011.

[6] J. Cordoba, M. Ventura-Cots, M. Simón-Talero et al., "Characteristics, risk factors, and mortality of cirrhotic patients hospitalized for hepatic encephalopathy with and without acute-on-chronic liver failure (ACLF)," *Journal of Hepatology*, vol. 60, no. 2, pp. 275–281, 2014.

[7] I. Merican, R. Guan, D. Amarapuka et al., "Chronic hepatitis B virus infection in Asian countries," *Journal of Gastroenterology and Hepatology*, vol. 15, no. 12, pp. 1356–1361, 2000.

[8] S. Sen, R. Williams, and R. Jalan, "The pathophysiological basis of acute-on-chronic liver failure," *Journal of Liver*, vol. 22, no. 2, pp. 5–13, 2002.

[9] P. S. Kamath and W. R. Kim, "The model for end-stage liver disease (MELD)," *Hepatology*, vol. 45, no. 3, pp. 797–805, 2007.

[10] J. Aguirre-Valadez, A. Torre, M. Vilatobã et al., "Indications for liver transplant," *Revista De Investigacion Clinica*, vol. 66, no. 6, pp. 534–546, 2014.

[11] Y.-M. Zhou, J.-M. Yang, B. Li et al., "Clinicopathologic characteristics of intrahepatic cholangiocarcinoma in patients with positive serum a-fetoprotein," *World Journal of Gastroenterology*, vol. 14, no. 14, pp. 2251–2254, 2008.

[12] K. Kakisaka, K. Kataoka, M. Onodera et al., "Alpha-fetoprotein: A biomarker for the recruitment of progenitor cells in the liver in patients with acute liver injury or failure," *Hepatology Research*, vol. 45, no. 10, pp. E12–E20, 2015.

[13] G. G. Karvountzis and A. G. Redeker, "Relation of alpha fetoprotein in acute hepatitis to severity and prognosis," *Annals of Internal Medicine*, vol. 80, no. 2, pp. 156–160, 1974.

[14] S. K. Jain, A. Rohatgi, K. K. Raman, and V. K. Sharma, "Study of serum prealbumin and serum alpha fetoprotein in cases of fulminant hepatic failure.," *Journal of the Association of Physicians of India*, vol. 43, no. 7, pp. 462-463, 1995.

[15] I. M. Murray-Lyon, A. H. Orr, B. Gazzard, J. Kohn, and R. Williams, "Prognostic value of serum alpha fetoprotein in fulminant hepatic failure including patients treated by charcoal haemoperfusion," *Gut*, vol. 17, no. 8, pp. 576–580, 1976.

[16] A. Varshney, R. Gupta, S. K. Verma, and S. Ahmad, "Alpha-fetoprotein as a prognostic marker in acute liver failure: a pilot study," *Tropical Doctor*, vol. 47, no. 3, pp. 202–205, 2017.

[17] H. Ohnishi, J. Sugihara, H. Moriwaki et al., "Acute-on-chronic liver failure," *Journal of Hepatology*, vol. 13, no. 12, pp. 2128–2139, 1995.

[18] A. Katoonizadeh, W. Laleman, C. Verslype et al., "Early features of acute-on-chronic alcoholic liver failure: A prospective cohort study," *Gut*, vol. 59, no. 11, pp. 1561–1569, 2010.

[19] S. Lin, J. Chen, M. Wang et al., "Prognostic nomogram for acute-on-chronic hepatitis B liver failure," *Oncotarget* , vol. 8, no. 65, pp. 109772–109782, 2017.

[20] S. M. Zhu, Y. Waili, X. T. Qi, Y. M. Chen, and Y. F. Lou, "Lymphocyte-monocyte ratio at admission predicts possible outcomes in patients with acute-on-chronic liver failure," *European Journal of Gastroenterology & Hepatology*, vol. 29, no. 1, pp. 31–35, 2017.

[21] B. Chen and S. Lin, "Albumin-bilirubin (ALBI) score at admission predicts possible outcomes in patients with acute-on-chronic liver failure," *Medicine (United States)*, vol. 96, no. 24, Article ID e7142, 2017.

[22] M.-H. Zheng, K.-Q. Shi, Y.-C. Fan et al., "A Model to Determine 3-Month Mortality Risk in Patients With Acute-on-Chronic Hepatitis B Liver Failure," *Clinical Gastroenterology and Hepatology*, vol. 9, no. 4, pp. 351–e3, 2011.

[23] J. Xin, W. Ding, S. Hao et al., "Serum macrophage inflammatory protein 3α levels predict the severity of HBV-related acute-on-chronic liver failure," *Gut*, vol. 65, no. 2, pp. 355–357, 2016.

[24] Y. Yan, L. Mai, Y.-B. Zheng et al., "What MELD score mandates use of entecavir for ACLF-HBV HBeAg-negative patients?" *World Journal of Gastroenterology*, vol. 18, no. 33, pp. 4604–4609, 2012.

[25] T. Wu, J. Li, L. Shao et al., "Development of diagnostic criteria and a prognostic score for hepatitis B virus-related acute-on-chronic liver failure," *Gut*, p. gutjnl-2017-314641.

[26] L. Chen, Y. Lou, Y. Chen, and J. Yang, "Prognostic value of the neutrophil-to-lymphocyte ratio in patients with acute-on-chronic liver failure," *International Journal of Clinical Practice*, vol. 68, no. 8, pp. 1034–1040, 2014.

[27] L. E. Schmidt and K. Dalhoff, "Alpha-fetoprotein is a predictor of outcome in acetaminophen-induced liver injury," *Hepatology*, vol. 41, no. 1, pp. 26–31, 2005.

[28] F. V. Schiodt, G. Ostapowicz, N. Murray et al., "Alpha-fetoprotein and prognosis in acute liver failure," *Liver Transplantation*, vol. 12, no. 12, pp. 1776–1781, 2006.

[29] G. I. Abelev, S. D. Perova, N. I. Khramkova, Z. A. Postnikova, and I. S. Irlin, "Production of embryonal α-globulin by transplantable mouse hepatomas," *Transplantation*, vol. 1, no. 2, pp. 174–180, 1963.

[30] Y. R. Krishna, V. A. Saraswat, K. Das et al., "Clinical features and predictors of outcome in acute hepatitis A and hepatitis E virus hepatitis on cirrhosis," *Liver International*, vol. 29, no. 3, pp. 392–398, 2009.

[31] H. Garg, A. Kumar, V. Garg, P. Sharma, B. C. Sharma, and S. K. Sarin, "Clinical profile and predictors of mortality in patients of acute-on-chronic liver failure," *Digestive and Liver Disease*, vol. 44, no. 2, pp. 166–171, 2012.

48-Week Outcome after Cessation of Nucleos(t)ide Analogue Treatment in Chronic Hepatitis B Patient and the Associated Factors with Relapse

Wen-xiong Xu,[1,2] Qian Zhang,[3] Xiang Zhu,[1,2] Chao-shuang Lin,[1,2] You-ming Chen,[1,2] Hong Deng,[1,2] Yong-yu Mei,[1,2] Zhi-xin Zhao,[1,2] Dong-ying Xie,[1,2] Zhi-liang Gao,[1,2] Chan Xie,[1,2] and Liang Peng[1,2]

[1]*Department of Infectious Diseases, Third Affiliated Hospital of Sun Yat-sen University, Guangzhou, Guangdong 510630, China*
[2]*Guangdong Key Laboratory of Liver Disease Research, Third Affiliated Hospital of Sun Yat-sen University, Guangzhou, Guangdong 510630, China*
[3]*Department of Infectious Diseases, Union Hospital, Tongji Medical College, Huazhong University of Science and Technology, Wuhan, Hubei 430022, China*

Correspondence should be addressed to Chan Xie; happyxiechan@hotmail.com and Liang Peng; pliang@mail.sysu.edu.cn

Wen-xiong Xu and Qian Zhang contributed equally to this work.

Academic Editor: Kevork M. Peltekian

Background and Aims. We aimed to ascertain the feasibility and safety of NA cessation, the status of patients after cessation, and the predictive factors for relapse and subsequent retreatment. *Methods.* A total of 92 patients were enrolled in this prospective study. Patients were monitored every month for the first 3 months after cessation and every 3 months thereafter. *Results.* Sixty-two patients finished 48 weeks of follow-up. None died or developed liver failure, cirrhosis, or HCC. The 62 patients could be divided into 4 categories according to the 48-week clinical development of relapse. Virologic relapses occurred in 39 (62.9%) patients, with 72.7% occurring in the first 24 weeks in origin HBeAg positive patients and 82.4% in the first 12 weeks in origin HBeAg negative patients. Age (OR = 1.06, 95% CI = 1.02–1.10; $p = 0.003$), the HBsAg level (OR = 2.21, 95% CI = 1.47–3.32; $p < 0.001$), and positive origin HBeAg status (OR = 0.32, 95% CI = 0.14–0.74; $p = 0.008$) were predictive factors to virologic relapse. HBV DNA level (OR = 1.34, 95% CI = 1.13–1.58; $p < 0.001$) was predictive factor to retreatment. *Conclusions.* NA cessation is safe under supervision. Age, HBsAg level, and origin HBeAg status can be predictive factors for virologic relapse. The study was submitted to ClinicalTrials.gov Protocol Registration and Results System with the assigned NCT ID NCT02883647.

1. Introduction

Chronic hepatitis B virus (HBV) infection is a major health problem, as approximately 240 million people are infected worldwide [1]. Nucleos(t)ide analogues (NA) have been developed to control HBV [2], and they can strongly inhibit reverse transcriptase to suppress the HBV DNA levels but cannot erase covalently closed circular DNA (cccDNA), as it integrates into the genome in the nuclei of the host hepatocytes [3]. Therefore, most patients require long-term NA therapy, even though HBV DNA levels are suppressed to undetectable levels in a short amount of time.

Long-term NA therapy can control chronic hepatitis B, but several problems remain. The first is the economical burden, especially in developing countries where health care and life insurance are poor. The second are poor adherence and retention in care of the patients, resulting from this high cost. The third is the side effect of the drugs, including renal and bone toxicity. The fourth are viral mutant and drug resistance which are further hindrances to drug efficacy.

Finite NA therapy has the advantages of solving the above problems. How to make finite NA therapy is what physicians and patients concern.

Guidelines of prevention and treatment of chronic hepatitis B (CHB) from China [4], Asian Pacific Association for the Study of the Liver (APASL) [5], European Association for the Study of the Liver (EASL) [6], American Association for the Study of Liver Diseases (AASLD) [7], and World Health Organization (WHO) [8] all make suggestions on NA cessation, including parameters like NA treatment duration and consolidation treatment duration. Although physicians follow these suggestions, recent studies still indicate high virologic relapse rates ranging from 40% to 95% in the first year after NA cessation [9–12]. Some authors in these studies presented predictive factors for relapse, such as age, consolidation treatment duration, NA treatment duration, and baseline HBV DNA level. But some authors had the opposite opinion. There are, as yet, difficulties of how to stop NA therapy without relapse. Otherwise, NA cessation without supervision may result in an unpredictable worsening of disease and the possible development of cirrhosis, fulminant hepatitis, or acute-on-chronic liver failure (ACLF). Safety of NA therapy cessation and NA retreatment efficacy after relapse are very important issues that should be found out. In this study, we aimed to determine the feasibility and safety of NA cessation, the therapeutic effect of retreatment in relapsed patients, the features of patients after cessation, and the predictive factors for relapse and retreatment.

2. Materials and Methods

2.1. Study Population. This prospective study recruited 92 Chinese HAN outpatients with chronic hepatitis B in Third Affiliated Hospital of Sun Yat-sen University from December 2013 to January 2017. All patients were treated with nucleos(t)ide analogues, such as entecavir (ETV), telbivudine (LDT), lamivudine (LAM), adefovir dipivoxil (ADV), or a combination of LAM and ADV. Informed consent from the patients was obtained.

2.2. Inclusion and Exclusion Criteria

Inclusion Criteria. They include the following: (1) CHB patients (hepatitis B surface antigen [HBsAg] and HBV DNA positive for at least 6 months [5]) receiving NA therapy; (2) age from 18 to 65 years; (3) patients who had been treated with NA for at least 2 years with undetectable HBV DNA levels on at least 3 separate occasions, 6 months apart, before the cessation of treatment (otherwise, hepatitis B e antigen (HBeAg) seroconversion was required and maintained for at least one year in origin HBeAg positive patients); (4) HBV DNA level that were "not detected" or "<20 IU/mL," as determined by Roche COBAS detection before cessation.

Exclusion Criteria. They include the following: (1) patients with liver cirrhosis, hepatocellular carcinoma (HCC), or other malignancies; (2) patients with other factors causing liver disease; (3) pregnant or lactating women; (4) patients with concomitant HIV infection or congenital immune deficiency diseases; (5) patients with diabetes or autoimmune diseases; (6) patients with important organ dysfunctions or serious complications (e.g., infection, ascites, hepatic encephalopathy, hepatorenal syndrome, or gastrointestinal bleeding).

2.3. Follow-Up Evaluation. All patients were monitored every month for the first 3 months after cessation and every 3 months thereafter. Symptoms (e.g., fatigue, poor appetite, and jaundice), occurrence of liver cirrhosis or HCC, and mortality were all recorded for the study. Blood cells (white blood cells, red blood cells, hemoglobin, and platelets), biochemical parameters (serum aspartate transaminase [AST], alanine transaminase [ALT], total bilirubin, blood urea nitrogen [BUN], and creatinine), virologic parameters (quantitative HBsAg, HBeAg, HBeAb, and HBV DNA), T lymphocytes (CD4 positive T lymphocytes [$CD4^+T$], CD8 positive T lymphocytes [$CD8^+T$], Type 1 helper T lymphocytes [Th1], and Type 2 helper T lymphocytes [Th2]), and ultrasound results were assessed at every visit.

Routine automated techniques were used for all biochemical tests at our clinical laboratories. Serum HBsAg levels were measured using Roche Elecsys HBsAg II quant assay (range 0.05–52000 IU/mL, Roche Diagnostics, Mannheim, Germany). Serum HBeAg and HBeAb were assayed using the EIA kit (Abbott Diagnostics, North Chicago, IL). Serum HBV DNA levels were measured with real-time PCR using the COBAS AmpliPrep/COBAS TaqMan HBV Test, version 2.0 (detection limit: 20 IU/mL, Roche Molecular Systems, Inc., Branchburg, NJ, USA). T lymphocytes were measured using flow cytometry analysis with a BD Accuri C6 flow cytometer according to the manufacturer's instructions.

2.4. Definition and Management of Relapse. According to guideline of prevention and treatment of chronic hepatitis B from APASL [5], virologic relapse was defined as HBV DNA > 2000 IU/mL, while clinical relapse was defined as HBV DNA > 2000 IU/mL and ALT > 2 times upper limit of normal (ULN).

Patients Management. (1) Patients with nonrelapse would go on for the next visit. (2) Patients with virologic relapse would go on for the next visit if ALT ≤ 2 times ULN. (3) Patients with clinical relapse would go on for the next visit if they have no symptoms and ALT ≤ 5 times ULN. (4) Patients with clinical relapse would be retreated with NA if they have symptoms and ALT ≤ 5 times ULN. (5) Patients with clinical relapse would be retreated with NA if ALT > 5 times ULN. Patients were monitored every month for the first 3 months after retreatment with NA and every 3 months thereafter.

2.5. Ethical Approval. Ethical approval was provided by the Ethics Committee of Medical Clinical Trials, the Third Affiliated Hospital of Sun Yat-sen University (March 20, 2015).

2.6. Statistical Analysis. Continuous data were indicated with mean ± SD while categorical data were reported as number and percentage (%). Spearman correlation coefficient was used to investigate the correlation among HBsAg, HBV DNA, and T lymphocytes. Nonparametric tests including Mann–Whitney U test and Wilcoxon signed-rank test were used to compare means between groups for data normality was not assumed.

The outcome variables included the occurrences of virologic relapse or retreatment at baseline (month 0) and 1, 2, 3, 6, and 12 months after cessation. Associations between independent variables and outcome variables were analyzed using univariate/multivariate generalized estimating equation (GEE) and binary logistic regression models. An independent working correlation matrix was adopted for the repeated measure data. ROC analysis was further used to assess the diagnostic effectiveness of independent variables which were found associated with outcome. The statistical significance level for all the tests was set at a p value < 0.05. Statistical analyses were performed using IBM SPSS Version 20 (SPSS Statistics V20, IBM Corporation, Somers, New York).

3. Results

3.1. Baseline Characteristics. A total of 92 patients treated with NA were recruited in this study. Nine of the patients were lost to follow-up, and 62 finished the 48 weeks of follow-up. Thirty-nine of the 62 patients were origin HBeAg positive before NA treatment; they gained HBeAg seroconversion before NA cessation. Twenty-three patients were origin HBeAg negative before NA treatment. Nineteen patients were treated with ETV for 4.55 ± 1.93 years before cessation, 23 patients were treated with LDT for 3.35 ± 1.34 years, 5 patients were treated with LAM for 5.02 ± 2.46 years, 7 patients were treated with ADV for 7.51 ± 2.65 years, and 8 patients were treated with combination of LAM and ADV for 4.94 ± 2.95 years. The flow of patient recruiting and clinical development was indicated in Figure 1. The baseline characteristics of the 62 patients were shown in Table 1.

3.2. Safety of NA Cessation. In the course of the 48 weeks of follow-up, none of the 62 patients died or developed liver failure, cirrhosis, or hepatocellular carcinoma. Twenty-one (33.9%) patients were retreated with NA (origin NA or ETV or TDF) and regained normal ALT and undetectable HBV DNA within 24 weeks.

3.3. Four Categories in Follow-Up. According to the development of patient's levels of HBV DNA and ALT across time (from 0 to 48 weeks) and features of relapse in the follow-up, the 62 patients could be divided into 4 categories (Figures 1 and 2): Category A, consisting of 23 patients in the nonrelapse group, for whom ALT remained normal and HBV DNA levels were not higher than 2000 IU/mL during the follow-up; Category B, consisting of 4 patients in the virologic relapse group, for whom ALT levels were not higher than 2 ULN and HBV DNA remained above 2000 IU/mL during the follow-up; Category C, consisting of 14 patients in the virologic relapse group, for whom HBV DNA levels decreased into no higher than 2000 IU/mL automatically without antiviral treatment during the follow-up, changing patient status to nonrelapse; Category D, consisting of 21 patients with high ALT levels and HBV DNA levels which were sufficiently elevated during the follow-up to necessitate retreatment with NA, in order to avoid fulminant hepatitis or cirrhosis.

3.4. Cumulative Relapse and Retreatment Rates. For all 62 patients who finished 48-week follow-up, the 48-week cumulative virologic relapse, clinical relapse, and retreatment rate were 62.9%, 38.7%, and 33.9%, respectively. For the 39 origin HBeAg positive patients, the 48-week cumulative virologic relapse, clinical relapse, and retreatment rate were 56.4%, 35.9%, and 30.8%, respectively. Sixteen of 22 (72.7%) virologic relapses and 11 of 14 (78.6%) clinical relapses occurred in the first 24 weeks in origin HBeAg positive patients. For the 23 origin HBeAg negative patients, the 48-week cumulative virologic relapse, clinical relapse, and retreatment rate were 73.9%, 43.5%, and 39.1%, respectively. Fourteen of 17 (82.4%) virologic relapses and 6 of 10 (60%) clinical relapses occurred in the first 12 weeks in origin HBeAg negative patients. The results were shown in Figure 3.

3.5. $CD4^+T$, $CD8^+T$, Th1, and Th2. To further investigate the association among HBsAg, HBV DNA, and flow cytometry results, correlation analyses were used. A negative correlation was found between HBsAg and $CD4^+T$ ($r = -0.37$, $p < 0.001$), a positive correlation was found between HBsAg and $CD8^+T$ ($r = 0.37$, $p < 0.001$), and no correlations at all were found between HBsAg and Th1 ($p = 0.832$) or Th2 ($p = 0.887$). A negative correlation was found between HBV DNA and $CD4^+T$ ($r = -0.44$, $p < 0.001$), and no correlations at all were found between HBV DNA and $CD8^+T$ ($p = 0.114$) or Th1 ($p = 0.243$) or Th2 ($p = 0.703$). The changes in these ratios over the course of follow-up in both nonrelapse and virologic relapse patients were shown in Figure 4. No statistical significance was found between any of the groups (all $p > 0.05$).

3.6. Predictive Factors for Virologic Relapse and Retreatment. Univariate and multivariate logistic regression under GEE models were used to investigate the possibly predictive factor for virologic relapse or retreatment. Independent variables which were not significant in univariate results would still be modeled in multivariate model as adjustment of covariates. Only the variables which reached significance in both univariate and multivariate models would be recognized as possibly predictive factor to virologic relapse or retreatment.

As shown in Table 2, age and the level of HBsAg were significant risk factors. As age and the level of HBsAg are increasing, the more likely patients would occur with virologic relapse. The estimated ORs (odds ratio) of age and the level of HBsAg were 1.06 (95% CI = 1.02–1.10; $p = 0.003$) and 2.21 (95% CI = 1.47–3.32; $p < 0.001$), respectively. On the contrary, positive status of origin HBeAg before NA treatment was a protective factor. The estimated OR was 0.32 (95% CI = 0.14–0.74; $p = 0.008$) which means lower risk to occur with virologic relapse.

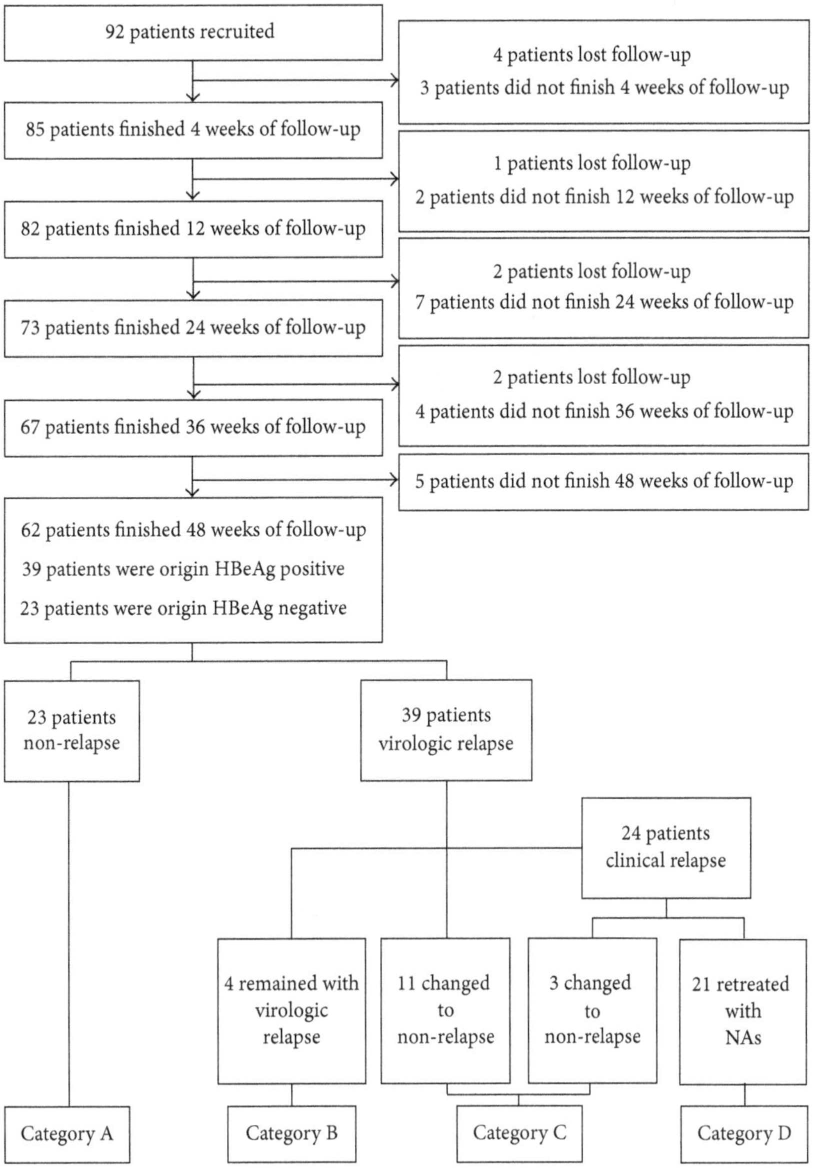

Figure 1: Flow chart of patient recruitment and clinical development.

Table 1: Baseline characteristics of 62 patients before NA treatment cessation.

	origin HBeAg positive ($n = 39$)	origin HBeAg negative ($n = 23$)	All ($n = 62$)
Age, year	33.18 ± 8.33	44.39 ± 8.99	37.34 ± 10.11
Gender, male (%)	26 (66.7)	19 (82.6)	45 (72.6)
BMI, kg/cm^2	21.31 ± 2.91	23.01 ± 3.12	21.95 ± 3.08
NA treatment, ratio of ETV : LDT : LAM : ADV : LAM + ADV*	10 : 17 : 3 : 5 : 4	9 : 6 : 2 : 2 : 4	19 : 23 : 5 : 7 : 8
Duration of NA treatment, year	4.64 ± 2.63	4.33 ± 1.74	4.52 ± 2.33
Duration of negative HBV DNA maintenance, year	3.83 ± 2.15	3.68 ± 1.31	3.78 ± 1.87
Duration of HBeAg seroconversion maintenance, year	3.19 ± 2.47	-	-
EOT HBsAg, log 10(IU/mL)#	2.65 ± 1.22	2.36 ± 1.38	2.54 ± 1.28

*NA: nucleos(t)ide analogues; ETV: entecavir; LDT: telbivudine; LAM: lamivudine; ADV: adefovir dipivoxil; #EOT: end of treatment.

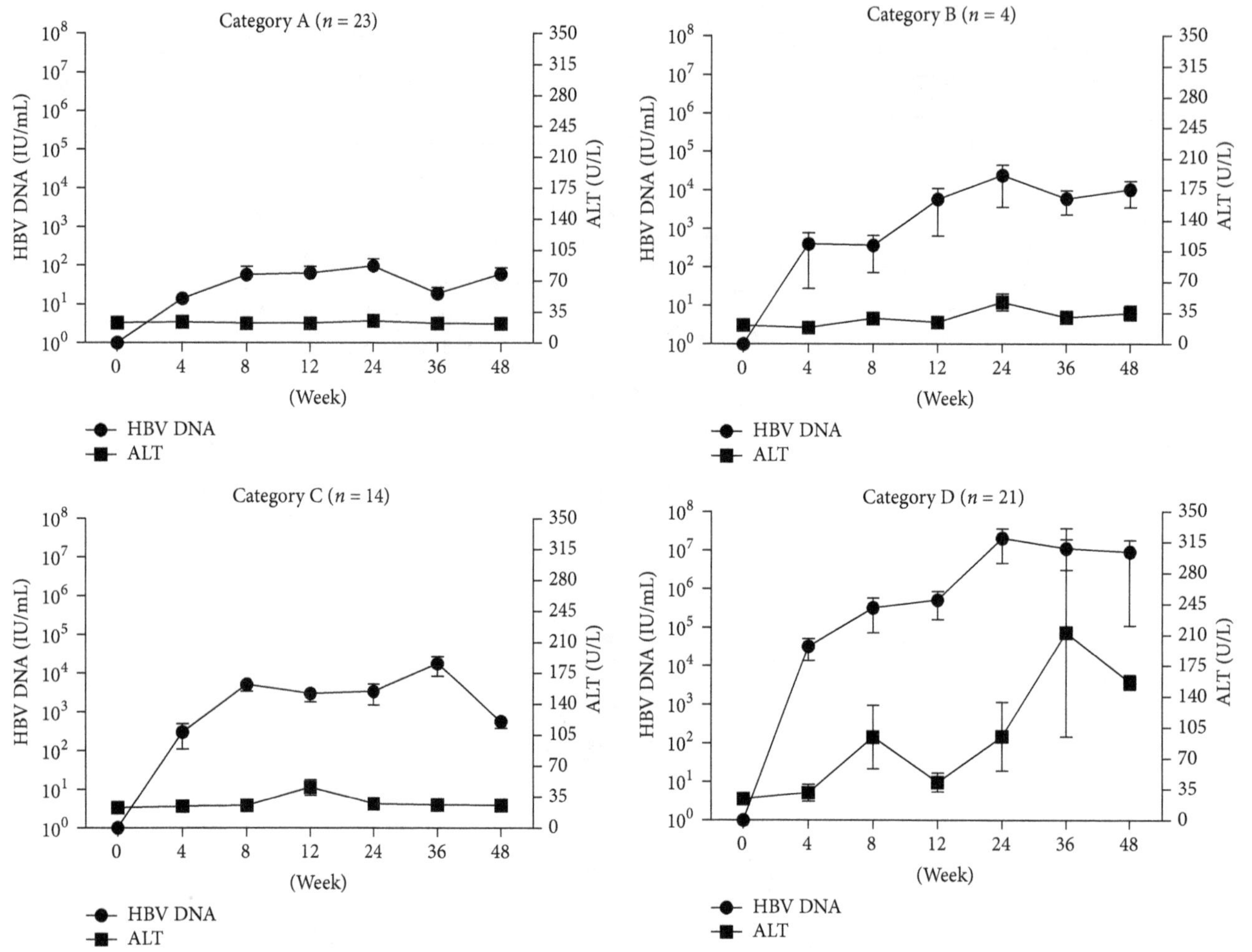

FIGURE 2: Change of levels of ALT and HBV DNA in four categories from 0 to 48 weeks.

TABLE 2: Independent variables associated with virologic relapse in GEE models.

Parameters	Univariate		Multivariate	
	OR (95% CI)	p	OR (95% CI)	p
Sex				
Male	Ref	-	Ref	-
Female	1.12 (0.51–2.49)	0.774	1.14 (0.59–2.19)	0.704
Age, year	1.05 (1.01–1.08)	0.009	1.06 (1.02–1.10)	0.003
BMI, kg/m^2	0.97 (0.87–1.09)	0.617	0.85 (0.75–0.95)	0.006
Duration of NA treatment, year	0.89 (0.74–1.08)	0.255	1.40 (1.14–1.73)	0.001
Duration of negative HBV DNA maintenance, year	0.81 (0.65–1.01)	0.066	0.52 (0.33–0.83)	0.005
HBsAg, log 10(IU/mL)	1.79 (1.32–2.45)	<0.001	2.21 (1.47–3.32)	<0.001
Origin HBeAg				
Negative	Ref	-	Ref	-
Positive	0.38 (0.19–0.79)	0.010	0.32 (0.14–0.74)	0.008

The results of retreatment were indicated in Table 3. The level HBV DNA was found to be the only variable which was significant in both univariate and multivariate models. The estimated OR of HBV DNA was 1.34 (95% CI = 1.13–1.58; $p < 0.001$) which means every unit increased would increase 1.34 times of odds of needing retreatment.

ROC analysis was further used to investigate the diagnostic effectiveness of these associated factors. As indicated in Figure 5, the results of age to virologic relapse (Figure 5(a)), the level of HBsAg to virologic relapse (Figure 5(b)), and the level of HBsAg to clinical relapse (Figure 5(c)) all showed significant diagnostic effectiveness (all $p < 0.05$). The optimal

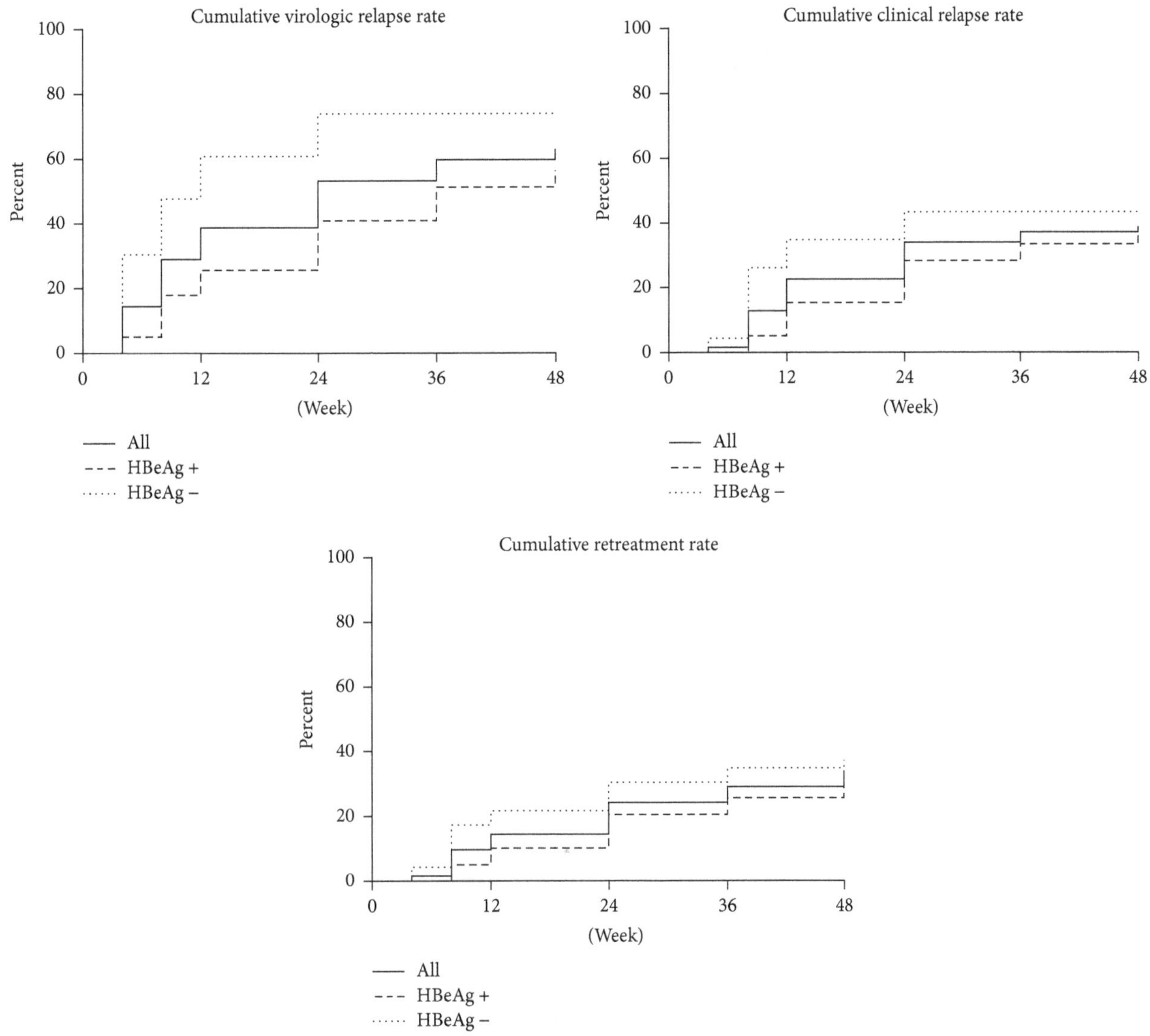

FIGURE 3: Forty-eight-week cumulative rates of virologic relapse, clinical relapse, and retreatment.

TABLE 3: Independent variables associated with retreatment in GEE models.

Parameters	Univariate		Multivariate	
	OR (95% CI)	*p*	OR (95% CI)	*p*
Sex				
Male	Ref	-	Ref	-
Female	1.75 (0.42–7.35)	0.445	2.17 (0.45–10.43)	0.332
Age, year	1.06 (0.98–1.14)	0.177	1.04 (0.92–1.18)	0.490
BMI, kg/m^2	1.00 (0.80–1.26)	0.975	1.02 (0.78–1.34)	0.878
Duration of NA treatment, year	1.25 (0.81–1.95)	0.314	1.08 (0.53–2.20)	0.830
Duration of negative HBV DNA maintenance, year	1.45 (0.90–2.33)	0.130	1.11 (0.42–2.91)	0.830
HBV DNA, log 10(IU/mL)	1.28 (1.08–1.50)	0.003	1.34 (1.13–1.58)	<0.001
HBsAg, log 10(IU/mL)	0.69 (0.26–1.83)	0.460	0.64 (0.24–1.72)	0.382
Origin HBeAg				
Negative	Ref	-	Ref	-
Positive	1.07 (0.30–3.80)	0.921	1.23 (0.17–8.93)	0.838

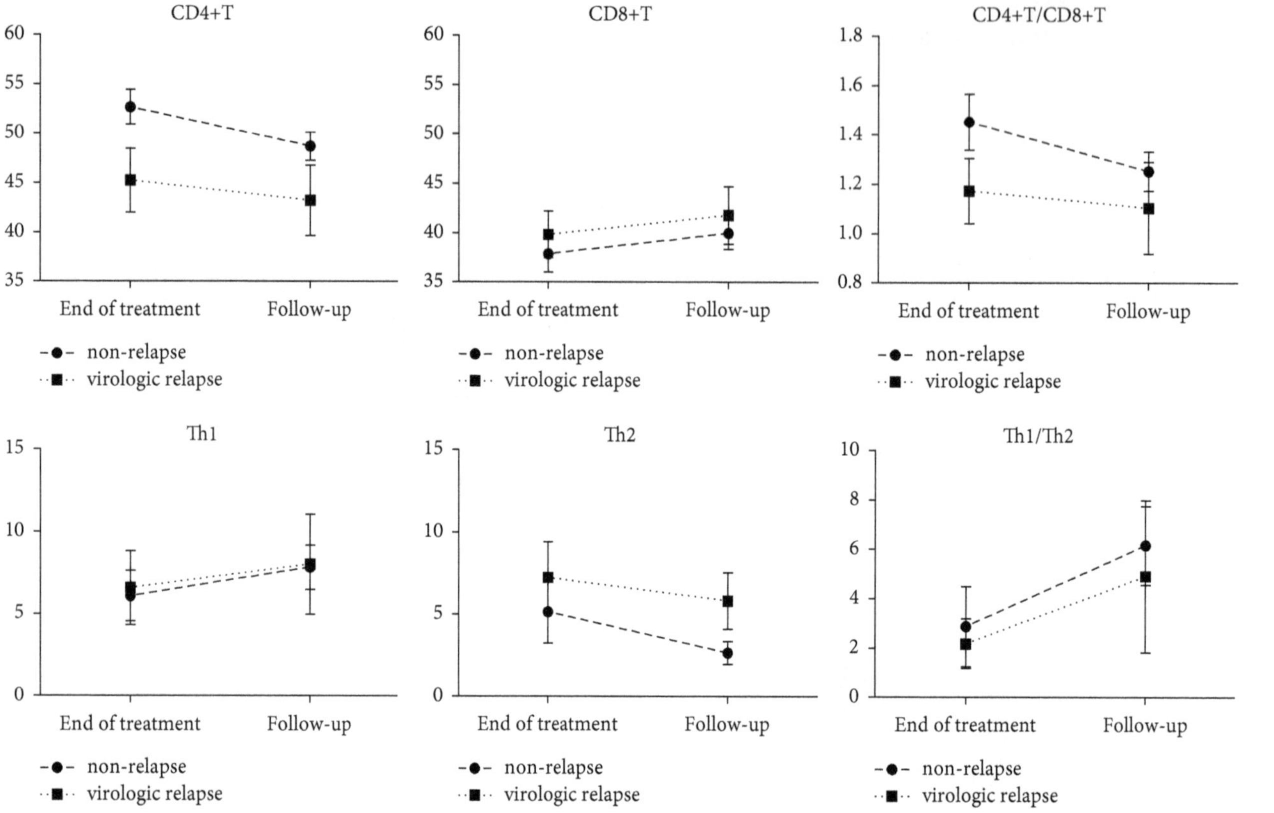

FIGURE 4: Changes in the ratios of $CD4^+T$, $CD8^+T$, Th1, and Th2 in nonrelapse and virologic relapse patients.

cutoffs chosen by Youden's index of age to virologic relapse, the level of HBsAg to virologic relapse, and the level of HBsAg to clinical relapse were 32.5 years, 2.05 log 10(IU/mL), and 2.30 log 10(IU/mL), respectively. All these three ROC results demonstrated good sensitivity (over 0.8) but lower specificity (lower than 0.5); however these results still indicated that age and HBsAg were potential factors in predicting relapse.

4. Discussion

In this study, under supervision, none of the patients in our study died or developed cirrhosis, liver failure, or hepatocellular carcinoma. The 48-week cumulative virologic relapse rates in origin HBeAg positive and negative CHB patients were 56.4% and 73.9%, respectively, which were similar results to a study [13] by Lee et al. and a systematic review [14] by Chang et al., although we strictly followed the 2012 APASL guidelines [5]. Twenty-one (39.1%) patients required retreatment with NAs. Fortunately, the virologic relapse was controlled by retreatment within 24 weeks.

Increased attention should be paid during the first 24 weeks of the follow-up after NA cessation in origin HBeAg positive patients, since 16 of 22 (72.7%) virologic relapses and 11 of 14 (78.6%) clinical relapses occurred in these first 24 weeks. Similarly, the first 12 weeks of follow-up after NA cessation also require increased vigilance in origin HBeAg negative patients, since 14 of 17 (82.4%) virologic relapses and 6 of 10 (60%) clinical relapses occurred in these first 12 weeks.

The 62 patients could be divided into four categories in this study. We designated Category A as "immune control," since no relapse occurred in the category. We designated Category B as "immune retolerance," since we assumed that the immune status of these patients is similar to "immune tolerance" in childhood during chronic HBV infection with a high load of HBV replication and normal ALT levels. We designated Category C as "immune recontrol," since we assumed that host immunity blocked HBV replication without help from the NA therapy. We designated Category D as "immune reactivation," since we assumed these patients were similar to naïve patients receiving NA therapy with elevated ALT and HBV DNA levels. The four different immune statuses may relate to the function of HBV-specific T cells, because the antiviral drug-induced attenuation of viremia provides a window for the reconstitution of the HBV-specific immune response [15]. Further study of HBV-specific T cell response should be conducted, in order to ascertain the differences between these four categories.

In this study, we found a negative correlation between HBsAg and $CD4^+T$, a positive correlation between HBsAg and $CD8^+T$, and a negative correlation between HBV DNA and $CD4^+T$. In patients with chronic HBV infection, cytotoxic T cell response is weak [16], especially for virus-specific T cell response [17]. $CD8^+T$ activity is inhibited by high levels of HBV DNA, microRNA-146a, and immunosuppressive cytokines such as interleukin-10 [18, 19]. Therefore, removal of viral antigens, allowing T cells to rest, is important for functional reconstitution of T cell immune response [20].

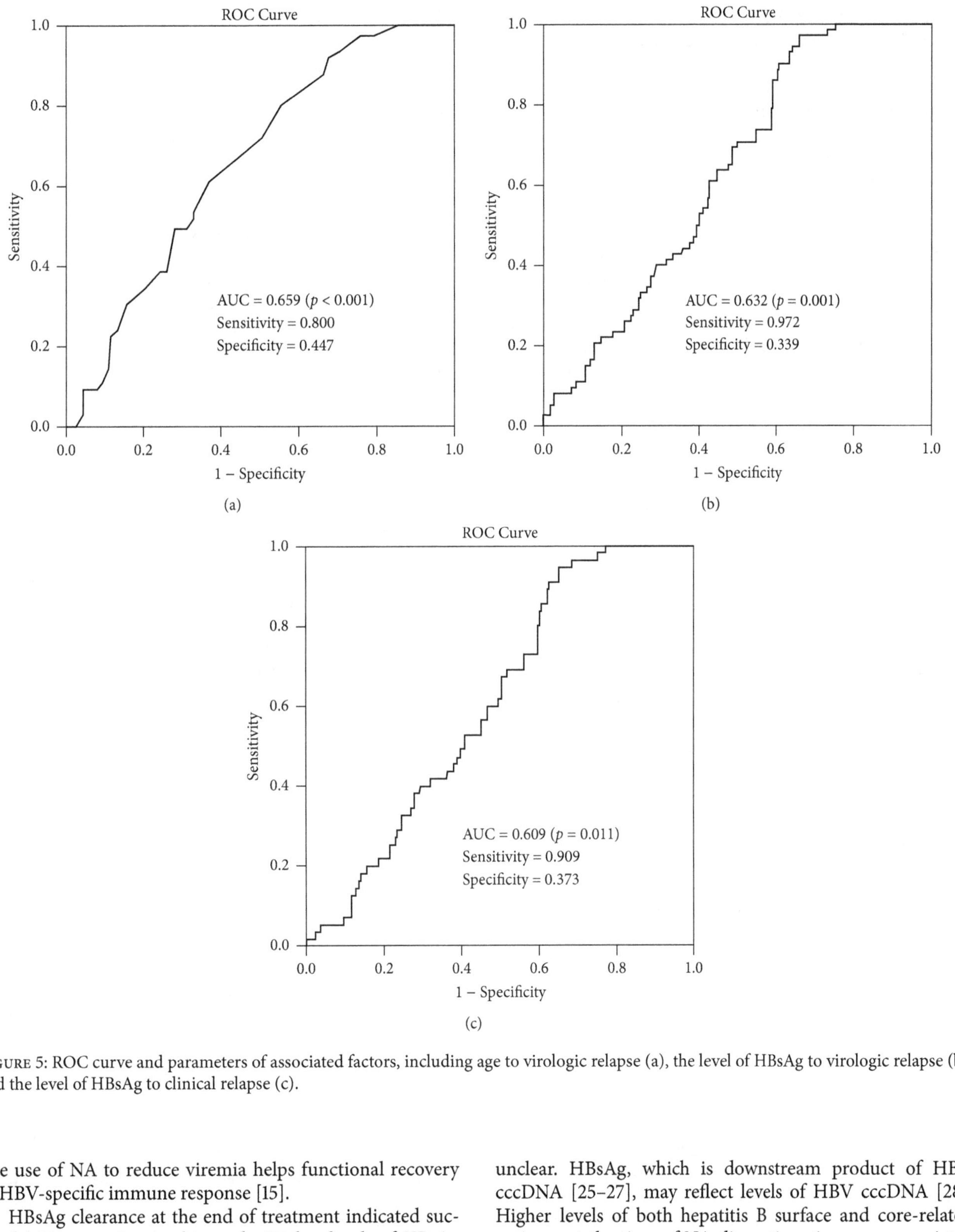

FIGURE 5: ROC curve and parameters of associated factors, including age to virologic relapse (a), the level of HBsAg to virologic relapse (b), and the level of HBsAg to clinical relapse (c).

The use of NA to reduce viremia helps functional recovery of HBV-specific immune response [15].

HBsAg clearance at the end of treatment indicated successful NA cessation in this study. Higher levels of HBsAg indicated increased risk of virologic relapse. Similar results were reported in some studies [21–23]. In contrast, Seto et al. reported that HBsAg levels at the beginning of entecavir treatment, entecavir cessation, and the subsequent rate of HBsAg reduction were not associated with virologic relapse [24]. The reason for these two opposite opinions is still unclear. HBsAg, which is downstream product of HBV cccDNA [25–27], may reflect levels of HBV cccDNA [28]. Higher levels of both hepatitis B surface and core-related antigens at the time of NA discontinuation were associated with relapse [28]. Lower end-of-treatment HBsAg levels may contribute to higher cumulative HBsAg loss rate after NA cessation [29]. A quite lengthy follow-up observation after NA cessation is necessary for evaluating the rate of HBsAg loss. A randomized controlled study from Berg T [30] found that HBsAg levels decreased in the 144 weeks follow-up after

TDF therapy stopped. Study from Hadziyannis et al. [31] showed 39% of patients lose HBsAg in the 6-year follow-up after ADV therapy cessation. But it is assumed that NA therapy requires 52.2 years in order to achieve HBsAg clearance and that a finite treatment duration is unlikely [32]. As HBsAg clearance is not easy to achieve, other predictive factors should be investigated in the clinical practice.

In this study, age was a predictive factor for virologic relapse. Some studies have shown that age > 40 years predicted relapse in origin HBeAg positive patients [9, 23, 33]. Age served as a predictor for virologic relapse in origin HBeAg negative patients in other studies [21, 23]. We found no other predictive factors for virologic relapse, such as NA treatment duration or duration of negative HBV DNA maintenance. Chaung et al. [10] reported that HBeAg seroconversion and consolidation duration were not predictors for relapse. Findings from Chen et al. suggest that there were no predictive factors for relapse [34]. It seems that prolonged NA treatment or prolonged consolidation treatment cannot reduce the virologic relapse rate, which is not in accordance with the new updates of guidelines, comparing to the old ones, from APASL [35], suggesting more than 3 years of consolidation treatment in origin HBeAg positive patients to stop NA, or from EASL [36], suggesting more than 3 years of virological suppression in origin HBeAg negative patients to stop NA. But a systematic review [37] suggests that on-therapy virological remission (VR) > 24 months offers higher chances of off-NA VR in patients with HBeAg negative chronic hepatitis B.

As mentioned above, there are difficulties to stop NA therapy without relapse. Discontinuation of NA therapy in CHB continues to be a hot topic with contrasting views in the recent liver meeting: patients may benefit from NA therapy cessation [38]; however there is no robust evidence to support treatment discontinuation [39].

This study has some limitations. First, the case number was small, since we recruited patients from only one center. Second, pretreatment HBV genotype results were not carried out, since diagnostic reagents were scarce and HBV genotype was not a routine test in the past ten years in China which is still a developing country. Third, further study on HBV-specific cytotoxic T lymphocytes immune response was not carried out.

5. Conclusion

NA cessation is safe under supervision. Increased vigilance was required in the first 24 weeks in origin HBeAg positive patients and the first 12 weeks in negative patients. Age, HBsAg level before NA cessation, and origin HBeAg status before NA treatment can be predictive factors for virologic relapse. HBV DNA can be predictive factor for retreatment.

Abbreviations

NA: Nucleos(t)ide analogues
HBV: Hepatitis B virus
CHB: Chronic hepatitis B
HCC: Hepatocellular carcinoma
ETV: Entecavir
LDT: Telbivudine
LAM: Lamivudine
ADV: Adefovir dipivoxil
TDF: Tenofovir disoproxil fumarate
HBsAg: Hepatitis B surface antigen
HBeAg: Hepatitis B e antigen
AST: Aspartate transaminase
ALT: Alanine transaminase
$CD4^+T$: CD4 positive T lymphocytes
$CD8^+T$: CD8 positive T lymphocytes
Thl: Type 1 helper T lymphocytes
Th2: Type 2 helper T lymphocytes
ULN: Upper limit of normal
EOT: End of treatment
VR: Virological remission.

Acknowledgments

Thanks are due to Pan Shun-wen and Li Wan-tao of the laboratory of Third Affiliated Hospital of Sun Yat-sen University. This study was supported by Plan of Science and Technology of Guangdong (nos. 411308023039 and 2016A020215221), Guangzhou Science and Technology Project (nos. 201508020118 and 2014Y2-00544), the National Natural Science Foundation of China (nos. 81570539 and 81370535), and the Fundamental Research Funds for the Central Universities (Precision Medicine and Biological Big Data) (no. 15ykjc21d).

References

[1] J. J. Ott, G. A. Stevens, J. Groeger, and S. T. Wiersma, "Global epidemiology of hepatitis B virus infection: new estimates of age-specific HBsAg seroprevalence and endemicity," *Vaccine*, vol. 30, no. 12, pp. 2212–2219, 2012.

[2] J. L. Dienstag, "Benefits and risks of nucleoside analog therapy for hepatitis B," *Hepatology*, vol. 49, no. 5, pp. S112–S121, 2009.

[3] B. Werle-Lapostolle, S. Bowden, S. Locarnini et al., "Persistence of cccDNA during the natural history of chronic hepatitis B and decline during adefovir dipivoxil therapy," *Gastroenterology*, vol. 126, no. 7, pp. 1750–1758, 2004.

[4] Chinese Society of Hepatology, Chinese Society of Infectious Diseases, and Chinese Medical Association, "The guideline of prevention and treatment for chronic hepatitis B (2010 version)," *Chinese Journal of Hepatology*, vol. 19, no. 1, pp. 13–24, 2011.

[5] Asian Pacific Association for the Study of the Liver, "Asian-Pacific consensus statement on the management of chronic hepatitis B: a 2012 update," *Hepatology International*, vol. 6, pp. 531–561, 2012.

[6] European Association for the Study of the Liver, "EASL clinical practice guidelines: management of chronic hepatitis B virus infection," *Journal of Hepatology*, vol. 57, no. 1, pp. 167–185, 2012.

[7] A. S. F. Lok and B. J. McMahon, "Chronic hepatitis B: update 2009," *Hepatology*, vol. 50, no. 3, pp. 661-662, 2009.

[8] World Health Organization, "Guidelines for the prevention, care and treatment of persons with chronic hepatitis B infection," 2015, http://www.who.int/hepatitis/publications/hepatitis-b-guidelines/en/.

[9] M. J. Song, D. S. Song, H. Y. Kim et al., "Durability of viral response after off-treatment in HBeAg positive chronic hepatitis B," *World Journal of Gastroenterology*, vol. 18, no. 43, pp. 6277–6283, 2012.

[10] K. T. Chaung, N. B. Ha, H. N. Trinh et al., "High frequency of recurrent viremia after hepatitis B e antigen seroconversion and consolidation therapy," *Journal of Clinical Gastroenterology*, vol. 46, no. 10, pp. 865–870, 2012.

[11] Y. J. Kim, K. Kim, S. H. Hwang et al., "Durability after discontinuation of nucleos(t)ide therapy in chronic HBeAg negative hepatitis patients.," *Clinical and Molecular Hepatology*, vol. 19, no. 3, pp. 300–304, 2013.

[12] W.-J. Jeng, I.-S. Sheen, Y.-C. Chen et al., "Off-therapy durability of response to entecavir therapy in hepatitis B e antigen-negative chronic hepatitis B patients," *Hepatology*, vol. 58, no. 6, pp. 1888–1896, 2013.

[13] I.-C. Lee, C.-K. Sun, C.-W. Su et al., "Durability of Nucleos(t)ide analogues treatment in patients with chronic hepatitis B," *Medicine (United States)*, vol. 94, no. 32, Article ID e1341, 2015.

[14] M.-L. Chang, Y.-F. Liaw, and S. J. Hadziyannis, "Systematic review: Cessation of long-term nucleos(t)ide analogue therapy in patients with hepatitis B e antigen-negative chronic hepatitis B," *Alimentary Pharmacology & Therapeutics*, vol. 42, no. 3, pp. 243–257, 2015.

[15] E. Zhang, A. Kosinska, M. Lu, H. Yan, and M. Roggendorf, "Current status of immunomodulatory therapy in chronic hepatitis B, fifty years after discovery of the virus: Search for the "magic bullet" to kill cccDNA," *Antiviral Research*, vol. 123, pp. 193–203, 2015.

[16] B. Rehermann, P. Fowler, J. Sidney et al., "The cytotoxic T lymphocyte response to multiple hepatitis B virus polymerase epitopes during and after acute viral hepatitis," *The Journal of Experimental Medicine*, vol. 181, no. 3, pp. 1047–1058, 1995.

[17] M. C. Jung, U. Spengler, W. Schraut et al., "Hepatitis B virus antigen-specific T-cell activation in patients with acute and chronic hepatitis B," *Journal of Hepatology*, vol. 13, no. 3, pp. 310–317, 1991.

[18] Y. Sobao, H. Tomiyama, K. Sugi et al., "The role of hepatitis B virus-specific memory CD8 T cells in the control of viral replication," *Journal of Hepatology*, vol. 36, no. 1, pp. 105–115, 2002.

[19] S. Wang, X. Zhang, Y. Ju et al., "MicroRNA-146a feedback suppresses T cell immune function by targeting Stat1 in patients with chronic hepatitis B," *The Journal of Immunology*, vol. 191, no. 1, pp. 293–301, 2013.

[20] A. Bertoletti and C. Ferrari, "Innate and adaptive immune responses in chronic hepatitis B virus infections: towards restoration of immune control of viral infection," *Gut*, vol. 61, no. 12, pp. 1754–1764, 2012.

[21] F. Liu, L. Wang, X. Y. Li et al., "Poor durability of lamivudine effectiveness despite stringent cessation criteria: a prospective clinical study in hepatitis B e antigen-negative chronic hepatitis B patients," *Journal of Gastroenterology and Hepatology*, vol. 26, no. 3, pp. 456–460, 2011.

[22] Y. Liang, J. Jiang, M. Su et al., "Predictors of relapse in chronic hepatitis B after discontinuation of anti-viral therapy," *Alimentary Pharmacology and Therapeutics*, vol. 34, pp. 344–352, 2011.

[23] C.-H. Chen, C.-H. Hung, T.-H. Hu et al., "Association between level of hepatitis B surface antigen and relapse after entecavir therapy for chronic hepatitis B virus infection," *Clinical Gastroenterology and Hepatology*, vol. 13, no. 11, pp. 1984–1992.e1, 2015.

[24] W.-K. Seto, A. J. Hui, V. W.-S. Wong et al., "Treatment cessation of entecavir in Asian patients with hepatitis B e antigen negative chronic hepatitis B: a multicentre prospective study," *Gut*, vol. 64, no. 4, pp. 667–672, 2015.

[25] E. Tanaka and A. Matsumoto, "Guidelines for avoiding risks resulting from discontinuation of nucleoside/nucleotide analogs in patients with chronic hepatitis B," *Hepatology Research*, vol. 44, no. 1, pp. 1–8, 2014.

[26] H.-C. Yang and J.-H. Kao, "Persistence of hepatitis B virus covalently closed circular DNA in hepatocytes: Molecular mechanisms and clinical significance," *Emerging Microbes and Infections*, vol. 3, no. 9, article e64, 2014.

[27] C.-M. Tang, T. O. Yau, and J. Yu, "Management of chronic hepatitis B infection: current treatment guidelines, challenges, and new developments," *World Journal of Gastroenterology*, vol. 20, no. 20, pp. 6262–6278, 2014.

[28] A. Matsumoto, E. Tanaka, Y. Suzuki et al., "Combination of hepatitis B viral antigens and DNA for prediction of relapse after discontinuation of nucleos(t)ide analogs in patients with chronic hepatitis B," *Hepatology Research*, vol. 42, no. 2, pp. 139–149, 2012.

[29] C. H. Chen, C. H. Hung, J. H. Wang, S. Lu, T. Hu, and C. Lee, "Long-term incidence and predictors of hepatitis B surface antigen loss after discontinuing nucleoside analogues in noncirrhotic chronic hepatitis B patients," *Clinical Microbiology and Infection*, 2017.

[30] T. Berg, K.-G. Simon, S. Mauss et al., "Long-term response after stopping tenofovir disoproxil fumarate in non-cirrhotic HBeAg-negative patients—FINITE study," *Journal of Hepatology*, vol. 67, no. 5, pp. 918–924, 2017.

[31] S. J. Hadziyannis, V. Sevastianos, I. Rapti, D. Vassilopoulos, and E. Hadziyannis, "Sustained responses and loss of HBsAg in HBeAg-negative patients with chronic hepatitis B who stop long-term treatment with adefovir," *Gastroenterology*, vol. 143, no. 3, pp. 629–636, 2012.

[32] S. Chevaliez, C. Hézode, S. Bahrami, M. Grare, and J.-M. Pawlotsky, "Long-term hepatitis B surface antigen (HBsAg) kinetics during nucleoside/nucleotide analogue therapy: Finite treatment duration unlikely," *Journal of Hepatology*, vol. 58, no. 4, pp. 676–683, 2013.

[33] H. W. Lee, H. J. Lee, J. S. Hwang et al., "Lamivudine maintenance beyond one year after HBeAg seroconversion is a major factor for sustained virologic response in HBeAg-positive chronic hepatitis B," *Hepatology*, vol. 51, no. 2, pp. 415–421, 2010.

[34] D.-B. Chen, Y.-M. Chen, J. Liu et al., "Durability of efficacy after telbivudine off-treatment in chronic hepatitis B patients," *Journal of Clinical Virology*, vol. 59, no. 1, pp. 50–54, 2014.

[35] Asian Pacific Association for the Study of the Liver, "Asian-Pacific clinical practice guidelines on the management of hepatitis B: a 2015 update," *Hepatology International*, vol. 10, pp. 1–98, 2016.

[36] European Association for the Study of the Liver, "EASL 2017 Clinical Practice Guidelines on the management of hepatitis B virus infection," *Journal of Hepatology*, vol. 67, no. 2, pp. 370–398, 2017.

16

The Value of Ozone in CT-Guided Drainage of Multiloculated Pyogenic Liver Abscesses

Bing Li, Chuan Liu, Lang Wang, Yang Li, Yong Du, Chuan Zhang, Xiao-xue Xu, and Han Feng Yang

Sichuan Key Laboratory of Medical Imaging, Department of Radiology, Affiliated Hospital of North Sichuan Medical College, Nanchong City, Sichuan Province 637000, China

Correspondence should be addressed to Han Feng Yang; yhfctjr@yahoo.com

Academic Editor: Pierluigi Toniutto

Objective. This study was designed to compare the effects of catheter drainage alone and combined with ozone in the management of multiloculated pyogenic liver abscess (PLA). *Methods.* The prospective study included 60 patients diagnosed with multiloculated PLA. All patients were randomly divided into two groups: catheter drainage alone (group I) and catheter drainage combined with ozone (group II). Drainage was considered successful when (1) the abscess cavity was drained and (2) clinical symptoms were resolved. Kruskal-Wallis nonparametric test was used to compare the success rates, length of stay (LOS), and need for further surgery of the two groups. $P < 0.05$ indicates significant difference. *Results.* All patients' catheters were successfully placed under CT guidance. Group I was treated with catheters alone and group II was treated with catheters and ozone. The success rates of groups I and II were 86% and 96%, respectively ($P < 0.05$). And compared with group II, the duration of fever in group I was longer ($P < 0.05$), and the LOS was also longer ($P < 0.05$). *Conclusion.* Catheter drainage combined with ozone is an effective and safe treatment in multiloculated PLA. The Clinical Registration Number is ChiCTR1800014865.

1. Introduction

Therapy of pyogenic liver abscess (PLA) includes antibiotics alone or in combination with percutaneous or surgical drainage [1, 2]. A number of studies have shown that percutaneous abscess drainage is effective and safe, and it is minimally invasive and does not require general anesthesia [3]. However, the optimal treatment of multiloculated abscesses is still a subject of debate, as the multiloculated PLA often contain viscid pus, or small locules of the abscesses cannot communicate with each other, which may make percutaneous drainage difficult [3–6].

Multiloculated liver abscess was defined as an abscess with enhancing internal septations [7]. Studies have been showed that the presence of multiloculated abscess lesions has been considered as one of the factors that increase the risk of percutaneous catheter drainage failure [7, 8]. And these literatures showed that the mortality rates for multiloculated pyogenic liver abscesses range from 44% to 22.1%, which was higher than single PLA [8, 9]. In addition, multiloculated PLA may need multiple percutaneous drains or surgical intervention in an attempt to achieve source control and hence some authors advocate surgical intervention [10]. Moreover, some patients with multiloculated PLA have various infections, where using antibiotics alone often has a poor effect [11]. Long-term use of antibiotics, in addition, can cause bacteria resistance [6].

Ozone can inactivate bacteria, viruses, yeasts, protozoa, and fungi and stimulate the immune system and oxygen metabolism, so ozone has been widely considered to be one of the best sterilization, antifungal, and antiviral agents [12]. For some chronic wounds, such as nutrition ulcers, ischemic ulcers, and diabetic wounds, ozone has also been empirically used as clinical therapeutic agent [13–15].

In order to improve the therapeutic effect of multiloculated PLA, this study intends to compare catheter drainage alone and its combination with ozone therapy in the treatment of multiloculated PLA.

2. Materials and Methods

This prospective study was approved by our Hospital Institutional Review Board (HIRB), which included 60 patients who were diagnosed with multiloculated PLA (32 males and 28 females, aged 37–71 years; median age of 47.4 years) between January 2014 and October 2017. All patients had given written consent for this study. Diagnosis of the pyogenic abscess was proved by aspiration or microbiologic findings in all patients. Patients with cancer or diabetes were excluded from this study.

Inclusion criteria were as follows:

(1) Multiloculated PLA more than 5 cm in size

(2) Multiloculated PLA in mature stage (a capsule was formed around the necrotic cavity)

Exclusion criteria were as follows:

(1) Multiple abscesses

(2) Abscess ruptured into thoracic and peritoneal cavity

All patients have been uniformly managed with antibiotics throughout the study period, usually a combination of a third-generation cephalosporin along with metronidazole. Subsequently antibiotic therapy is tailored according to culture and sensitivity results of blood or pus.

Patients were randomly allocated into two groups with the help of a computer-generated table of random numbers: catheter drainage alone (group I) and catheter drainage combined with ozone (group II). Contrast-enhanced CT scans were performed in all patients to determine the size, location, and extent of the lesion and choose transhepatic route to avoid injuring other organs, blood vessel, and biliary systems. All catheters were placed by CT guidance, performed under local anesthesia. 10F pigtail catheters were placed into the patients by using the Seldinger technique. Attention should be taken to ensuring the side holes of catheter were placed within the abscess cavity. In this way, we avoid secondary liver infection. Abdominal CT images were obtained immediately after abscess drainage to assess the catheter location, abscess cavity, and complications such as bleeding. Then the valve of catheter was unclamped for open drainage.

In group II, in addition to drainage, according to the size of the abscess cavity, 10.0–20.0 mL oxygen-ozone gas mixture (ozone concentration 25 μg/ml, based on our previous experiments [12]) was given through catheter, until the amount of drainage was less than 20 mL per day. We used an ozone generator (Herrmann, Kleinwallstadt, Germany) to produce oxygen-ozone gas mixtures prior to injection. After oxygen-ozone gas mixture injection, the catheter was clamped for one hour and then left unclamped for 23 hours to allow for open drainage.

The drainage was considered successful when clinical symptoms of patients were resolved and the abscess cavities were drained. And the patients were referred for further surgical treatment when (1) the abscess failed to resolve, (2) the follow-up imaging (ultrasound or CT) showed that the abscess wall becomes thicker and cannot be aspirated, or (3) the patients have ongoing sepsis after drainage.

We evaluated the patient characteristics differences between the two groups and the technical success of catheter placement, as well as the length of hospital stay (LOS). Clinical details such as patients with ongoing sepsis, duration of fever (morning oral temperature of >37.5°C), and patients who converted into further surgery treatment were also written down.

We used SPSS software (version 20.0; SPSS Corporation, New York, USA) for statistical analyses of the two groups. The mean and standard deviation (SD) of each variable from two groups were calculated. Kruskal-Wallis nonparametric test was used to calculate statistical differences between two groups, with a P value of less than 0.05 considered significant. And the descriptive statistical analysis was calculated too.

TABLE 1: Comparison of preadmission variables among treatment groups.

Variable, mean (SD)	Group I	Group II
Number of patients	30	30
Average age (yr)	41.4 (10.4)	38.2 (13.6)
Duration of symptoms (d)	14.5 (8.9)	14.3 (7.9)
Initial WBC (×103)	14.9 (9.4)	15.4 (9.2)
Total lymphocytes (×103)	11.4 (6.7)	10.9 (6.9)
Abscess size (cm)	6.8 (2.6)	6.7 (2.5)
Catheter size (Fr)	10	10

TABLE 2: Positive results of bacterial culture among treatment groups.

Variable, mean	Group I	Group II
Bacterial culture	17	16
Streptococcus species	7	6
Enterococcus species	5	6
Escherichia coli	4	4
Klebsiella species	3	2

3. Results

All of the 60 patients' catheters were successfully placed under CT guidance. Group I was treated with catheters alone (Figure 1) and group II was treated with catheters and ozone (Figure 2). Different variables of the two groups are all shown in Table 1. Mean age, abscess sizes, and number of two groups were not significantly different ($P = 0.437$; $P = 0.471$; Table 1). Among the 60 patients, bacteriologic study of cultures had positive findings in 100% of patients; some patients have mixed infection (Table 2). The remaining abscesses were diagnosed based on increased white blood cell count in the aspirated fluid but had negative findings on culture. Streptococcus species were the main bacteria isolated, followed by *Enterococcus* species, *Escherichia coli*, and *Klebsiella* species.

Initial white blood cell count (WBC), lymphocytes, and duration of symptoms were different in two groups but were not significant ($P > 0.05$). Success rates of groups I and II were 86% and 96%, respectively. And compared with group II, the duration of fever in group I was longer ($P < 0.05$), and the LOS was also longer ($P < 0.05$). Furthermore, there were significant differences when comparing patients who

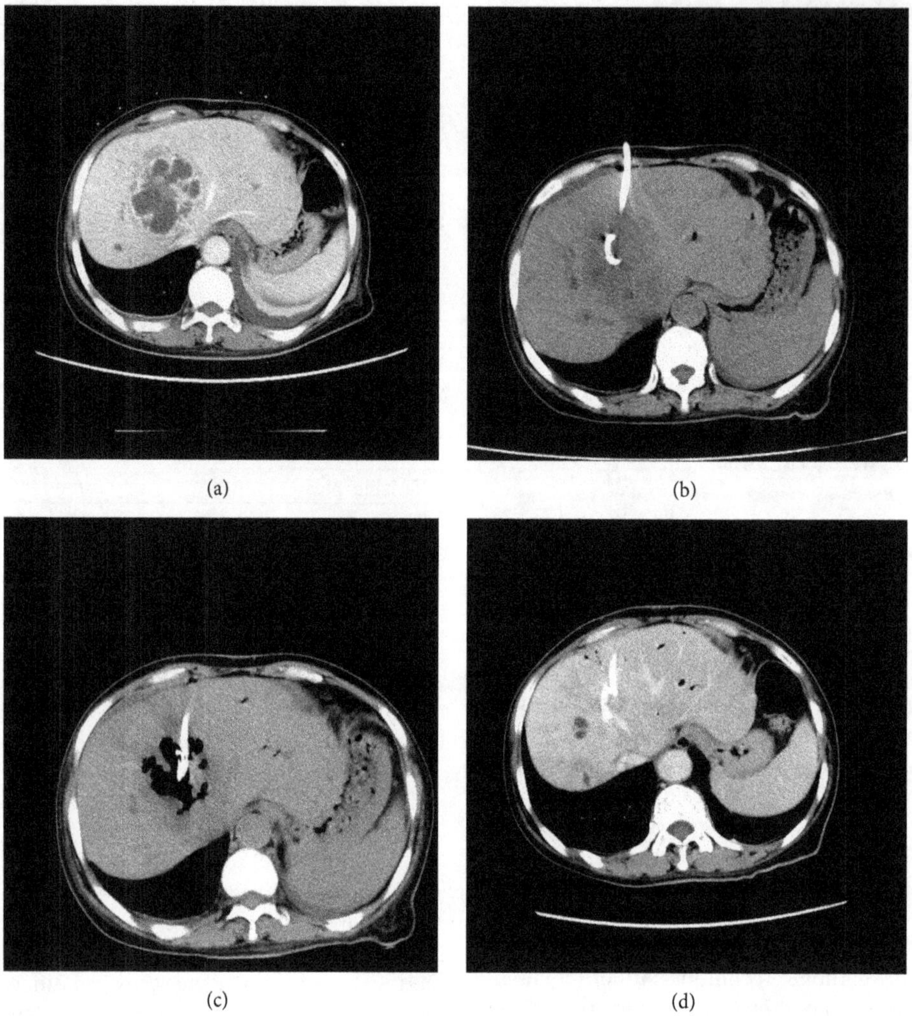

Figure 1: A 49-year-old male presented with fever and right back pain for one week. (a) A lager multiloculated liver abscess in the right hepatic lobes was shown by enhanced CT, and small amount of fluid can be seen in the left chest. (b) Catheter was placed under CT guidance, without injection of oxygen-ozone gas. (c) Three-week follow-up showing that abscess was not fully absorbed. (d) Abscess was fully absorbed after eight weeks.

converted into further surgery between the two groups (14% versus 4%; $P < 0.05$) (Table 3). Complications included three patients with minimal perihepatic bleeding. No other complications were founded.

4. Discussion

Despite advances in diagnostic technology and new strategies for treatment, PLA remains a big therapeutic challenge. Conventional treatment of PLA is antibiotic therapy and image-guided percutaneous drainage or aspiration [16]. However, the study reported that percutaneous catheter drainage still has high failure rates, especially in patients with multiloculated PLA [8, 17]. The possible reason behind such high failure rate is either the presence of viscid pus within the abscesses or the inability of multiple small locals of the abscesses to fuse together and communicate with each other [2]. And no matter any intervention type for an abscess was used, the bacteria may release into the bloodstream [18]. Some studies have showed the chance of postprocedure sepsis after liver abscess drainage [7, 16, 19].

Our study used catheter drainage combined with ozone to improve the effects of treatment for multiloculated PLA and achieved relatively higher success rates (96%) than when using catheter drainage only [16, 20]. And the rates of ongoing sepsis and LOS were decreased significantly.

The operation of this study was carried out under CT guidance. CT imaging can more accurately display the lesion and the septae of the abscess, which is critical to the success rate of treatment. And we used a Seldinger technique which a guide wire was placed through abscess cavities; in this way, the septae of abscess may disrupt, and then the abscess can be drained more effectively. Through this method, compared with the standard catheter drainage treatment, we can get a better therapeutic effect. Abscesses with small collections and with presence of air as well as those closely abutting the

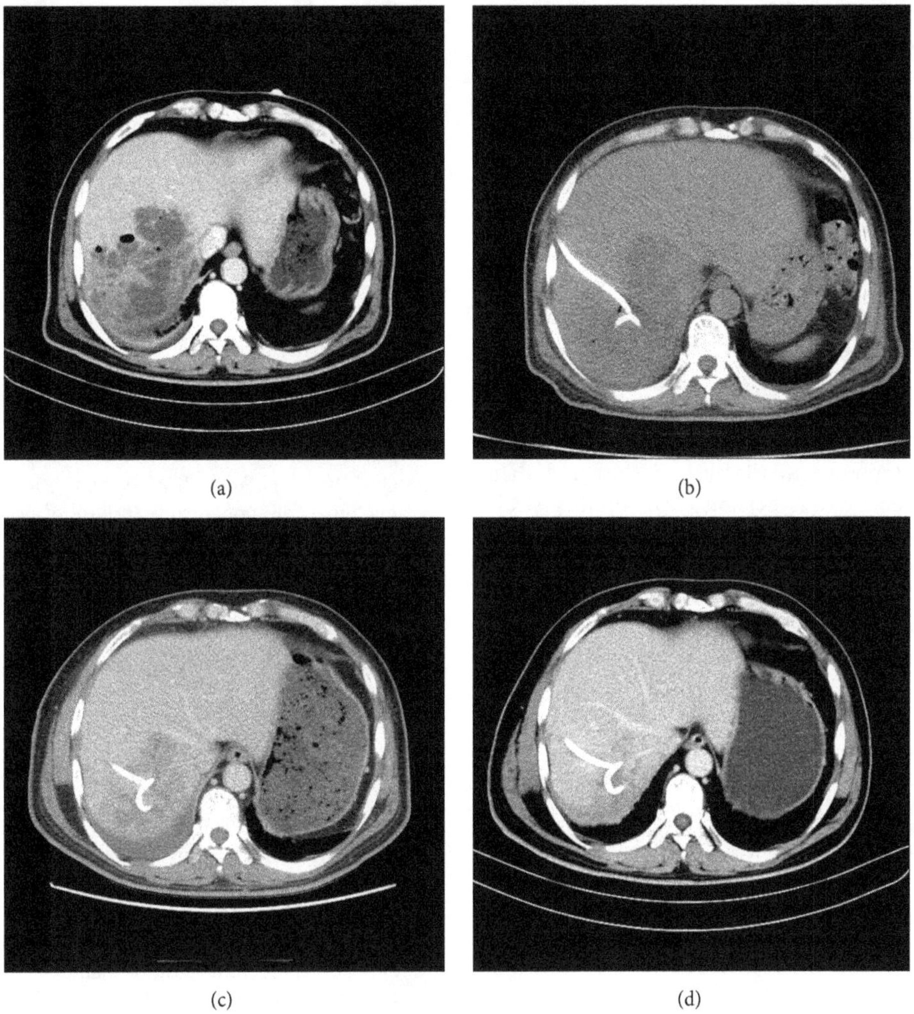

FIGURE 2: A 43-year-old male presented with fever and right abdominal pain for five days. (a) Enhanced CT shows a lager multiloculated liver abscess in the right hepatic lobe. The abscess cavity has gas formation, which is associated with mortality. (b) Catheter was placed under CT guidance. (c) After the pus was pulled out, oxygen-ozone gas mixture was given through catheter and filled the small locules of the abscesses; some separation was broken. (d) Abscess was absorbed after three weeks.

TABLE 3: Comparison of hospitalization and outcome variables among treatment groups.

Variable, mean (SD)	Group I	Group II
Technical success of catheter placement	100%	100%
Success rate of management	86%	96%
LOS (d)	26.1 (10.3)	21.4 (8.2)
Duration of fever (d)	5.5 (3.0)	3.5 (2.1)
Converted into further surgery	4 (14%)	1 (4%)
With ongoing sepsis	6 (20%)	1 (4%)

diaphragm are poorly defined on US. CT imaging was found to be superior in depicting such abscesses [21].

Clinical application has proven that ozone is a powerful and reliable antimicrobial agent and can inactivate bacteria, fungi, protozoa, and viruses [12, 22, 23]. From a century ago, ozone therapy has been widely used and studied. Its mechanism action is through stimulating the oxygen metabolism and the immune system of bacteria, viruses, fungi, yeast, and protozoa, to achieve inactivation [12, 22, 23].

Using antibiotics only sometimes cannot achieve satisfactory results as most multiloculated PLA patients have mixed infections. In addition, long-term use of antibiotics can lead to bacterial resistance [2, 6, 24]. And the excess and indiscriminate use of antimicrobial drugs appears to be the most significant factor in the emergence of resistant microorganisms in recent years. In 2016, a global alliance consists of a multidisciplinary task force from 79 different countries developing a consensus on the rational use of antimicrobials for patients with intra-abdominal infections (IAIs). The consensus demonstrates the necessity of a multidisciplinary and collaborative approach in the battle against antimicrobial resistance in surgical infections. The use of ozone as a secondary antibacterial agent to treat multiloculated PLA has achieved a better effect.

Identifying pathogenic organisms has a great clinical importance. Experiences, however, have shown that this was not always possible because many patients were treated before fluid was obtained for culture [2]. Therefore, the blood culture of some patients in two groups of our study was negative. We observe that commonest organism in our study is neither *Klebsiella* nor *E. coli* and this is contradictory to global reports [25]. Prophylactic antibiotics for *E. coli* are usually used in clinical practice in our institution. This may result in negative bacteria culture in some patients who were originally infected with *E. coli*. There was a decreased mortality in culture negative PLA patients who receive percutaneous drainage. And there was no difference in outcomes of percutaneous drainage between *E. coli* PLA and *Klebsiella* PLA.

The study found that the beneficial effects of ozone on the wound healing might be assumed due to increased oxygen tension by ozone exposure in the wound area and then ameliorated impaired wounds healing [23]. Another study reported that ozone exposure could activate transcription factors. And this is important to adjust inflammatory reactions and eventually the whole process of wounds healing [22]. Therefore, ozone has also been used empirically as a clinical therapeutic agent for chronic wounds, such as ischemic ulcers, trophic ulcers, and diabetic wounds [26]. Furthermore, ozone can be dispersed into the cavity of the abscess, causing abscess wall dehydration [15]. Moreover, injection of ozone can break the septae of abscess and separate the adhesion in abscess cavity to make the drainage more effective (Figure 2) [12]. So the use of drainage combined with ozone has a synergistic effect on the management of liver abscess.

The categories of PLA often included biliary infection, portal vein seeding, direct extension, hepatic arterial seeding, penetrating trauma, and cryptogenic cause [25]. In our study, the biliary obstruction with cholangitis is the most common cause of PLA. Some complications from catheter drainage, such as hemorrhage owing to intercostal vessel and liver parenchyma injury, catheter-related pain, and subcutaneous emphysema, have been reported [11]. In this study, we did not encounter any serious complications. And there was no significant clinical bleeding noted in any patient in groups I and II.

5. Conclusions

In short, combined treatment of catheter drainage and ozone is a safe and valid therapeutic procedure in multiloculated PLA. This technology can decrease the ratio of surgical interventions and the LOS and should be confirmed with a larger patient series in other medical institutions.

Abbreviations

PLA: Pyogenic liver abscess
LOS: Length of stay
PCD: Percutaneous drainage catheter
WBC: White blood cell count.

Authors' Contributions

Han Feng Yang and Bing Li designed the study. Bing Li performed percutaneous drainage. Bing Li, Yang Li, Chuan Zhang, Lang Wang, and Chuan Liu performed examinations and collected the date. Han Feng Yang, Yong Du, and Xiao-xue Xu contributed to the analysis and supervised the report. Bing Li and Han Feng Yang wrote this paper together. Bing Li, Xiao-xue Xu, and Chuan Liu revised the paper.

References

[1] G. Dulku, G. Mohan, S. Samuelson, J. Ferguson, and J. Tibballs, "Percutaneous aspiration versus catheter drainage of liver abscess: A retrospective review," *Australasian Medical Journal*, vol. 8, no. 1, pp. 7–18, 2015.

[2] C. H. Jun, J. H. Yoon, J. W. Wi et al., "Risk factors and clinical outcomes for spontaneous rupture of pyogenic liver abscess," *Journal of Digestive Diseases*, vol. 16, no. 1, pp. 31–36, 2015.

[3] S. Ahmed, C. L. K. Chia, S. P. Junnarkar, W. Woon, and V. G. Shelat, "Percutaneous drainage for giant pyogenic liver abscess - Is it safe and sufficient?" *The American Journal of Surgery*, vol. 211, no. 1, pp. 95–101, 2016.

[4] K.-C. Lai, K.-S. Cheng, L.-B. Jeng et al., "Factors associated with treatment failure of percutaneous catheter drainage for pyogenic liver abscess in patients with hepatobiliary-pancreatic cancer," *The American Journal of Surgery*, vol. 205, no. 1, pp. 52–57, 2013.

[5] W.-I. Liao, S.-H. Tsai, C.-Y. Yu et al., "Pyogenic liver abscess treated by percutaneous catheter drainage: MDCT measurement for treatment outcome," *European Journal of Radiology*, vol. 81, no. 4, pp. 609–615, 2012.

[6] A. Srivastava, S. K. Yachha, V. Arora, U. Poddar, R. Lal, and S. S. Baijal, "Identification of high-risk group and therapeutic options in children with liver abscess," *European Journal of Pediatrics*, vol. 171, no. 1, pp. 33–41, 2012.

[7] C.-H. Liu, D. A. Gervais, P. F. Hahn, R. S. Arellano, R. N. Uppot, and P. R. Mueller, "Percutaneous Hepatic Abscess Drainage: Do Multiple Abscesses or Multiloculated Abscesses Preclude Drainage or Affect Outcome?" *Journal of Vascular and Interventional Radiology*, vol. 20, no. 8, pp. 1059–1065, 2009.

[8] F.-F. Chou, S.-M. Sheen-Chen, Y.-S. Chen, and M.-C. Chen, "Single and multiple pyogenic liver abscesses: Clinical course, etiology, and results of treatment," *World Journal of Surgery*, vol. 21, no. 4, pp. 384–389, 1997.

[9] A. Giorgio, G. De Stefano, A. Di Sarno, G. Liorre, and G. Ferraioli, "Percutaneous needle aspiration of multiple pyogenic abscesses of the liver: 13-Year single-center experience," *American Journal of Roentgenology*, vol. 187, no. 6, pp. 1585–1590, 2006.

[10] M. Luo, X.-X. Yang, B. Tan et al., "Distribution of common pathogens in patients with pyogenic liver abscess in China: a meta-analysis," *European Journal of Clinical Microbiology & Infectious Diseases*, vol. 35, no. 10, pp. 1557–1565, 2016.

[11] L. Cioffi, A. Belli, P. Limongelli et al., "Laparoscopic Drainage as First Line Treatment for Complex Pyogenic Liver Abscesses," *Hepato-Gastroenterology*, vol. 61, no. 131, pp. 771–775, 2014.

[12] B. Li, C. Liu, Y. Li et al., "Computed tomography-guided catheter drainage with urokinase and ozone in management of empyema," *World Journal of Radiology*, vol. 9, no. 4, pp. 212–216, 2017.

[13] C. Andreula, "Ozone therapy," *Neuroradiology*, vol. 53, Supplement 1, pp. S207–S209, 2011.

[14] B. Li, X. X. Xu, Y. Du et al., "CT-guided chemonucleolysis combined with psoas compartment block in lumbar disc herniation: A randomized controlled study," *Pain Medicine*, vol. 15, no. 9, pp. 1470–1476, 2014.

[15] L. Re, R. Rowen, and V. Travagli, "Ozone Therapy and Its Use in Medicine: Further Comments," *Cardiology (Switzerland)*, vol. 136, no. 4, p. 269, 2017.

[16] J. Thomas, S. R. Turner, R. C. Nelson, and E. K. Paulson, "Postprocedure sepsis in imaging-guided percutaneous hepatic abscess drainage: How often does it occur?" *American Journal of Roentgenology*, vol. 186, no. 5, pp. 1419–1422, 2006.

[17] S.-C. Chen, Y.-T. Lee, S.-J. Tsai et al., "Clinical Outcomes and Prognostic Factors of Cancer Patients with Pyogenic Liver Abscess," *Journal of Gastrointestinal Surgery*, vol. 15, no. 11, pp. 2036–2043, 2011.

[18] N. Sharma, H. Kaur, N. Kalra, A. Bhalla, S. Kumar, and V. Singh, "Complications of Catheter Drainage for Amoebic Liver Abscess," *Journal of Clinical and Experimental Hepatology*, vol. 5, no. 3, pp. 256–258, 2015.

[19] K. Kusumoto, A. Hamada, T. Kusaka et al., "A patient with sepsis and a gas-forming liver abscess caused by Clostridium perfringens treated with continuous perfusion drainage," *Nihon Shokakibyo Gakkai Zasshi*, vol. 111, no. 7, pp. 1416–1423, 2014.

[20] S. Bari, K. A. Sheikh, A. A. Malik, R. A. Wani, and S. H. Naqash, "Percutaneous aspiration versus open drainage of liver abscess in children," *Pediatric Surgery International*, vol. 23, no. 1, pp. 69–74, 2007.

[21] Y. Takeuchi, H. Okabe, S. Myojo, and S. Fujimoto, "CT-guided drainage of a mediastinal pancreatic pseudocyst with a transhepatic transdiaphragmatic approach," *Hepato-Gastroenterology*, vol. 49, no. 43, pp. 271-272, 2002.

[22] A. M. Elvis and J. S. Ekta, "Ozone therapy: a clinical review," *Journal of Natural Science, Biology and Medicine*, vol. 2, no. 1, pp. 66–70, 2011.

[23] G. Gupta and B. Mansi, "Ozone therapy in periodontics.," *Journal of Medicine and Life*, vol. 5, no. 1, pp. 59–67, 2012.

[24] J. Z. W. Lo, J. J. J. Leow, P. L. F. Ng et al., "Predictors of therapy failure in a series of 741 adult pyogenic liver abscesses," *Journal of Hepato-Biliary-Pancreatic Sciences*, vol. 22, no. 2, pp. 156–165, 2015.

[25] G. J. Webb, T. P. Chapman, P. J. Cadman, and D. A. Gorard, "Pyogenic liver abscess," *Frontline Gastroenterology*, vol. 5, no. 1, pp. 60–67, 2013.

[26] G. Yu, X. Liu, and Z. Chen, "Ozone therapy could attenuate tubulointerstitial injury in adenine-induced CKD rats by mediating Nrf2 and NF-kappaB," *Iranian Journal of Basic Medical Sciences*, vol. 19, no. 10, pp. 1136–1143, 2016.

17

Portal Hypertensive Polyposis in Advanced Liver Cirrhosis: The Unknown Entity?

David Kara,[1] Anna Hüsing-Kabar,[1] Hartmut Schmidt,[1] Inga Grünewald,[2] Gursimran Chandhok,[1,3] Miriam Maschmeier,[1] and Iyad Kabar[1]

[1]*Department of Gastroenterology and Hepatology, University Hospital Muenster, 48149 Muenster, Germany*
[2]*University Hospital Muenster, Gerhard-Domagk-Institute of Pathology, 48149 Muenster, Germany*
[3]*Department of Anatomy and Developmental Biology, and Neuroscience Program, Monash Biomedicine Discovery Institute, Monash University, Clayton, Melbourne, VIC 3800, Australia*

Correspondence should be addressed to Iyad Kabar; iyad.kabar@ukmuenster.de

Academic Editor: Andrea Mancuso

Background. Portal hypertension is a serious complication of liver cirrhosis. *Objective.* To identify relevant endoscopic findings in patients with advanced cirrhosis and consecutive portal hypertension. *Methods.* This was a retrospective study of liver transplant candidates who underwent upper gastrointestinal endoscopy between April 2011 and November 2015. *Results.* A total of 1,045 upper endoscopies were analyzed. Portal hypertensive gastric and duodenal polyps were frequently observed and were associated with thrombocytopenia ($p = 0.040$; OR: 2.4, 95% CI 1.04–5.50), Child-Pugh score > 6 ($p = 0.033$; OR: 2.3, 95% CI 1.07–4.92), Model for End Stage Liver Disease score > 16 ($p = 0.030$; OR: 4.1, 95% CI 1.14–15.00), and previous rubber band ligation ($p < 0.001$; OR = 5.2, 95% CI 2.5–10.7). These polyps often recurred after polypectomy; however, no malignant transformation occurred during the observational time until October 2017. The most common endoscopic finding was esophageal varices, observed in more than 90% of patients. *Conclusion.* Portal hypertensive polyposis is common in patients with advanced cirrhosis. Our data suggest that these polyps have benign characteristics.

1. Introduction

Portal hypertension is a common consequence and major complication of cirrhosis [1]. Portal hypertension is defined by an elevated portal pressure gradient caused by increased resistance to portal blood flow due to architectural changes in the cirrhotic liver, contraction of intrahepatic components as a result of decreased intrahepatic nitric oxide production, and increased splanchnic blood flow [1, 2]. Portal hypertension is a syndrome that involves several organ systems, leading to the formation of portosystemic collaterals, esophageal and gastric varices, gastropathy, enteropathy, colopathy, and splenomegaly with consecutive blood abnormalities including thrombocytopenia caused by hypersplenism [1].

In cirrhotic patients, endoscopy not only is used to detect esophageal varices but can also detect further gastrointestinal complications of portal hypertension such as portal hypertensive gastropathy or gastric varices. There have also been a few recent reports of polyposis related to portal hypertension [3–15]. The clinical relevance of this so-called portal hypertensive polyposis (PHP) remains unclear.

The present study was performed at a tertiary center and aimed to identify pathological findings during upper gastrointestinal endoscopy in patients with advanced cirrhosis who were under consideration for liver transplantation (LT) or who were already on the waiting list for LT in general and to explore the clinical characteristics of PHP in these patients.

2. Patients and Methods

This was an investigator-initiated, single center, retrospective analysis. All patients with cirrhosis who were under the care of the Department for Transplant Medicine at the University Hospital of Muenster and who underwent upper gastrointestinal endoscopy between April 2011 and November 2015 were considered for inclusion in this study. Inclusion criteria

TABLE 1: Demographic data and clinical and laboratory characteristics.

	n = 407
Age [years], median (range)	60 (21–88)
Females/males, n (%)	127 (31.2%)/280 (68.8%)
Ethanol (active or past substantial consumption)	111 (27.3%)
Hepatitis C	77 (18.9%)
Non-alcoholic fatty liver disease	63 (15.4%)
Cryptogenic	40 (9.8%)
Hepatitis B	23 (5.7%)
Primary sclerosing cholangitis	21 (5.2%)
Autoimmune hepatitis	15 (3.7%)
Hemochromatosis	9 (2.2%)
Wilson's disease	7 (1.7%)
Primary biliary cirrhosis	5 (1.2%)
Miscellaneous	36 (8.8%)
Splenomegaly	328 (82.8%)
Ascites	228 (56.4%)
Encephalopathy	118 (29.0%)
I–II	103 (25.3% of all patients)
III–IV	15 (3.7% of all patients)
Thrombocyte count	101 (18–630) thousand/μl
International normalized ratio	1.3 (0.86–4.80)
Creatinine	1 (0.10–16.60) mg/dL
Albumin	3.3 (0.20–4.80) g/dL
Bilirubin	3.9 (0.2–40.1) mg/dL
Child-Pugh score	
≤ 6	142 (34.9%)
> 6	265 (65.1%)
Child-Pugh class	
A	142 (34.9%)
B	158 (38.8%)
C	107 (26.3%)
Model for End Stage Liver Disease score, mean ± SD/ median (range)	15.2 ± 7.3/ 13 (6–40)
Portal vein thrombosis	35 (8.6%)
Hepatocellular carcinoma	78 (19.2%)
Beta-blocker	299 (73.5%)
Proton-pump inhibitor	378 (92.9%)

were the presence of liver cirrhosis, patient age 18 years or above, and available patient data. Patients' clinical and demographic data were collected from electronic healthcare files. All patients were regularly followed up at our outpatient clinic until October 2017. This study was approved by the Ethics Committee of the University Hospital of Muenster on April 28, 2016, and was carried out in accordance with the standards in the Declaration of Helsinki. Written informed consent was given by all patients prior to intervention.

2.1. Statistical Analysis. Statistical analysis was performed using IBM SPSS® Statistics 24 for Windows (IBM Corporation, Somers, NY, USA). Data are presented in both absolute and relative frequencies. Continuous variables with normal distribution are expressed as the mean ± standard deviation, whereas variables that do not follow normal distribution are shown as the median and maximal range.

Stepwise variable selection using univariable binary logistic regression analysis was performed to explore potential single risk factors for endoscopic findings. All variables that reached a significance level of $p \leq 0.1$ were included in the multivariable binary logistic regression analysis to identify independent risk factors for the endoscopic finding being investigated.

3. Results

3.1. Study Population and Clinical Data. A total of 1,045 upper endoscopies performed in 407 cirrhotic patients were eligible for statistical analysis. The demographic data and clinical and laboratory characteristics of these patients are summarized in Table 1. Most of the patients were male. Mean patient age was 59 ± 11.2 years. The most common Child-Pugh category was B, followed by A and then C.

Table 2: Endoscopic findings.

Gastroscopy	n = 407
Esophageal varices	373 (91.6%)
Grade I	145 (38.9%)
Grade II	137 (36.7%)
Grade III	91 (24.4%)
Barrett‘s esophagus	28 (6,9%)
Gastric varices	40 (9.8%)
Portal hypertensive gastropathy	373 (91.6%)
Gastric polyps	38 (9.5%)
Histopathology of endoscopically obtained biopsies (n = 36)	
Hyperplastic	29 (80.6%)
Foveolar hyperplasia	3 (8.3%)
Tubular adenoma	1 (2.8%)
Inflammatory	3 (8.3%)
Helicobacter pylori	23 (10.5%) (n = 219)*
Duodenal polyps	32 (7.9%)
Histopathology of endoscopically obtained biopsies (n = 22)	
Hyperplastic	10 (45.5%)
Tubular adenoma	2 (9.1%)
Inflammatory	1 (4.5%)
Brunner glands	4 (18.2%)
Lipoma	2 (9.1%)
Endocrine tumor	2 (9.1%)
LGIEN	1 (4.5%)
Colonoscopy	n = 363
Colon polyps	135 (37.2%)
Histopathology of endoscopically obtained biopsies (n = 113)	
Hyperplastic	34 (30.1%)
Hyperplastic and LGIEN	16 (14.2%)
LGIEN	55 (48.7%)
Sessile adenoma	2 (1.8%)
Adenocarcinoma	4 (3.5%)
Leiomyoma	2 (1.8%)

*Only tested in 219 patients.
LGIEN = low grade intraepithelial neoplasia.

3.2. Endoscopic Findings. The endoscopic findings are summarized in Table 2. Esophageal varices were present in most patients. Grade I and II varices were present in 35.6% and 33.6% of cases, respectively, while grade III varices were found in 22.4% of patients. Gastric varices were found in approximately 10% of patients. Portal hypertensive gastropathy was as prevalent as esophageal varices and was observed in about 90% of patients. *Helicobacter pylori* was detected in 23 of the 219 patients (11%) in whom a biopsy was performed. Gastric polyps were present in about 10% of patients; these polyps mainly had the histologic characteristics of hyperplastic polyps, with foveolar hyperplasia and markedly proliferating, ectatic capillaries in the lamina propria. These portal hypertensive polyps were the most commonly found gastric polyps on biopsy and comprised more than 80% of all detected polyps. Adenomas were very rare (2.8%). Duodenal polyps were present in 8% of patients; these were also mostly hyperplastic. However, hyperplastic polyps were less frequent in the duodenum than in the stomach. Tubular adenoma and endocrine tumors were seen in two patients, with one patient showing a low-grade intraepithelial neoplasia.

An additional colonoscopy was performed in 363 of the 407 included patients. A total of 135 patients (37.2%) had evident colon polyps, of which 113 polyps were endoscopically removed. Of these 113 removed colon polyps, 71 (62.8%) were adenoma with low-grade intraepithelial neoplasia, 34 (30.1%) were hyperplastic, two (1.8%) were sessile adenoma, four (3.5%) were adenocarcinoma, and two (1.8%) were leiomyoma (Table 2).

3.3. Portal Hypertensive Gastric Polyposis. More than one polypoid lesion was present in the stomach in 79% of PHP cases. A total of 19 polypectomies were performed in 16 patients. There was no bleeding or perforation observed in

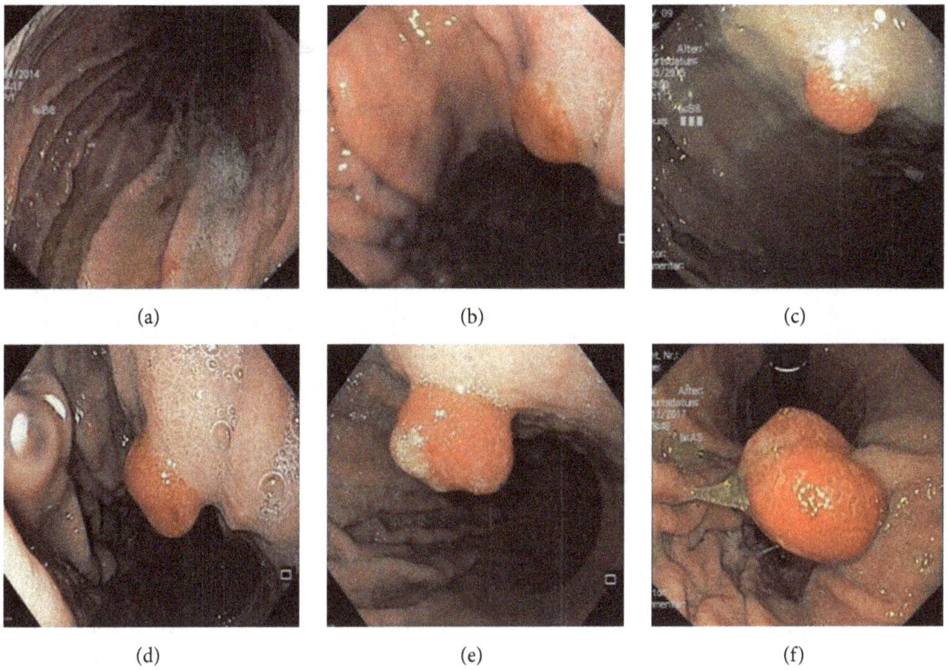

FIGURE 1: Chronological evolution of a portal hypertensive polyp in one patient after rubber band ligation of esophageal varices between 2014 and 2017 (a-f).

any of the cases. Of the resected portal hypertensive polyps, 15 polyps (79%) recurred after polypectomy and were detectable in subsequent endoscopies. Notably, 55% of hyperplastic polyps with typical signs of PHP first arose or progressed following rubber band ligation (Figure 1).

During a mean follow-up of 44.6 ± 14.7 months, none of the polyps degenerated into malignant carcinoma. No episodes of spontaneous bleeding related to portal hypertensive polyps were observed during the time of the study. All polyps were localized in the distal part of the stomach (antrum and prepyloric region). Using multivariable binary regression analysis, thrombocytopenia (defined as platelet count $< 130 \times 10^3/\mu l$) was shown to be an independent risk factor of PHP ($p = 0.040$; OR = 2.4, 95% CI 1.04–5.50). The other independent predictors of the occurrence of PHP were Child-Pugh score > 6 ($p = 0.033$; OR = 2.3, 95% CI 1.07–4.92), MELD score > 16 ($p = 0.030$; OR = 4.1, 95% CI 1.14–15.00), and previous rubber band ligation ($p < 0.001$; OR = 5.2, 95% CI 2.5–10.7) (Figures 2 and 3).

In multivariable analysis, male sex ($p = 0.01$; OR 1.9, 95% CI 1.2-3.2), evidence of duodenal polyps ($p = 0.02$; OR 2.5, 95% CI 1.4-5.3), and HCC ($p = 0.04$; OR 1.8, 95% CI 1.0-3.1) were found to be significantly associated with colonic polyps.

Statistical analysis showed no association between proton-pump inhibitors and PHP ($p = 0.680$; OR = 0.946). However, it should be pointed out that the majority of patients received PPI. Therefore, the analysis regarding the role of PPIs may be limited by this fact.

Binary regression analysis showed no association between beta-blockers and PHP ($p = 0.460$; OR = 0.968)

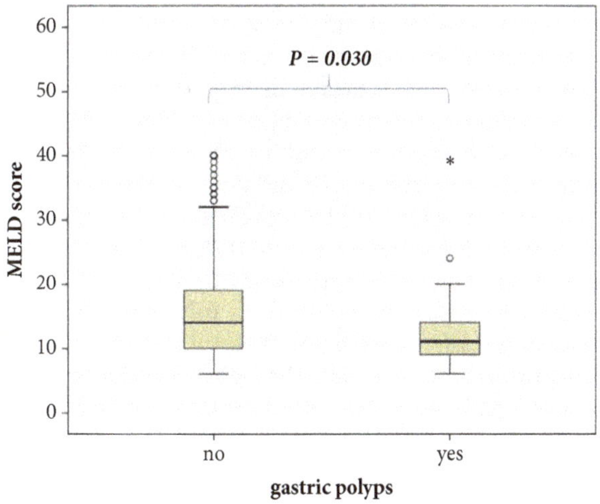

FIGURE 2: Distribution of gastric polyps with regard to MELD score. Higher MELD score was associated with the presence of hypertensive polyposis of the stomach, suggesting a higher prevalence of gastric polyps in advanced cirrhosis. MELD: Model for End Stage Liver Disease.

4. Discussion

To the best of our knowledge, the present study is the largest study investigating upper gastrointestinal endoscopy findings in LT candidates with advanced cirrhosis. The present study identified a very high prevalence (> 90%) of esophageal varices and portal hypertensive gastropathy. Previous studies have estimated the prevalence of esophageal varices at the

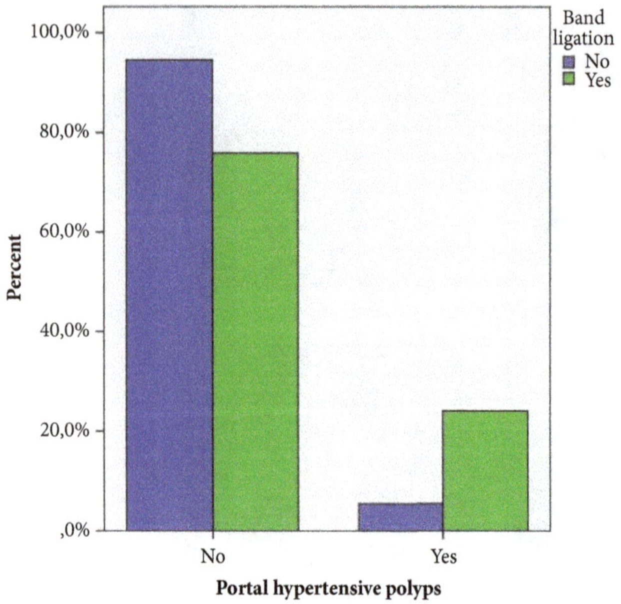

FIGURE 3: Bar chart showing the distribution of portal hypertensive polyposis with regard to rubber band ligation.

time of diagnosis of liver cirrhosis as about 35% in patients with compensated cirrhosis and 60% in patients with decompensated cirrhosis [1], while portal hypertensive gastropathy is reportedly seen in 11–80% of cirrhotic patients [1, 16–18]. Our patients underwent endoscopy at the time of referral to a tertiary center, which probably explains the greater frequencies of varices and portal hypertensive gastropathy. One study on LT candidates undergoing screening endoscopy reported incidences of varices and portal hypertensive gastropathy of 73% and 62%, respectively [17]. The higher prevalence of these findings in our study may be explained by the presence of more advanced disease in our cohort (Child-class C in 26% in our study versus 17% in the study by Zaman et al. [17]). The prevalence of both portal hypertensive gastropathy and variceal progression is strongly correlated with the increasing severity of cirrhosis [1, 17, 18]. The higher prevalence of these complications in our study may also partly be explained by the extensive experience of our endoscopists in endoscopic examination of patients with cirrhosis, as our center is highly specialized in this field, allowing the detection of early endoscopic alterations. The detection of grade I varices in nearly 40% of cases may be consistent with this assumption.

In our study, splenomegaly (83%) and ascites (56%) were also highly prevalent findings. This is consistent with another study on LT candidates [19].

4.1. Portal Hypertensive Polyposis. Apart from the expected cirrhosis-related pathologies such as esophagogastric varices and portal hypertensive gastropathy, there was a noticeable high prevalence of gastroduodenal polyposis observed in our patients. The prevalence of gastroduodenal polyps in the general population reportedly ranges from 0.5% to 6.35% [3, 4]. In contrast, gastroduodenal polyps were far more frequent in our study; almost 10% of patients had gastric polyps, and 8% had duodenal polyps.

Gastric and duodenal hypertension has been associated with the presence of portal hypertensive polyps, but this has mostly been reported in case reports and a few small case series [5–10, 12–15]. In our study, we comprehensively evaluated the clinical appearance of PHP. These polyps are typically localized in the stomach; however, they can be found all through the intestine [8, 11, 14]. Macroscopically, portal hypertensive polyps cannot be distinguished from normal hyperplastic polyps but frequently present with small ulcerations [7, 9]. Even histologically, there are similarities between hyperplastic and portal hypertensive polyps [6]. There are still no clear diagnostic criteria for portal hypertensive polyps [11]. However, typical features of portal hypertensive polyps reportedly include foveolar hyperplasia of the epithelium as well as proliferating, ectatic capillaries in the lamina propria; this indicates their portal hypertensive nature and distinguishes them from inflammatory polyps (Figure 4) [3, 7, 8, 11, 14].

In our cohort, polyps were pathologically classified as "hyperplastic" in the majority of cases, even though they showed the abovementioned histological criteria of portal hypertensive polyps. One notable characteristic of these polyps in our study was that they almost always occurred in multiples. Other studies including cirrhotic patients have reported a PHP frequency of 0.9–1.3% [6, 8, 11]. As portal hypertensive polyps are still relatively unknown by both endoscopists and pathologists, they may be considerably underdiagnosed. The pathogenic mechanism of PHP remains unknown, but increased congestion caused by increased portal pressure may play an important role in inducing proliferation and angiogenesis. Some observations suggest that these polyps may respond to the treatment of portal hypertension [8–10]. Therefore, the presence of these portal hypertensive polyps may have been particularly high in the present study due to the advanced stage of cirrhosis in our cohort. Accordingly, the independent risk factors for PHP were identified as thrombocytopenia (platelet count $< 130 \times 10^3/\mu l$), Child-Pugh score > 6, and MELD score > 16. Of note, the strongest risk factor for the development of these polyps was previous rubber band ligation. This may be because band ligation of the esophageal varices leads to increased formation of portosystemic shunts, including the gastric wall. This hypothesis is also consistent with the histological finding of proliferating ectatic vessels in the gastric mucosa and strongly supports our hypothesis of an evident proliferation stimulus of the increased portal blood flow on the gastric mucosa.

PHP is still poorly understood, and little is known about the risks and benefits of endoscopic resection. Although endoscopic resection was performed in all cases without complications in our study, the necessity of polypectomy should be critically considered, as portal hypertensive polyps frequently recurred and not one malignant transformation was observed during follow-up of 44.6 ± 14.7 months.

In our study, the incidence of colon polyps and the frequency of adenoma within these polyps were similar to those reported in another cohort of LT candidates (37% versus 42% for colon polyps and 54.1% versus 53.6% for adenoma within colon polyps) [20]. In contrast to the polyps

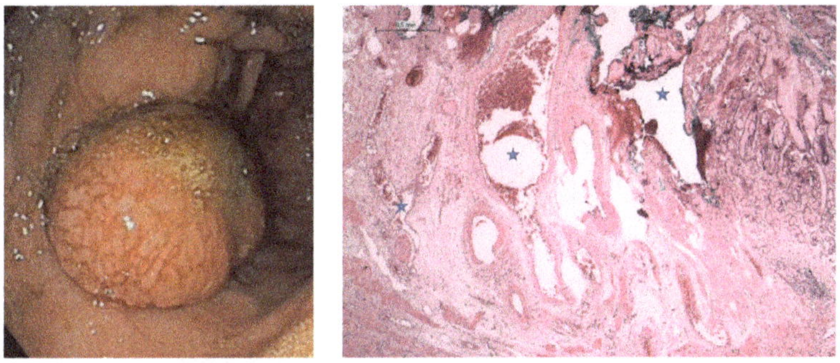

(a) (b)

FIGURE 4: Images of hypertensive polyps. (a) Macroscopic aspect of a portal hypertensive antral polyp. (b) Histological image of a hypertensive gastric polyp showing proliferating ectatic vessels (starlets).

found in the upper gastrointestinal tract, adenomas are the most common detected entity of colon polyps. As this entity represents a preliminary stage of adenocarcinoma, colon polyps should always be resected and studied histopathologically to assess their potential for malignant transformation. Subsequent endoscopic surveillance of colonic polyps depends on number, size, and histopathology of polyps, as well as the prevalence of hereditary conditions [21]. The Paris classification of gastrointestinal lesions can be used to classify colon lesions into polypoid, nonpolypoid, and depressed or excavated, where the latter is more likely to show high-grade dysplasia or malignancy (the Paris endoscopic classification of superficial neoplastic lesions: esophagus, stomach, and colon).

Some data indicate a positive association between higher levels of sex hormones in men and the development of colorectal carcinoma, while estradiol seems to have protective effects [22]. Given the adenoma-carcinoma-sequence, these findings may give an explanation for the higher rate of colon polyps in men in our patient cohort.

The higher prevalence of colon neoplasia in patients with the evidence of incidental duodenal polyps emphasizes the recommendation for colonoscopy in patients with sporadic duodenal neoplasia that has been stated in former studies [23, 24].

One interesting finding of our study was the positive association between HCC and the prevalence of colon polyps. This fact may be explained by the results of several studies indicating a higher rate of colorectal polyps in patients with liver cirrhosis, while liver cirrhosis is also the main risk factor of HCC [20, 25].

5. Conclusions

PHP is a common finding in patients with advanced liver cirrhosis, which until now may have been underestimated by both endoscopists and pathologists. These PHP lesions are typically localized in the antrum of the stomach, are mostly multiple, and show typical microscopic findings. Portal hypertension seems to play a crucial role in the pathogenesis of PHP, as these lesions are mostly seen in advanced cirrhosis, frequently after rubber ligation of preexistent esophageal varices. There is currently no evidence of these polyps having malignant potential. In our opinion and based on these findings, both polypectomy and endoscopic surveillance are dispensable in case of PHP.

Authors' Contributions

Miriam Maschmeier and Iyad Kabar contributed equally to this work.

Acknowledgments

The authors thank Kelly Zammit, BVSc, from Edanz Group (http://www.edanzediting.com/ac), for editing a draft of this manuscript.

References

[1] J. Bosch, A. Berzigotti, J. C. Garcia-Pagan, and J. G. Abraldes, "The management of portal hypertension: rational basis, available treatments and future options," *Journal of Hepatology*, vol. 48, no. supplement 1, pp. S68–S92, 2008.

[2] J. Bosch and J. C. García-Pagán, "Complications of cirrhosis. I. Portal hypertension," *Journal of Hepatology*, vol. 32, no. 1, supplement, pp. 141–156, 2000.

[3] A. D. Amarapurkar, D. Amarapurkar, M. Choksi, N. Bhatt, and P. Amarapurkar, "Portal hypertensive polyps: Distinct entity," *Indian Journal of Gastroenterology*, vol. 32, no. 3, pp. 195–199, 2013.

[4] S. Elhanafi, M. Saadi, W. Lou et al., "Gastric polyps: association with Helicobacter pylori status and the pathology of the surrounding mucosa, a cross sectional study," *World Journal of Gastrointestinal Endoscopy*, vol. 7, no. 10, pp. 995–1002, 2015.

[5] A. Gurung, P. E. Jaffe, and X. Zhang, "Duodenal polyposis secondary to portal hypertensive duodenopathy," *World Journal of Gastrointestinal Endoscopy*, vol. 7, no. 17, pp. 1257–1261, 2015.

[6] M. C. W. Lam, S. Tha, D. Owen et al., "Gastric polyps in patients with portal hypertension," *European Journal of Gastroenterology & Hepatology*, vol. 23, no. 12, pp. 1245–1249, 2011.

[7] T. H. Lee, J. Y. Jang, S. W. Jeong, and S. Y. Jin, "Gastric polyposis associated with portal hypertension," *Korean Journal of Internal Medicine*, vol. 28, no. 2, p. 261, 2013.

[8] A. Lemmers, S. Evrard, P. Demetter et al., "Gastrointestinal polypoid lesions: a poorly known endoscopic feature of portal hypertension," *United European Gastroenterology Journal*, vol. 2, no. 3, pp. 189–196, 2014.

[9] V. Martin Dominguez, A. Diaz Mendez, C. Santander, and L. Garcia-Buey, "Portal hypertensive polyps, a new entity?" *Revista Espanola de Enfermedades Digestivas*, vol. 108, no. 5, pp. 279-280, 2016.

[10] S. J. S. Nagpal, C. Macaron, R. K. Pai, and N. Alkhouri, "Gastric polyposis: a rare cause of iron deficiency anemia in a patient with portal hypertension," *ACG Case Reports Journal*, vol. 2, no. 2, pp. 89–91, 2015.

[11] C. G. Pai, "Portal hypertensive polyp—what is in a name?" *Indian Journal of Gastroenterology*, vol. 32, no. 3, pp. 163-164, 2013.

[12] C. Panackel, H. Joshy, B. Sebastian, R. Thomas, and S. K. Mathai, "Gastric antral polyps: A manifestation of portal hypertensive gastropathy," *Indian Journal of Gastroenterology*, vol. 32, no. 3, pp. 206-207, 2013.

[13] S. B. Pillai, V. R. Ram Ganesh, A. Mohanakrishnan, and V. Nirmala, "Portal duodenopathy presenting as polyposis," *Indian Journal of Pathology & Microbiology*, vol. 53, no. 3, pp. 558-559, 2010.

[14] K. Sawada, T. Ohtake, N. Ueno et al., "Multiple portal hypertensive polyps of the jejunum accompanied by anemia of unknown origin," *Gastrointestinal Endoscopy*, vol. 73, no. 1, pp. 179–182, 2011.

[15] J.-D. Zeitoun, A. Chryssostalis, B. Terris, F. Prat, M. Gaudric, and S. Chaussade, "Portal hypertensive duodenal polyp: a case report," *World Journal of Gastroenterology*, vol. 13, no. 9, pp. 1451-1452, 2007.

[16] M. Primignani, L. Carpinelli, P. Preatoni et al., "Natural history of portal hypertensive gastropathy in patients with liver cirrhosis. The New Italian Endoscopic Club for the study and treatment of esophageal varices (NIEC)," *Gastroenterology*, vol. 119, no. 1, pp. 181–187, 2000.

[17] A. Zaman, R. Hapke, K. Flora, H. Rosen, and K. Benner, "Prevalence of upper and lower gastrointestinal tract findings in liver transplant candidates undergoing screening endoscopic evaluation," *American Journal of Gastroenterology*, vol. 94, no. 4, pp. 895–899, 1999.

[18] K. W. Burak, S. S. Lee, and P. L. Beck, "Portal hypertensive gastropathy and gastric antral vascular ectasia (GAVE) syndrome," *Gut*, vol. 49, no. 6, pp. 866–872, 2001.

[19] G. Gravante, D. Delogu, and D. Venditti, "Upper and lower gastrointestinal diseases in liver transplant candidates," *International Journal of Colorectal Disease*, vol. 23, no. 2, pp. 201–206, 2008.

[20] B. D. Bhatt, T. Lukose, A. B. Siegel, R. S. Brown, and E. C. Verna, "Increased risk of colorectal polyps in patients with non-alcoholic fatty liver disease undergoing liver transplant evaluation," *Journal of Gastrointestinal Oncology*, vol. 6, no. 5, pp. 459–468, 2015.

[21] S. Tanaka, Y. Saitoh, T. Matsuda et al., "Evidence-based clinical practice guidelines for management of colorectal polyps," *Journal of Gastroenterology*, vol. 50, no. 3, pp. 252–260, 2015.

[22] J. H. Lin, S. M. Zhang, K. M. Rexrode et al., "Association between sex hormones and colorectal cancer risk in men and women," *Clinical Gastroenterology and Hepatology*, vol. 11, no. 4, pp. 419–424.e1, 2013.

[23] M. A. Murray, M. J. Zimmerman, and H. C. Ee, "Sporadic duodenal adenoma is associated with colorectal neoplasia," *Gut*, vol. 53, no. 2, pp. 261–265, 2004.

[24] D. Apel, R. Jakobs, U. Weickert, and J. Ferdinand Riemann, "High frequency of colorectal adenoma in patients with duodenal adenoma but without familial adenomatous polyposis," *Gastrointestinal Endoscopy*, vol. 60, no. 3, pp. 397–399, 2004.

[25] S. Naveau, J. C. Chapnut, P. Bedossa et al., "Cirrhosis as an independent risk factor for colonic adenomas," *Gut*, vol. 33, no. 4, pp. 535–540, 1992.

18

The Expanding Role of Systemic Therapy in the Management of Hepatocellular Carcinoma

Omar Abdel-Rahman[1,2] and Winson Y. Cheung[2]

[1]Clinical Oncology Department, Faculty of Medicine, Ain Shams University, Cairo, Egypt
[2]Department of Oncology, University of Calgary, Tom Baker Cancer Centre, Calgary, Alberta, Canada

Correspondence should be addressed to Winson Y. Cheung; winson.cheung@ahs.ca

Academic Editor: Alexandros Giakoustidis

Hepatocellular carcinoma (HCC) represents a global health problem, with the majority of patients presenting at an advanced or incurable stage. The development of effective systemic therapy options for this disease has been challenging because many HCC patients suffer from underlying liver cirrhosis that precludes the safe delivery of systemic therapy. The current review seeks to provide an overview of the current systemic therapeutic approaches for advanced HCC as well as some of the novel management strategies that are currently being evaluated.

1. Introduction

Primary liver cancer represents a global health problem since it is the sixth most common cause of cancer as well as the second most common cause of cancer mortality worldwide [1]. Hepatocellular carcinoma (HCC) represents more than 90% of cases of primary liver cancer [2].

The development of cirrhosis precedes tumor formation in most cases and as expected most causes of cirrhosis represent the main risk factors for developing HCC. These include mainly hepatitis B and C, chronic alcoholism, aflatoxin exposure, and other rarer causes of cirrhosis such as hemochromatosis [3]. The association between all etiologic forms of cirrhosis and HCC is illustrative of geographic imbalance in the incidence of HCC worldwide. For example, hepatitis B is endemic to parts of Asia [3].

According to international guidelines focusing on the management of HCC, the diagnosis of HCC should be based on well-defined imaging criteria and/or histological confirmation. A number of screening programs have been implemented worldwide in order to detect cases of HCC at an earlier stage anticipating that this strategy can lead to improvements in patient outcomes [4].

Effective HCC management relies on multidisciplinary involvement in the decision-making process and takes into account the various patient-related, disease-related, and treatment-related factors [5]. This is reflected in the various staging systems for clinical decision-making in HCC where in contrast to the majority of solid tumors, the traditional TNM staging system is not commonly utilized [6]. The staging system validated and used most frequently for outcome prediction and treatment allocation is the Barcelona Clinic Liver Cancer (BCLC) staging system [7]. For early-stage cases among fit patients, potentially curative treatments (e.g., resection, transplantation, and ablation) represent the standard of care [8]. For intermediate-stage cases, transarterial chemoembolization and other locoregional therapies might be used [9, 10]. Conversely, for advanced-stage disease (portal vein invasion or extrahepatic disease) in patients with preserved liver function, systemic therapy options represent the primary treatment modality.

Unfortunately, most cases of HCC are detected at an advanced or incurable stage. In the context of currently available treatment modalities, overall survival for many of these cases does not exceed one year [11]. Improvement in the outcomes of advanced-stage disease is thus the focus of most current scientific efforts.

The current review aims to provide an overview of the available standard of care systemic treatments for HCC, as well as offering some insights into new investigational approaches.

2. Current First-Line Therapy of Advanced-Stage Disease (Stage C BCLC)

Systemic therapy is the current standard of care for advanced-stage disease. Sorafenib (a multikinase inhibitor) was the first agent to demonstrate overall survival and received regulatory approval in 2007. Its approval was based principally on two landmark international phase III studies, the SHARP study and the Asia-Pacific study [12, 13]. Both studies randomized patients with advanced HCC into either treatment with sorafenib or placebo. Both studies limited their inclusion to patients with good performance status, adequate liver function, and minimal comorbidity. In the SHARP study, there was a statistically significant improvement in overall survival with sorafenib compared to placebo (median overall survival was 10.7 months in the sorafenib group and 7.9 months in the placebo group; HR, 0.69; 95% CI, 0.55 to 0.87; P=0.00058). Similarly, in the Asia-Pacific study, there was a statistically significant, albeit smaller, benefit in overall survival with sorafenib compared to placebo (median overall survival was 6.5 months in patients treated with sorafenib, compared with 4.2 months in the placebo group; HR 0.68; 95% CI 0.50-0.93; P=0.014).

Subsequent secondary analyses of phase III studies have shown that lower ALBI (albumin/bilirubin) score, ECOG (Eastern Cooperative Oncology Group) performance score of 0, BMI (Body Mass Index) ≥ 25, AFP (Alpha-fetoprotein) < 200 ng/ml, and no extrahepatic spread are associated with better overall survival among patients treated with sorafenib [14]. Interestingly, sorafenib appears to be of greater benefit for HCC patients with underlying hepatitis C virus infection compared to hepatitis B virus infection [15].

Subsequently, several other studies have been conducted in order for other targeted agents (e.g., brivanib and sunitinib) to be studied in comparison to sorafenib. However, it was demonstrated that the studied agents were nonsuperior or equal to sorafenib and additionally had a less favorable side effects profile and poorer tolerability [16, 17]. Other studies have also evaluated different sorafenib-based combinations (e.g., sorafenib plus erlotinib, sorafenib plus doxorubicin); however, there was no superiority in terms of survival [18, 19].

An important caveat for the interpretation of the above is the fact that the vast majority of patients included into the two landmark studies had well-preserved liver function (Child-Pugh class A) and good performance status. This is very important as the majority of HCC patients encountered in routine clinical practice are typically significantly frailer. They usually have advanced cirrhosis, poor liver function, and a compromised functional status. Accordingly, extrapolation of these data from clinical trials into the real world should be done cautiously. More recently, lenvatinib (multikinase inhibitor) was compared in a phase III study to sorafenib in the first-line treatment of unresectable HCC. This study showed that lenvatinib was noninferior to sorafenib with regard to overall survival [20].

3. Current Second-Line Therapy of Advanced HCC (after Failure of Sorafenib)

Several other cytotoxic and targeted agents have also been tested as second-line treatment. However, most of these studies have not proven to be successful due to lack of efficacy and/or poor tolerability [21–23]. In 2016 regorafenib, another multikinase inhibitor became approved in this setting. The approval of regorafenib was based on a landmark phase III study which compared regorafenib versus placebo in patients who tolerated and progressed on sorafenib. Regorafenib improved overall survival (HR 0·63; 95% CI 0·50-0·79; P<0·0001); median overall survival was 10·6 months for the regorafenib group versus 7·8 months for the placebo group [24]. However, it should be noted that patients included in the above study were also highly selected (i.e., good performance status and Child A liver function), which is in contrast to the vast majority of advanced HCC, post-sorafenib patients encountered in routine clinical practice. Furthermore, regorafenib has significant toxicities which may preclude its use in most real-world patients. Specific side effects include hand-foot syndrome, fatigue, and hypertension. Overall, the use of regorafenib in this fragile patient population with borderline liver function needs to be cautiously approached.

More recently, the results of another landmark trial (CELESTIAL study) comparing cabozantinib versus placebo as second-line treatment were published. Cabozantinib is a multikinase inhibitor with potent inhibitory activity against c-MET [25]. In the CELESTIAL phase III study, cabozantinib improved overall survival compared to placebo. Median overall survival was 10.2 months for cabozantinib versus 8.0 months for placebo (HR 0.76, 95% CI 0.63-0.92; P=0.0049) [26]. It is expected that cabozantinib will be soon adopted as an alternative second-line treatment for advanced HCC following progression on sorafenib. The favorable outcomes in the placebo-treated group likely underscore the fact that trial patients were probably highly selected. Thus, caution should again be exercised when generalizing these results into routine clinical practice.

A third agent which has recently drawn much attention in the second-line treatment of advanced HCC is nivolumab which is a PD-1 inhibitor. The results of a phase 1/2, open-label, noncomparative, dose escalation, and expansion trial (CheckMate 040) were recently published [27]. In this study, previous sorafenib treatment was allowed. The objective response rate was 20% (95% CI 15–26%) in patients treated with nivolumab 3 mg/kg in the dose-expansion phase and 15% (95% CI 6–28%) in the dose-escalation phase. As a consequence, the FDA has granted nivolumab conditional approval as a second-line agent. The results of a phase III study (CHECKMATE 459) comparing nivolumab versus sorafenib in treatment-naïve HCC are anticipated, alongside a number of other ongoing studies.

Following the favorable results of nivolumab, a number of other immune checkpoint inhibitors are currently being evaluated. The interest in immune checkpoint inhibitors was stimulated by several preclinical findings suggesting that HCC is an immunogenic tumor with numerous tumor-associated antigens [28]. Moreover, there has been work focusing on elucidating the HCC tumor microenvironment with early suggestions of the presence of an upregulated PD(L)1 pathway in HCC [29]. This has led to a plethora of ongoing clinical trials investigating PD(L)1 inhibitors (alone or in combination with other treatments) in the management of HCC. As of April 2018 and on the clinicaltirals.gov registry, there are 23 open clinical trials investigating nivolumab and 19 investigating pembrolizumab in the management of HCC.

Before adopting the use of immune checkpoint inhibitors in the management of these patients, it is noteworthy that these agents are also known to produce a wide spectrum of immune-related adverse events including cutaneous, hepatic, gastrointestinal, endocrine, and pulmonary adverse events [30–34]. Given the impaired liver function seen in the majority of patients with HCC, appropriate and thorough assessment of the tolerability and pattern of adverse events among these patients (particularly with respect to hepatic and gastrointestinal adverse events) needs to be conducted. Previous reports have suggested that the use of immune checkpoint inhibitors may potentially lead to viral hepatitis reactivation [35]. The extent to which immune checkpoint inhibitors can be safely administered in HCC patients is not yet known with certainty.

4. Investigational Role of Systemic Therapy in Earlier Stages of HCC

4.1. Adjuvant Systemic Therapy. The use of adjuvant systemic therapy following resection, transplantation, or locoregional ablation drew attention among oncologists and hepatologists treating patients with HCC. However, all relevant studies to date have failed to provide a convincing benefit to justify their routine use in clinical practice [36].

4.2. Systemic Therapy in Combination with Locoregional Transarterial Treatments. Several studies have also evaluated various combinations of systemic therapy (particularly sorafenib) with locoregional treatments (including transarterial (chemo)-embolization and radio-embolization). The stated rationale for such combinations is the potential of transarterial treatments to induce a consequent surge in VEGF levels following the procedure, and this was presumed to be the main pathogenetic process behind treatment failure [37]. Thus, this resulted in significant interest towards the concurrent administration of VEGF-VEGFR targeted agents, which was hypothesized to decrease the rates of failure by countering this mechanism. Despite some interesting preliminary findings, the overall evidence provided is not yet convincing enough to justify the widespread use of this approach [38, 39].

5. Conclusions and Future Directions

Outcomes of patients with advanced HCC are still very poor. The development of novel therapeutic approaches to improve overall survival and quality of life is an unmet need. The introduction of sequential targeted therapeutics including sorafenib as first-line treatment and regorafenib, cabozantinib, and nivolumab as second-line treatment could contribute to improved outcomes for these patients. Nevertheless, severe side effects and poor tolerability pose a real challenge and the vast majority of advanced HCC patients in clinical practice have compromised performance status and/or poor liver function. To date, prevention of liver cirrhosis remains the most effective way to prevent development of HCC. For instance, there has been significant reduction of hepatitis B-related HCC following the introduction of hepatitis B vaccination. Future research should be directed towards a better understanding of the biology of the disease and of the complexity of the biological process within its microenvironment. Agents targeting a single pathway or a single pathogenetic process within HCC have not been very successful in combating this disease. We are in need for more unique and strategic approaches which may include various combinations of treatments or modalities.

References

[1] J. Ferlay, I. Soerjomataram, R. Dikshit et al., "Cancer incidence and mortality worldwide: sources, methods and major patterns in GLOBOCAN 2012," *International Journal of Cancer*, vol. 136, no. 5, pp. E359–E386, 2014.

[2] S. Mittal and H. B. El-Serag, "Epidemiology of hepatocellular carcinoma: consider the population," *Journal of Clinical Gastroenterology*, vol. 47, no. 1, pp. S2–S6, 2013.

[3] R. X. Zhu, W.-K. Seto, C.-L. Lai, and M.-F. Yuen, "Epidemiology of hepatocellular carcinoma in the Asia-Pacific region," *Gut and Liver*, vol. 10, no. 3, pp. 332–339, 2016.

[4] D. Kansagara, J. Papak, A. S. Pasha et al., "Screening for hepatocellular carcinoma in chronic liver disease: a systematic review," *Annals of Internal Medicine*, vol. 161, no. 4, pp. 261–269, 2014.

[5] O. Abdel-Rahman, "Systemic therapy for hepatocellular carcinoma (HCC): from bench to bedside," *Journal of the Egyptian National Cancer Institute*, vol. 25, no. 4, pp. 165–171, 2013.

[6] O. Abdel-Rahman, "Assessment of the discriminating value of the 8th AJCC stage grouping for hepatocellular carcinoma," *HPB*, vol. 20, no. 1, pp. 41–48, 2018.

[7] S. P. Choo, W. L. Tan, B. K. P. Goh, W. M. Tai, and A. X. Zhu, "Comparison of hepatocellular carcinoma in Eastern versus Western populations," *Cancer*, vol. 122, no. 22, pp. 3430–3446, 2016.

[8] H. Oweira, U. Petrausch, D. Helbling et al., "Early stage hepatocellular carcinoma in the elderly: a SEER database analysis," *Journal of Geriatric Oncology*, vol. 8, no. 4, pp. 277–283, 2017.

[9] O. Abdel-Rahman and Z. Elsayed, "External beam radiotherapy for unresectable hepatocellular carcinoma," *Cochrane Database of Systematic Reviews*, vol. 2017, no. 3, 2017.

[10] O. M. Abdel-Rahman and Z. Elsayed, "Yttrium-90 microsphere radioembolisation for unresectable hepatocellular carcinoma," *Cochrane Database of Systematic Reviews*, vol. 2016, no. 2, 2016.

[11] O. Abdel-Rahman and M. Fouad, "Sorafenib-based combination as a first line treatment for advanced hepatocellular carcinoma: a systematic review of the literature," *Critical Review in Oncology/Hematology*, vol. 91, no. 1, pp. 1–8, 2014.

[12] A. Cheng, Y. Kang, Z. Chen et al., "Efficacy and safety of sorafenib in patients in the Asia-Pacific region with advanced hepatocellular carcinoma: a phase III randomised, double-blind, placebo-controlled trial," *The Lancet Oncology*, vol. 10, no. 1, pp. 25–34, 2009.

[13] J. M. Llovet, S. Ricci, V. Mazzaferro et al., "Sorafenib in advanced hepatocellular carcinoma," *The New England Journal of Medicine*, vol. 359, no. 4, pp. 378–390, 2008.

[14] O. Abdel-Rahman, "Impact of baseline characteristics on outcomes of advanced HCC patients treated with sorafenib: a secondary analysis of a phase III study," *Journal of Cancer Research and Clinical Oncology*, pp. 1–8, 2018.

[15] J. Bruix, J.-L. Raou, and M. Sherman, "Efficacy and safety of sorafenib in patients with advanced hepatocellular carcinoma: subanalyses of a phase III trial," *Journal of Hepatology*, vol. 57, no. 4, pp. 821–829, 2012.

[16] P. J. Johnson, S. Qin, J. W. Park, R. T. Poon, J. L. Raoul, and P. A. Philip, "Brivanib versus sorafenib as first-line therapy in patients with unresectable, advanced hepatocellular carcinoma: results from the randomized phase III BRISK-FL study," *Journal of Clinical Oncology*, vol. 31, no. 28, pp. 3517–3524, 2013.

[17] A.-L. Cheng, Y.-K. Kang, D.-Y. Lin et al., "Sunitinib versus sorafenib in advanced hepatocellular cancer: results of a randomized phase III trial," *Journal of Clinical Oncology*, vol. 31, no. 32, pp. 4067–4075, 2013.

[18] A. X. Zhu, O. Rosmorduc, T. R. J. Evans et al., "Search: a phase III, randomized, double-blind, placebo-controlled trial of sorafenib plus erlotinib in patients with advanced hepatocellular carcinoma," *Journal of Clinical Oncology*, vol. 33, no. 6, pp. 559–566, 2015.

[19] G. K. Abou-Alfa, P. Johnson, J. J. Knox et al., "Doxorubicin plus sorafenib vs doxorubicin alone in patients with advanced hepatocellular carcinoma: a randomized trial," *Journal of the American Medical Association*, vol. 304, no. 19, pp. 2154–2160, 2010.

[20] M. Kudo, R. S. Finn, S. Qin et al., "Lenvatinib versus sorafenib in first-line treatment of patients with unresectable hepatocellular carcinoma: a randomised phase 3 non-inferiority trial," *The Lancet*, vol. 391, no. 10126, pp. 1163–1173, 2018.

[21] J. M. Llovet, T. Decaens, J.-L. Raoul et al., "Brivanib in patients with advanced hepatocellular carcinoma who were intolerant to sorafenib or for whom sorafenib failed: results from the randomized phase III BRISK-PS study," *Journal of Clinical Oncology*, vol. 31, no. 28, pp. 3509–3516, 2013.

[22] A. X. Zhu, A. D. Baron, P. Malfertheiner et al., "Ramucirumab as second-line treatment in patients with advanced hepatocellular carcinoma analysis of REACH trial results by child-pugh score," *JAMA Oncology*, vol. 3, no. 2, pp. 235–243, 2017.

[23] O. Abdel-Rahman and M. Fouad, "Second line systemic therapy options for advanced hepatocellular carcinoma; A systematic review," *Expert Review of Anticancer Therapy*, vol. 15, no. 2, pp. 165–182, 2015.

[24] J. Bruix, S. Qin, P. Merle et al., "Regorafenib for patients with hepatocellular carcinoma who progressed on sorafenib treatment (RESORCE): a randomised, double-blind, placebo-controlled, phase 3 trial," *The Lancet*, vol. 389, no. 10064, pp. 56–66, 2017.

[25] R. K. Kelley, C. Verslype, A. L. Cohn et al., "Cabozantinib in hepatocellular carcinoma: results of a phase 2 placebo-controlled randomized discontinuation study," *Annals of Oncology*, vol. 28, no. 3, pp. 528–534, 2017.

[26] G. K. Abou-Alfa, T. Meyer, A. L. Cheng et al., "Cabozantinib in patients with advanced and progressing hepatocellular carcinoma," *New England Journal of Medicine*, vol. 379, no. 1, pp. 54–63, 2018.

[27] A. B. El-Khoueiry, B. Sangro, T. Yau et al., "Nivolumab in patients with advanced hepatocellular carcinoma (CheckMate 040): an open-label, non-comparative, phase 1/2 dose escalation and expansion trial," *The Lancet*, vol. 389, no. 10088, pp. 2492–2502, 2017.

[28] N. Schmidt and R. Thimme, "Role of immunity in pathogenesis and treatment of hepatocellular carcinoma," *Digestive Diseases*, vol. 34, no. 4, pp. 429–437, 2016.

[29] A. D. Pardee and L. H. Butterfield, "Immunotherapy of hepatocellular carcinoma: unique challenges and clinical opportunities," *OncoImmunology*, vol. 1, no. 1, pp. 48–55, 2012.

[30] O. Abdel-Rahman, H. ElHalawani, and M. Fouad, "Risk of cutaneous toxicities in patients with solid tumors treated with immune checkpoint inhibitors: a meta-analysis," *Future Oncology*, vol. 11, no. 17, pp. 2471–2484, 2015.

[31] O. Abdel-Rahman, H. Elhalawani, and M. Fouad, "Risk of elevated transaminases in cancer patients treated with immune checkpoint inhibitors: a meta-analysis," *Expert Opinion on Drug Safety*, vol. 14, no. 10, pp. 1507–1518, 2015.

[32] O. Abdel-Rahman, H. Elhalawani, and M. Fouad, "Risk of endocrine complications in cancer patients treated with immune check point inhibitors: a meta-analysis," *Future Oncology*, vol. 12, no. 3, pp. 413–425, 2016.

[33] O. Abdel-Rahman, H. Elhalawani, and M. Fouad, "Risk of gastrointestinal complications in cancer patients treated with immune checkpoint inhibitors: a meta-analysis," *Immunotherapy*, vol. 7, no. 11, pp. 1213–1227, 2015.

[34] O. Abdel-Rahman and M. Fouad, "Risk of pneumonitis in cancer patients treated with immune checkpoint inhibitors: a meta-analysis," *Therapeutic Advances in Respiratory Disease*, vol. 10, no. 3, pp. 183–193, 2016.

[35] D. B. Johnson, R. J. Sullivan, and A. M. Menzies, "Immune checkpoint inhibitors in challenging populations," *Cancer*, vol. 123, no. 11, pp. 1904–1911, 2017.

[36] J. Bruix, T. Takayama, V. Mazzaferro et al., "Adjuvant sorafenib for hepatocellular carcinoma after resection or ablation (STORM): a phase 3, randomised, double-blind, placebo-controlled trial," *The Lancet Oncology*, vol. 16, no. 13, pp. 1344–1354, 2015.

[37] R. S. Finn and A. X. Zhu, "Targeting angiogenesis in hepatocellular carcinoma: focus on VEGF and bevacizumab," *Expert Review of Anticancer Therapy*, vol. 9, no. 4, pp. 503–509, 2009.

[38] A. Erhardt, F. Kolligs, M. Dollinger et al., "TACE plus sorafenib for the treatment of hepatocellular carcinoma: results of the multicenter, phase II SOCRATES trial," *Cancer Chemotherapy and Pharmacology*, vol. 74, no. 5, pp. 947–954, 2014.

[39] Y.-H. Chung, G. Han, J.-H. Yoon et al., "Interim analysis of START: study in asia of the combination of TACE (transcatheter arterial chemoembolization) with sorafenib in patients with hepatocellular carcinoma trial," *International Journal of Cancer*, vol. 132, no. 10, pp. 2448–2458, 2013.

19

Immunotherapy in Advanced Gastric Cancer: An Overview of the Emerging Strategies

Helena Magalhães, Mário Fontes-Sousa, and Manuela Machado

Medical Oncology Department, Portuguese Institute of Oncology of Porto (IPO Porto), Porto, Portugal

Correspondence should be addressed to Helena Magalhães; hmmagalhaes88@gmail.com,
Mário Fontes-Sousa; mario_fontes_sousa@hotmail.com, and Manuela Machado; m.machado.fn@gmail.com

Academic Editor: Lintao Jia

Gastric cancer (GC) remains a public health problem, being the fifth most common cancer worldwide. In the western countries, the majority of patients present with advanced disease. Additionally, 65 to 75% of patients treated with curative intent will relapse and develop systemic disease. In metastatic disease, systemic treatment still represents the state of the art, with less than a year of median overall survival. The new molecular classification of GC was published in 2014, identifying four distinct major subtypes of gastric cancer, and has encouraged the investigation of new and more personalized treatment strategies. This paper will review the current evidence of immunotherapy in advanced gastric cancer.

1. Introduction

GC is the 5th most common cancer diagnosed worldwide, and it represents one of the major causes of malignant disease morbidity and mortality, with almost 107,000 deaths in Europe in 2012 [1, 2].

The majority of the patients are diagnosed with locally advanced disease not suitable for surgery or metastatic disease. For these patients, chemotherapy is the standard of care in patients with clinical conditions, with median overall survival (OS) of less than 12 months. When compared to best supportive care (BSC), systemic treatment showed a clear advantage in OS [3, 4].

Currently, a combination of a platinum and fluoropyrimidine doublet is the mainstay of chemotherapy. The addition of a taxane or an anthracycline to this combination in human epidermal growth factor receptor 2 (HER-2) negative population increases response rate and survival outcomes but also generally implies higher toxicity, so the risks versus benefits should be well balanced. In the phase III ToGA trial, the addition of trastuzumab to cisplatin and fluoropyrimidine backbone improved median overall survival (OS), progression free survival (PFS), and response rate (RR) in Her-2 positive advanced or metastatic gastric cancer and established this regimen as standard of care in those patients [5, 6].

Second line chemotherapy, is an option for patients with good performance status. Docetaxel, irinotecan, and paclitaxel have all demonstrated improved survival compared to BSC in this setting. Additionally, ramucirumab, a vascular endothelial growth factor receptor (VEGFR-2) antibody, was the first biological treatment given as a single drug or in combination with paclitaxel in patients with advanced gastric or gastroesophageal junction (GEJ) adenocarcinoma progressing after first-line chemotherapy that demonstrated survival benefits in two randomized trials [7–11].

Despite these treatment options, the prognosis of advanced and metastatic GC is still poor and novel treatment strategies and patient selection tools are needed.

In the "era of the revolution" in cancer management with immunotherapy, it appears that a new hope is also arising for patients with advanced GC, as it has in other malignancies where this class of drugs demonstrated benefit.

Evidence and rationale for the use of immunotherapy in gastric cancer GC is a heterogeneous disease which can be divided into 4 major subtypes based on molecular signature according to Cancer Genome Atlas Research Network (TCGA): Epstein Barr virus (EBV) positive, microsatellite unstable (MSI), and genomically stable (GS) and chromosomal instability (CIN) tumours [12].

Two subtypes, EBV positive and MSI GC, are considered to be most potentially responsive to immunotherapy drugs.

The EBV positive GC that represents 9% of all GC is more prevalent in younger patients, in males (a twofold ratio in male/female), with no difference between intestinal and diffuse histology. EBV positive GC is associated with programmed death-ligand 1 (PD-L1) gene amplification, which suggests higher immunogenicity, and might therefore be more likely to respond to immune checkpoint inhibition. It is known that PD-L1 is highly predictive in lung cancer, but yet controversial in gastric cancer.

MSI tumours seem to occur in 15–30% of GC and are related more commonly with female gender, older patients, and intestinal histology and tumours arising from the distal stomach. This category of gastric cancer is characterized by increased lymphocytic infiltrate, which may reflects activation of T-cells against tumour antigens and genomic changes in tumour cells that are linked to PD-L1 expression, indicating a potential role for immunotherapy [13].

Both MSI and EBV positive GCs have a high somatic mutational burden which also is a feature that has been associated with response to immunotherapy.

2. Checkpoint Inhibition

Given the success of checkpoint inhibitors in melanoma, non-small-cell lung cancer, renal cell cancer, urothelial carcinoma, and head and neck cancer it seemed logical to investigate the role of these agents in gastric cancer.

Cytotoxic T lymphocyte protein 4 (CTLA-4) and programmed cell death protein-1 (PD-1) are immune checkpoints that inhibit the T-cell response, which provide the escape mechanism of the tumour cells to T-cell antitumour activity [14].

The B7-H1, also known as PD-L1, in positive tumours interacts with its receptor PD-1 and this consequently leads to inhibition of the T-cells migration, proliferation, resulting in an antiapoptotic signal, preventing overactivation of the immune system, escaping from destruction [15].

In GC, some studies evaluate the expression and clinical significance of PD-1/PD-L1 pathway. Wu et al. found that PD-L1 was expressed in 42,2% of GC tissues and was not found in normal tissue. The immunodetection of PD- L1 was significantly associated with tumour size, invasion, lymph node metastasis, and survival time of patients [16].

In another study, Hou et al. found the expression of PD-L1 in 63% of the 111 GC patients analyzed and that its overexpression was linked to lymph node metastasis, an advanced clinicopathological stage, and lower overall survival rate [17].

Therefore, immunologic checkpoint blockade with antibodies that target CTLA-4 and PD-1/PD-L1 seemed promising strategies that could improve the outcomes in GC and deserved more specific studies (Figure 1).

We tried to summarize the relevant clinical data about specific immune checkpoints agents and the possible future applications in treatment of advanced gastric cancer.

3. Anti-CTLA4

Ipilimumab and tremelimumab are two anti-CTLA4 antibodies that were evaluated in GC.

A phase II trial evaluated the efficacy of ipilimumab immediately following 1st line chemotherapy in unresectable or metastatic adenocarcinoma of the gastric and GEJ compared with BSC. From 143 patients screened, 57 were randomized to each arm, and in an interim analysis, no differences were seen in PFS between groups, and the study ended early. At study closeout (8 months after interim analysis), the median OS was 12.7 months in BSC versus 12.1 months for the arm with ipilimumab [18].

Tremelimumab was investigated in a phase II trial as 2nd line treatment for patients with metastatic gastric and oesophageal adenocarcinomas. The response rate was only 5%, but there was a clinical benefit with evidence of stable disease in 4 of the 18 patients, and one patient showed a durable response, receiving 32.7 months of treatment after trial enrollment [19].

4. Anti-PD-1

Nivolumab is a PD-1 blocking antibody approved for the treatment of advanced melanoma, advanced non-small-cell lung cancer (NSCLC), advanced renal cell carcinoma, advanced squamous cell carcinoma of the head and neck (SCCHN), and urothelial carcinoma.

Two randomized trials showed efficacy and safety for nivolumab alone in both Asian and western populations in gastric cancer.

The phase I/II CHECKMATE 032 trial, a multicohort study, included patients with metastatic gastric or GEJ cancer, treated with nivolumab in monotherapy (3 mg/kg IV every 2 weeks) or in combination with ipilimumab, irrespective of PD-L1 status [20].

In the single-arm (the cohort with 59 patients), the objective response rate, defined as the proportion of patients who achieved a complete response or a partial response (ORR), with nivolumab was 14% (including 1 complete response and 7 partial responses). Moreover, the stable disease rate was 19%, for a total disease control rate of 32%. The median time to response was 1.6 months and the median duration of response was 7.1 months. The median OS was 5.0 months with nivolumab (95% CI, 3.4–12.4). The 12-month OS rate was 36%. The median PFS was 1.36 months (95% CI, 1.3–1.5) and the 6-month PFS rate was 18%. In the subgroup with PD-L1 expression on ≥1% of cells (n = 15), the ORR was 27% with nivolumab. In those with PD-L1 expression on <1% (n = 25), the ORR was 12%.

The combination of nivolumab with ipilimumab was also evaluated in this trial, with two separate dose levels: nivolumab 1 mg/kg and ipilimumab 3 mg/kg (n = 49) or nivolumab 3 mg/kg plus ipilimumab 1 mg/kg (n = 52). The ORR was 26% for the first arm and 10% for the second. Six-month PFS was 24% and 9%, respectively. The 12-month OS was 34% in first cohort and not available in the second. Grade 3 or greater adverse effects (AEs) were seen in 27 and 45%

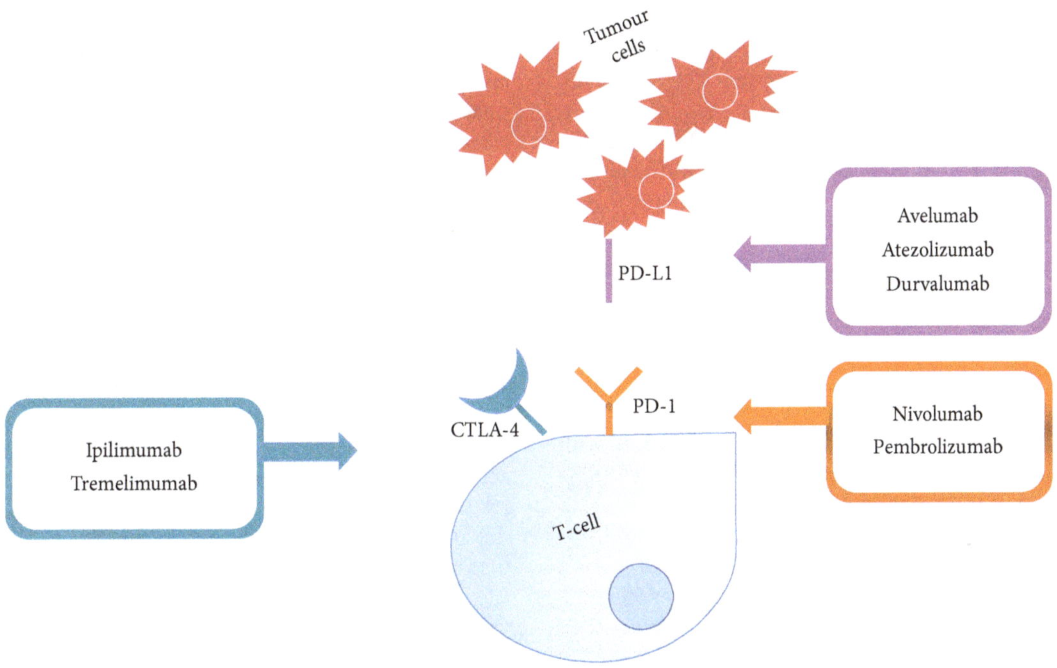

FIGURE 1: Immune checkpoint blockade with different monoclonal antibodies.

of the patients, respectively, which was higher than in the nivolumab alone arm (17%).

The ONO-4538-12 ATTRACTION-2 trial evaluated the efficacy and safety of nivolumab in Asian patients with unresectable advanced or recurrent gastric cancer (including GEJ) who progressed after two or more chemotherapy lines of treatment [21].

Median OS was 5.26 months (95% CI = 4.60–6.37) for patients treated with nivolumab, compared to 4.14 months (95% CI = 3.42–4.86) for those treated with placebo.

In addition, the 12-month OS in the nivolumab group was 26.2% (95% CI = 20.7–32.0) versus 10.9% (95% CI = 6.2–17.0) in the placebo group. Patients treated with nivolumab had an ORR of 11.2% (95% CI 7.7–15.6) compared to 0% (95% CI 0.0–2.8) with placebo. Patients with confirmed response to nivolumab had a median duration of response of 9.53 months (95% CI 6.14–9.82). Grade 3 or greater AEs occurred in 10% of nivolumab arm and 4% of placebo arm.

There were divergent results according to tumour negative PD-L1 expression versus ≥1%. In tumour with negative PD-L1 expression, median OS was 6.05 months in nivolumab arm (versus 4.19 months in the placebo arm; hazard ratio 0.72); in patients with PD-L1 expression ≥1%, median OS was 5.22 months in the arm of nivolumab (versus 3.83 months in the placebo arm; hazard ratio 0.51).

Currently, an important milestone marked the oncology community: pembrolizumab, a humanized IgG4 monoclonal anti-PD1 antibody, had accelerated approval by FDA (Food and Drug Administration) for the treatment of adult patients with unresectable or metastatic solid tumours that have been identified as having a biomarker referred to as microsatellite instability-high (MSI-H) or mismatch repair deficient (dMMR). This indication includes patients that have progressed following prior treatment and who have no satisfactory alternative treatment options.

Results on safety and efficacy from pembrolizumab specifically in gastric cancer were first presented at ESMO Congress 2014 by Muro et al. (KEYNOTE-012) and published in 2016 [22, 23]. Of the 39 patients included in gastric cancer cohort, the ORR was 22% (95% CI 10–39) by central review, all partial responses. Median time to response was 8 weeks (range 7–16), with median response duration of 24 weeks. The 6-month PFS rate was 26% (95% CI 13–41) and OS rate was 66% (95% CI 49–78) and 42% (95% CI 25–59) at 6 and 12 months, respectively. The toxicity was manageable, with only 5 patients experiencing grade 3 or greater adverse effects.

KEYNOTE-059 is a phase II trial multicohort study in advanced gastric or GEJ adenocarcinoma. In cohort 1, patients who have received at least two prior therapies received pembrolizumab as monotherapy. In cohort 2 patients who have not received any previous therapy for their disease received pembrolizumab in combination with cisplatin and 5-FU (in Japan capecitabine could be used instead of 5 FU). In Cohort 3, participants who did not received any previous therapy and who had PD-L1 positive tumours received monotherapy with pembrolizumab.

The results of cohort 1 were presented at ASCO 2017 and the updated data was also presented at ESMO 2017 [24, 25]. From 259 patients in cohort 1, 76.4% were male, and median age was 62.0 years, with patients from United States (47.9%), East Asia (13.1%), and the rest of the world (39.0%); 51.7% and 29% of the patients received pembrolizumab as 3rd line (3L) and 4th line therapy, respectively.

PD-L1 positive patients had expression in ≥1% tumour or stromal cells using immunohistochemistry (IHC). In this cohort 57.1% had PD-L1 positive tumours.

The ORR with pembrolizumab in all patients was 11.6% (95% CI 8.0–16.1). In PD-L1-positive ORR was 15.5% (95% CI 10.1–22.4) and in PD-L1 negative tumours ORR was 6.4% (95% CI 2.6–12.8). The median duration of response (DOR) in all patients was 8.4 months. The median DOR in the PD-L1–positive group was 16.3 versus 6.9 months in those with PD-L1–negative disease.

In the 7 patients with MSI-H tumours, ORR was 57.1%; in comparison with 167 patients with non-MSI-H tumours, ORR was 9.0%.

The median PFS was 2.0 months and the median OS was 5.6 months. Treatment was well tolerated, but 2 treatment-related grade 5 AEs were reported (acute kidney injury and pleural effusion).

In 3rd line the ORR was 16.4% (95% CI 10.6–23.8), with 3% of CR and 13.4% of PR; in 4th line the ORR was 6.4% (95% CI 2.8–12.2).

The cohort 2 was presented in ASCO 2017 and the updated data was also presented at ESMO 2017 [25, 26]. From 25 enrolled patients, 64% were men, median age was 64 years, 68% were Asian, and 64% had PD-L1 positive tumours. In PD-L1-expressing patients, ORR was 68.8% versus 37.5% in PD-L1-negative patients. Median duration of response was 4.6 months in overall population, 4.6 months in PD-L1-positive patients, and 5.4 months in PD-L1-negative patients. Investigators observed grade 3/4 AEs in 76% of patients.

The cohort 3 was presented at ESMO congress in September 2017 [25]. In the 31 patients included, with a median follow-up of 17.5 months, the ORR was 26% and the DCR 36%. The median PFS was 3.3 months and the median OS 20.7 months.

Several randomized clinical trials are currently ongoing to evaluate pembrolizumab and nivolumab in earlier lines of therapy in monotherapy and in combination with chemotherapy regimens or biologic agents for patients with advanced gastric/gastroesophageal cancer (Table 1).

5. Anti-PD-L1

Avelumab is a fully human anti-PD-L1 IgG1 antibody, and its efficacy and safety were first investigated in a phase 1b trial, in patients with advanced gastric or GEJ in first line as maintenance and in second line (2L) of treatment. Patients received avelumab at 10 mg/kg IV every 2 weeks until progression, unacceptable toxicity, or withdrawal [27].

The ORR, until now unconfirmed, in maintenance and 2L was 7.3% (with 1 complete response, 3 partial responses) and 15%, respectively. The disease control rate (DCR) was 54.5% and 50%, and median PFS was 14,1 and 11,6 weeks in two arms (maintenance and 2L respectively). A trend towards longer PFS was observed in patients with PD-L1-positive tumours. Grade ≥ 3 AEs were documented in 9.9% patients, which included fatigue, asthenia, increased gamma-glutamyl transferase (GGT), thrombocytopenia, and anaemia. There was 1 treatment-related death (hepatic failure/autoimmune hepatitis).

With these encouraging results, two randomized trials with avelumab were envisaged: JAVELIN Gastric 300 (NCT02625623) that will compare avelumab plus BSC in third line treatment versus physician's choice of chemotherapy plus BSC and JAVELIN Gastric 100 (NCT02625610), a phase 3 trial, whose purpose is to demonstrate the superiority of treatment with avelumab as maintenance versus continuation of first-line chemotherapy with oxaliplatin-fluoropyrimidine doublet.

Durvalumab is a humanized IgG-1κ monoclonal antibody that blocks PD-L1.

Segal et al. reported durvalumab clinical activity in an expansion study in multiple cancer types, including NSCLC, melanoma (cutaneous and ocular), gastroesophageal, hepatocellular carcinoma, pancreatic, SCCHN, and triple negative breast cancer. Durvalumab was administered as 10 mg/kg IV every 2 weeks for 12 months. This agent showed clinical activity in gastric cancer with an ORR of 25% (4 partial responses). Treatment-related AEs occurred in one-third of the patients, with ≥Grade 3 AEs in 7% and none led to discontinuation of study drug [28].

Durvalumab, as maintenance, as in combination with a variety of immunomodulators and targeted agents is ongoing in gastric cancer field (Table 2).

Atezolizumab is another human monoclonal antibody that contains an engineered Fc-domain that targets PD-L1, blocking PD-L1 from binding to PD-1 and B7.1, and demonstrated clinical activity in locally advanced and metastatic cancers. In a phase I trial, atezolizumab was administered as a single agent to patients with locally advanced or metastatic solid tumours or hematologic malignancies, and 175 patients were evaluated by RECIST v1.1 and confirmed that complete and partial responses were observed in 18% of patients with all tumour types, 21% in NSCLC, 26% in melanoma, 13% in renal cell carcinoma, and 13% of patients with other tumours including colorectal cancer, gastric cancer (only one patient), and head and neck squamous cell carcinoma. A statistical association between tumours expressing high levels of PD-L1 was observed, especially PD-L1 expressed by tumour-infiltrating immune cells and response to atezolizumab treatment [29, 30].

6. Discussion

After a long time of stagnation in GC treatment, with only two molecular target agents providing modest results in OS and PFS (trastuzumab and ramucirumab), maybe a new paradigm shift in oncology is arising: instead of targeting cancer cells, we can target immune cells, thus stimulating the host immune system against its own cancer cells [31].

Gastric cancer is a heterogeneous condition stratified in 4 molecular subtypes, based on genomic changes [12]. The molecular classification improved our knowledge about the biologic behavior of this disease and offered potential actionable oncogenic drivers. With this deep understanding, we will maximize treatment efficacy.

Certainly, MSI and EBV subtype are of particular interest, deriving from their high immunogenicity and potential greater response with immunotherapy agents.

Table 1: Ongoing trials with anti-PD1 in advanced gastric cancer.

Study ID	Study phase	Treatment	Population	Status
NCT02901301	Ib/II	Pembrolizumab + trastuzumab + cisplatin + capecitabine	HER2 positive advanced gastric cancer	Recruiting
CP-MGAH22-05 (NCT02689284)	Ib/II	Margetuximab in combination with pembrolizumab	Relapsed/refractory advanced HER2+ GEJ or gastric cancer	Recruiting
NCT02318901	Ib/II	Pembrolizumab and monoclonal antibody therapy	Patients with advanced cancer (one cohort for patients with unresectable HER2 overexpressing gastric or GEJ cancers)	Active, not recruiting
NCT03095781	Ib	Pembrolizumab and XL888	Patients with stage IV or locally advanced unresectable gastrointestinal adenocarcinomas who have failed at least one prior therapy	Recruiting
NCT02178722	I/II	Pembrolizumab in combination with epacadostat	Patients with selected cancers (including gastric cancer)	Recruiting
NCT03342937	II	Pembrolizumab + oxaliplatin and capecitabine	First-line treatment of patients with gastroesophageal cancer	Not yet recruiting
NCT02954536	II	Pembrolizumab in combination with trastuzumab, capecitabine/cisplatin	First-line stage IV HER2-positive metastatic esophagogastric (EG) cancer	Recruiting
NCT03196232	II	Epacadostat and pembrolizumab	Metastatic or unresectable GEJ or gastric cancer that progressed at least first line of prior therapy	Recruiting
KEYNOTE KN-463 (NCT03122548)	II	CRS-207 and pembrolizumab	Recurrent or metastatic gastric, GEJ, or esophageal cancer who have received 2 prior systemic chemotherapy treatment	Recruiting
KEYNOTE-063 (NCT03019588)	III	Pembrolizumab versus paclitaxel	Asian subjects with advanced gastric or GEJ adenocarcinoma who progressed after first-line therapy with platinum and fluoropyrimidine	Recruiting
KEYNOTE-062 (NCT02494583)	III	Pembrolizumab as monotherapy and in combination with cisplatin + 5-fluorouracil versus placebo + cisplatin + 5-fluorouracil	As first-line treatment in subjects with advanced gastric or GEJ adenocarcinoma	Active, not recruiting
KEYNOTE-061 (NCT02370498)	III	Pembrolizumab versus paclitaxel	Advanced gastric or GEJ adenocarcinoma who progressed after first-line therapy with platinum and fluoropyrimidine	Active, not recruiting
ONO4538 (NCT02267343)	III	Nivolumab versus placebo	Unresectable advanced or recurrent gastric cancer (including esophagogastric junction cancer) refractory to or intolerant of standard therapy	Active, not recruiting
CA209-929 (NCT03342417)	II	Combination of nivolumab and ipilimumab in breast, ovarian, and gastric cancer patients	In gastric cancer arm: advanced gastric cancer patients who are recurrent/refractory to a prior therapy not involving herceptin	Recruiting
ONO-4538-37 (NCT02746796)	II/III	Nivolumab and chemotherapy versus placebo and chemotherapy	Unresectable advanced or recurrent gastric cancer (including esophagogastric junction cancer) not previously treated with the first-line therapy	Recruiting
CheckMate 649 (NCT02872116)	III	Nivolumab plus ipilimumab or nivolumab in combination with oxaliplatin plus fluoropyrimidine versus oxaliplatin plus fluoropyrimidine	Patients with previously untreated advanced or metastatic gastric or gastroesophageal junction cancer	Recruiting
FRACTION-GC (NCT02935634)	II	Nivolumab plus ipilimumab versus nivolumab plus relatlimab versus nivolumab and BMS-986205	Patients with advanced gastric cancer	Recruiting
NCCH-1611 NCT02999295	I/II	Ramucirumab plus nivolumab	Second-line therapy in Participants with gastric or GEJ cancer	Recruiting

Table 1: Continued.

Study ID	Study phase	Treatment	Population	Status
AIO-STO-0217 (NCT03409848)	II	Ipilimumab or FOLFOX in combination with nivolumab and trastuzumab	Previously untreated HER2 positive locally advanced or metastatic esophagogastric adenocarcinoma	Not yet recruiting
INCAGN 1876-201 (NCT03126110)	I/II	INCAGN01876 combined with nivolumab versus INCAGN01876 combined with ipilimumab versus INCAGN01876 combined with nivolumab and ipilimumab	Subjects with advanced or metastatic malignancies	Recruiting

Table 2: Ongoing trials with anti-PD-L1 in advanced gastric cancer.

Study ID	Study phase	Treatment	Population	Status
YO39609 (NCT03281369)	I/II	Multiple immunotherapy-based treatment combinations, including atezolizumab as immunotherapeutic agent	Patients with locally advanced unresectable or metastatic gastric or gastroesophageal junction cancer	Recruiting
JAVELIN Gastric 300 (NCT02625623)	III	Avelumab + best supportive care (BSC) versus physician's choice chemotherapy + BSC or BSC alone	Unresectable, recurrent, locally advanced, or metastatic gastric or gastroesophageal junction adenocarcinoma gastric cancer third line	Active, not recruiting
JAVELIN Gastric 100 (NCT02625610)	III	Avelumab (MSB0010718C) versus continuation of first-line chemotherapy	Unresectable, locally advanced, or metastatic adenocarcinoma of the stomach or of the gastroesophageal junction	Active, not recruiting
JAVELIN MEDLEY (NCT02554812)	Ib/II	Avelumab (MSB0010718C) in combination with other cancer immunotherapies	Patients with locally advanced or metastatic solid tumors	Recruiting
MEDIOLA (NCT02734004)	I/II	MEDI4736 in combination with olaparib	Patients with advanced solid tumors, selected based on a rationale for response to olaparib	Active, not recruiting
I4T-MC-JVDJ (NCT02572687)	I	Ramucirumab plus MEDI4736	Participants with locally advanced and unresectable or metastatic gastrointestinal or thoracic malignancies including gastric or gastroesophageal junction (GEJ) adenocarcinoma, non-small-cell lung cancer (NSCLC) or hepatocellular carcinoma (HCC)	Active, not recruiting
PLATFORM (NCT02678182)	II	Maintenance therapies following completion of standard first-line chemotherapy: placebo versus capecitabine versus durvalumab versus trastuzumab versus rucaparib	Patients with locally advanced or metastatic HER-2 positive or HER-2 negative oesophagogastric adenocarcinomas	Recruiting
D419SC00001 (NCT02658214)	Ib	Durvalumab and tremelimumab in combination with first-line chemotherapy	Patients with advanced solid tumors	Recruiting

MEDI4736 also known as durvalumab.

As detailed before, immune checkpoint blockade with antibodies targeting CTLA-4, PD-1, and PD-L1 has revealed clinical activity in gastric cancer. While anti-CTLA4 showed only slight activity in gastric cancer, and PD-1 and PD-L1 inhibitors showed promising results and will probably take place in gastric cancer management in the near future.

We would like to highlight the phase III KEYNOTE-059 trial, as it showed antitumour activity and durable responses in patients with advanced gastric/GEJ cancer progression after more than 2 lines of therapy. Until now there was no evidence for 3rd and 4th lines in gastric cancer, and based on the cohort 1 results, pembrolizumab was approved by the FDA recently [24].

In the cohort 2, patients received pembrolizumab and chemotherapy with cisplatin and 5- fluorouracil, with favourable clinical activity and manageable toxicity, though more data is needed to draw conclusions [25, 26].

Also, a question to consider is if the results of nivolumab in Asian patients will be reproduced in western patients? [20, 21]

Results from phase I/II CheckMate 032 trial, which included heavily pretreated European and North American population, revealed long-term overall survival and responses with nivolumab. These findings suggest a possible benefit with nivolumab in Asian and western patients, although we need more studies to make a definitive conclusion.

This and much more questions remain to be answered: which gastric cancer subpopulation does benefit more from immune checkpoints inhibitors? In which stage of the disease should we use immunotherapy, in earlier lines or after progression of more than 2 lines of therapy?

We look forward at the ongoing phase III trials and wait with hope for their results. Besides, more studies are needed to validate predictive and prognostic biomarkers to immunotherapy agents in gastric cancer.

Additionally, integration of immune checkpoints combined with targeted agents, chemotherapy, or radiotherapy appears to be exciting multimodal approaches and randomized trials are also ongoing.

In conclusion, some progress has been reached in the treatment of advanced gastric cancer in the last years.With the recent biologic and molecular knowledge, we have recognized that gastric cancer is a group of distinct molecular entities rather than a single disease. This molecular characterization will allow achieving a better selection of patients that can benefit from a treatment strategy.

The field is unquestionably moving towards a more precise medicine, and the progressing accomplishments will transform the clinical practice in the management of advanced gastric cancer in the near future.

Additional Points

Core Tip. GC is a highly heterogeneous disease and the recent molecular characterization will help us to better select patients who might benefit from immune checkpoint inhibitors and other agents. There are encouraging results with agents that target programmed death 1 (PD-1) and its ligands in gastric cancer; however more trials are needed to identify predictive and prognostic biomarkers to select patients most appropriately for this treatment. In this review, we explore the current evidence supporting the use of immunotherapy in advanced GC.

References

[1] M. Arnold, H. E. Karim-Kos, J. W. Coebergh et al., "Recent trends in incidence of five common cancers in 26 European countries since 1988: Analysis of the European Cancer Observatory," *European Journal of Cancer*, vol. 51, no. 9, article no. 8948, pp. 1164–1187, 2015.

[2] J. Ferlay, I. Soerjomataram, R. Dikshit et al., "Cancer incidence and mortality worldwide: sources, methods and major patterns in GLOBOCAN 2012," *International Journal of Cancer*, 2014.

[3] A. DIgklia and A. D. Wagner, "Advanced gastric cancer: Current treatment landscape and future perspectives," *World Journal of Gastroenterology*, vol. 22, no. 8, pp. 2403–2414, 2016.

[4] B. Glimelius, K. Ekström, K. Hoffman et al., "Randomized comparison between chemotherapy plus best supportive care with best supportive care in advanced gastric cancer," *Annals of Oncology*, vol. 8, no. 2, pp. 163–168, 1997.

[5] N. Haj Mohammad, E. ter Veer, L. Ngai, R. Mali, M. G. H. van Oijen, and H. W. M. van Laarhoven, "Optimal first-line chemotherapeutic treatment in patients with locally advanced or metastatic esophagogastric carcinoma: triplet versus doublet chemotherapy: a systematic literature review and meta-analysis," *Cancer and Metastasis Reviews*, vol. 34, no. 3, pp. 429–441, 2015.

[6] Y.-J. Bang, E. Van Cutsem, A. Feyereislova et al., "Trastuzumab in combination with chemotherapy versus chemotherapy alone for treatment of HER2- positive advanced gastric or gastro-oesophageal junction cancer (ToGA): a phase 3, open-label, randomised controlled trial," *The Lancet*, vol. 376, no. 9742, pp. 687–697, 2010.

[7] P. C. Thuss-Patience, A. Kretzschmar, D. Bichev et al., "Survival advantage for irinotecan versus best supportive care as second-line chemotherapy in gastric cancer—a randomised phase III study of the Arbeitsgemeinschaft Internistische Onkologie (AIO)," *European Journal of Cancer*, vol. 47, no. 15, pp. 2306–2314, 2011.

[8] H. E. R. Ford, A. Marshall, J. A. Bridgewater et al., "Docetaxel versus active symptom control for refractory oesophagogastric adenocarcinoma (COUGAR-02): an open-label, phase 3 randomised controlled trial," *The Lancet Oncology*, vol. 15, no. 1, pp. 78–86, 2014.

[9] J. H. Kang, S. Lee, D. H. Lim et al., "Salvage chemotherapy for pretreated gastric cancer: a randomized phase III trial comparing chemotherapy plus best supportive care with best supportive care alone," *Journal of Clinical Oncology*, vol. 30, pp. 1513–1518, 2012.

[10] C. S. Fuchs, J. Tomasek, C. J. Yong et al., "Ramucirumab monotherapy for previously treated advanced gastric or gastro-oesophageal junction adenocarcinoma (REGARD): an international, randomised, multicentre, placebo-controlled, phase 3 trial," *The Lancet*, vol. 383, no. 9911, pp. 31–39, 2014.

[11] H. Wilke, K. Muro, and E. van Custem, "Ramucirumab plus paclitaxel versus placebo plus paclitaxel in patients with previously treated advanced gastric or gastro-oesophageal junction adenocarcinoma (RAINBOW): a double-blind, randomised phase 3 trial," *The Lancet Oncology*, vol. 15, no. 11, pp. 1224–1235, 2014.

[12] A. J. Bass, V. Thorsson, I. Shmulevich et al., "Comprehensive molecular characterization of gastric adenocarcinoma," *Nature*, vol. 513, pp. 202–209, 2014.

[13] S. K. Garattini, D. Basile, M. Cattaneo et al., "Molecular classifications of gastric cancers: Novel insights and possible future applications," *World Journal of Gastrointestinal Oncology*, vol. 9, no. 5, pp. 194–208, 2017.

[14] F. Lordick, K. Shitara, and Y. Y. Janjigian, "New agents on the horizon in gastric cancer," *Annals of Oncology*, vol. 28, no. 8, Article ID mdx051, pp. 1767–1775, 2017.

[15] S. Su and B. Liu, "Immune checkpoint blockade and gastric cancer," in *Personalized Management of Gastric Cancer: Trans-*

lational and Precision Medicine, pp. 115–127, Springer, 2017.

[16] C. Wu, Y. Zhu, J. Jiang, J. Zhao, X.-G. Zhang, and N. Xu, "Immunohistochemical localization of programmed death-1 ligand-1 (PD-L1) in gastric carcinoma and its clinical significance," *Acta Histochemica*, vol. 108, no. 1, pp. 19–24, 2006.

[17] J. Hou, Z. Yu, R. Xiang et al., "Correlation between infiltration of FOXP3+ regulatory T cells and expression of B7-H1 in the tumor tissues of gastric cancer," *Experimental and Molecular Pathology*, vol. 96, no. 3, pp. 284–291, 2014.

[18] M. H. Moehler, J. Y. Cho, Y. H. Kim et al., "A randomized, open-label, two-arm phase II trial comparing the efficacy of sequential ipilimumab versus best supportive care (BSC) following first line chemotherapy in patients with unresectable, locally advanced/metastic gastric or gastro-esophageal junction cancer," *ASCO Meet. Abstr*, vol. 34, p. 4011, 2016.

[19] C. Ralph, E. Elkord, D. J. Burt et al., "Modulation of lymphocyte regulation for cancer therapy: a phase II trial of tremelimumab in advanced gastric and esophageal adenocarcinoma," *Clinical Cancer Research*, vol. 16, no. 5, pp. 1662–1672, 2010.

[20] Y. Y. Janjigian, J. C. Bendell, E. Calvo, J. Kim, P. Ascierto, P. Sharma et al., "CheckMate-032: Phase I/II, open-label study of safety and activity of nivolumab (nivo) alone or with ipilimumab (ipi) in advanced and metastatic (A/M) gastric cancer (GC)," *Journal of Clinical Oncology*, vol. 34, 15, p. 4010, 2016.

[21] Y.-K. Kang, N. Boku, T. Satoh et al., "Nivolumab in patients with advanced gastric or gastro-oesophageal junction cancer refractory to, or intolerant of, at least two previous chemotherapy regimens (ONO-4538-12, ATTRACTION-2): a randomised, double-blind, placebo-controlled, phase 3 trial," *The Lancet*, vol. 390, no. 10111, pp. 2461–2471, 2017.

[22] K. Muro, Y. Bang, V. Shankaran et al., "LBA15: a phase 1B study of pembrolizumab (pembro; MK-3475) in patients (PTS) with advanced gastric cancer," *Annals of Oncology*, vol. 25, supplement 4, pp. 1–41, 2014.

[23] K. Muro, H. C. Chung, V. Shankaran et al., "Pembrolizumab for patients with PD-L1-positive advanced gastric cancer (KEYNOTE-012): a multicentre, open-label, phase 1b trial," *The Lancet Oncology*, vol. 17, no. 6, pp. 717–726, 2016.

[24] C. S. Fuchs, T. Doi, R. W.-J. Jang et al., "KEYNOTE-059 cohort 1: Efficacy and safety of pembrolizumab (pembro) monotherapy in patients with previously treated advanced gastric cancer," *Journal of Clinical Oncology*, vol. 35, 4003, no. 15, 2017.

[25] Z. Wainberg, S. Jalal, K. Muro et al., "LBA28_PRKEYNOTE-059 Update: Efficacy and safety of pembrolizumab alone or in combination with chemotherapy in patients with advanced gastric or gastroesophageal (G/GEJ) cancer," *Annals of Oncology*, vol. 28, no. suppl_5, pp. v605–v649, 2017.

[26] Y. J. Bang, K. Muro, C. S. Fuchs et al., "KEYNOTE-059 cohort 2: Safety and efficacy of pembrolizumab (pembro) plus 5-fluorouracil (5-FU) and cisplatin for first-line (1L) treatment of advanced gastric cancer," *Journal of Clinical Oncology*, vol. 35, 2017.

[27] H. C. Chung, H. Arkenau, L. Wyrwicz et al., "Safety, PD-L1 expression, and clinical activity of avelumab (MSB0010718C), an anti-PD-L1 antibody, in patients with advanced gastric or gastroesophageal junction cancer.," *Journal of Clinical Oncology*, vol. 34, no. 4_suppl, pp. 167-167, 2016.

[28] N. H. Segal, S. J. Antonia, Brahmer. J. R. et al., "Preliminary data from a multi- arm expansion study of MEDI4736, an anti-PD-L1 antibody," *Journal of Clinical Oncology*, vol. 32, 2014.

[29] R. S. Herbst, M. S. Gordon, G. D. Fine et al., "A study of MPDL3280A, an engineered PD-L1 antibody in patients with locally advanced or metastatic tumors," *Journal of Clinical Oncology*, vol. 31, 2013.

[30] R. S. Herbst, J. C. Soria, and M. Kowanetz, "Predictive correlates of response to the anti-PD-L1 antibody MPDL3280A in cancer patients," *Nature*, vol. 515, no. 7528, pp. 563–567, 2014.

[31] T. Shekarian, S. Valsesia-Wittmann, C. Caux, and A. Marabelle, "Paradigm shift in oncology: Targeting the immune system rather than cancer cells," *Mutagenesis*, vol. 30, no. 2, pp. 205–211, 2015.

20

Analysis of the Patient Information Quality and Readability on Esophagogastroduodenoscopy (EGD) on the Internet

P. Priyanka ,[1] Yousaf B. Hadi,[1] and G. J. Reynolds [2]

[1]*Department of Medicine, West Virginia University Hospitals, Morgantown, WV, USA*
[2]*Department of Medicine, Section of Digestive diseases, West Virginia University Hospitals, Morgantown, WV, USA*

Correspondence should be addressed to P. Priyanka; priyanka.priyanka@hsc.wvu.edu

Academic Editor: Raffaele Pezzilli

Objective. Patients are increasingly using the Internet to inform themselves of health-related topics and procedures, including EGD. We analyzed the quality of information and readability of websites after a search on 3 different search engines. *Methods.* We used an assessment tool for website quality analysis that we developed in addition to using validated instruments for website quality, Global Quality Score (GQS) and Health on Net (HON) certification. The readability was assessed using Flesch-Kincaid Reading Ease (FRE) and Flesch-Kincaid Grade level (FKG). 30 results of each search terms 'EGD' and 'Upper Endoscopy' from Google and 15 each from Bing and Yahoo were analyzed. A total of 45 websites were included from 100 URLs after removing duplicates, video links, and journal articles. *Results.* Only 3 websites were found to have good quality and comprehensive and authentic information. These websites were https://www.healthline.com, https://www.uptodate.com, and https://www.emedicine.medscape.com. There were additional 13 sites with moderate quality of information. The mean Flesch-Kincaid Reading Ease (FRE) score was 46.92 (range 81.6-6.5). The mean Flesch-Kincaid Grade level (FKG) was 11th grade, with a range of 6th grade to 12th grade and above making them difficult to read. *Conclusions.* Our study shows that there are quite a few websites with moderate quality content. We recommend 3 comprehensive and authentic websites out of 45 URLs analyzed for information on Internet for EGD. In addition, the readability of the websites was consistently at a higher level than recommended by AMA at 11th grade level. In addition, we identified 3 websites with moderate quality content written at 8th grade and below readability level. We feel that gastroenterologists can help their patients better understand this procedure by directing them to these comprehensive websites.

1. Introduction

There were 4.1 billion Internet users worldwide and 286 million within United States as of 2017, with 87.9% Americans having access to the Internet [1]. In one estimate, about 60% of the individuals with online access admitted going online to seek health-related information in 2013 [2]. This rapidly increasing use of web to seek information has made it possible for the patients to supplement their knowledge of medical conditions in a way that would not have been possible before the age of Internet. At the same time, the world wide web is still a largely unregulated place with a few rules to check the reliability or the accuracy of the information available. The content on the Internet is growing exponentially every year. This leads to the concern of either information overload where it is hard to determine relevant information from a barrage of sources or that patients may acquire information that might not be completely accurate and may affect the way they make important treatment decisions. A very few studies are available on the magnitude of this problem affecting gastroenterology patients seeking healthcare. The previously conducted studies on colorectal screening and non-GI conditions like knee arthroscopy, scoliosis, and ureteral stents have indicated that the online information available on these topics is highly variable in quality and mostly has suboptimal suitability and uniformly higher readability levels than AMA recommended 6th grade level for health information [3–8].

Esophagogastroduodenoscopy (EGD) is a widely performed gastrointestinal (GI) procedure since it first became available about a century ago [9]. In general, it is physicians' responsibility to explain the details of this procedure when it is warranted for either diagnostic or therapeutic purposes.

But many times, patients turn towards Internet to get a better understanding of the various aspects of this procedure. About 6.9 million EGD procedures were performed in 2009 alone at an estimated cost of $12.3 billion [10]. A 50% increase in EGD utilization was noted among Medicare recipients from 2000 to 2010 and this trend continues to grow [11]. Currently, there is no exact information on the quality and readability of the web resources providing patient information on the topic of EGD. In this study, we tried to assess the quality and readability level of the online resources available to the patients on the topic of EGD. We also compared the results obtained from different search engines in an attempt to establish the most efficient search strategy.

2. Methods

2.1. Search Strategy. We used 3 different search engines for the purpose of this study, Google, Bing, and Yahoo. This was based on the popularity of the search engines with these three search engines cited to be among the most popular among the individuals seeking healthcare information [2]. The search terminology was "EGD" and "Upper Endoscopy" and typed as a phrase in each individual search engine. For the purpose of this study, we included the first 30 URLs from Google with each search term separately to obtain a total of 60 search results. We included first 15 URLs each from Bing and Yahoo with each search terminology. Overall, 100 search results were obtained and analyzed from these 3 different search engines. Of these 100 URLs, duplicates, video links, and research papers were excluded. Overall, 45 websites were selected for web resource quality and readability analysis.

2.2. Quality Assessment. The quality analysis was performed by using a comprehensive modified quality assessment questionnaire that was designed based on the methods used in previous similar studies (Table 1). Health on net (HON) certification and global quality score (GQS) were added to further refine the quality standards. HON Foundation is a nonprofit organization that grants certification to the websites with health-related information if they are in compliance with certain quality standards [12]. Each website was analyzed separately by 2 blinded observers using the above-mentioned questionnaire. Each item on the questionnaire was previously discussed and well-defined among the observers. For the adequacy of the content part, there were 6 subheadings and for each subheading the scores of 0, 3, and 5 could be given. Score of 0 indicated no information available on that subheading, 3 meant some information was available but suboptimal in content, and 5 was given if most of the information on that subheading was present. Similarly, authenticity scores of 0, 3, 5, and 10 were given if there were no references at all, website references, textbook references, or both textbook and scientific articles' references, respectively. HON certification, if present, was noted separately. GQS of 1-5 as mentioned in Table 1 was awarded separately by each observer. GQS has previously been used in similar studies to evaluate the overall quality and usefulness of a website [5, 13]. A final decision on the recommendation of a website was based on a score of at least 3 on all the subheadings under adequacy, at least 5 on authenticity, and a GQS of at least 4 and ideally had HON certification. We did not use HON certification as a final criterion for the recommending a website because only 3 websites we analyzed had HON certification and none of these 3 websites met our other quality criteria completely. For the items where the responses were different for each observer, a consensus was reached by discussion with the senior author, who was blinded with regard to the nature of the study. The mean interobserver reliability of the questionnaire was 0.94 (range 0.88-0.98). All the subcomponents of the quality assessment tool had interobserver reliability of >0.90 except GQS that had interobserver reliability of 0.88.

2.3. Readability Assessment. The readability of the websites was evaluated using Flesch-Kincaid Reading Ease (FRE) and Flesch-Kincaid grade level (FKG). FRE and FKG are widely used readability assessment tools validated for this purpose [14]. FRE is graded out of 100 and the easier text scores higher based on the sentence length and average number of syllables per word. The scores were calculated using Microsoft Word (Redmond, Washington) word processing software. The headings, web-links, illustrations, and foot notes were removed for the purpose of the readability assessment.

2.4. Statistical Analysis. Statistical analysis was performed using IBM SPSS software, version 22.0. Descriptive statistics were used for the quality and readability analysis of websites. Interobserver reliability was calculated to evaluate the quality of the questionnaire.

3. Results

3.1. Quality Analysis. Of 100 URLs, 45 were included in the final quality analysis. The remaining links were excluded as they were either video links, journal articles, PDF files, or duplicates. The search on Bing yielded 3 additional websites, and a search on Yahoo did not yield any unique website that was not previously identified on Google (Tables 2 and 3).

3.2. Information Update. The date of the most recent update of information was available only on 17 (38%) websites. Among these 17 sites, the median time since update was 14 months (range 0-76 months).

3.3. Content Presentation and Accessibility. All the 45 websites were easily accessible, except only 1 URL being inaccessible (page not found). None of the sites required user registration or were password protected. 15 of the 45 websites (33%) utilized illustrations or pictures to assist in the understanding of the procedure. Only 10 websites (22.2%) contained authorship information, with 9 of the 10 being either authored or reviewed by the physicians. Out of the 45 included websites, 20 (44.44%) contained promotional messages, 10 contained product related marketing messages, and 9 advertised for services. The target audience was recognized as the general

Table 1: Assessment tool for the website quality analysis.

Search Engine Google Bing Yahoo
Website description
URL address
Type of ownership
Position in search result
Accessibility Easy Page not found No longer exists Password-protected
Illustrations and pictures Y / N
Quality
Last information update Y / N If yes, how old?
Authorship information available, Y/ N If yes, easy to find Y / N
If yes, is author identified as - General Public, Educational institution, Club,
Prof organization, For-profit organization., physician.
Promotional message Y / N
What is being promoted? Product / service / advertisement / procedure
Target audience information Y/N
Type of target audience General public / HCPs
Adequacy of content (0, No information, 3, Some information, 5, adequate information)

Indications	0	3	5
Pre-procedure preparation	0	3	5
Procedure	0	3	5
Post procedure protocol	0	3	5
Complications	0	3	5
Warning signs of complications	0	3	5

Total
Authenticity of the content 0 3 5 10
0-No referencing at all, 3-Good quality website referenced, 5-textbook referenced
10-Textbook and scientific articles referenced
HON certification Yes / No
Global Quality Score: ___
1 Poor quality, poor flow of the site, most information missing, not at all useful for patients.
2 Generally poor quality and poor flow, some information listed but many important topics missing, of very limited use to patients.
3 Moderate quality, suboptimal flow, some important information is discussed adequately but other information is poorly discussed, somewhat useful for patients.
4 Good quality and generally good flow, most of the relevant information is listed, but some topics are not covered, useful for patients.
5 Excellent quality and excellent flow, very useful for patients.
Would you recommend the site Y / N
Readability: FRE: ___ FKS grade level: ___

public explicitly on 14 (31%) websites and no website identified its intended users as healthcare professionals. A total of 3 (6.6%) websites included in the final cohort were owned by the government agencies, 2 (4.4%) identified themselves as nonprofit, open access general information websites, 7 (15.5%) were for-profit strictly online resources, 3 (6.6%) were run by professional healthcare bodies, 13 (28.88%) were operated by educational healthcare institutions, and 15 (33.3%) were operated by private healthcare systems.

3.4. Content Quality Analysis. Out of the 45 websites analyzed, only 3 URLs were found to be adequate for the content per the predefined study criteria (Table 4). The rest of the 42 websites failed to satisfy the adequacy of content as criteria outlined previously. At least some mention of preprocedure, procedure-related, and postprocedure details was noted on 36 (91%), 41 (95%), and 38(84%) of the URLs. The complications were discussed only in 18 (40%), and the postprocedure warning signs were mentioned on 22 websites (48.9%). Only 5 (11%) websites had references available for the information presented and therefore could be considered authentic. HON certification was available only for 3 (7%) websites. Additionally, 13 more sites had a GQS > or equal to 4. Four websites were owned by professional bodies, 5 each were from educational institutions, private health systems, and for-profit online health information portals (Table 5). Of these, the search rank did not correlate with the chances of having better quality content.

Table 2: Search results with website URLs.

Website urls	Website number
https://medlineplus.gov/ency/article/003888.htm	1
https://www.healthline.com/health/egd-esophagogastroduodenoscopy	2
http://ddc.musc.edu/public/procedures/upper-endoscopy.html	3
https://en.wikipedia.org/wiki/Esophagogastroduodenoscopy	4
https://www.hopkinsmedicine.org/gastroenterology_hepatology/clinical_services/basic_endoscopy/esophagogastroduodenoscopy.html	5
https://www.cancercenter.com/treatments/esophagogastroduodenoscopy/	6
https://www.webmd.com/digestive-disorders/upper-endoscopy#1	7
https://www.scripps.org/articles/273-egd-esophagogastroduodenoscopyhttps://www.scripps.org/articles/273-egd-esophagogastroduodenoscopy	8
https://www.northshore.org/gastroenterology/procedures/egd-test/	9
https://emedicine.medscape.com/article/1851864-overview	10
http://ohiogi.com/procedurespreps/procedures/upper-endoscopy-esophagogastroduodenoscopy-egd/	11
https://www.valleyhealth.com/gastrointestinal_services.aspx?id=2690	12
https://www.aurorahealthcare.org/services/gastroenterology-colorectal-surgery/esophagogastroduodenoscopy	13
https://www.uofmhealth.org/conditions-treatments/digestive-and-liver-health/upper-endoscopy-egd	14
https://medicine.yale.edu/intmed/digestivediseases/clinical/Egd%20STENT%20pt%20handout%207.17_270191_1095_23162_v2.pdf	15
https://www.gihealthcare.com/egd/	16
https://www.gastrorockies.com/preps/colonoscopy-egd-prep-instructions	17
http://gastroarkansas.com/egd-esophagogastroduodenoscopy/	18
http://www.arizonadigestivehealth.com/procedures-services/upper-gi-endoscopy/	19
http://www.riverviewmedicalcenter.com/RMC/services/Endoscopy/UpperEndoscopy.cfm	20
https://www.michigangastro.com/upper-gi	21
https://www.drugs.com/mcp/upper-endoscopy	22
https://medical-dictionary.thefreedictionary.com/EGD	23
http://www.gastroenterology.com/procedures/egd	24
https://www.mayoclinic.org/tests-procedures/endoscopy/about/pac-20395197	25
https://www.asge.org/home/for-patients/patient-information/understanding-upper-endoscopy	26
https://www.niddk.nih.gov/health-information/diagnostic-tests/upper-gi-endoscopy	27
https://www.cancer.net/navigating-cancer-care/diagnosing-cancer/tests-and-procedures/upper-endoscopy	28
https://www.medicinenet.com/endoscopy/article.htm	29
https://www.uptodate.com/contents/upper-endoscopy-beyond-the-basics	30
https://www.sages.org/publications/patient-information/patient-information-for-upper-endoscopy-from-sages/	31
https://www.gastro.org/practice-guidance/patientInfo/procedures	32
http://www.jerseyshoreuniversitymedicalcenter.com/JSUMC/services/gastroenterology/UpperEndoscopy.cfm	33
https://stanfordhealthcare.org/medical-conditions/cancer/stomach-cancer/stomach-cancer-diagnosis/upper-endoscopy.html	34
http://www.mountsinai.org/patient-care/service-areas/digestive-disease/endoscopy-suite/types-of-endoscopy-procedures/egd-or-upper-endoscopy	35
https://www.mskcc.org/cancer-care/patient-education/about-your-upper-endoscopy	36
https://www.gikids.org/content/59/en/endoscopy/upper	37
http://www.chp.edu/our-services/transplant/intestine/education/patient-procedures/upper-endoscopy	38
https://www.cincinnatichildrens.org/health/u/upper-endoscopy	39
https://www.cancer.gov/publications/dictionaries/cancer-terms/def/upper-endoscopy	40
http://www.morethanheartburn.com/testsandtreatments/upper-endoscopy	41
http://health.usf.edu/medicine/internalmedicine/digestive/upperendoscopy	42
http://www.gandhofcny.com/procedures/upper-endoscopy/	43
https://www.gastro.org/practice-guidance/patientInfo/procedures	44

TABLE 3: Results of website content analysis and readability assessment.

Website number	Adequacy total	Authenticity	Overall content	Recommended	FRE	FKS	HON	GQS
1	21	10	good	yes	81.6	6	yes	5
2	30	10	good	yes	57.3	9	no	5
3	25	10	good	yes	58.6	9	no	4
4	19	3	fair	no	49.3	10	no	3
5	16	0	fair	no	51	9.3	no	3
6	9	0	fair	no	46.6	12	no	3
7	30	0	good	yes	57.4	9	no	5
8	16	0	fair	no	74.4	6	yes	4
9	16	0	fair	no	57.5	9	no	3
10	30	10	good	yes	-6.5	12	no	5
11	30	0	good	yes	46	11	no	5
12	18	0	fair	no	46.2	12	no	3
13	9	0	poor	no	63.3	8	no	2
14	26	0	good	yes	46.9	11	no	4
15	23	0	fair	no	57.1	10	no	3
16	18	0	fair	no	48.7	12	no	3
17	15	0	poor	no	59.7	10	no	3
18	14	0	poor	no	50.5	11	no	3
19	25	0	good	yes	33.6	12	no	4
20	21	0	fair	no	44.6	11	no	4
21	30	0	good	yes	26.9	12	no	5
22	30	0	good	yes	36.4	13	yes	5
23	15	0	poor	no	35.9	13	no	2
24	16	0	fair	no	46	12	no	3
25	30	0	good	yes	38.2	12	no	5
26	24	0	fair	yes	37.4	12	no	4
27	28	0	fair	yes	29.6	13.2	no	4
28	18	0	fair	no	56	8	no	4
29	15	0	fair	no	21	16.3	no	3
30	30	10	good	yes	38.2	13.3	no	5
31	26	0	good	yes	35	12.1	no	5
32	18	0	fair	no	38.9	13	no	3
33	3	0	poor	no	61.2	8	no	2
34	26	0	good	yes	37.1	15.6	no	5
35	16	0	fair	no	58	10	no	3
36	17	0	fair	no	43	12.73	no	3
37	19	0	fair	no	50	11	no	3
38	6	0	poor	no	50	10	no	2
39	6	0	poor	no	64	8	no	2
40	14	0	fair	no	43	12	no	3
41	17	0	fair	no	45	12	no	3
42	11	0	fair	no	61	8	no	3
43	23	0	good	no	48	10	no	4
44	PNF	PNF	PNF	PNF	PNF	PNF	PNF	PNF

GQS: global quality score, HON: health on net certification, FRE: Flesch-Kincaid Reading Ease (FRE), FKG: Flesch-Kincaid grade level, and PNF: page not found.

TABLE 4: Websites found to have adequate content on EGD.

https://www.healthline.com/health/egd-esophagogastroduodenoscopy
https://emedicine.medscape.com/article/1851864-overview
https://www.uptodate.com/contents/upper-endoscopy-beyond-the-basics

Table 5: Websites with moderate quality content on EGD (GQS of 4 or more).

https://medlineplus.gov/ency/article/003888.htm
http://ddc.musc.edu/public/procedures/upper-endoscopy.html
https://www.webmd.com/digestive-disorders/upper-endoscopy#1
http://ohiogi.com/procedurespreps/procedures/upper-endoscopy-esophagogastroduodenoscopy-egd/
https://www.uofmhealth.org/conditions-treatments/digestive-and-liver-health/upper-endoscopy-egd
http://www.arizonadigestivehealth.com/procedures-services/upper-gi-endoscopy/
https://www.michigangastro.com/upper-gi
https://www.drugs.com/mcp/upper-endoscopy
https://www.mayoclinic.org/tests-procedures/endoscopy/about/pac-20395197
https://www.asge.org/home/for-patients/patient-information/understanding-upper-endoscopy
https://www.niddk.nih.gov/health-information/diagnostic-tests/upper-gi-endoscopy
https://www.sages.org/publications/patient-information/patient-information-for-upper-endoscopy-from-sages/
https://stanfordhealthcare.org/medical-conditions/cancer/stomach-cancer/stomach-cancer-diagnosis/upper-endoscopy.html

Table 6: Websites with moderate quality content and readability level of 8th grade and less.

https://medlineplus.gov/ency/article/003888.htm
https://www.scripps.org/articles/273-egd-esophagogastroduodenoscopy
https://www.cancer.net/navigating-cancer-care/diagnosing-cancer/tests-and-procedures/upper-endoscopy

3.5. Readability. The overall readability level of the websites was high, with mean Flesch-Kincaid Reading Ease (FRE) score of 46.92 (range 81.6-6.5). The mean Flesch-Kincaid grade level (FKG) was 11th grade, with a range of 6th grade to 12th grade and above. Only 2 websites had a reading grade level of 6 and below (medlineplus.gov, scripps.org) as recommended by AMA, and a total of 6 websites were written at the level of 8th grade and below (Table 6).

4. Discussion

In our study, we analyzed a sample of 100 web-links using 3 leading search engines. After the exclusion of the video links, journal articles, and repetitions 45 websites were identified to be included in our study for quality and readability analysis. Out of these 45 websites, only 3 were found to be recommendable, based on the adequacy criteria that comprised authenticity, content quality, and GQS (Table 2). Based on these results, our analysis shows that enormous amount of information is available regarding the EGD procedure on the Internet, mostly of moderate quality that may not be updated regularly. Although we intended to use HON as a criterion for website adequacy for recommendation, only 3 websites in our sample were found to have HON certification, and while all three had a GQS of 4, they were found to be deficient in one or more content quality subcomponents and could not be included in the final list of recommendable websites. Only less than one-third of the sites had clearly identified target audience as patients and less than a quarter websites had authorship information available, prompting a concern about the source of information about the rest of three-quarters of the content. About half of the sites included in this study were using their website for promotional messages or advertisements that may lead to potential conflicts of interest and undermine their seriousness about the patients' well-being. After the subheading analysis of content quality analysis, although most websites discussed indications, preprocedure, procedure, and postprocedure somewhat adequately (80-95%), only about less than half mentioned the possible complications of the procedure (40%) and warning signs to recognize them (48.9%). This pattern was noted for both for-profit and nonprofit websites like educational institutions and government owned websites, though it was seen more frequently with the privately owned websites. This trend is worrisome as these websites seemed to make patients aware of the procedure without educating them adequately of the associated risks and even worse, to recognize the complications if they occurred. This also speaks somewhat about us as a medical community where we sometimes underinform our patients of the possible risks of the procedures in a subconscious attempt to not scare patients by discussing the complications in detail. 13 websites with GQS of at least 4 that did not fulfill all the quality criteria could still be considered as reliable with at least moderate quality content (Table 5). Not surprisingly, most of these websites were owned by nonprofit organizations like professional bodies, government, and educational institutions.

For the readability analysis, the median FRE score was 46.92, consistent with an 11th grade reading level. None of these websites were determined to be having adequate content per our quality criteria. The two websites written at the 6th grade level were both HON certified but failed to meet our adequacy criteria due to absent information in one or two subcategories. These findings emphasize the challenges faced by the low education achievement patients seeking good quality information presented in a manner appropriate for their reading skills. We were able to recognize at least 3 websites with readability level of 8th grade or below and GQS of 4 in an attempt to help this cohort of patients. (Table 6)

It can be safely assumed that the trend of using the Internet is going to be ever expanding in the medical decision-making for many of our patients. The use of Internet by the patients has been a topic of debate in various medical and surgical specialties. As early as 1997, a study reviewed the websites on the cancer treatments in an attempt to recommend those sites to the patients [15]. A few other studies have examined the quality and readability of the topic specific information on the world wide web [4–7, 16]. In a study in 2001 on online information on intersex anomalies, 6 different general search engines were used and first 50 search results were included [16]. They concluded that of the 300 websites analyzed, only 45 were found to have patient related information and only 5 were recommendable (1.6%). This was similar to our study, where we used 3 different search engines with 100 website links and 45 were analyzed and 3 were found to have high-quality information but none of these having readability levels of 8th grade and below. Similarly, John et al. in 2016 analyzed 80 articles using different search terms for colorectal cancer screening including colonoscopy, flexible sigmoidoscopy, fecal occult blood test and CT colonography for the readability and overall quality [4]. Similar to our study results, they found that these 80 sites were written at 11.7 grade level in contrast to the recommended 3rd to 7th grade levels by AMA and NIH. This study also found reliability, accessibility, and usability of these websites to be moderate.

We did not find false or misleading information on EGD in the web pages that we searched. No portals or discussion forums were encountered among the search results obtained using our search strategy. Therefore, there was a general lack of subjectivity in the web pages that were obtained. EGD is a commonly performed procedure and is likely to be searched more than other GI procedures except perhaps colonoscopy. The conclusions from this study regarding the quality of information available on the Internet for EGD, therefore, cannot be extrapolated for other GI procedures.

It remains to be studied, however, if the patients prefer to use other applications like social media including Twitter, Reddit, and Facebook as important resources for health information. Either large organizations or healthcare institutions operated most of the web sites that were included in our analysis. While the search engines like Google and Bing have developed complex algorithms, and the web pages that are suggested to users appear in a sequence that is in part generated by the relevance and authenticity of the web site, searches on social media may be more liable to subjective opinion. This concern has recently been studied by Stock et al., who found while studying cleft lip and palate that although social media groups provided an avenue for real-time health discussion and were frequently used, they suffered from the disadvantage of reliance on opinion and subjective experience [17]. Regardless, as a growing avenue for obtaining health information on the Internet, this aspect of the world wide web needs further investigation.

Our study highlights the challenges faced by the patients in successfully navigating the Internet when making important healthcare decisions involving the use of EGD. Our analysis shows that most of the information available online is moderate quality with some comprehensive and reliable websites, but it can be difficult to find these resources and cause confusion to the readers. This puts gastroenterologists in a unique situation where we need to encourage our patients to make informed decisions and balance it with the information available online. We believe gastroenterologists should be more aware of the quality of the resources available on the Internet for EGD and other procedures to provide better patient experience. We feel that the role of physicians here could be in directing the patients to high-quality websites to supplement their knowledge of the EGD procedure. We envision that physicians should be able to use these resources to facilitate the thorough understanding of the procedure and make informed decisions when patients elect to have EGD. This may require closing the loop of communication with the patients by encouraging patients to get back to the physicians after they had a chance to go through these high-quality recommendable websites.

The strengths of our study are that we have targeted an extremely common GI procedure for which no current data on the quality of online resources exists in the scientific literature. We used multiple search engines in an attempt to come up with the best search strategy on this topic. Our study showed that there was not much added benefit to using different search engines for obtaining the high-quality results. Another unique feature of our study was that we were able to identify 3 overall good quality content websites and another 3 websites for lower readability level patients to better assist them in understanding this procedure.

We recognize that our study had some limitations as well. We are aware that the order of the search results obtained by the individual patients may not be strictly the same as those obtained by us due to geographical location variations, previous search history, and cookies on individual computers. We are also cognizant of the dynamic nature of the Internet and the fact that this study was cross-sectional in design. Our search was limited to English language results and there are many users on the Internet who prefer languages other than English and the results of this study may not be applicable to these patients.

5. Conclusions

Our study shows that there is a wide variation in the content of the websites available on EGD on the Internet. There are quite a few websites with moderate quality content but authenticity of the content remains a challenge. We could analyze 3 comprehensive and authentic websites out of 45 URLs and 13 other moderate quality websites. In addition, the readability of the websites was consistently at higher level than recommended by AMA. We identified 3 websites with moderate quality content written at 8th grade and below readability level. We feel that the active involvement of gastroenterologists in directing their patients to superior information quality websites will help their patients understand the EGD procedure better and help prevent miscommunication regarding its nature and risks.

Disclosure

An earlier version of this study has been presented as a Poster presentation at 'ACG 2018 Annual Scientific Meeting Abstracts Philadelphia, Pennsylvania: American College of Gastroenterology' in October 2018.

References

[1] Internet users in the world,.

[2] Majority of Adults Look Online for Health Information,.

[3] S. Mathur, N. Shanti, M. Brkaric et al., "Surfing for scoliosis: The quality of information available on the internet," *The Spine Journal*, vol. 30, no. 23, pp. 2695–2700, 2005.

[4] E. S. John, A. M. John, D. R. Hansberry et al., "Colorectal cancer screening patient education materials—how effective is online health information?" *International Journal of Colorectal Disease*, vol. 31, no. 12, pp. 1817–1824, 2016.

[5] E. H. Schreuders, E. J. Grobbee, E. J. Kuipers, M. C. W. Spaander, and S. J. O. Veldhuyzen van Zanten, "Variable Quality and Readability of Patient-oriented Websites on Colorectal Cancer Screening," *Clinical Gastroenterology and Hepatology*, vol. 15, no. 1, pp. 79–85.e3, 2017.

[6] C. Tian, S. Champlin, M. Mackert, A. Lazard, and D. Agrawal, "Readability, suitability, and health content assessment of web-based patient education materials on colorectal cancer screening," *Gastrointestinal Endoscopy*, vol. 80, no. 2, pp. 284–e2, 2014.

[7] S. N. Sambandam, V. Ramasamy, P. Priyanka, and B. Ilango, "Quality Analysis of Patient Information About Knee Arthroscopy on the World Wide Web," *Arthroscopy - Journal of Arthroscopic and Related Surgery*, vol. 23, no. 5, pp. 509–e2, 2007.

[8] S. Mozafarpour, B. Norris, J. Borin, and B. H. Eisner, "Assessment of readability, quality and popularity of online information on ureteral stents," *World Journal of Urology*, pp. 1–8, 2018.

[9] J. M. Edmonson, "History of the instruments for gastrointestinal endoscopy," *Gastrointestinal Endoscopy*, vol. 37, pp. S27–S56, 1991.

[10] W. G. Park, N. J. Shaheen, J. Cohen et al., "Quality indicators for EGD," *Gastrointestinal Endoscopy*, vol. 81, no. 1, pp. 17–30, 2015.

[11] A. F. Peery, E. S. Dellon, J. Lund et al., "Burden of gastrointestinal disease in the United States: 2012 update," *Gastroenterology*, vol. 143, no. 5, pp. 1179.e3–1187.e3, 2012.

[12] C. Boyer, M. Selby, and R. D. Appel, "The health on the net code of conduct for medical and health web sites," in *Proceedings of the 9th World Congress on Medical Informatics, MedInfo 1998*, pp. 1163–1166, August 1998.

[13] A. Bernard, M. Langille, S. Hughes, C. Rose, D. Leddin, and S. V. van Zanten, "A systematic review of patient inflammatory bowel disease information resources on the world wide web," *American Journal of Gastroenterology*, vol. 102, no. 9, pp. 2070–2077, 2007.

[14] R. Flesch, "A new readability yardstick," *Journal of Applied Psychology*, vol. 32, no. 3, pp. 221–233, 1948.

[15] R. Sikorski and R. Peters, "Oncology ASAP: Where to find reliable cancer information on the Internet," *Journal of the American Medical Association*, vol. 277, no. 18, pp. 1431-1432, 1997.

[16] C. A. Corpron and J. L. Lelli Jr., "Evaluation of pediatric surgery information on the internet," *Journal of Pediatric Surgery*, vol. 36, no. 8, pp. 1187–1189, 2001.

[17] N. M. Stock, A. Martindale, and C. Cunniffe, "CleftProud: A Content Analysis and Online Survey of 2 Cleft Lip and Palate Facebook Groups," *The Cleft Palate-Craniofacial Journal*, Article ID 1055665618764737, 2018.

21

Dynamic Changes of the Frequency of Classic and Inflammatory Monocytes Subsets and Natural Killer Cells in Chronic Hepatitis C Patients Treated by Direct-Acting Antiviral Agents

Gang Ning, Yi-ting Li, You-ming Chen, Ying Zhang, Ying-fu Zeng, and Chao-shuang Lin

Department of Infectious Diseases, The Third Affiliated Hospital of Sun Yat-Sen University, Guangzhou 510630, China

Correspondence should be addressed to Chao-shuang Lin; shuangss@21cn.com

Academic Editor: José L. Mauriz

Objective. Up to now, little was known about the immunological changes of chronic hepatitis C (CHC) patients treated with direct-acting antiviral agents (DAAs); we try to explore the effect of DAAs on the frequency of monocytes, NK cells, and cytokines that promote their activation. *Methods.* 15 treatment-naive CHC patients and 10 healthy controls were recruited. Patients were examined before DAAs therapy (0 w) and at week 4 (4 w) and week 12 (12 w) of therapy. Percentage of monocytes and NK cells of the peripheral blood was analyzed by flow cytometry. Serum cytokines IL-12, IL-18, CXCL10, CXCL11, sCD14, and sCD163 were measured by enzyme linked immunosorbent assay. *Results.* The frequency of $CD3^{-}CD16^{+}CD56^{+}$ NK cells and classic $CD14^{++}CD16^{-}$ monocytes decreased, while $CD14^{+}CD16^{+}$ monocytes and cytokines IL-12, IL-18, CXCL10, CXCL11, sCD14, and sCD163 increased at 0 w compared to healthy controls. During DAAs treatment, the decreased NK cells and classic monocytes gradually increased to normal levels; the increased inflammatory monocytes and cytokines IL-12 and CXCL11 decreased to normal levels, but the increased cytokines IL-18, CXCL10, sCD14, and sCD163 still remained at high levels at 12 w though they decreased rapidly from 0 w. *Conclusion.* Our results showed that DAAs treatment attenuated the activation of monocytes and NK cells in CHC patients. Trial registration number is NCT03063723.

1. Introduction

Treatment of hepatitis C virus (HCV) infection has greatly advanced with the advent of the new direct-acting antivirals (DAAs) in the past 5 years. More than 90% of chronic hepatitis C (CHC) patients could achieve a sustained viral response (SVR) using DAAs after 12 weeks of treatment [1–3]. Among all the DAAs regimens, daclatasvir/sofosbuvir and ledipasvir/ sofosbuvir are recommended for all of the genotypes except for patients with genotype 3 infection with cirrhosis by WHO. Now, these two DAAs regimens are included in voluntary licensing agreements signed between the originator companies and generics companies. In fact, daclatasvir/sofosbuvir and ledipasvir/sofosbuvir are already available in generic formulations in some countries. The introduction of generic formulations results in lower prices. It has been report reported that the price for a 12-week regimen of generic sofosbuvir would be less than US$ 500/patient in India, and no doubt, the wide-scale implementation of HCV treatment will be facilitated by this rapid reduction in the price of daclatasvir/sofosbuvir and ledipasvir/sofosbuvir [4].

Previous studies have shown that suppression or eradication of HCV infection has been related to a reduced risk of developing hepatocellular carcinoma (HCC) and improved outcomes in CHC patients [5–7]. In one recent meta-analysis study, the estimated relative risk of HCC development in CHC patients with all stages of fibrosis who achieved SVR by interferon therapy was 0.24, meaning that interferon therapy was able to reduce the risk of HCC occurrence by 76% [8]. Considering high rates of SVR achieved in patients with CHC treated with DAAs, it is reasonable to raise the hope of a drastic decline in HCC occurrence and even a decline in HCC recurrence.

Surprisingly and unexpectedly, increased aggressiveness and high rates of HCC recurrence (28% (16/58) and 29%

(17/59), resp.) have been reported in patients who cleared HCV with DAAs after achieving a complete response to resection or local ablation within only 6 months of therapy [9, 10]. The authors hypothesized that the rapid eradication of HCV and control of liver inflammation would impact antitumoral immune control, which in turn might contribute to the neoplastic cells proliferation. Conversely, three independent prospective French cohorts failed to reveal an increased risk of HCC recurrence after DAAs treatment in CHC patients after receiving curative cancer treatments [11]. The conflicting results have raised commentaries and criticism which are a controversial issue with potential clinical implications [12–14].

Although the impact of DAAs treatment on the rate of HCC occurrence or recurrence still remain unclear, it would be more important to pay attention to the immunological changes of CHC patients treated with DAAs. Until now, however, only a few studies were performed to explore the changes of immunological milieu of CHC patients during DAAs treatment [15–17]. Hengst et al. and Carlin et al. explored the effect of DAAs treatment on the inflammatory cytokines and chemokines of CHC patients; they found that DAAs-induced HCV clearance could only partially restore the altered inflammatory mediators [15, 16]. Martin et al. found that DAAs therapy improved the proliferation of HCV-specific T cells, but it still remained unknown to which extent cytokine production of HCV-specific T cells could be recovered [17]. In spite of this, little is known about the influence of DAAs treatment on monocytes.

Here in our study, we aim to explore the effect of antiviral treatment of CHC patients with DAAs on the frequency of monocytes (classic $CD14^{++}CD16^{-}$ monocytes and inflammatory $CD14^{+}CD16^{+}$ monocytes) [18], NK cells ($CD3^{-}CD16^{+}CD56^{+}$) [19], and cytokines IL-12, IL-18, CXCL10, and CXCL11, which are necessary to activation of NK cells, and soluble CD14 (sCD14) and soluble CD163 (sCD163), which reflect monocytes activation.

2. Material and Methods

2.1. Patients and Samples. 15 treatment-naive CHC patients (6 males and 9 females) and 10 healthy controls (6 males and 4 females) were recruited at the third affiliated hospital of Sun Yat-Sen university (Guangzhou, China) from January 2016 to November 2016. The mean age of CHC patients was 48.06 ± 3.82 years and the mean age of healthy controls was 27.30 ± 3.40 years. Eight CHC patients were treated with sofosbuvir (400 mg, qd)/ledipasvir (90 mg, qd) for 12 weeks and 7 CHC patients were treated with sofosbuvir (400 mg, qd)/daclatasvir (60 mg, qd) for 12 weeks. Basic characteristics of all the subjects were shown in Table 1. Patients coinfected with HAV, HBV, HDV, HEV, and human immunodeficiency virus were excluded. Besides, pregnant patients or patients with psychiatric disorder were also excluded. This study protocol was approved by the Ethics Review Board of the third affiliated hospital of Sun Yat-Sen university and written informed consent was obtained from the patients before enrollment.

Table 1: Basic characteristics of subjects.

Index	CHC Patients	Healthy Controls
Number	15	10
Age (y)	48.06 ± 3.82	27.30 ± 3.40
Gender (M/f)	6/9	6/4
ALT (U/L, mean ± SE)	49.29 ± 7.47	NA
AST (U/L, mean ± SE)	52.78 ± 9.39	NA
HCV-RNA (log 10 IU/mL)	6.02 ± 0.30	NA
HCV-RNA genotype	1b (42%)/6a (30%)/2a (28%)	NA
Treatment	Sofosbuvir + ledipasvir (8/15), sofosbuvir + daclatasvir (7/15)	NA
RVR/SVR	100%	NA

CHC patients: chronic hepatitis C patients; RVB: ribavirin; RVR: rapid virological response; SVR: sustained virological response.

2.2. Peripheral Blood Mononuclear Cells (PBMC) Isolation and Storage. All CHC patients were monitored before, during and after DAAs treatment at the out patients clinic of department of infectious diseases. Peripheral blood samples (10 mL) were collected from CHC patients before therapy (0 w), at 4 weeks (4 w), and at the end of treatment (12 w) and from healthy controls with EDTA anticoagulation tubes (Invitrogen, BD). Then PBMC were isolated from peripheral blood samples and cryopreserved at −80°C and 72 hours later were transferred to the liquid nitrogen as previously described [20].

2.3. Measurement of Viral Load, ALT, and AST. Serum HCV RNA was quantified by COBAS Taqman assay (Roche Diagnostic, Basel, Switzerland). ALT and AST were measured with Hitachi 7170 automatic biochemistry analyzer in the laboratory center of the third affiliated hospital.

2.4. Flow Cytometry. In order to examine the phenotype and frequency of classic $CD14^{++}CD16^{-}$ monocytes, nonclassic/intermediate $CD14^{+}CD16^{+}$ monocytes and $CD3^{-}CD16^{+}CD56^{+}$ NK cells, relevant labeled multicolor fluorescence anti-human monoclonal antibodies (mAbs) purchased from eBioscience (San Diego, CA, US) were used for surface staining: anti-CD14-FITC, anti-CD16-PERCP-Cy7, anti-CD3-PERCP, anti-CD56-PERCP-Cy7, and anti-CD16-PE. PBMC was first thawed and then resuspended in flow staining buffer (PBS plus 1% FBS); after being washed twice, PBMC was resuspended again and incubated with the above labeled multicolor fluorescence anti-human monoclonal antibodies. Then the stained PBMC was washed with flow staining buffer and centrifuged. Finally, the stained PBMC were diluted and analyzed on a flow cytometer (BD LSR II) (BD Biosciences). Data was acquired as the fraction of labeled cells within a cell gate set for 20,000 events. The detailed procession was described in our previous study [20].

2.5. Enzyme Linked Immunosorbent Assay (ELISA). Measurement of serum IL-12p70, IL-18, CXCL10, CXCL11, sCD14, and sCD163 were performed with the ProcartaPlex™ Multiplex Immunoassay (eBioscience) according to the manufacturer's protocol using a BD FACSCanto™ II flow cytometer. The Flowlogic™ and Beadlogic™ software (Inivai Technologies, Mentone, Vic., Australia) were used for data analysis.

2.6. Statistical Analysis. Normally distributed quantitative data were presented as mean ± standard, while the non-normally distributed data were expressed as interquartile range. 1-way ANOVA test was used for assessment of the differences among values during the course of treatment, and Mann–Whitney U tests or unpaired t-test was used for comparison between patients and healthy controls. All data were analyzed by SPSS Statistics 20 and all figures were made by Prizm5.0 statistical analysis software (GraphPad Software). P value less than 0.05 was considered to be statistically significant.

3. Results

3.1. Effect of DAAs Treatment on HCV Viremia and Liver Inflammation. All 15 treatment-naive CHC patients had achieved a rapid virological response (RVR), defined as undetectable HCV RNA <15 U/mL, at the first 4 weeks of sofosbuvir/ledipasvir or sofosbuvir/daclatasvir treatment (Table 1). What is more, none of them experienced virological breakthrough at week 12. Similarly, serum ALT and AST levels had also decreased significantly within the 4 weeks of DAAs treatment and none experienced ALT or AST rebound.

3.2. Dynamic Changes of the Frequency of Monocytes Subsets and Natural Killer Cells during DAAs Treatment. We used flow cytometry to analyze the dynamic changes of the frequency of monocytes subsets and NK cells in the peripheral blood of CHC patients during DAAs treatment, and representative flow cytometry plots of $CD14^{++}CD16^{-}$ monocyte, $CD14^{+}CD16^{+}$ monocyte, $CD3^{-}CD16^{+}CD56^{+}$ NK cells were presented in Figure 1(a). The frequency of classic $CD14^{++}CD16^{-}$ monocytes was less than healthy controls at baseline (0 w) (59.14 ± 0.54% versus 72.75 ± 1.31%, $P < 0.001$) and then gradually increased to HC levels (71.54 ± 2.99% versus 72.75 ± 1.31%, $P > 0.05$) during DAAs treatment (12 w). Conversely, the levels of inflammatory $CD14^{+}CD16^{+}$ monocyte were higher than HC levels at 0 w (18.49 ± 1.54% versus 10.65 ± 0.83%, $P < 0.0001$) but then rapidly decreased to normal levels of HC (12.42 ± 1.60% versus 10.65 ± 0.83, $P > 0.05$) at 12 w. The changes of the frequency of $CD3^{-}CD16^{+}CD56^{+}$ NK cells were similar to classic $CD14^{++}CD16^{-}$ monocytes. The frequency of $CD3^{-}CD16^{+}CD56^{+}$ NK cells decreased compared to that of HC level at baseline (13.29 ± 0.85% versus 18.72 ± 1.91%, $P < 0.001$), and after treatment with DAAs, it gradually increased to normal levels of HC at 12 w (14.44 ± 1.60% versus 18.72 ± 1.91, $P > 0.05$) (Figures 1(b)–1(d)). The detailed information about dynamic changes of the frequency of monocytes subsets and natural killer cells was shown in Table 2.

3.3. Kinetics of the Levels of Serum sCD14, sCD163, IL-12, IL-18, CXCL10, and CXCL11 during DAAs Treatment. To further explored the effect of DAAs treatment on the function of monocytes subsets and natural killer cells, we next analyzed the kinetics of the levels of serum sCD14 and sCD163, which reflected monocytes activation and serum IL-12, IL-18, CXCL10, and CXCL11, which promoted NK cells activation during DAAs treatment. Consistent with the above results, all the levels of serum sCD14, sCD163, IL-12, IL-18, CXCL10, and CXCL11 were higher than that of HC at baseline, and during DAAs treatment, sCD14, serum sCD163, and CXCL10 decreased rapidly while IL-12, IL-18, and CXCL11 decreased gradually. However, plasma IL-12 and CXCL11 levels decreased to normal levels of HC, but serum sCD14, sCD163, CXCL10, and IL-18 still remained at high levels (Figures 2(a)–2(f)). The detailed information about dynamic changes of the levels of serum sCD14, sCD163, IL-12, IL-18, CXCL10, and CXCL11 during DAAs treatment was shown in Table 2.

4. Discussion

The development of highly effective interferon-free DAAs regiments has revolutionized the treatment of HCV infection and may thus lead to complete eradication of HCV worldwide. However, little was known about the immunological changes of CHC patients during DAAs treatment. So, here in our study, we explored the impact of DAAs treatment on the frequency of monocytes subsets and NK cells.

NK cells are the main innate immune cells of the liver in healthy human and their frequency decreases in the blood but increases in the liver in chronic HCV infection [21]. NK cells from CHC patients are activated by low levels of HCV-induced interferon-α, and they expressed increased cytotoxic functions and TNF-related apoptosis-inducing ligand (TRAIL) but decreased antiviral cytokine interferon-γ production. Besides, these NK cells also expressed higher levels of activated receptors, such as NKp30, NKp44, NKp46, NKG2C, NKG2D, and CD122, and inhibitory receptor NKG2A than those from healthy controls [22, 23]. Previous studies had explored the effect of interferon therapy on the NK cells. It has been shown that CHC patients with SVR by interferon therapy exhibited greater levels of NK cell degranulation and enhanced NK cytotoxicity and thus, NK cell responses can be used as an indicator of a patient's interferon responsiveness [24, 25]. Recently, Spaan et al. explored the effect of DAAs therapy on NK cells; they found that DAAs therapy increased the percentage of $CD3^{+}CD56^{dim}$ NK cells, downregulated surface NKp30, NKp46, and NKG2A expression on NK cells to a phenotype resembling healthy controls, and decreased NK cell-related cytokines (IL-12, IL-18) and TRAIL expression of CHC patients during DAAs treatment [26]. In line with Spaan's study, we also found that NK cells frequency of peripheral blood decreased before DAAs treatment but then gradually increased to normal levels of healthy controls. The changes of serum IL-12, IL-18, CXCL10, and CXCL11 were consistent with the changes of NK cells. They were higher than healthy controls at baseline but then diminished during DAAs treatment. IL-12, IL-18,

TABLE 2: The kinetics of the immunological parameters during the treatment of patients with chronic hepatitis C and their comparison with healthy controls.

Parameter	CHC patients			Healthy controls	*P* value				
	0 w	4 w	12 w		0 W–HC	4 W–0 W	12 W–0 W	4 W–12 W	12 W–HC
$CD14^{++}CD16^{-}$ monocyte cells (%)	59.14 ± 0.54	67.59 ± 1.98	71.54 ± 2.99	72.75 ± 1.31	**	ns	**	ns	ns
$CD14^{+}CD16^{+}$ monocyte cells (%)	18.49 ± 1.54	13.39 ± 1.07	12.42 ± 1.60		***	*	*	ns	ns
$CD3^{-}CD16^{+}CD56^{+}$ NK cells (%)	13.29 ± 0.85	12.68 ± 1.09	14.44 ± 1.60	18.72 ± 1.91	**	ns	ns	ns	ns
Serum sCD14 (pg/mL)	64407.38 ± 5778.49	51639.83 ± 5778.49	44390.06 ± 3330.17	28370.76 ± 2357.68	***	ns	*	ns	**
Serum sCD163 (pg/mL)	22853.80 ± 4137.61	11975.35 ± 1795.91	11494.79 ± 1836.97	2934.41 ± 223.31	***	*	*	ns	**
Serum IL-12 (pg/mL)	2.98 ± 0.13	2.61 ± 0.13	2.51 ± 0.10	2.49 ± 0.1	**	ns	*	ns	ns
Serum IL-18 (pg/mL)	76.51 ± 11.01	52.73 ± 5.00	40.63 ± 3.72	11.45 ± 1.77	***	ns	**	ns	***
Serum CXCL-10 (pg/mL)	64.41 ± 6.16	37.64 ± 5.22	29.09 ± 3.49	10.48 ± 0.43	***	**	***	ns	***
Serum CXCL-11 (pg/mL)	23.64 ± 3.54	15.53 ± 2.07	9.64 ± 1.77	8.27 ± 2.19	**	ns	**	ns	ns

CHC patients: chronic hepatitis C patients; $^{*}P < 0.05$; $^{**}P < 0.01$; $^{***}P < 0.001$; ns: no significance.

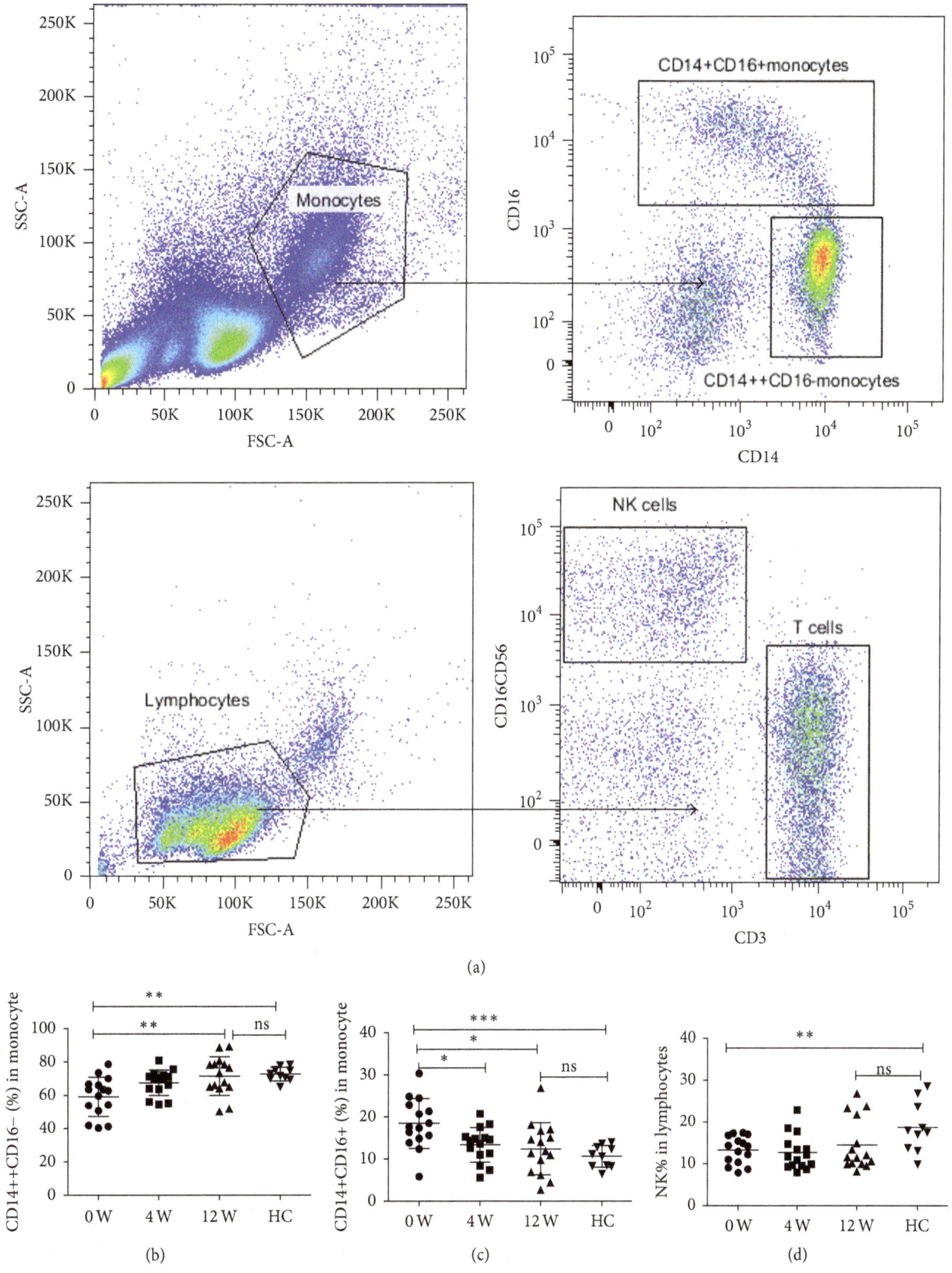

FIGURE 1: *Dynamic changes of the frequency of monocytes subsets and natural killer cells during DAAs treatment.* (a) Representative flow cytometry plots of $CD14^{++}CD16^{-}$ monocytes, $CD14^{+}CD16^{+}$ monocytes, and $CD3^{-}CD16^{+}CD56^{+}$ NK cells; (b) dynamic changes of the frequency of $CD14^{++}CD16^{-}$ monocytes; (c) dynamic changes of the frequency of $CD14^{+}CD16^{+}$ monocytes; (d) dynamic changes of the frequency of $CD3^{-}CD16^{+}CD56^{+}$ NK cells. $^{*}p < 0.05$; $^{**}p < 0.01$; $^{***}p < 0.001$.

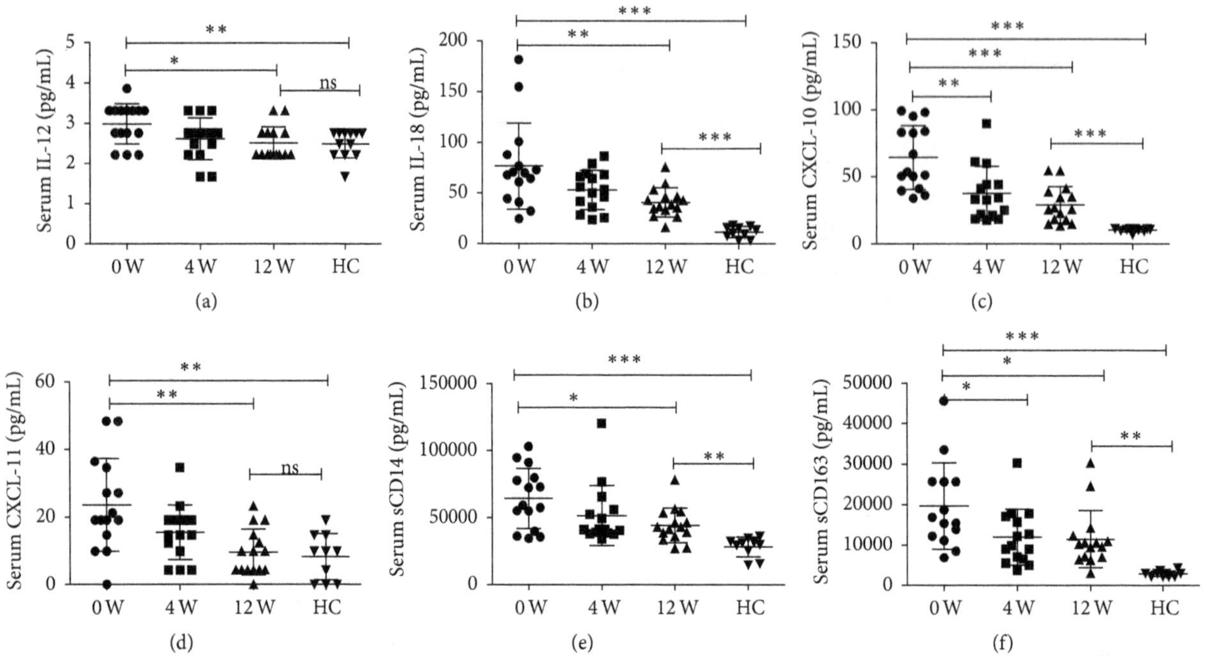

FIGURE 2: *Kinetics of the levels of serum cytokines during DAAs treatment.* (a) Dynamic changes of the levels of IL-12; (b) dynamic changes of the levels of IL-18; (c) dynamic changes of the levels of CXCL10; (d) dynamic changes of the levels of CXCL11; (e) dynamic changes of the levels of sCD14; (f) dynamic changes of the levels of sCD163. $^{*}p < 0.05$; $^{**}p < 0.01$; $^{***}p < 0.001$.

CXCL10, and CXCL11 are important for NK cells activation. IL-12 and IL-18 could promote interferon-γ production of NK cells, and CXCL10 and CXCL11 could activate NK cells to express higher levels of STAT1 and pSTAT1, which are an essential part of signaling downstream of the interferon receptor [27]. Serti et al. demonstrated that DAAs treatment decreased serum levels of CXCL10 and CXCL11, leading to decreased expression of the STAT1 and pSTAT1 of NK cells, and the decreased expression of STAT1 and pSTAT1 was associated with normalization of NK cells phenotype observed in Spaan's study [26, 27]. Furthermore, Serti et al. had also found that DAAs treatment-induced normalization of NK cells phenotype and function may follow a hierarchy. Briefly speaking, significant decrease in HCV titer by DAAs treatment first induced decrease in activation surface HLA-DR expression of NK cells and then reversed the alter cytokine production by NK cells and last normalized the alter cytotoxicity of NK cells.

Similar to NK cells, monocytes are also an important part of the first line of defense against HCV infection. During HCV infection, peripheral blood monocytes are attracted to the liver and differentiate into macrophages and Kupffer cells. Monocytes/macrophages play an important role in initiating the adaptive immune response and influencing the Th1/Th2 polarization by producing excessive inflammatory and immune-modulatory cytokines, such as IL-10 and IL-12. These cytokines may also impair the ability of antigen presenting cells to activate naive T cells and thus help to HCV replication and establish persistent infection [28]. Zheng et al. found that circulating $CD14^{++}CD16^{-}$ monocytes decreased while $CD14^{+}CD16^{+}$ monocytes increased in CHC patients when compared to HCV spontaneous resolved and healthy controls, and $CD14^{+}CD16^{+}$ monocytes were negatively correlated with HCV viremia but PD-L1/CD86 ratio in $CD14^{+}CD16^{+}$ monocytes was closely correlated with HCV viremia [29]. Similarly, in our study, we also found that $CD14^{++}CD16^{-}$ monocytes decreased but $CD14^{+}CD16^{+}$ monocytes increased at baseline in CHC patients. Furthermore, we also found that $CD14^{++}CD16^{-}$ monocytes increased to levels of healthy controls while $CD14^{+}CD16^{+}$ monocytes decreased to the levels which was similar to healthy controls during DAAs treatment. Up to now, however, little is known about the effect of DAAs treatment on the function of monocytes. In our study, we found that the changes of serum sCD14 and sCD16 which reflected the monocytes activation were similar to the changes of $CD14^{+}CD16^{+}$ monocytes, indirectly indicating a decrease in the monocyte activation. Recently, Bility et al. found that HCV-induced M2 macrophages activation was associated with liver fibrosis during HCV infection and supernatant of HCV-infected cells could polarize human monocytes to a M2-like phenotype. What is more, DAAs treatment attenuated M2 macrophages activation and associated liver fibrosis [30]. Interestingly, Gambato et al. found that DAAs treatment did not have obvious effect on the phagocytic and oxidative burst capacity of monocytes in patients with advanced liver fibrosis [31]. Therefore, further studies are needed to explore the impact of DAAs treatment on the changes of the function of monocytes.

There are several limitations in our study. First, the impact of DAAs treatment on the frequency of monocytes and NK cells was only evaluated at the first 12 weeks of treatment and therefore, the long-term effects still remain unknown. However, we would continue the study and explore the long-term effects by DAAs treatment. Second, CHC patients were not treated with the same DAAs regimen and the HCV genotypes were different; this may have an impact on our results. Finally, we did not evaluate the functional status of circulating monocytes and NK cells which could have been associated with the observed decrease in serum sCD14, sCD163, IL-12, IL-18, CXCL10, and CXCL11.

In conclusion, our results show that DAAs treatment attenuated the activation of monocytes and NK cells in CHC patients during DAAs treatment, indicated by decreased levels of sCD14, sCD163, IL-12, IL-18, CXCL10, and CXCL11 and normalization of the frequency of monocytes and NK cells, but the effect of DAAs treatment on their function still needs further research.

Abbreviations

HCV: Hepatitis C virus
DAAs: Direct-acting antivirals
CHC: Chronic hepatitis C
SVR: Sustained viral response
HCC: Hepatocellular carcinoma
RVR: Rapid virological response
TRAIL: TNF-related apoptosis-inducing ligand.

Acknowledgments

This research is supported by grants of National Natural Science Foundation of China (Grant no. 31370907). The authors are grateful to the patients for their participation in this study.

References

[1] S. A. Alqahtani, N. Afdhal, S. Zeuzem et al., "Safety and tolerability of ledipasvir/sofosbuvir with and without ribavirin in patients with chronic hepatitis C Virus genotype 1 infection: analysis of phase III ION trials," *Hepatology*, vol. 62, no. 1, pp. 25–30, 2015.

[2] E. Lawitz, M. Makara, U. S. Akarca et al., "Efficacy and safety of ombitasvir, paritaprevir, and ritonavir in an open-label study of patients with genotype 1b chronic hepatitis C virus infection with and without cirrhosis," *Gastroenterology*, vol. 149, no. 4, pp. 971–980.e1, 2015.

[3] K. R. Reddy, M. Bourlière, M. Sulkowski et al., "Ledipasvir and sofosbuvir in patients with genotype 1 hepatitis C virus infection and compensated cirrhosis: an integrated safety and efficacy analysis," *Hepatology*, vol. 62, no. 1, pp. 79–86, 2015.

[4] WHO, *Guidelines for the Screening, Care and Treatment of Persons with Chronic Hepatitis C Infection Updated Version*, World Health Organization, 2016.

[5] H. B. El-Serag, F. Kanwal, P. Richardson, and J. Kramer, "Risk of hepatocellular carcinoma after sustained virologic response in veterans with HCV-infection," *Hepatology*, vol. 64, no. 1, pp. 130–137, 2016.

[6] A. J. van der Meer, B. J. Veldt, J. J. Feld et al., "Association between sustained virological response and all-cause mortality among patients with chronic hepatitis C and advanced hepatic fibrosis," *The Journal of the American Medical Association*, vol. 308, no. 24, pp. 2584–2593, 2012.

[7] M. Manns, D. Samuel, E. J. Gane et al., "Ledipasvir and sofosbuvir plus ribavirin in patients with genotype 1 or 4 hepatitis C virus infection and advanced liver disease: a multicentre, open-label, randomised, phase 2 trial," *The Lancet Infectious Diseases*, vol. 16, no. 6, pp. 685–697, 2016.

[8] R. L. Morgan, B. Baack, B. D. Smith, A. Yartel, M. Pitasi, and Y. Falck-Ytter, "Eradication of hepatitis C virus infection and the development of hepatocellular carcinoma: a meta-analysis of observational studies," *Annals of Internal Medicine*, vol. 158, no. 5, part 1, pp. 329–337, 2013.

[9] M. Reig, Z. Mariño, C. Perelló et al., "Unexpected high rate of early tumor recurrence in patients with HCV-related HCC undergoing interferon-free therapy," *Journal of Hepatology*, vol. 65, no. 4, pp. 719–726, 2016.

[10] F. Conti, F. Buonfiglioli, A. Scuteri et al., "Early occurrence and recurrence of hepatocellular carcinoma in HCV-related cirrhosis treated with direct-acting antivirals," *Journal of Hepatology*, vol. 65, no. 4, pp. 727–733, 2016.

[11] S. Pol, "Lack of evidence of an effect of Direct Acting Antivirals on the recurrence of hepatocellular carcinoma: The ANRS collaborative study group on hepatocellular carcinoma (ANRS CO22 HEPATHER, CO12 CIRVIR and CO23 CUPILT cohorts)," *Journal of Hepatology*, vol. 65, no. 4, pp. 734–740, 2016.

[12] C. Cammà, G. Cabibbo, and A. Craxì, "Direct antiviral agents and risk for HCC early recurrence: much ado about nothing," *Journal of Hepatology*, vol. 65, no. 4, pp. 861–862, 2016.

[13] H. A. Torres, J. N. Vauthey, M. P. Economides, P. Mahale, and A. Kaseb, "Hepatocellular carcinoma recurrence after treatment with direct-acting antivirals: first, do no harm by withdrawing treatment," *Journal of Hepatology*, vol. 65, no. 4, pp. 862–864, 2016.

[14] J.-C. Nault and M. Colombo, "Hepatocellular carcinoma and direct acting antiviral treatments: controversy after the revolution," *Journal of Hepatology*, vol. 65, no. 4, pp. 663–665, 2016.

[15] J. Hengst, V. Schlaphoff, K. Deterding et al., "DAA-induced HCV clearance does not restore the altered cytokine and chemokine milieu in patients with chronic hepatitis C," *Journal of Hepatology*, vol. 64, no. 2, pp. S417–S418, 2016.

[16] A. F. Carlin, P. Aristizabal, Q. Song et al., "Temporal dynamics of inflammatory cytokines/chemokines during sofosbuvir and ribavirin therapy for genotype 2 and 3 hepatitis C infection," *Hepatology*, vol. 62, no. 4, pp. 1047–1058, 2015.

[17] B. Martin, N. Hennecke, V. Lohmann et al., "Restoration of HCV-specific CD8+ T cell function by interferon-free therapy," *Journal of Hepatology*, vol. 61, no. 3, pp. 538–543, 2014.

[18] F. L. van de Veerdonk and A. M. G. Netea, "Diversity: a hallmark of monocyte society," *Immunity*, vol. 33, no. 3, pp. 289–291, 2010.

[19] M. A. Caligiuri, "Human natural killer cells," *Blood*, vol. 112, no. 3, pp. 461–469, 2008.

[20] G. Ning, L. She, L. Lu et al., "Analysis of monocytic and granulocytic myeloid-derived suppressor cells subsets in patients with hepatitis c virus infection and their clinical significance," *BioMed Research International*, vol. 2015, Article ID 385378, 8 pages, 2015.

[21] B. Oliviero, S. Varchetta, E. Paudice et al., "Natural killer cell functional dichotomy in chronic hepatitis B and chronic hepatitis C virus infections," *Gastroenterology*, vol. 137, no. 3, pp. 1151–1160.e7, 2009.

[22] G. Ahlenstiel, R. H. Titerence, C. Koh et al., "Natural killer cells are polarized toward cytotoxicity in chronic hepatitis C in an interferon-alfa-dependent manner," *Gastroenterology*, vol. 138, no. 1, pp. 325.e2–335.e2, 2010.

[23] P. Bonorino, M. Ramzan, X. Camous et al., "Fine characterization of intrahepatic NK cells expressing natural killer receptors in chronic hepatitis B and C," *Journal of Hepatology*, vol. 51, no. 3, pp. 458–467, 2009.

[24] B. Edlich, G. Ahlenstiel, A. Z. Azpiroz et al., "Early changes in interferon signaling define natural killer cell response and refractoriness to interferon-based therapy of hepatitis C patients," *Hepatology*, vol. 55, no. 1, pp. 39–48, 2012.

[25] G. Ahlenstiel, B. Edlich, L. J. Hogdal et al., "Early changes in natural killer cell function indicate virologic response to interferon therapy for hepatitis C," *Gastroenterology*, vol. 141, no. 4, pp. 1231–1239.e2, 2011.

[26] M. Spaan, G. Van Oord, K. Kreefft et al., "Immunological analysis during interferon-free therapy for chronic Hepatitis C virus infection reveals modulation of the natural killer cell compartment," *Journal of Infectious Diseases*, vol. 213, no. 2, pp. 216–223, 2016.

[27] E. Serti, X. Chepa-Lotrea, Y. J. Kim et al., "Successful interferon-free therapy of chronic hepatitis C virus infection normalizes natural killer cell function," *Gastroenterology*, vol. 149, no. 1, pp. 190–200.e2, 2015.

[28] G. Szabo, S. Chang, and A. Dolganiuc, "Altered innate immunity in chronic hepatitis C infection: cause or effect?" *Hepatology*, vol. 46, no. 4, pp. 1279–1290, 2007.

[29] J. Zheng, H. Liang, C. Xu et al., "An unbalanced PD-L1/CD86 ratio in CD14 ++ CD16 + monocytes is correlated with HCV viremia during chronic HCV infection," *Cellular and Molecular Immunology*, vol. 11, no. 3, pp. 294–304, 2014.

[30] M. T. Bility, K. Nio, F. Li et al., "Chronic hepatitis C infection–induced liver fibrogenesis is associated with M2 macrophage activation," *Scientific Reports*, vol. 6, article 39520, 2016.

[31] M. Gambato, N. Caro-Pérez, P. González et al., "Neutrophil and Monocyte function in patients with chronic hepatitis C undergoing antiviral therapy with regimens containing protease inhibitors with and without interferon," *PLoS ONE*, vol. 11, no. 11, Article ID e0166631, 2016.

22

Evaluation of Adrenal Function in Nonhospitalized Patients with Cirrhosis

Maryam Moini,[1] Mitra Yazdani Sarvestani,[2] Mesbah Shams,[3] and Masood Nomovi[4]

[1] *Gastroenterohepatology Research Center, Shiraz University of Medical Sciences, Nemazee Hospital, Zand Street, Shiraz 71935-1311, Iran*
[2] *Department of Internal Medicine, Fasa University of Medical Sciences, Ebne Sina Square, Fasa, Iran*
[3] *Endocrinology and Metabolism Research Center, Shiraz University of Medical Sciences, Shiraz, Iran*
[4] *Department of Internal Medicine, Shiraz University of Medical Sciences, Shiraz, Iran*

Correspondence should be addressed to Maryam Moini; dornam@hotmail.com

Academic Editor: Emmanuel Tsochatzis

Background. Patients with cirrhosis and advancing hepatic insufficiency may show various degrees of other organ malfunction, including brain, kidney, and lung. Several studies have also shown a high prevalence of adrenal insufficiency in cirrhotic patients that may cause hemodynamic instability. *Materials and Methods.* In this study we prospectively evaluated adrenal function in a population of nonhospitalized cirrhotic patients. Categorization of liver disease severity was done according to model for end-stage liver disease (MELD) score. Adrenocorticotropic hormone stimulation testing was performed on subjects using 250 μg of synthetic short acting hormone; radio immunoassay was used to measure plasma cortisol levels. *Results.* Of 105 cirrhotic patients, 15.23% had evidence of adrenal insufficiency. These patients were not statistically different from those with normal adrenal function in levels of serum creatinine or bilirubin, MELD score, or presence of cirrhosis related complications. Significant differences were seen in mean international normalized ratio and serum sodium. Patients with a sodium level < 135 mEq/L had a higher rate (31.25%) of adrenal insufficiency. *Conclusion.* Adrenal dysfunction was identified in a population of stable nonhospitalized cirrhotic patients. Our results suggest a possible role for adrenal dysfunction as a contributing factor in hyponatremia in cirrhosis independent of other known factors of neurohormonal activation secondary to systemic vasodilation.

1. Introduction

Liver cirrhosis has increasingly become a common cause of mortality and disease worldwide [1]. There are a wide variety of complications resulting from extrahepatic organ malfunction in the setting of liver cirrhosis. Hemodynamic derangements, frequently observed in more advanced stages of liver disease, are among the most challenging to treat. Circulatory failure resulting from decreased peripheral vascular resistance and systemic vasodilation, low mean arterial pressure, and poor response to vasopressors could be terminal events in advanced cirrhosis. These homodynamic alterations in cirrhosis share many features with adrenal dysfunction in critically ill patients referred to as "critical illness-related corticosteroid insufficiency" [2, 3].

Adrenal insufficiency has been revealed to be a common complication among critically ill patients with liver disease [4–6]. However, even among patients with stable liver cirrhosis, adrenal dysfunction (if investigated) may not be a rare finding [7, 8]. Proposed as "hepatoadrenal syndrome" [4], adrenal insufficiency in the setting of liver disease is shown to be associated with a high mortality rate [9, 10]. Cirrhotic patients with relative adrenal insufficiency are demonstrated to be at greater risks of circulatory derangement, severe sepsis, renal function impairment, and even hepatorenal syndrome type 1 [9].

The exact mechanism of adrenal insufficiency in cirrhosis is not well understood; however, several mechanisms are suggested. One of these proposed mechanisms is the role of cholesterol and its synthesis impairment in liver disease.

Cholesterol is an essential precursor for cortisol synthesis by adrenal gland. In cirrhosis the metabolism of lipoproteins is impaired and low levels of total cholesterol, high-density lipoprotein, and low-density lipoprotein are frequent findings [11, 12]. Low substrate level can lead to the decrease in the production of cortisol by the adrenal in cirrhosis especially in stress conditions. As another mechanism, there could be a possible role for negative feedback of proinflammatory cytokines (which are shown to have increased circulatory level in cirrhosis) on hypothalamic-pituitary-adrenal axis [13]. Adrenal hemorrhage in the setting of impaired coagulation in liver disease also has been implicated as a rare cause of adrenal insufficiency [13].

Prevalence of adrenal insufficiency in studies of patients with liver disease is found to be very variable, perhaps due to the heterogenicity of index cases in addition to different definitional criteria and methods of diagnosis [14, 15]. Most of these studies were on critically ill or decompensated cirrhotic patients, most during hospitalization. The present study is among the few that have evaluated adrenal function and associated factors in stable cirrhotic patients in an outpatient setting.

2. Material and Methods

The study included patients with liver cirrhosis referred to the outpatient liver clinics of Shiraz University of Medical Sciences. A diagnosis of cirrhosis was made based on liver histology, clinical manifestations and complications of cirrhosis, imaging findings, and/or a combination of these. Patients with a diagnosis of autoimmune hepatitis and those who had received steroid therapy for any reason during the last 6 months before study were excluded from the study. Critical illness, sepsis, and active infection were among other exclusion criteria. These included recent hospitalization for any critical illness or history of documented bacterial infection or receiving oral or parenteral antibiotic therapy within last 30 days before enrolment. The study was approved by the ethics committee of Shiraz University of Medical Sciences with reference number of EC-91-6369. Every patient gave informed consent prior to their participation in this study.

A total number of 105 patients were included in the study. Demographic data, physical findings, and the results of routine laboratory tests were recorded. Severity of liver disease was graded using model for end-stage liver disease (MELD). Patients were also classified at study entry according to their Child-Turcotte-Pugh (CTP) score and class using laboratory and clinical data. Patients were also classified into compensated cirrhosis and decompensated cirrhosis groups. Decompensation was defined as presence of any of the following conditions: history of ascites, variceal bleeding, or encephalopathy.

For evaluation of adrenal function, adrenocorticotropic hormone (ACTH) stimulation testing was performed on every subject in the Endocrinology and Metabolism Research Center lab. The test was done in the morning between 7:00 and 8:00 am after a 12 hr fast. Baseline cortisol level testing was performed on 2 cc blood drawn from each patient by venipuncture and stored in a colt tube. Then 250 μg of synthetic short acting ACTH was injected intravenously, and, after 60 minutes, another blood sample (2 cc) was taken for cortisol level measurement. Radio immunoassay (RIA) kit was used to measure the level of cortisol in collected plasma samples.

As our patients were not in critically ill condition, adrenal insufficiency was defined as a post ACTH stimulating serum cortisol level of less than 20 mcg/dl (550 nmol/L) [13–15].

Test results were divided into two groups: group 1 included patients with normal adrenal function and group 2 those with adrenal insufficiency.

Statistical analyses were conducted using Statistical Package for Social Sciences (SPSS, Chicago, IL, USA) release 16.0 for Windows. Nonparametric Mann–Whitney test was applied for comparing means of the two groups. Chi square test was used to determine whether the frequency of variables such as presence of ascites, history of gastrointestinal bleeding, encephalopathy, and spontaneous bacterial peritonitis are statistically significant across the two groups. Univariate analysis was used to define the factors associated with adrenal insufficiency. Multiple logistic regression models with backward elimination method were also employed to investigate the correlation of variables with adrenal insufficiency. Covariates with p values less than 0.05 were considered to have significant correlation. A receiver operator characteristic (ROC) curve was used to determine a cut-off value for serum sodium level to predict adrenal insufficiency. Area under the curve (AUC) more than 0.6 was considered acceptable. All p values less than 0.05 were considered significant.

3. Results

The study subjects were consisted of 105 cirrhotic patients, 74 males, ages 15 to 68 years, with a mean age of 40.5 ± 12.4 (±SD) years. Of the patients, 14 were Child class A, 50 were Child class B, and 41 were Child C. The mean MELD score was 18.19 ± 5.46 SD in all cases. Eighty-three patients (79%) had MELD scores of 15 or higher and were considered to be listed for liver transplant. Of all studied patients, 94 were classified as decompensated cirrhosis and only 11 were in the compensated cirrhosis group.

According to defined criteria, adrenal insufficiency was detected in 16 patients (15.23%).

Patients with normal adrenal function (group 1) were not different from group 2 in mean age and sex distribution. The two groups were not different with respect to levels of albumin, creatinine, total bilirubin, or CTP score and MELD score. However, group 2 patients had statistically significantly higher mean INR and lower mean serum sodium levels (see Table 1). Other factors such as presence and severity of ascites, encephalopathy, and history of spontaneous bacterial peritonitis or gastrointestinal bleeding were also investigated for the two groups (Table 1).

Patients with compensated cirrhosis were not statistically different from decompensated ones in the prevalence of adrenal insufficiency (18.2% versus 14.9% $p = 0.673$),

TABLE 1: Demographic data and clinical characteristics of all patients, patients with normal adrenal function (group 1) and adrenal insufficiency (group 2).

	All patients	Group 1 (Normal Adrenal Function)	Group 2 (Adrenal Insufficiency)	p values for differences between group 1 and 2
Age	40.5 ± 12.4	40.53 ± 12.97	40.38 ± 11.84	0.963
Male sex (%)	74 (70.48%)	60 (67.4%)	14 (87.5%)	0.141
MELD score	18.19 ± 5.46	17.88 ± 5.38	19.94 ± 5.73	0.188
CTP score	8.70 ± 1.67	8.61 ± 1.69	9.25 ± 1.53	0.193
Total bilirubin (mg/dl)	3.49 ± 3.04	3.55 ± 3.22	3.15 ± 1.7	0.64
Albumin (mg/dl)	3.4 ± 0.61	3.45 ± 0.59	3.13 ± 0.68	0.095
Creatinine (mg/dl)	1.11 ± 0.65	1.1 ± 0.69	1.17 ± 0.25	0.099
INR	1.97 ± 0.94	1.88 ± 0.81	2.52 ± 1.35	0.032
Sodium (mEq/L)	137.06 ± 7.43	137.88 ± 7.16	132.5 ± 7.53	0.012
Hyponatremia (%)	32 (30.5%)	10 (62.5%)	22 (27.8%)	0.006
Potassium (mEq/L)	4.2 ± 0.54	4.15 ± 0.51	4.5 ± 0.59	0.045
Encephalopathy (%)	79 (75.2%)	70 (78.7%)	9 (56.3%)	0.067
Ascites (%)	34 (32.4%)	32 (36%)	2 (12.5%)	0.065
History of GIB (%)	55 (52.4%)	45 (50.6%)	10 (62.5%)	0.379
History of SBP (%)	46 (43.8%)	41 (46.1%)	5 (31.25%)	0.271

Data are presented as mean ± standard deviation; MELD: model for end stage liver disease; CTP: Child-Turcotte-Pugh; INR: international normalized ratio; GIB: gastrointestinal bleeding; SBP: spontaneous bacterial peritonitis.

although the number of compensated patients was too small for separate analysis.

According to univariate analysis, while serum albumin, total bilirubin, CTP score, and MELD score were not associated with adrenal insufficiency, serum sodium and INR level showed significant associations ($p < 0.05$). The lack of association with adrenal insufficiency was also true for presence of ascites and history of gastrointestinal bleeding, encephalopathy, and spontaneous bacterial peritonitis. Using ROC curve analysis, the cut-off level of serum sodium with optimal sensitivity and specificity for association with adrenal insufficiency was determined to be 133 mEq/L (sensitivity: 0.625, specificity: 0.787) with AUC of 0.697. (Figure 1). To provide a better interpretation of the effect of serum sodium level, subjects were subsequently categorized to two groups, those below and those above 133 mEq/L. As expected, the group with lower sodium showed significant correlation with adrenal insufficiency (OR, 6.41 [95% CI, 1.980–19.047], p = 0.02). It was shown that, for every 1 mEq/L sodium level less than 133, there was a 6 times chance of adrenal insufficiency in our patients. However, categorization of the serum sodium level did not change our findings principally. Accordingly, in the multiple logistic model including both INR and serum sodium as categorical variable using cut-off of 133 mEq/L, INR was removed ($p = 0.001$).

The two variables, serum sodium level and serum potassium level, showed significant correlation but in reverse direction (p = 0.001) where the two variables moved in opposite directions. Regarding this correlation and in order to prevent colinearity, potassium was not entered in the multiple logistic model while sodium was present.

Regarding these results we decided to evaluate the rate of adrenal insufficiency in hyponatremic patients in our study group and compare them with those who did not have hyponatremia. Serum sodium level less than 135 mEq/L was regarded as hyponatremia [16]. Thirty-two of 105 patients (30.5%) were hyponatremic versus 73 (69.5%) with serum sodium levels ≥ 135 mEq/L. Patient with hyponatremia had significantly higher prevalence of adrenal insufficiency (31.25% versus 8.22% and p = 0.003) (Figure 2).

4. Discussion

The present study revealed that impaired adrenal function was present in 15.23% of nonhospitalized patients with liver cirrhosis, a population where adrenal function is not routinely tested. The considerable prevalence of this complication among critically ill patients with liver cirrhosis has been established by previous studies. In an intensive care unit (ICU) based study, the rate of adrenal insufficiency was reported to be 66% among patients with decompensated cirrhosis and 33% among those with acute liver failure [4]. In another study, again in an ICU setting, a rate of 29.9% was reported in cirrhotic patients with gastroesophageal variceal bleeding [3]. Rates as high as 68% and 51% were reported in cirrhosis with severe sepsis or septic shock, by others [5, 6]. The rate for adrenal insufficiency in our patients is lower than for those in studies of hospitalized cirrhotics. However, our study is one of only a few that was done in stable cirrhotic patients [15]. Adrenal insufficiency is reported to be a more common complication in cirrhosis with variceal bleeding compared with stable hospitalized cirrhotic

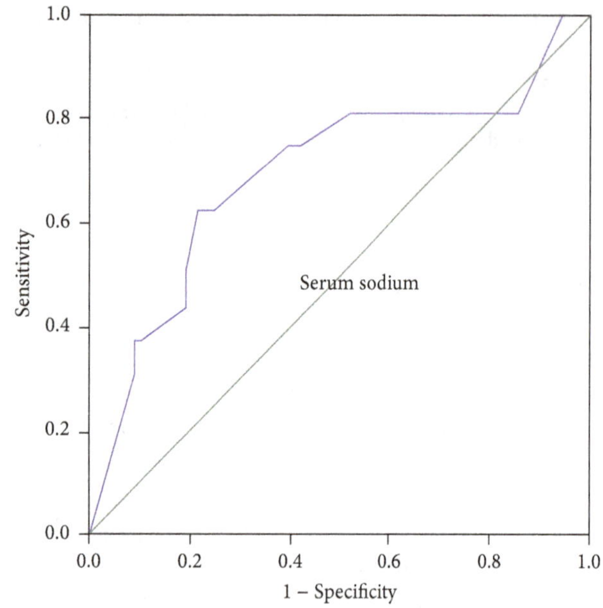

FIGURE 1: Receiver operator characteristic (ROC) curve for serum sodium in cirrhotic patients tested for adrenal insufficiency.

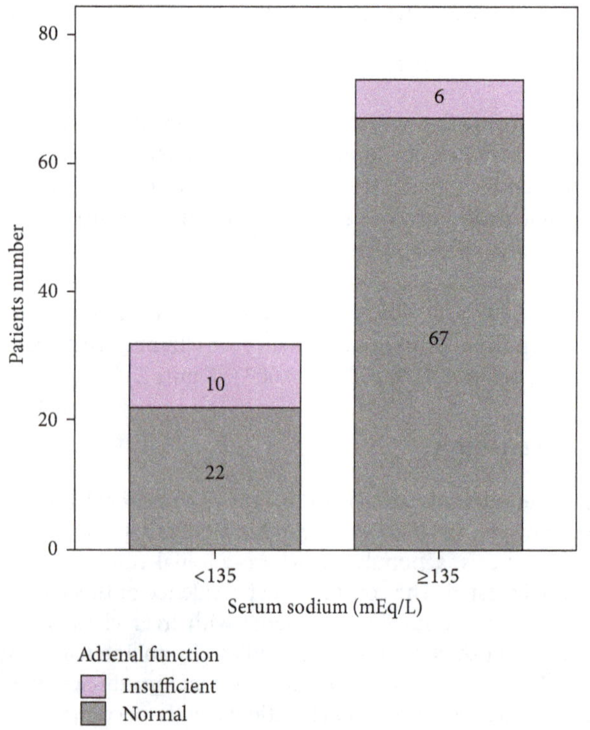

FIGURE 2: Adrenal function in cirrhotic patients with hyponatremia versus nonhyponatremic ones.

patients [8]. Even in studies conducted on patients with stable cirrhosis, variable rates have been reported for this complication. Different methods of testing, inhomogeneity of aimed patient population regarding the etiology of liver disease and presence of complications, and status of hospitalization are among the factors contributing to this difference. In contrast with most of the similar studies, all of the patients we included in this study were selected from outpatient clinics and were not hospitalized. Patients were from both sexes and included patients with a wide variety of severity of liver disease (MELD scores: 6 to more than 40) and many etiologies, except for autoimmune hepatitis where steroid use would have been a confounding factor.

In this study the indices of severity of liver disease, MELD and CPT score, although higher in the group with adrenal insufficiency, did not significantly differ from patients with normal adrenal function. A similar finding was reported in the study by Acevedo et al. who did not find any correlation between disease severity and relative adrenal insufficiency in their hospitalized patients with acute decompensation of cirrhosis but who were not critically ill [9]. However, significantly higher levels of INR in our patients with adrenal insufficiency may be indicative of more impaired liver function. High INR is an index of impaired synthetic function of liver and is one of the three variable components in the MELD formula, and the one with the highest coefficient [17, 18].

The major finding of our study is the association of hyponatremia with adrenal dysfunction in our patient population. In logistic models, serum sodium level (whether continuous or categorical) was shown to have the highest relation with adrenal insufficiency among other evaluated factors. This finding was also similar to the finding reported by Acevedo et al. [9]. Hyponatremia is a known complication in advanced cirrhosis and harbors a grave prognosis [19–21]. The mechanism of development of hyponatremia in liver cirrhosis is similar to what happens in heart failure [22]. Arterial underfilling resulting from systemic vasodilation in cirrhosis plays a key role in compensatory activation of neurohormonal system [23]. Nonosmotic release of arginine vasopressin (AVP), activation of sympathetic nervous system, and rennin-angiotensin are among these compensatory mechanisms [22, 24]. The result of action of these mechanisms is sodium and water retention and dilutional hyponatremia.

Glucocorticoid deficiency, on the other hand, may be associated with hyponatremia. With glucocorticoid deficiency, the hypotonic suppression of the osmostat for AVP release is impaired. The results of persistent secretion of AVP are clinical features similar to the syndrome of inappropriate secretion of antidiuretic hormone (SIADH). Although the exact mechanism for this phenomenon is not well defined, the lack of tonically inhibitory effect of glucocorticoids on AVP which responds to glucocorticoid administration may be contributing to this [22, 25].

Our finding of high rate of hyponatremia in patients with cirrhosis and adrenal insufficiency and its reverse (high rate of adrenal insufficiency in cirrhosis with hyponatremia) might be attributed to adrenal dysfunction itself rather than just a symptom of more advanced circulatory dysfunction in patients. It was suggested that adrenal dysfunction may play a role in the development of cardiomyopathy and hepatorenal syndrome in cirrhosis [26]. High plasma renin activity and norepinephrine concentration and also a high probability of hepatorenal syndrome type 1 have been shown in cirrhotic patients with relative adrenal insufficiency [9]. According to the results of ours and similar studies, it can be concluded that adrenal dysfunction could be considered as one of the factors contributing to pathogenesis of hemodynamic alteration in cirrhosis.

5. Conclusion

In summary, our study showed that adrenal insufficiency is not a rare complication in cirrhosis, even in nonhospitalized patients. The relation of adrenal insufficiency with low serum sodium level points to the possible role for adrenal dysfunction in hemodynamic instability observed in cirrhosis. The effect of medical treatment of adrenal insufficiency on the management of hyponatremia, circulatory failure, and prevention of resultant complications in cirrhosis such as hepatorenal syndrome could be the subject of future studies.

Abbreviations

ACTH: Adrenocorticotropic hormone
AUC: Area under the curve
AVP: Arginine vasopressin
CTP: Child-Turcotte-Pugh
ICU: Intensive care unit
INR: International normalized ratio
MELD: Model for end-stage liver disease
RIA: Radio immunoassay
ROC: Receiver operator characteristic
SIADH: Inappropriate secretion of antidiuretic hormone.

Disclosure

Preliminary result of this study was presented as an abstract in 24th annual conference of Asian Pacific Association for the Study of the Liver.

Authors' Contributions

Maryam Moini designed the work, referred patients, collected and analyzed data, and wrote the paper. Mitra Yazdani Sarvestani followed patients and collected data. Mesbah Shams designed methods and visited and followed patients as endocrine consultant. Massod Nomovi collected and analyzed data.

References

[1] E. A. Tsochatzis, J. Bosch, and A. K. Burroughs, "Liver cirrhosis," *The Lancet*, vol. 383, no. 9930, pp. 1749–1761, 2014.

[2] P. E. Marik, S. M. Pastores, D. Annane et al., "Recommendations for the diagnosis and management of corticosteroid insufficiency in critically ill adult patients: consensus statements from an international task force by the American college of critical care medicine," *Critical Care Medicine*, vol. 36, no. 6, pp. 1937–1949, 2008.

[3] M.-H. Tsai, H.-C. Huang, Y.-S. Peng et al., "Critical illness-related corticosteroid insufficiency in cirrhotic patients with acute gastroesophageal variceal bleeding: risk factors and association with outcome," *Critical Care Medicine*, vol. 42, no. 12, pp. 2546–2555, 2014.

[4] P. E. Marik, T. Gayowski, and T. E. Starzl, "The hepatoadrenal syndrome: a common yet unrecognized clinical condition," *Critical Care Medicine*, vol. 33, no. 6, pp. 1254–1259, 2005.

[5] J. Fernández, A. Escorsell, M. Zabalza et al., "Adrenal insufficiency in patients with cirrhosis and septic shock: effect of treatment with hydrocortisone on survival," *Hepatology*, vol. 44, no. 5, pp. 1288–1295, 2006.

[6] M.-H. Tsai, Y.-S. Peng, Y.-C. Chen et al., "Adrenal insufficiency in patients with cirrhosis, severe sepsis and septic shock," *Hepatology*, vol. 43, no. 4, pp. 673–681, 2006.

[7] G. Fede, L. Spadaro, T. Tomaselli et al., "Assessment of adrenocortical reserve in stable patients with cirrhosis," *Journal of Hepatology*, vol. 54, no. 2, pp. 243–250, 2011.

[8] C. K. Triantos, M. Marzigie, G. Fede et al., "Critical illness-related corticosteroid insufficiency in patients with cirrhosis and variceal bleeding," *Clinical Gastroenterology and Hepatology*, vol. 9, no. 7, pp. 595–601, 2011.

[9] J. Acevedo, J. Fernández, V. Prado et al., "Relative adrenal insufficiency in decompensated cirrhosis: relationship to short-term risk of severe sepsis, hepatorenal syndrome, and death," *Hepatology*, vol. 58, no. 5, pp. 1757–1765, 2013.

[10] R. Harry, G. Auzinger, and J. Wendon, "The clinical importance of adrenal insufficiency in acute hepatic dysfunction," *Hepatology*, vol. 36, no. 2, pp. 395–402, 2002.

[11] C. Cicognani, M. Malavolti, A. M. Morselli-Labate, L. Zamboni, C. Sama, and L. Barbara, "Serum lipid and lipoprotein patterns in patients with liver cirrhosis and chronic active hepatitis," *Archives of Internal Medicine*, vol. 157, no. 7, pp. 792–796, 1997.

[12] M. Trieb, A. Horvath, R. Birner-Gruenberger et al., "Liver disease alters high-density lipoprotein composition, metabolism and function," *Biochimica et Biophysica Acta - Molecular and Cell Biology of Lipids*, vol. 1861, no. 7, pp. 630–638, 2016.

[13] A. K. A. Karagiannis, T. Nakouti, C. Pipili, and E. Cholongitas, "Adrenal insufficiency in patients with decompensated cirrhosis," *World Journal of Hepatology*, vol. 7, no. 8, pp. 1112–1124, 2015.

[14] A. Trifan, S. Chiriac, and C. Stanciu, "Update on adrenal insufficiency in patients with liver cirrhosis," *World Journal of Gastroenterology*, vol. 19, no. 4, pp. 445–456, 2013.

[15] G. Fede, L. Spadaro, T. Tomaselli et al., "Adrenocortical dysfunction in liver disease: a systematic review," *Hepatology*, vol. 55, no. 4, pp. 1282–1291, 2012.

[16] G. Spasovski, R. Vanholder, B. Allolio et al., "Clinical practice guideline on diagnosis and treatment of hyponatraemia," *Nephrology Dialysis Transplantation*, vol. 29, supplement 2, pp. i1–i39, 2014.

[17] M. Malinchoc, P. S. Kamath, F. D. Gordon, C. J. Peine, J. Rank, and P. C. J. Ter Borg, "A model to predict poor survival in patients undergoing transjugular intrahepatic portosystemic shunts," *Hepatology*, vol. 31, no. 4, pp. 864–871, 2000.

[18] R. B. Freeman Jr., R. H. Wiesner, A. Harper et al., "The new liver allocation system: moving toward evidence-based transplantation policy," *Liver Transplantation*, vol. 8, no. 9, pp. 851–858, 2002.

[19] S. W. Biggins, H. J. Rodriguez, P. Bacchetti, N. M. Bass, J. P. Roberts, and N. A. Terrault, "Serum sodium predicts mortality in patients listed for liver transplantation," *Hepatology*, vol. 41, no. 1, pp. 32–39, 2005.

[20] W. R. Kim, S. W. Biggins, W. K. Kremers et al., "Hyponatremia and mortality among patients on the liver-transplant waiting list," *The New England Journal of Medicine*, vol. 359, no. 10, pp. 1018–1026, 2008.

[21] M. Moini, M. K. Hoseini-Asl, S. A. Taghavi et al., "Hyponatremia a valuable predictor of early mortality in patients with cirrhosis listed for liver transplantation," *Clinical Transplantation*, vol. 25, no. 4, pp. 638–645, 2011.

[22] R. W. Schrier, S. Sharma, and D. Shchekochikhin, "Hyponatraemia: more than just a marker of disease severity?" *Nature Reviews Nephrology*, vol. 9, no. 1, pp. 37–50, 2013.

[23] S. John and P. J. Thuluvath, "Hyponatremia in cirrhosis: pathophysiology and management," *World Journal of Gastroenterology*, vol. 21, no. 11, pp. 3197–3205, 2015.

[24] J. H. Henriksen, F. Bendtsen, A. L. Gerbes, N. J. Christensen, H. Ring-Larsen, and T. I. A. Sorensen, "Estimated central blood volume in cirrhosis: relationship to sympathetic nervous activity, β-adrenergic blockade and atrial natriuretic factor," *Hepatology*, vol. 16, no. 5, pp. 1163–1170, 1992.

[25] K. Kamoi, T. Tamura, K. Tanaka, M. Ishibashi, and T. Yamaji, "Hyponatremia and osmoregulation of thirst and vasopressin secretion in patients with adrenal insufficiency," *Journal of Clinical Endocrinology and Metabolism*, vol. 77, no. 6, pp. 1584–1588, 1993.

[26] M. Egerod Israelsen, L. L. Gluud, and A. Krag, "Acute kidney injury and hepatorenal syndrome in cirrhosis," *Journal of Gastroenterology and Hepatology*, vol. 30, no. 2, pp. 236–243, 2015.

23

The Relationship between Gender, Severity of Disease, Treatment Type, and Employment Outcome in Patients with Inflammatory Bowel Disease in Israel

Timna Naftali,[1] Adi Eindor-Abarbanel ,[2] Nahum Ruhimovich,[1] Ariella Bar-Gil Shitrit,[3] Fabiana Sklerovsky-Benjaminov,[1] Fred Konikoff,[1] Shay Matalon ,[2] Haim Shirin ,[2] Yael Milgrom,[3] Tomer Ziv-Baran,[4] and Efrat Broide [2]

[1]Department of Gastroenterology and Hepatology, Meir Medical Center, affiliated with the Sackler School of Medicine, Tel Aviv University, Tel Aviv, Israel
[2]The Kamila Gonczarowski Institute for Gastroenterology and Liver Diseases, Assaf Harofeh Medical Center, affiliated with the Sackler School of Medicine, Tel Aviv University, Tel Aviv, Israel
[3]Digestive Diseases Institute, Shaare Zedek Medical Center, Jerusalem, Israel
[4]Department of Epidemiology and Preventive Medicine, School of Public Health, Sackler Faculty of Medicine, Tel Aviv University, Tel Aviv, Israel

Correspondence should be addressed to Adi Eindor-Abarbanel; adiabarbanel@gmail.com

Academic Editor: Kevork M. Peltekian

Introduction. Since individuals with IBD typically experience symptoms during their prime years of employment, it raises the question about IBD impact on employment status. Most studies concentrated on absenteeism from work with varying results in different populations. However, absenteeism reflects only one dimension of the ability to work and does not expose the problem of inability to hold a full-time job. *Aims.* To evaluate the influence of IBD on unemployment and working hours in Israel. Secondary aims were to investigate the correlation between working hours and the type of medical treatment and the impact of severity of disease. *Patients and Methods.* Demographic data, employment status, number of weekly working hours, and disease parameters. The data was compared to that of the general Israeli population extracted from the website of the Central Bureau of Statistics. *Results.* 242 IBD patients were interviewed. Patients median age was 37.04(IQR 30.23-44.68) years and 88 (36.4%) were men and 154 (63.6%) women. Diagnosis of CD was established in 167 (69%) patients and UC in 65 (26.9%). There was no significant reduction in employment rates or working hours among the IBD patients comparing to the general population. Immunosuppressive or biologic treatment did not influence employment status. The unemployed patients had higher disease severity (median 7.33, IQR 5-10.66) compared to employed patients (median 6, IQR 3.66-7.66; p=0.003). *Conclusions.* Although IBD patients in Israel do not have higher unemployment, those with severe disease have lower proportion of employment.

1. Introduction

Inflammatory bowel diseases (IBD) are characterized by episodic and continuous symptoms including diarrhea, abdominal discomfort, and fatigue among many other complaints. These symptoms can interfere with the ability to perform daily routine activities [1]. Although few people with IBD experience permanent disability [2], the relapsing-remitting nature of the disease may lead to recurrent hospitalization and periods of disability [3–5]. Additionally, some patients need routine intravenous treatments such as biologics [6, 7] and iron supplementation [8, 9]. These are time-consuming and can challenge IBD patients' ability to meet their obligations to their place of employment.

The onset of IBD can occur at any age [10], but Crohn's disease (CD) is most often diagnosed in patients in their third decade of life and ulcerative colitis (UC) in patients in their fourth decade [11], corresponding with productive work years. Since individuals with IBD typically experience symptoms during their prime years of employment, we evaluated the impact of IBD on employment status. Previous studies have concentrated on absenteeism from work with varying results among different populations [3, 12]. However, absenteeism reflects only one dimension of the ability to work and does not expose the problem of inability to hold a full-time job. Other studies explored employment status of patients, but did not refer to the number of hours worked [3]. Furthermore, only one study investigated the long-term impact of the disease on the ability of IBD patients to work [13].

Israel has the third highest prevalence of IBD in the world and this has nearly doubled in the past decade [14]. At the end of 2015, 38,291 IBD patients were residing in Israel, with a prevalence of 459 per 100,000 (0.46%). Despite this high prevalence, data on its effect on employment status in the Israeli population is lacking. In this study, we evaluated the influence of IBD on unemployment and working hours in Israel. Secondary aims were to investigate the correlation between working hours and the type of medical treatment and disease severity.

2. Methods

2.1. Participants. Between November 2015 and May 2017, consecutive ambulatory patients, ages 25 to 65 years, with an established diagnosis of IBD were enrolled in the study. Diagnosis of Crohn's disease (CD) and ulcerative colitis (UC) were previously confirmed by established criteria based on clinical, endoscopic, histopathological, and radiological findings. Patients were recruited from three university-affiliated hospitals in Israel: Assaf Harofeh, Meir Medical Center, and Shaare Zedek Medical Center.

All patients completed questionnaires regarding demographic data, employment status, number of weekly working hours, and disease parameters. The study was approved by the Ethics Committee of each hospital. All patients provided signed informed consent.

Data about employment rates and working hours of the general population was extracted from the website of the Central Bureau of Statistics (CBS) of Israel, which was updated in 2016.

Clinical disease severity was calculated based on a scale modified from a study by the GETAID [15] group. This scale was developed by a panel of 20 IBD experts from the "Groupe d'Etudes Thérapeutiques des Affections Inflamma- toires du tube Digestif" (GETAID) who selected the most relevant criteria for discriminating a severe from a mild-to-moderate CD course during a 15-year period. The severity scale was calculated based on an average of disease severity as reported by the physician. The scale was graded on a scale from 0 to 5 (0, no symptoms; 1, mild symptoms; 2, medium symptoms; 3, active disease; 4, hospitalization in the past year; 5, surgery in the past year or current stoma). Another component of severity was based on medical treatment, based on the total score of a scale varying from 0 to 5 (0, no treatment; 1, 5-ASA or antibiotics; 2, less than 10 mg per day dose steroids; 3, steroids in a regular dose; 4, immunomodulatory treatment; 5, biological treatment). These scales were calculated for each year of the last three years. The final score was the average of the score from each year over the last three years (the Appendix).

2.2. Data Analysis. Categorical variables were described using frequency and percentage. Continuous variables were evaluated for normal distribution using histograms and Q-Q plots. One sample T- test was used to compare working hours to those reported by the CBS. Working status was compared to the CBS using one sample binomial test. Within the cohort, categorical variables were compared using chi-squared test and Fisher's exact test. Continuous variables were compared using independent simple t-test. Spearman's rank correlation coefficient was used to describe the association between continuous variables.

All statistical analyses were performed using IBM SPSS Statistics for Windows, Version 23.0 (Released 2015,IBM Corp. Armonk, NY).

3. Results

3.1. Patient Population. From November 2015 through May 2017, 242 consecutive IBD patients attending outpatient clinics in the participating hospitals were interviewed. Patients' median age was 37.04(IQR 30.23-44.68) years and 88 (36.4%) were men and 154 (63.6%) women. A total of 167 (69%) patients were diagnosed with CD, 65(26.9%) with UC and 10 (4.1%) with IBD-U and 50 (20%) with perianal disease. Demographic and disease characteristics are listed in Table 1. Four patients did not report employment status. Because of the low rates of refusal, these patients were not analyzed separately.

3.2. Employment and Working Hours. Employment status and working hours, according to gender are compared in Table 2. Table 3 compares working hours between the study patients and the Israeli population according to gender. There were 79 patients on immunosuppressive drugs, and 19% were unemployed, while the rate of unemployment in the other patients was 16.5% (p=0.625). There was no significant difference in the weekly hours worked between these two groups (40.08 ±12.97) and (39.56 ± 13.51, respectively; p=0.809).

Among 116 patients receiving biologic treatment, the unemployment rate was 20.7%, as compared to the other patients whose unemployment rate was 13.9% (p=0.168). There was no significant difference in the working hours between these two groups (39.99 ± 12.58 vs. 39.49 ± 13.89, respectively; p=0.801).

There was a significant difference in disease severity scores between the unemployed patients (median 7.33, IQR 5-10.66) as compared to the employed patients (median 6, IQR 3.66-7.66; p=0.003). There was also a medium correlation between working hours and disease severity (Spearman correlation = 0.368).

TABLE 1: Demographic and disease characteristics.

Characteristic	Patients N=242
Age median(IQR)	37.04(30.23-44.68)
Gender n(%)	
Male	88(36.4)
Female	154 (63.2)
Education >12 yrs	154(63.3)
Marital status n(%)	
Single	52(21.5)
In a relationship	171(70.7)
Past relationship	17(7)
Income level n(%)	
Low	126(54.3)
Medium	46(19.8)
High	60(25.9)
Disease type	
Crohn's	167(69)
UC	65(26.9)
IBDU	10(4.1)
Other diseases n(%)	
Diabetes	10(4.1)
Cardiovascular	4(1.7)
Hypertension	10(4.1)
Cancer	2(0.8)
Lung	3(1.2)
Hyperlipidemia	13(5.4)
Other disease	26(10.7)
Disease severity score	6(3.66-8)
Medications n(%)	
Topical 5_ASA	24(9.9)
Tab 5_ASA	80(33.1)
Budesonide	12(5)
Prednisone	19(7.9)
Immunosuppressive	80(33.2)
Biologics	118(48.8)
Cannabis	22(9.1)
More than 3 medications	53 (21.9)

4. Discussion

Crohn's disease and UC affect nearly 0.5% of the Israeli population [5]. The relapsing-remitting disease course and the complications are major sources of morbidity [3, 16]. The diseases are associated with work absenteeism and constitute substantial economic burden to employers [17].

Surprisingly, we found that both employment status and working hours of IBD patients did not differ from those of the general population. These results are similar to the findings of the Danish cohort published by Vester-Andersen et al. [3], but were in contrast with the study of Mahlich et al. [4] from Japan who described a lower employment rate in IBD patients as compared to the general population. When divided according to age groups, Malich [4] observed that older IBD patients have lower employment rates than does the general population. Vester-Andersen also demonstrated that patients with IBD were at higher risk for work disability, particularly male patients older than 55 years-of-age. We also found that older male patients worked fewer hours per week, although this trend did not reach statistical significance because of the small sample size.

Although employment among IBD patients overall equaled that of the general population, this was not true for the subgroup of patients with severe disease. Disease severity was significantly correlated with rates of unemployment and with fewer hours worked per week. Perianal Crohn's disease as a separate severity measure was recently reported to be associated with unemployment in Crohn's disease. When correcting for age, disease duration, inflammatory bowel disease-related surgery, and faecal incontinence, active perianal disease was independently affecting employment (OR 0.67; 95% CI 0.50–0.91; $P = 0.01$). Although in our study we did not consider any perianal disease, we did include complicated perianal disease requiring surgery as a component in the disease severity scale [18].

This study used a comprehensive method to evaluate disease severity by using a modified calculator from the GETAID [6] group. It considers the 3-year course of the disease instead of a certain time frame. We preferred this approach because of the assumption that employment status is influenced by a long period of time prior to that currently being investigated. Therefore, a score that reflects disease severity over a prolonged period is superior to a score that reflects disease activity over one week [19].

Although we demonstrated that more severe disease is correlated with unemployment, immunosuppressive or biologic treatment was not correlated with unemployment among IBD patients. Biologic treatment sometimes entails IV administration and may therefore cause absenteeism. However, it may induce remission and prevent permanent compromise of work ability.

The current study has some limitations. Only ambulatory patients were included; thus, there is a possibility of selection bias, because adherent patients who attend outpatients clinics may have better rates of employment than nonadherent patients do. Also, we included only patients 25 years and older because we wanted to compare the results with the data available from the CBS. Finally, we did not differentiate between patients receiving medications intravenously [20, 21] or subcutaneously [22] because the groups were too small to analyze separately. As this study investigated permanent effects on unemployment rather than absenteeism, we assumed all biologic treatments can have an effect due to adverse reactions [23–25] and the inconvenience of the route of administration.

This study is the first to investigate the roll of IBD on work habits among Israeli IBD patients. We demonstrated that although these patients do not have higher rates of unemployment, those with severe disease have a lower proportion of employment. In addition, the type of drug administered did not affect employment rates. Therefore, health providers in Israel should pay more attention to evaluating disease severity and increase their treatment efforts when facing a patient with sever disease. The aim of treatment should be not only to

TABLE 2: Comparison of the proportion of employment among IBD patients and the general Israeli population.

Gender	Israeli citizen	Study patients	p-value	Crohn's	p-value	UC	p-value
Men	81.4	89.5	<0.001	92.1	<0.001	78.9	0.482
Women	72	78.9	0.043	76.2	0.201	86.7	0.021

TABLE 3: Comparison of hours worked per week between patients and the general population.

Age group	Men				Women			
	Patients, mean (SD)	N	General population, mean	P-value	Patients mean (SD)	N	General population, mean	P-value
25-34.9	43.85 (10.74)	32	43.9	0.9	37.44 (11.7)	55	36.4	0.51
35-44.9	46.75 (12.31)	24	46.9	0.953	37.67 (15.42)	34	37.5	0.947
45-54.9	40 (19.27)	10	46.5	0.314	33.33 (13.58)	15	36.9	0.327
55-64.9	38.33 (9.31)	6	44.1	0.19	39 (9.76)	7	34.5	0.268

TABLE 4: Disease severity questionnaire.

	Year:		
Disease activity:	**This year**	**One year ago**	**Two years ago**
No Symptoms-0			
Mild Symptoms-1			
Medium Symptoms-2			
Active Disease- 3			
Hospitalization- 4			
Surgery- 5			
Stoma- 5			
(a) Highest score			
Treatment:			
No Treatment-0			
5-ASA or Antibiotics-1			
Low dose steroids-2			
Steroids-3			
Immunosuppresive-4			
Biologics-5			
(b) Sum of treatments			
Total year score (a+b)			

improve patients' symptoms, but also to lower unemployment rates.

Appendix

See Table 4.

Authors' Contributions

Adi Eindor-Abarbanel, Timna Naftali, Nahum Ruhimovich, and Efrat Broide performed the research and analyzed the data. Adi Eindor-Abarbanel, Timna Naftali, Nahum Ruhimovich, Efrat Broide, Ariella Bar-Gil Shitrit, Yael Milgrom, Haim Shirin, Shay Matalon, Fred Konikoff, and Fabiana Sklerovsky-Benjaminov collected the data. Timna Naftali, Nahum Ruhimovich, Efrat Broide designed the research study. Adi Eindor-Abarbanel, Nahum Ruhimovich, Timna Naftali, Efrat Broide wrote the paper. Adi Eindor-Abarbanel, Haim Shirin, Shay Matalon, Fabiana Sklerovsky-Benjaminov, Fred Konikoff, Yael Milgrom, and Ariella Bar-Gil Shitrit contributed to the study design. Tomer Ziv-Baran statistical analysis and wrote parts of the manuscript. All authors had full access to all the data in the study, approved the final draft submitted, and had final responsibility for the decision to submit for publication. Timna Naftali and Adi Eindor-Abarbanel contributed equally to this study.

References

[1] J. H. Sellin, "Deconstructing disability in inflammatory bowel disease," *Clinical Gastroenterology and Hepatology*, vol. 12, no. 8, pp. 1338–1341, 2014.

[2] M. van der Have, H. H. Fidder, M. Leenders et al., "Self-reported disability in patients with inflammatory bowel disease largely determined by disease activity and illness perceptions," *Inflammatory Bowel Diseases*, vol. 21, no. 2, pp. 369–377, 2015.

[3] M. K. Vester-Andersen, M. V. Prosberg, I. Vind, M. Andersson, T. Jess, and F. Bendtsen, "Low risk of unemployment, sick leave, and work disability among patients with inflammatory bowel disease: a 7-year follow-up study of a danish inception cohort," *Inflammatory Bowel Diseases*, vol. 21, no. 10, pp. 2296–2303, 2015.

[4] F. Balzola, G. Cullen, H. O. GT, R. K. Russell, and J. Wehkamp, "Work disability in inflammatory bowel disease patients 10 years after disease onset: Results from the IBSEN Study," *Inflamm Bowel Dis Monit*, vol. 13, pp. 18-19, 2012.

[5] B. Lo, M. V. Prosberg, L. L. Gluud et al., "Systematic review and meta-analysis: assessment of factors affecting disability in inflammatory bowel disease and the reliability of the inflammatory bowel disease disability index," *Alimentary Pharmacology & Therapeutics*, vol. 47, no. 1, pp. 6–15, 2018.

[6] F. Magro and F. Portela, "Management of inflammatory bowel disease with infliximab and other anti-tumor necrosis factor alpha therapies," *BioDrugs*, vol. 24, 1, no. 1, pp. 3–14, 2010.

[7] O. H. Nielsen, K. Bendtzen, and J. Pedersen, "Anti-TNF-α therapy for extraintestinal manifestations of inflammatory bowel disease," *Anti-Tumor Necrosis Factor Therapy in Inflammatory Bowel Disease*, pp. 206–213, 2015.

[8] R. Evstatiev and C. Gasche, "Diagnosis and management of anemia in IBD," *Inflammatory Bowel Disease Monitor*, vol. 11, no. 4, pp. 152–159, 2011.

[9] M. F. Neurath, "Current and emerging therapeutic targets for IBD," *Nature Reviews Gastroenterology & Hepatology*, vol. 14, no. 5, pp. 269–278, 2017.

[10] J. Ruel, D. Ruane, S. Mehandru, C. Gower-Rousseau, and J.-F. Colombel, "IBD across the age spectrum—is it the same disease?" *Nature Reviews Gastroenterology & Hepatology*, vol. 11, no. 2, pp. 88–98, 2014.

[11] J. Cosnes, C. Gowerrousseau, P. Seksik, and A. Cortot, "Epidemiology and natural history of inflammatory bowel diseases," *Gastroenterology*, vol. 140, no. 6, pp. 1785–1794, 2011.

[12] T. B. Gibson, E. Ng, and R. J. Ozminkowski, "The direct and indirect cost burden of Crohns disease and ulcerative colitis," *Journal of Occupational and Environmental Medicine*, vol. 50, no. 11, pp. 1261–1272, 2008.

[13] J. Mahlich, K. Matsuoka, Y. Nakamura, and R. Sruamsiri, "The relationship between socio-demographic factors, health status, treatment type, and employment outcome in patients with inflammatory bowel disease in Japan," *BMC Public Health*, vol. 17, no. 1, article no. 623, 2017.

[14] "A switch in the prevalence ratio of Crohn's disease vs".

[15] J. Y. Mary and R. Modigliani, "Development and validation of an endoscopic index of the severity for Crohn's disease: a prospective multicentre study. Groupe d'Etudes Therapeutiques des Affections Inflammatoires du Tube Digestif (GETAID)," *Gut*, vol. 30, no. 7, pp. 983–989, 1989.

[16] S. Danese and C. Fiocchi, "Ulcerative colitis," *The New England Journal of Medicine*, vol. 365, no. 18, pp. 1713–1725, 2011.

[17] C. Gunnarsson, J. Chen, J. A. Rizzo, J. A. Ladapo, A. Naim, and J. H. Lofland, "The employee absenteeism costs of inflammatory bowel disease: Evidence from US national survey data," *Journal of Occupational and Environmental Medicine*, vol. 55, no. 4, pp. 393–401, 2013.

[18] P. F. Vollebregt, A. A. van Bodegraven, T. M. Markus-de Kwaadsteniet, D. van der Horst, and R. J. Felt-Bersma, "Impacts of perianal disease and faecal incontinence on quality of life and employment in 1092 patients with inflammatory bowel disease," *Alimentary Pharmacology & Therapeutics*, vol. 47, no. 9, pp. 1253–1260, 2018.

[19] J.-M. Chen, T. Liu, S. Gao, X.-D. Tong, F.-H. Deng, and B. Nie, "Efficacy of noninvasive evaluations in monitoring inflammatory bowel disease activity: A prospective study in China," *World Journal of Gastroenterology*, vol. 23, no. 46, pp. 8235–8247, 2017.

[20] L. Guidi, C. Felice, M. Marzo, and A. Armuzzi, "Infliximab in inflammatory bowel diseases: Pharmacology, uses and limitations," *Infliximab: Pharmacology, Uses and Limitations*, pp. 99–118, 2012.

[21] M. A. Kamm, "Safety issues relating to biological therapies, with special reference to infliximab therapy," *Ibd and Salicylates*, vol. 24, pp. 79–86, 2001.

[22] G. Fiorino, L. Peyrin-Biroulet, A. Repici, A. Malesci, and S. Danese, "Adalimumab in ulcerative colitis: Hypes and hopes," *Expert Opinion on Biological Therapy*, vol. 11, no. 1, pp. 109–116, 2011.

[23] W. Blonski and G. R. Lichtenstein, "Safety of biologic therapy," *Inflammatory Bowel Diseases*, vol. 13, no. 6, pp. 769–796, 2007.

[24] M. Chandler and M. Borum, "Discontinuation of biologic therapy may be required for treatment of Clostridium difficile in Crohn's patients: A case of Adalimumab complicating treatment of relapsing C. difficile infection," *Inflammatory Bowel Diseases*, vol. 17, pp. S41–S42, 2011.

[25] I. Grimes, A. Soni, and F. Caldera, "Reactivation of latent tuberculosis after treatment with biologic therapy," *Inflammatory Bowel Diseases*, vol. 18, p. S14, 2012.

24

Laparoscopy-Assisted versus Open Hepatectomy for Live Liver Donor

Bin Zhang,[1,2] Yu Pan,[1,2] Ke Chen,[1,2] Hendi Maher,[2] Ming-Yu Chen,[1,2] He-Pan Zhu,[1,2] Yi-Bin Zhu,[1,2] Yi Dai,[1] Jiang Chen,[1] and Xiu-jun Cai[1]

[1] *Department of General Surgery, Sir Run Run Shaw Hospital, School of Medicine, Zhejiang University, 3 East Qingchun Road, Hangzhou, Zhejiang Province 310016, China*
[2] *School of Medicine, Zhejiang University, 866 Yuhangtang Road, Hangzhou, Zhejiang Province 310058, China*

Correspondence should be addressed to Xiu-jun Cai; srrsh_cxj@zju.edu.cn

Academic Editor: Kevork M. Peltekian

Objective. To assess the feasibility, safety, and potential benefits of laparoscopy-assisted living donor hepatectomy (LADH) in comparison with open living donor hepatectomy (ODH) for liver transplantation. *Background*. LADH is becoming increasingly common for living donor liver transplant around the world. We aim to determine the efficacy of LADH and compare it with ODH. *Methods*. A systematic search on PubMed, Embase, Cochrane Library, and Web of Science was conducted in May 2017. *Results*. Nine studies were suitable for this analysis, involving 979 patients. LADH seemed to be associated with increased operation time (WMD = 24.85 min; 95% CI: −3.01~52.78, $P = 0.08$), less intraoperative blood loss (WMD = −59.92 ml; 95% CI: −94.58~−25.27, $P = 0.0007$), similar hospital stays (WMD = −0.47 d; 95% CI: −1.78~0.83, $P = 0.47$), less postoperative complications (RR = 0.70, 95% CI: 0.51~0.94, $P = 0.02$), less analgesic use (SMD = −0.22; 95% CI: −0.44~−0.11, $P = 0.04$), similar transfusion rates (RR = 0.82; 95% CI: 0.24~3.12, $P = 0.82$), and similar graft weights (WMD = 7.31 g; 95% CI: −23.45~38.07, $P = 0.64$). *Conclusion*. Our results indicate that LADH is a safe and effective technique and, when compared to ODH.

1. Introduction

Liver transplantation from living donors is a potential treatment for end-stage liver disease. And due, in part, to the limited number of available livers from deceased patients, living donor liver transplantation (LDLT) has become an established solution. Since the first successful LDLT for a child in 1989 [1], this life-saving procedure has developed rapidly, providing similar or even better outcomes, especially in children, in comparison with cadaver liver grafts [2]. Living donors are typically healthy adults; therefore the donor's safety is paramount.

Over the past two decades, laparoscopic surgery has been widely applied to liver surgery. In 2002, Cherqui et al. [3] reported the first case of laparoscopic living donor left lobectomy and laparoscopic LDLT was increasingly used in some centers. However, owing to technical difficulties, this procedure developed relatively slowly. The first case of laparoscopic-assisted hybrid living donor hepatectomy (LADH) was reported by Koffron et al. [4] in 2006, in which hands were introduced into the abdomen while still maintaining the pneumoperitoneum. In this procedure, a laparoscopic technique is employed for mobilization of liver and hilar dissection; however, the parenchymal transection is performed as an open procedure. As a result, this hybrid procedure achieved the advantage of avoiding a large subcostal incision while retaining the safety and familiarity of an open dissection and resection. In addition, laparoscopic-assisted surgeries offered surgeons an opportunity to accumulate expertise before converting to complete laparoscopic living donor hepatectomies.

Several studies have compared the outcome of laparoscopic-assisted living donor hepatectomy (LADH) with widely used open living donor hepatectomy (ODH). However, no consensus has been reached on this topic; it is still not clear which method is of more benefit to the donor. In this setting, we comprehensively collected relevant data and conducted a systematic review with meta-analysis to assess the feasibility, safety, and potential benefits of laparoscopic-assisted living donor hepatectomy.

2. Materials and Methods

2.1. Systematic Literature Search. This meta-analysis was finished by searching electronic databases of PubMed, Embase, Cochrane Library, and Web of Science and scanning reference lists of articles in *May 2017* by Two investigators (B. Zhang and Y. Pan) independently. Strategies included the terms "laparoscopy", "laparoscopic", "minimally invasive", "hybrid", "hand-assisted", "hepatectomy", "liver resection", "hepatic resection", "living donor", and "liver donor". All eligible studies in English were retrieved, and their bibliographies were checked for potential relevant publications.

2.2. Eligibility Criteria. Studies comparing laparoscopy-assisted and open living liver donor hepatectomy are included for the systematic review and meta-analysis including prospective or retrospective case series. Studies were excluded if they met any of the following criteria: (1) case reports, letters, reviews, editorials, and studies lacking control groups; (2) studies that did not report the type of surgery or operation data; (3) if dual (or multiple) studies were reported by the same institution and/or authors, only the most recent publication or the highest quality of studies was included. However, articles from the same authors or centers but with different patient cohorts were included.

2.3. Data Extraction and Quality Assessment. Two investigators (M. Y. Chen and H. P. Zhu) independently assessed publications for inclusion and extracted data from eligible studies, including the baseline characteristics, such as first author, publication year, country of region, study type, sample size, and operation outcomes (operation time and intraoperative estimated blood loss) and postoperative outcomes (overall complications and length of hospital stay). The primary outcomes of the study include blood loss, complications, and analgesic use. The secondary outcomes are operation time, transfusion, length of stay, and graft weights. We made attempts to contact corresponding authors for missing data points. Only one author provided requested data for analysis [5].

The quality of the researches was evaluated by The Newcastle-Ottawa Quality Assessment Scale (NOS). The scale ranged from 0 to 9 stars: studies achieving more than or equal to 6 are deemed as good methodologically.

2.4. Statistical Analysis. All analyses were performed with Review Manager Version 5.3 (The Cochrane Collaboration, Oxford, United Kingdom). Risk ratio (RR) with a 95% confidence interval (CI) was used for the comparison analysis of dichotomous variables. The same continuous parameters were expressed as weighted mean difference (WMD) in the same unit or standard mean difference (SMD) for different unit with 95% CI. When data in individual studies was presented as median and a range, the means and standard deviations (SDs) were estimated by Hozo et al. [6]. The test of heterogeneity, which indicated between-study variance, was evaluated according to Cochran's test and Higgins-squared statistic [7]. Pooled effects were calculated using a random-effects model, unless heterogeneity was less than 50% or $P < 0.05$. Graphical funnel plots were generated to determine visual inspections for publication bias.

We conduct subgroup analyses in the studies focusing on right lobe hepatectomies (RH) and left lobe hepatectomies (LH).

3. Results

3.1. Study Eligibility. A flowchart of the search strategies, containing reasons for excluding studies, is shown in Figure 1. No randomized controlled trials were identified in the records. Nine studies were selected for the final meta-analysis. Five studies [8, 10, 12, 14, 15] compared laparoscopy-assisted and open donor right hepatectomy and one study [11] compared left hepatectomy. Two studies [5, 13] had data for both right hepatectomy and left hepatectomy comparisons. One study [9] evaluated the safety and feasibility of mixed laparoscopic-assisted donor right and left hepatectomies by comparing them with open donor hepatectomies.

A total of 979 patients were included in the analysis with 309 undergoing LADH (31.5%) and 670 undergoing OH (53.2%). Characteristics of included studies are summarized in Table 1. Four papers were conducted in Japan [5, 10, 11, 13], two in the United States [8, 9], one in China [15], one in Korea [14], and one in India [12]. Seven of the studies graded morbidity according to the Clavien-Dindo Classification. Four studies reported conversion in 10 cases, including diaphragmatic rupture (1 case), right hepatic vein injury (1 case), and IVC injury (1 case). And the other conversions were not documented in their respective studies. Three studies reported quality of life for donor in the follow-up period [11, 12, 14].

The quality of the research included was generally moderate to satisfactory. NOS shows that one out of the nine studies observed had 6 stars, six had 7 stars, and two had 8 stars. Table 2 shows the evaluation of quality according to NOS.

3.2. Meta-Analysis Results

3.2.1. Primary Outcome

Blood Loss. Intraoperative blood loss during surgery was significantly less for laparoscopy-assisted procedures compared to open ones (WMD = −59.92 ml; 95% CI: −94.58~−25.27, $P = 0.0007$) (Figure 2). In the subgroup analysis, LADH was a protective effect against blood loss compared with ODH in RH (WMD = −57.56 ml; 95% CI: −94.26~−20.87, $P = 0.002$). For the LH group, the results also show that LADH incurred lower blood loss (WMD = −91.50 ml; 95% CI: −198.68~15.67, $P = 0.08$). Furthermore, the difference was not significant in the mixed group (WMD = 300 ml; 95% CI: −300.93~900.93, $P = 0.33$).

Complication. All of the included studies reported complication rate. A reduced postoperative complication rate was

Table 1: Summary of studies included in the meta-analysis of laparoscopy-assisted versus open living donor hepatectomy.

Author	Region	Study design	Year	Study period	Lobe	Incision	Approach	Sample size	Age (year)	BMI	Sex (M/F)	Follow-up (month)	Parenchyma dissection	Graft weight (g)	Wound infection rate (%)	Incisional hernia rate (%)	Dindo-Clavien
Baker et al. [8]	USA	OCS (R)	2009	2006–2008	Ri	UMI	LA	33	37.0 ± 10.3	25.8 ± 4.1	15/18	3	—	900 ± 215	3.0	—	Yes
							Open	33	39.1 ± 11.1	25.9 ± 4.3	13/20		—	914 ± 160	—	—	
Thenappan et al. [9]	USA	OCS (R)	2011	2005–2009	Le, Ri	UMI	LA	15	33.9 ± 9.0	—	7/8	—	—	—	6.7	6.7	No
							Open	15	35.7 ± 8.1	—	6/9		—	—	0	13.3	
Choi et al. [10]	Japan	OCS (R)	2012	2008–2011	Ri	TI	LA	20	29.7 ± 10.1	23.6 ± 2.8	12/8	—	CUSA	—	10	0	No
							Open	90	36.8 ± 12.0	23.6 ± 2.9	58/32		CUSA	—	5.5	1.1	
Marubashi et al. [11]	Japan	OCS (P)	2013	2009–2012	Le	UMI	LA	31	35.8 ± 8.4	21.3 ± 3.6	13/18	13.9 ± 9.8	—	—	—	—	Yes
							Open	79	37.8 ± 10.1	22.6 ± 3.1	54/25		—	—	—	—	
Makki et al. [12]	India	OCS (P)	2014	2011–2013	Ri	UMI	LA	26	27.5 ± 9.4	24.2 ± 3.6	13/13	14 (6–22)	—	755.5 ± 87.9	11.5	—	Yes
							Open	24	32.4 ± 8.5	24.5 ± 4.4	18/6		—	725.8 ± 134.4	4.2	—	
Soyama et al. [13]	Japan	OCS (R)	2015	1997–2014	Le, Ri	UMI	LA	67	41 (26–65)	21.6 (16.9–29.0)	33/34	27	—	—	0	0	Yes
							Open	137	39 (19–67)	22.1 (16.4–34.7)	57/80	21–86	—	—	1.5	0	
Suh et al. [14]	Korea	OCS (P)	2014	2010–2013	Ri	TI	LA	14	24.9 ± 8.7	20.9 ± 2.9	206/62	32.6 (6.4–55.4)	—	—	0	0	Yes
							Open	268	34 ± 9.7	23.2 ± 3.0	1/13		—	—	1.1	0	
Shen et al. [15]	China	OCS (R)	2016	2011–2014	Ri	UMI	LA	28	40.4 ± 11.1	23.1 ± 1.8	15/13	—	CUSA	634.2 ± 124.2	0	0	Yes
							Open	20	38.3 ± 11.4	21.9 ± 1.9	13/7		CUSA	572.9 ± 122.5	0	0	
Kitajima et al. [5]	Japan	OCS (R)	2017	2011–2016	Le, Ri	UMI	LA	153	42 (20–67)	22.4 (16.5–28.7)	36/40	36.6 (1.4–66)	—	668 (460–1100)*	0	0	Yes
							Open	77	43 (21–64)	22.7 (16.8–29.8)	43/34		—	655 (505–1025)*	1.3	0	

OCS, observational clinical study; P, prospectively collected data; R, retrospectively collected data; LA: laparoscopy-assisted; O: open; Le, left lobe; Ri, right lobe; UMI, upper median incision; TI, transverse incision; CUSA, Cavitron Ultrasonic Surgical Aspirator; *right.

Table 2: Quality assessment based on the NOS for observational studies.

Author	Matched factors	Selection (out of 4)				Comparability (out of 2)	Outcomes (out of 3)			Total (out of 9)
		①	②	③	④		⑤	⑥	⑦	
Baker et al. [8]	abcdef	*	*	*	*	**	*			7
Thenappan et al. [9]	abcdef	*	*	*	*	**	*			7
Choi et al. [10]	abcdefghijkl	*	*	*	*	**	*			7
Marubashi et al. [11]	—	*	*	*	*	**	*	*		8
Makki et al. [12]	abcd	*	*	*	*	*	*			6
Soyama et al. [13]	abcd	*	*	*	*	**	*			7
Suh et al. [14]	—	*	*	*	*	*	*	*	*	8
Shen et al. [15]	abcd	*	*	*	*	**	*			7
Kitajima et al. [5]	—	*	*	*	*	**	*			7

Factors matched between groups: a: age; b: gender; c: body mass index; d: hepatic artery anomalies; e: portal vein anomalies; f: biliary anomalies; g: ALT; h: AST; i: hemoglobin; j: prothrombin time prothrombin time; k: prothrombin rate; l: international normalized ratio.

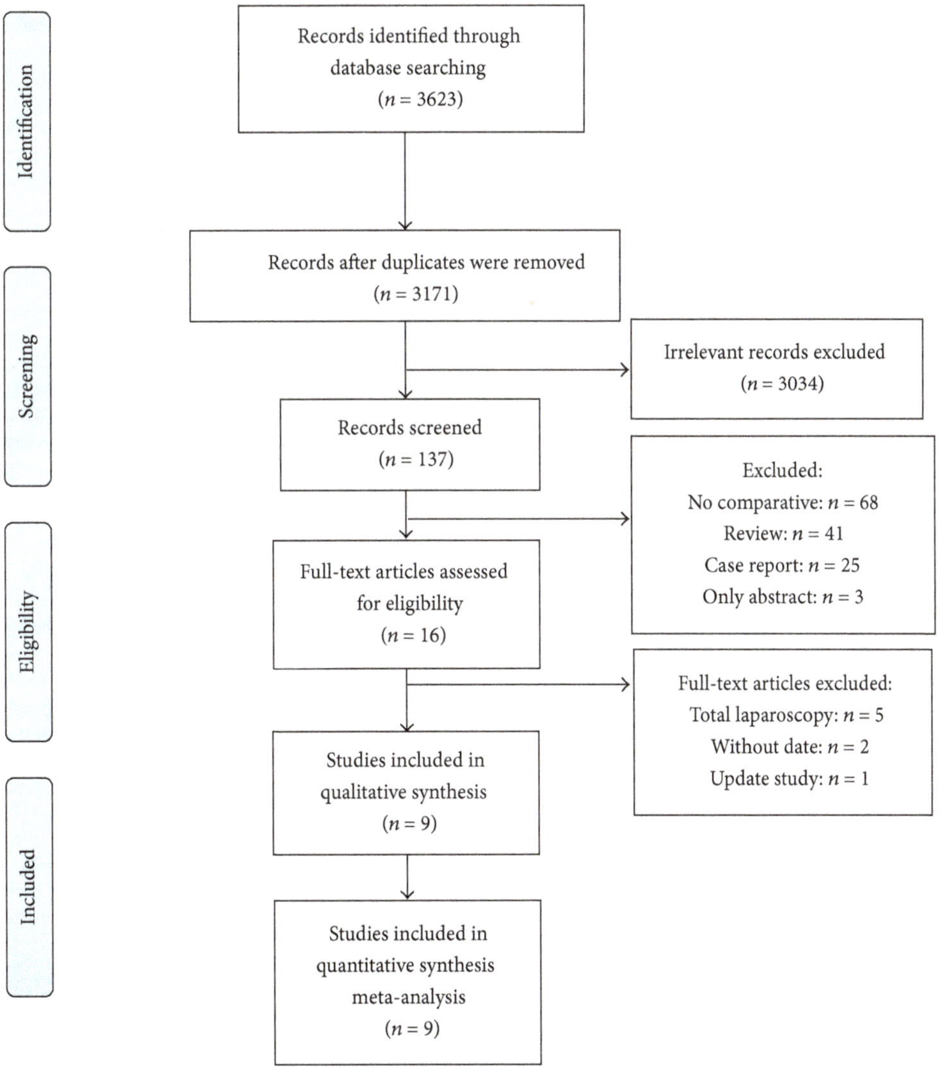

Figure 1: Flow diagram of included studies.

Study or subgroup	Lap Mean	Lap SD	Lap Total	Open Mean	Open SD	Open Total	Weight	Mean difference IV, fixed, 95% CI	Year
RH									
Baker et al., 2009	417	217	33	550	305	33	7.4%	−133.00 [−260.71, −5.29]	2009
Choi et al., 2012	870	653	20	531.7	322.6	90	1.4%	338.30 [44.46, 632.14]	2012
Makki et al., 2014	336.5	89.4	26	395.8	125.7	24	32.4%	−59.30 [−120.21, 1.61]	2014
Sub, 2014	298.3	118.8	14	333	215.2	268	26.5%	−34.70 [−102.05, 32.65]	2014
Soyama et al.,-R 2015	477	130.2	25	828.5	479.2	25	3.2%	−351.50 [−546.15, −156.85]	2015
Shen et al., 2016	383.5	180.4	28	416.5	163.6	20	12.5%	−33.00 [−131.01, 65.01]	2016
Kitajima et al.,-R 2017	286	309	41	330	339	39	5.9%	−44.00 [−186.36, 98.36]	2017
Subtotal (95% CI)			*187*			*499*	*89.2%*	*−57.56 [−94.26, −20.87]*	
Heterogeneity: χ^2 = 17.79, df = 6 (P = 0.007); I^2 = 66%									
Test for overall effect: Z = 3.07 (P = 0.002)									
LH									
Marubashi et al., 2013	353	396	31	456	347	79	4.7%	−103.00 [−262.02, 56.02]	2013
Soyama et al.,-L 2015	1,087.5	952.7	41	1,130	860.3	39	0.8%	−42.50 [−439.92, 354.92]	2015
Kitajima et al.,-L 2017	347	336	35	435	343	38	4.9%	−88.00 [−243.83, 67.83]	2017
Subtotal (95% CI)			*107*			*156*	*10.5%*	*−91.50 [−198.68, 15.67]*	
Heterogeneity: χ^2 = 0.08, df = 2 (P = 0.96); I^2 = 0%									
Test for overall effect: Z = 1.67 (P = 0.09)									
RH+LH									
Thenappan et al., 2011	1,033	1,096	15	733	457	15	0.3%	300.00 [−300.93, 900.93]	2011
Subtotal (95% CI)			*15*			*15*	*0.3%*	*300.00 [−300.93, 900.93]*	
Heterogeneity: Not applicable									
Test for overall effect: Z = 0.98 (P = 0.33)									
Total (95% CI)			*309*			*670*	*100.0%*	*−59.92 [−94.58, −25.27]*	
Heterogeneity: χ^2 = 19.60, df = 10 (P = 0.03); I^2 = 49%									
Test for overall effect: Z = 3.39 (P = 0.0007)									
Test for subgroup differences: χ^2 = 1.73, df = 2 (P = 0.42), I^2 = 0%									

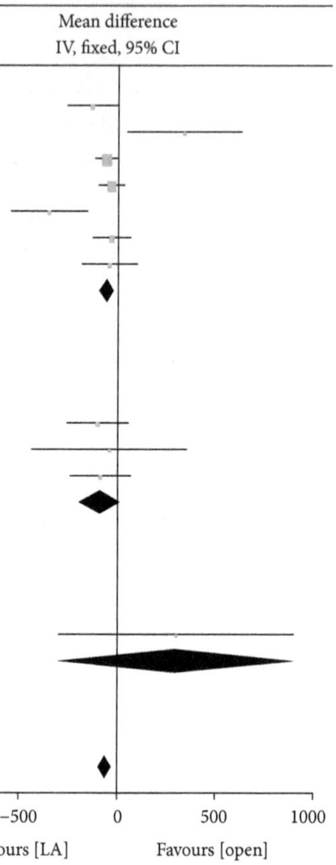

Figure 2: Forest plot of subgroup analyses—intraoperative blood loss. Lap: laparoscopy-assisted living donor hepatectomy, Open: open donor hepatectomy, RH: right lobe hepatectomy, LH: left lobe hepatectomy, and RH + LH: mixed group.

observed in the LADH group (RR = 0.70, 95% CI: 0.51~0.94, P = 0.02) (Figure 3(a)). In the subgroup analysis, LADH was comparable to ODH in RH group (RR = 0.95, 95% CI: 0.63~1.43, P = 0.80) and mixed group (RR = 0.59, 95% CI: 0.29~1.19, P = 0.14). However, complications were significantly decreased in LADH for LH procedures (RR = 0.43, 95% CI: 0.23~0.79, P = 0.007). There are no differences between the two groups regarding the Clavien grades I to IV and V complications (Figures 3(b), 3(c), and 3(d)). Postoperative complications included in this study are summarized in Table 3.

Analgesic Use. There are five studies that gave relevant information on analgesic use after surgery and postoperative pain was evaluated by the number of days of analgesic use or the dosage of analgesic. We found that analgesic use was significantly less in the LADH group (SMD = −0.22; 95% CI: −0.44~−0.11, P = 0.04) (Figure 4).

3.2.2. Secondary Outcomes

Operative Time. Nine of the included studies [5, 8–15] reported operation times and mean operation time tended to be longer in LADH compared to ODH (WMD = 24.85 min; 95% CI: −3.01~52.78, P = 0.08) (Figure 5). Two of the studies [5, 13] provided data for right lobe hepatectomy (RH) and left lobe hepatectomy (LH), respectively, and we then did a subgroup analysis of RH, LH, and mixed group. The subgroup analysis shows that there was no significant difference in operation time in LADH and ODH groups in RH (WMD = 23.86 min; 95% CI: −13.72~61.44, P = 0.21), LH (WMD = 20.92 min; 95% CI: −26.85~68.69, P = 0.39), and mixed (WMD = 52 min; 95% CI: −11.89~68.894, P = 0.11) subgroup.

Transfusion. Five studies reported transfusion information, with similar outcomes in both LADH and ODH (RR = 0.82; 95% CI: 0.24~3.12, P = 0.82) (Figure 6).

Length of Hospital Stay. Length of hospital stay was similar between LADH and ODH (WMD = −0.47 d; 95% CI: −1.78~0.83, P = 0.47) (Figure 7). For the subgroup analysis, there were no significant difference between LADH and ODH in the RH group (WMD = −0.84 d; 95% CI: −2.58~0.91, P = 0.35), LH (WMD = 1.00 d; 95% CI: −1.64~3.64, P = 0.46), or the mixed group (WMD = −0.40 d; 95% CI: −2.52~1.72, P = 0.71).

3.2.3. Graft Weight. A total of 4 studies reported graft weight, showing no difference between the two groups (WMD = 7.31 g; 95% CI: −23.45~38.07, P = 0.64) (Figure 8).

3.2.4. Publication Bias. A funnel plot for studies reporting RRs of postoperative overall complications was used to detect publication bias. The plots standing for the studies distributed

Table 3: Systematic review of postoperative complications.

Author	Group	n	Event	Specified complications	Complication (%)			
					1	2	3	4
Baker et al. [8]	LA	33	7	Small bowel injury × 1, biloma × 1, wound infection × 1	15.2	6.1	0	0
	O	33	7	Biloma × 1, pleural effusion × 1, bowel obstruction × 1	15.2	6.1	0	0
Thenappan et al. [9]	LA	15	2	Wound infection × 1, incisional hernia × 1	—	—	—	—
	O	15	3	Biliary leakage × 1, incisional hernia × 2	—	—	—	—
Choi et al. [10]	LA	20	6	Wound complication × 2, diaphragmatic hernia × 1, pleural effusion × 2, biliary stricture × 1	—	—	—	—
	O	90	21	Wound complication × 5, ventral hernia × 1, pleural effusion × 4, bile leak × 8, bleeding × 1, portal versus thrombosis × 2	—	—	—	—
Marubashi et al. [11]	LA	31	3	—	3.2	0	6.5	0
	O	79	17	—	8.9	1.3	11.3	0
Makki et al. [12]	LA	26	4	—	11.5	0	3.8	0
	O	24	5	—	3.8	7.7	7.7	0
Soyama et al. [13]	LA	67	7	Biliary leakage × 2, postoperative bleeding × 2, bleeding of duodenal ulcer × 1, PV thrombus × 1, ileus × 1	6.0	0	4.5	0
	O	137	25	Biliary leakage × 10, pleural effusion × 2, infectious complication × 3, nerve paralysis × 2, postoperative bleeding × 1, acute pancreatitis × 1, skin necrosis × 1, gastric stasis × 4, PV thrombus × 1	9.5	1.5	6.6	0.7
Suh et al. [14]	LA	14	0	0	0	0	0	0
	O	268	22	Hyperbilirubinemia × 1, pleural effusion × 6, ileus × 5, wound seroma × 2, bleeding × 3, wound infection × 3, biliary stricture × 2	5.2	2.2	0.7	0
Shen et al. [15]	LA	28	5	Pleural effusion × 2, pulmonary infection × 1, ileus × 1, intra-abdominal hemorrhage × 1	7.1	7.1	0	0
	O	20	1	Pulmonary infection × 1	0	5	0	0
Kitajima et al. [5]	LA	76	17	Wound dehiscence × 2, intra-abdominal fluid collection × 4; hyperbilirubinemia × 1, fever × 2, renal failure × 1, small bowel obstruction × 1, atelectasis × 1, pleural effusion × 2, bile leakage × 3	10.5	7.9	3.9	0
	O	77	23	Wound dehiscence × 5, pleural effusion × 2, ascites, × 1, portal venous thrombosis × 3, bile leakage × 5, drug-induced hepatotoxicity × 5, intraabdominal fluid collection × 1	19.5	3.9	6.5	0

LA: laparoscopy-assisted living donor hepatectomy; open: open living donor hepatectomy.

Study or subgroup	Lap Events	Lap Total	Open Events	Open Total	Weight	Risk ratio M-H, fixed, 95% CI	Year
RH							
Baker et al., 2009	7	33	7	33	8.5%	1.00 [0.39, 2.53]	2009
Choi et al., 2012	6	20	21	90	9.3%	1.29 [0.60, 2.77]	2012
Sub, 2014	0	14	19	268	2.5%	0.46 [0.03, 7.25]	2014
Makki et al., 2014	4	26	5	24	6.3%	0.74 [0.22, 2.43]	2014
Shen et al., 2016	5	28	1	20	1.4%	3.57 [0.45, 28.27]	2016
Kitajima et al.,-R 2017	9	41	13	39	16.2%	0.66 [0.32, 1.36]	2017
Subtotal (95% CI)		*162*		*474*	*44.2%*	*0.95 [0.63, 1.43]*	
Total events	31		66				
Heterogeneity: $\chi^2 = 3.59$, df = 5 ($P = 0.61$); $I^2 = 0\%$							
Test for overall effect: $Z = 0.25$ ($P = 0.80$)							
LH							
Marubashi et al., 2013	3	26	17	26	20.6%	0.18 [0.06, 0.53]	2013
Kitajima et al.,-L 2017	8	35	10	38	11.6%	0.87 [0.39, 1.95]	2017
Subtotal (95% CI)		*61*		*64*	*32.3%*	*0.43 [0.23, 0.79]*	
Total events	11		27				
Heterogeneity: $\chi^2 = 5.45$, df = 1 ($P = 0.02$); $I^2 = 82\%$							
Test for overall effect: $Z = 2.72$ ($P = 0.007$)							
RH + LH							
Thenappan et al., 2011	2	15	3	15	3.6%	0.67 [0.13, 3.44]	2011
Soyama et al., 2015	7	67	25	137	19.9%	0.57 [0.26, 1.26]	2015
Subtotal (95% CI)		*82*		*152*	*23.6%*	*0.59 [0.29, 1.19]*	
Total events	9		28				
Heterogeneity: $\chi^2 = 0.03$, df = 1 ($P = 0.87$); $I^2 = 0\%$							
Test for overall effect: $Z = 1.47$ ($P = 0.14$)							
Total (95% CI)		*305*		*690*	*100.0%*	*0.70 [0.51, 0.94]*	
Total events	51		121				
Heterogeneity: $\chi^2 = 12.07$, df = 9 ($P = 0.21$); $I^2 = 25\%$							
Test for overall effect: $Z = 2.34$ ($P = 0.02$)							
Test for subgroup differences: $\chi^2 = 4.84$, df = 2 ($P = 0.09$), $I^2 = 58.7\%$							

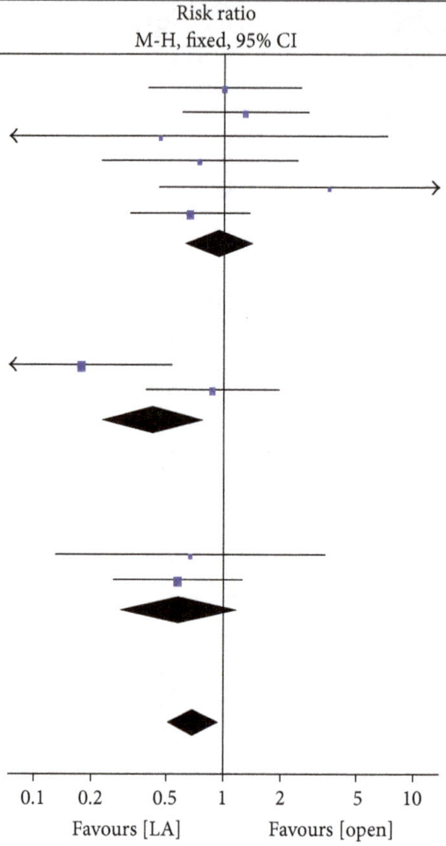

(a)

Study or subgroup	Lap Events	Lap Total	Open Events	Open Total	Weight	Risk ratio M-H, fixed, 95% CI	Year
RH							
Baker et al., 2009	5	33	5	33	14.1%	1.00 [0.32, 3.13]	2009
Sub, 2014	0	14	14	268	4.3%	0.62 [0.04, 9.88]	2014
Makki et al., 2014	3	26	1	24	2.9%	2.77 [0.31, 24.85]	2014
Shen et al., 2016	2	28	0	20	1.6%	3.62 [0.18, 71.57]	2016
Kitajima et al.,-R 2017	5	41	8	39	23.1%	0.59 [0.21, 1.66]	2017
Subtotal (95% CI)		*142*		*384*	*46.0%*	*0.97 [0.50, 1.86]*	
Total events	15		28				
Heterogeneity: $\chi^2 = 2.60$, df = 4 ($P = 0.63$); $I^2 = 0\%$							
Test for overall effect: $Z = 0.10$ ($P = 0.92$)							
LH							
Marubashi et al., 2013	1	31	7	79	11.1%	0.36 [0.05, 2.84]	2013
Kitajima et al.,-L 2017	3	35	7	38	18.9%	0.47 [0.13, 1.66]	2017
Subtotal (95% CI)		*66*		*117*	*30.0%*	*0.43 [0.14, 1.27]*	
Total events	4		14				
Heterogeneity: $\chi^2 = 0.04$, df = 1 ($P = 0.84$); $I^2 = 0\%$							
Test for overall effect: $Z = 1.53$ ($P = 0.13$)							
RH + LH							
Soyama et al., 2015	4	67	13	137	24.0%	0.63 [0.21, 1.86]	2015
Subtotal (95% CI)		*67*		*137*	*24.0%*	*0.63 [0.21, 1.86]*	
Total events	4		13				
Heterogeneity: Not applicable							
Test for overall effect: $Z = 0.84$ ($P = 0.40$)							
Total (95% CI)		*275*		*638*	*100.0%*	*0.72 [0.44, 1.19]*	
Total events	23		55				
Heterogeneity: $\chi^2 = 3.97$, df = 7 ($P = 0.78$); $I^2 = 0\%$							
Test for overall effect: $Z = 1.28$ ($P = 0.20$)							
Test for subgroup differences: $\chi^2 = 1.69$, df = 2 ($P = 0.43$), $I^2 = 0\%$							

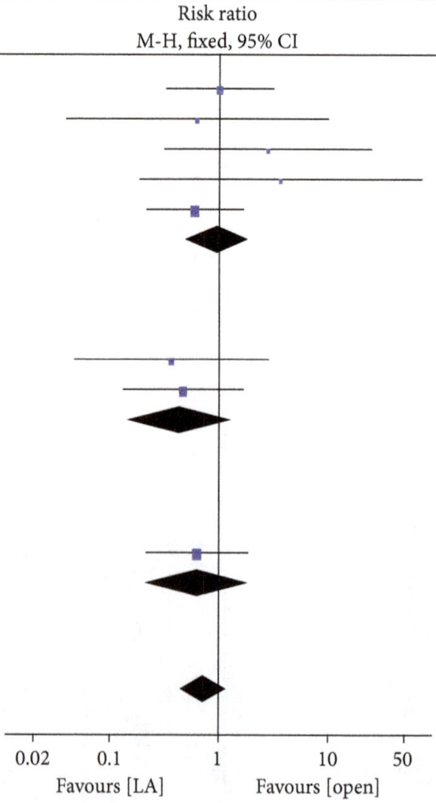

(b)

Figure 3: Continued.

Study or subgroup	Lap Events	Lap Total	Open Events	Open Total	Weight	Risk ratio M-H, fixed, 95% CI	Year
RH							
Baker et al., 2009	2	33	2	33	16.7%	1.00 [0.15, 6.68]	2009
Sub, 2014	0	14	6	268	5.7%	1.38 [0.08, 23.35]	2014
Makki et al., 2014	0	26	2	24	21.7%	0.19 [0.01, 3.67]	2014
Shen et al., 2016	2	28	1	20	9.7%	1.43 [0.14, 14.70]	2016
Kitajima et al.,-R 2017	4	41	2	39	17.1%	1.90 [0.37, 9.81]	2017
Subtotal (95% CI)		*142*		*384*	*71.0%*	*1.06 [0.43, 2.62]*	
Total events	8		13				
Heterogeneity: $\chi^2 = 1.90$, df = 4 ($P = 0.75$); $I^2 = 0\%$							
Test for overall effect: $Z = 0.12$ ($P = 0.90$)							
LH							
Marubashi et al., 2013	0	31	1	79	7.2%	0.83 [0.03, 19.92]	2013
Kitajima et al.,-L 2017	2	35	1	38	8.0%	2.17 [0.21, 22.91]	2017
Subtotal (95% CI)		*66*		*117*	*15.2%*	*1.54 [0.24, 9.73]*	
Total events	2		2				
Heterogeneity: $\chi^2 = 0.23$, df = 1 ($P = 0.63$); $I^2 = 0\%$							
Test for overall effect: $Z = 0.46$ ($P = 0.65$)							
RH + LH							
Soyama et al., 2015	0	67	2	137	13.8%	0.41 [0.02, 8.34]	2015
Subtotal (95% CI)		*67*		*137*	*13.8%*	*0.41 [0.02, 8.34]*	
Total events	0		2				
Heterogeneity: Not applicable							
Test for overall effect: $Z = 0.58$ ($P = 0.56$)							
Total (95% CI)		*275*		*638*	*100.0%*	*1.04 [0.48, 2.27]*	
Total events	10		17				
Heterogeneity: $\chi^2 = 2.68$, df = 7 ($P = 0.91$); $I^2 = 0\%$							
Test for overall effect: $Z = 0.10$ ($P = 0.92$)							
Test for subgroup differences: $\chi^2 = 0.55$, df = 2 ($P = 0.76$), $I^2 = 0\%$							

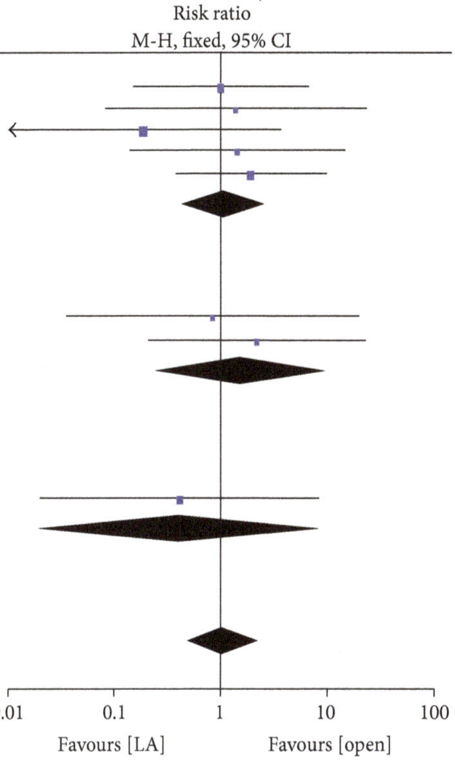

(c)

Study or subgroup	Lap Events	Lap Total	Open Events	Open Total	Weight	Risk ratio M-H, fixed, 95% CI	Year
RH							
Baker et al., 2009	0	33	0	33		Not estimable	2009
Makki et al., 2014	0	26	2	24	13.0%	0.19 [0.01, 3.67]	2014
Sub, 2014	0	14	2	268	1.3%	3.59 [0.18, 71.43]	2014
Shen et al., 2016	1	28	0	20	2.9%	2.17 [0.09, 50.74]	2016
Kitajima et al.,-R 2017	0	41	3	39	18.0%	0.14 [0.01, 2.55]	2017
Subtotal (95% CI)		*142*		*384*	*35.3%*	*0.45 [0.13, 1.60]*	
Total events	1		7				
Heterogeneity: $\chi^2 = 3.78$, df = 3 ($P = 0.29$); $I^2 = 21\%$							
Test for overall effect: $Z = 1.23$ ($P = 0.22$)							
LH							
Marubashi et al., 2013	2	31	9	79	25.5%	0.57 [0.13, 2.47]	2013
Kitajima et al.,-L 2017	3	35	2	38	9.6%	1.63 [0.29, 9.18]	2017
Subtotal (95% CI)		*66*		*117*	*35.1%*	*0.86 [0.29, 2.55]*	
Total events	5		11				
Heterogeneity: $\chi^2 = 0.83$, df = 1 ($P = 0.36$); $I^2 = 0\%$							
Test for overall effect: $Z = 0.28$ ($P = 0.78$)							
RH + LH							
Soyama et al., 2015	3	67	9	137	29.7%	0.68 [0.19, 2.44]	2015
Subtotal (95% CI)		*67*		*137*	*29.7%*	*0.68 [0.19, 2.44]*	
Total events	3		9				
Heterogeneity: Not applicable							
Test for overall effect: $Z = 0.59$ ($P = 0.56$)							
Total (95% CI)		*275*		*638*	*100.0%*	*0.66 [0.33, 1.32]*	
Total events	9		27				
Heterogeneity: $\chi^2 = 4.67$, df = 6 ($P = 0.59$); $I^2 = 0\%$							
Test for overall effect: $Z = 1.18$ ($P = 0.24$)							
Test for subgroup differences: $\chi^2 = 0.57$, df = 2 ($P = 0.75$), $I^2 = 0\%$							

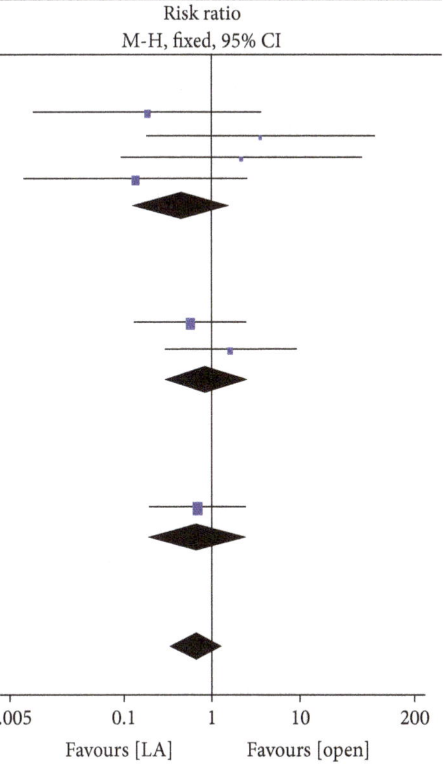

(d)

FIGURE 3: Forest plot of subgroup analyses. (a) Overall postoperative complications. (b) Clavien grade I complication. (c) Clavien grade II complication. (d) Clavien grade III complication. Lap: laparoscopy-assisted living donor hepatectomy, Open: open donor hepatectomy, RH: right lobe hepatectomy, LH: left lobe hepatectomy, and RH + LH: mixed group.

Study or subgroup	Lap Mean	Lap SD	Lap Total	Open Mean	Open SD	Open Total	Weight	Mean difference IV, fixed, 95% CI	Year
Thenappan et al., 2011	47.6	23.2	15	56.8	40.2	15	8.7%	−0.27 [−0.99, 0.45]	2011
Choi et al., 2012	2.5	1.1	20	2.55	1.1	90	19.2%	−0.05 [−0.53, 0.44]	2012
Makki et al., 2014	140.76	27.92	26	172.71	52.24	24	13.6%	−0.76 [−1.34, −0.18]	2014
Shen et al., 2016	2.8	0.9	28	3	0.7	20	13.6%	−0.24 [−0.81, 0.34]	2016
Kitajima et al., 2017	255	227.5	76	279	161.7	77	44.9%	−0.12 [−0.44, 0.20]	2017
Total (95% CI)			*165*			*226*	*100.0%*	*−0.22 [−0.44, −0.01]*	

Heterogeneity: $\chi^2 = 4.27$, df = 4 ($P = 0.37$); $I^2 = 6\%$

Test for overall effect: $Z = 2.05$ ($P = 0.04$)

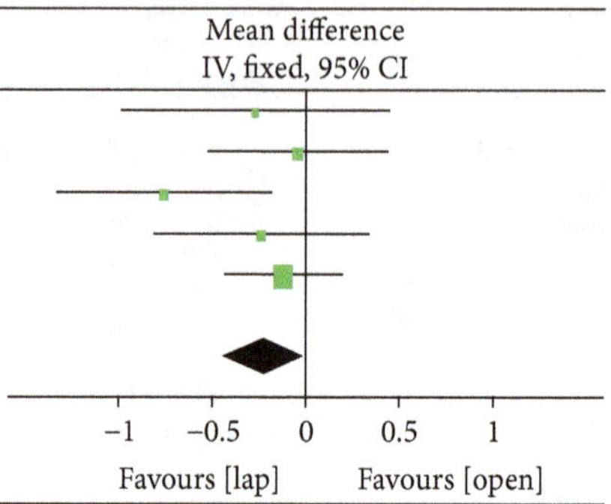

FIGURE 4: Forest plot of meta analyses—analgesic use.

Study or subgroup	Lap Mean	Lap SD	Lap Total	Open Mean	Open SD	Open Total	Weight	Mean difference IV, random, 95% CI	Year
RH									
Baker et al., 2009	265	48	33	316	61	33	10.2%	−51.00 [−77.48, −24.52]	2009
Choi et al., 2012	383.55	41.73	20	303.22	61.49	90	10.5%	80.33 [58.06, 102.60]	2012
Makki et al., 2014	702.5	124.1	26	675.2	117.5	24	6.8%	27.30 [−39.67, 94.27]	2014
Sub, 2014	338.8	61.7	14	275.9	45.7	268	9.7%	62.90 [30.12, 95.68]	2014
Soyama et al.,-R 2015	431.75	74.2	25	425.75	49.95	25	9.5%	6.00 [−29.06, 41.06]	2015
Shen et al., 2016	386.1	49.5	28	366.4	45.3	20	10.1%	19.70 [−7.32, 46.72]	2016
Kitajima et al.,-R 2017	432	74	41	410	68	39	9.8%	22.00 [−9.12, 53.12]	2017
Subtotal (95% CI)			*187*			*499*	*66.7%*	*23.86 [−13.72, 61.44]*	
Heterogeneity: $\tau^2 = 2248.10$; $\chi^2 = 61.72$, df = 6 ($P < 0.00001$); $I^2 = 90\%$									
Test for overall effect: $Z = 1.24$ ($P = 0.21$)									
LH									
Marubashi et al., 2013	435	103	31	383	73	79	9.1%	52.00 [12.33, 91.67]	2013
Soyama et al.,-L 2015	438.25	111.2	41	478	142.1	39	7.7%	−39.75 [−95.85, 16.35]	2015
Kitajima et al.,-L 2017	444	79	35	406	80	38	9.4%	38.00 [1.50, 74.50]	2017
Subtotal (95% CI)			*107*			*156*	*26.3%*	*20.92 [−26.85, 68.69]*	
Heterogeneity: $\tau^2 = 1279.48$; $\chi^2 = 7.29$, df = 2 ($P = 0.03$); $I^2 = 73\%$									
Test for overall effect: $Z = 0.86$ ($P = 0.39$)									
RH + LH									
Thenappan et al., 2011	435	103	15	383	73	15	7.1%	52.00 [−11.89, 115.89]	2011
Subtotal (95% CI)			*15*			*15*	*7.1%*	*52.00 [−11.89, 115.89]*	
Heterogeneity: Not applicable									
Test for overall effect: $Z = 1.60$ ($P = 0.11$)									
Total (95% CI)			*309*			*670*	*100.0%*	*24.85 [−3.09, 52.78]*	

Heterogeneity: $\tau^2 = 1813.35$; $\chi^2 = 69.61$, df = 10 ($P < 0.00001$); $I^2 = 86\%$

Test for overall effect: $Z = 1.74$ ($P = 0.08$)

Test for subgroup differences: $\chi^2 = 0.67$, df = 2 ($P = 0.71$), $I^2 = 0\%$

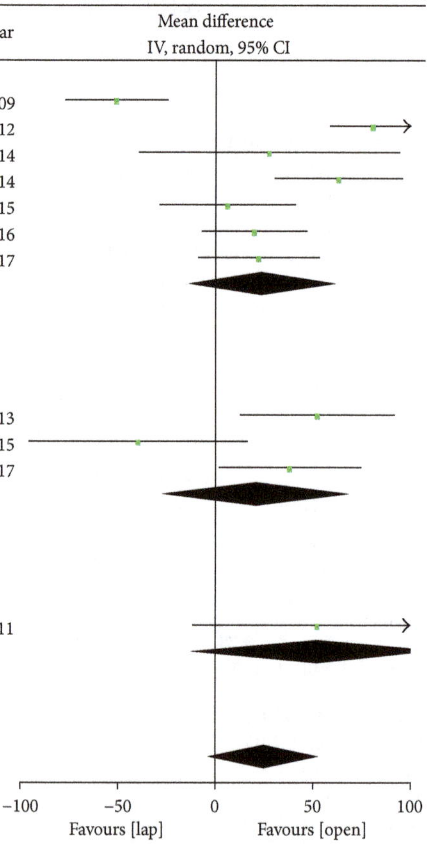

FIGURE 5: Forest plot of subgroup analyses—operation time. Lap: laparoscopy-assisted living donor hepatectomy, Open: open donor hepatectomy, RH: right lobe hepatectomy, LH: left lobe hepatectomy, and RH + LH: mixed group.

symmetrically. This result suggested that the publication bias was acceptable (Figure 9).

4. Discussion

Minimally invasive donor surgery was developed to reduce the morbidity and decrease the impact on the donor, minimizing tissue trauma, and improving postoperative pain and cosmesis for patients. LADH with manual hand manipulation in the abdominal cavity, giving the surgeon enhanced tactile feedback of the liver, allowed for more precise mobilization and dissection of the targeted lobe. This technique is combined with smaller incision while preserving the maneuverability and safety of an open liver resection. LADH apparently leads to less wound-related morbidity and the best cosmetic result [16]. In a recent review, Xu et al. [17] examined laparoscopic versus open liver resection for liver transplantation, showing less blood loss, shortened hospital stay, and longer operation time. However, this review did not attempt to clarify the different types of laparoscopic

Study or subgroup	Lap Events	Lap Total	Open Events	Open Total	Weight	Risk ratio M-H, fixed, 95% CI	Year
Thenappan et al., 2011	0	15	0	15		Not estimable	2011
Makki et al., 2014	1	26	3	24	65.2%	0.31 [0.03, 2.76]	2014
Shen et al., 2016	2	28	1	20	24.4%	1.43 [0.14, 14.70]	2016
Kitajima et al., 2017	1	76	0	77	10.4%	3.04 [0.13, 73.45]	2017
Total (95% CI)		*145*		*136*	*100.0%*	*0.86 [0.24, 3.12]*	
Total events	4		4				

Heterogeneity: $\chi^2 = 1.63$, df = 2 ($P = 0.44$); $I^2 = 0\%$
Test for overall effect: $Z = 0.22$ ($P = 0.82$)

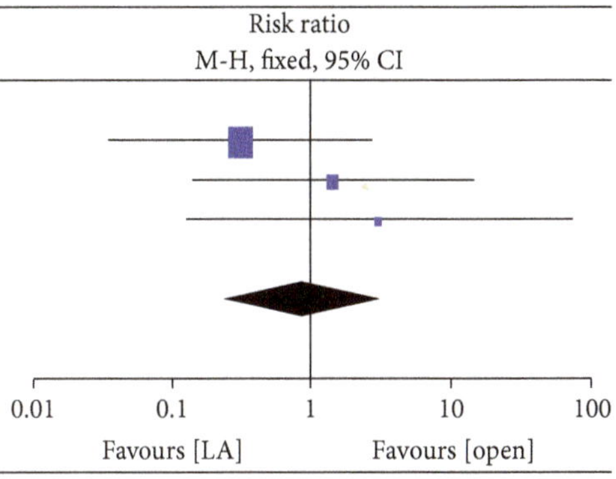

FIGURE 6: Forest plot of meta analyses—transfusion. Lap: laparoscopy-assisted living donor hepatectomy, Open: open donor hepatectomy.

Study or subgroup	Lap Mean	Lap SD	Lap Total	Open Mean	Open SD	Open Total	Weight	Mean difference IV, random, 95% CI	Year
RH									
Baker et al., 2009	4.3	4.4	33	3.9	16.7	33	4.0%	0.40 [−5.49, 6.29]	2009
Choi et al., 2012	12.1	2.81	20	12	3.61	90	18.1%	0.10 [−1.34, 1.54]	2012
Marubashi et al., 2013	10.3	3.3	31	18.3	16.7	79	7.6%	−8.00 [−11.86, −4.14]	2013
Sub, 2014	10.2	4.4	14	9.2	3.3	268	13.3%	1.00 [−1.34, 3.34]	2014
Shen et al., 2016	7.4	2.5	28	7.3	1.6	20	19.6%	0.10 [−1.06, 1.26]	2016
Kitajima et al.,-R 2017	13	4	41	14	8	39	11.2%	−1.00 [−3.79, 1.79]	2017
Subtotal (95% CI)			*167*			*529*	*73.8%*	*−0.84 [−2.58, 0.91]*	
Heterogeneity: $\tau^2 = 2.90$; $\chi^2 = 17.46$, df = 5 ($P = 0.004$); $I^2 = 71\%$									
Test for overall effect: $Z = 0.94$ ($P = 0.35$)									
LH									
Kitajima et al.,-L 2017	14	7	35	13	4	38	11.8%	1.00 [−1.64, 3.64]	2017
Subtotal (95% CI)			*35*			*38*	*11.8%*	*1.00 [−1.64, 3.64]*	
Heterogeneity: Not applicable									
Test for overall effect: $Z = 0.74$ ($P = 0.46$)									
RH + LH									
Thenappan et al., 2011	6	2	15	6.4	3.68	15	14.4%	−0.40 [−2.52, 1.72]	2011
Subtotal (95% CI)			*15*			*15*	*14.4%*	*−0.40 [−2.52, 1.72]*	
Heterogeneity: Not applicable									
Test for overall effect: $Z = 0.37$ ($P = 0.71$)									
Total (95% CI)			*217*			*582*	*100.0%*	*−0.47 [−1.78, 0.83]*	

Heterogeneity: $\tau^2 = 1.90$; $\chi^2 = 18.27$, df = 7 ($P = 0.01$); $I^2 = 62\%$
Test for overall effect: $Z = 0.72$ ($P = 0.47$)
Test for subgroup differences: $\chi^2 = 1.30$, df = 2 ($P = 0.52$), $I^2 = 0\%$

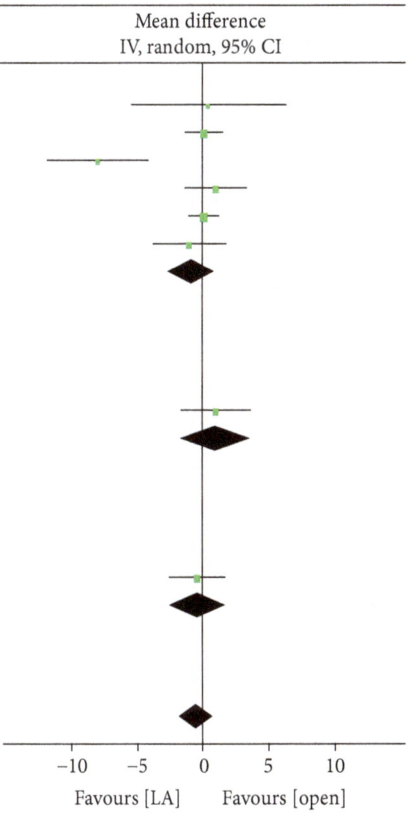

FIGURE 7: Forest plot of subgroup analyses—length of hospital stay. Lap: laparoscopy-assisted living donor hepatectomy, Open: open donor hepatectomy, RH: right lobe hepatectomy, LH: left lobe hepatectomy, and RH + LH: mixed group.

Study or subgroup	Lap Mean	Lap SD	Lap Total	Open Mean	Open SD	Open Total	Weight	Mean difference IV, fixed, 95% CI	Year
Baker et al., 2009	900	215	33	914	160	33	11.3%	−14.00 [−105.44, 77.44]	2009
Makki et al., 2014	755.5	87.94	26	725.8	134.4	24	23.5%	29.70 [−33.81, 93.21]	2014
Shen et al., 2016	634.2	124.2	28	572.9	122.5	20	18.9%	61.30 [−9.40, 132.00]	2016
Kitajima et al.,-R 2017	724	184.8	41	710	150.1	39	17.5%	14.00 [−59.61, 87.61]	2017
Kitajima et al.,-L 2017	413	99.6	35	455	147.2	38	28.8%	−42.00 [−99.26, 15.26]	2017
Total (95% CI)			*163*			*154*	*100.0%*	*7.31 [−23.45, 38.07]*	

Heterogeneity: $\chi^2 = 5.81$, df = 4 ($P = 0.21$); $I^2 = 31\%$
Test for overall effect: $Z = 0.47$ ($P = 0.64$)

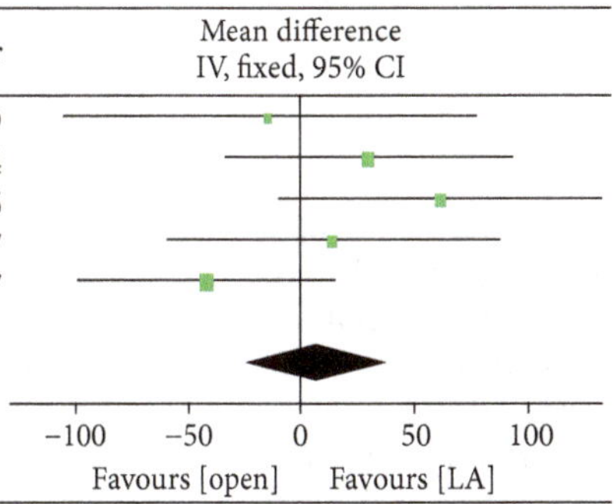

FIGURE 8: Forest plot of meta analyses—graft weight.

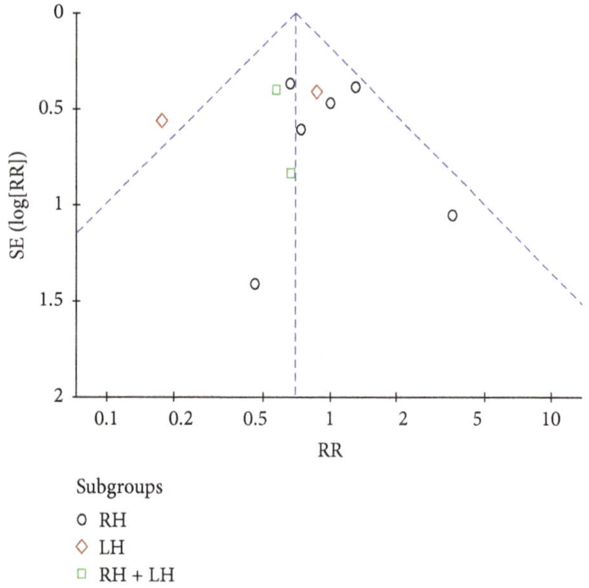

FIGURE 9: Funnel plot of overall postoperative complications. RH: right lobe hepatectomy, LH: left lobe hepatectomy, and RH + LH: mixed group.

surgery. In our meta-analysis, we only included the studies of laparoscopy-assisted (hybrid) surgery. Our further subgroup analysis was done to learn how LADH affects surgery in different areas of the liver.

Our result confirms that blood loss was significantly less in the LADH group than in the ODH group. This is consistent with published results for laparoscopic hepatectomies, even when laparoscopy is only used for the hepatic mobilization [18]. In the subgroup analysis of single types of hepatectomy to minimize the bias, there was no difference between the types of donor hepatectomy. LADH is a potential technique to decrease blood loss, confirmed by the colorectal surgery [19] and prior analysis [20]. Hand-assisted surgery has been promoted by its advocates in decreased complication rate in the colorectal surgery [19]. Our analysis of LADH demonstrated favourable overall complication rates compared to ODH, similar to the previous analysis [20]. In the subgroup analysis, LH shows a significantly lower rate of complications in the LADH group, which accounts for the lower complication rate in the total group. However, the case volume is small in the left hepatectomy subgroup. In theory, it is easier to mobilize the right lobe from the diaphragm by laparoscopic technique and inferior vena cava with the help of manual manipulation. Adequate mobilization, improved visualization, and better manipulation contribute to the enhanced safety of the operation. Living donor mortality in ODH was reported as 0.2% (23/1153), mostly related to surgical procedure [21]. There was no mortality to be reported in the studies both in laparoscopy-assisted and open group for donor. In other words, LADH shows a better tendency toward in the outcome of morbidity to ODH.

Smaller and midline incisions in the supraumbilical area resulted in reduced disruption of abdominal muscles, deceased scar discomfort, and less postoperative analgesic use in our analysis, raising the possibility of better cosmetic results and, possibly, faster return to work and normal physical activities. However, it tended to have an increased operative time associated with hand-assisted surgery, though it did not reach statistical significance. The result could be explained by the application of laparoscopic instruments for the meticulous mobilization in the liver surgery. Furthermore, the transfusion rate was comparable between LADH and ODH in this analysis. Additionally, LOS demonstrated no inferiority for LADH. Interestingly, the prior meta-analysis of laparoscopic versus open hepatectomy for live liver donor has shown the significantly shorter hospital stay in the LADH group [17, 20]. This may be ascribed to the methods of surgery and postoperation protocols and insurance policy. Regarding hospital cost, it was higher in the LADH. From published data, the overall cost of laparoscopic liver resection was lower than open liver resection [22].

After comparing laparoscopic-assisted operation and open operation, there was a high heterogeneity in the analysis, even in the subgroup analyses by type of surgery. These may result from differences in study designs, number of participants, donors' baseline characteristics, surgical techniques, and surgical types. In addition, some of the data estimated the mean and SD from median and range, which may result in inaccuracy. No random trials were included and most of the studies were cohort studies or case-control studies. Because of high-risk in the donor hepatectomy, a relative surgical abstention may present in the enrolled patients and their families. Based on these limitations, larger prospective studies and randomized trials are needed.

5. Conclusion

According to our data, laparoscopy-assisted living donor hepatectomy (LADH) is equally safe and effective technique. There was no increased risk of morbidity compared to ODH patients in our examined groups. Benefits of laparoscopy-assisted donor hepatectomy compared to open surgery have demonstrated improved short-term outcomes, especially lower intraoperative blood loss and complications. We conclude that LADH is an appropriate minimally invasive procedure for living donor hepatectomies, which needs to be selected by patients' and surgery' preferences.

Abbreviations

LADH: Laparoscopy-assisted living donor hepatectomy
ODH: Open donor hepatectomy
LLR: Laparoscopic liver resection
WMD: Weighted mean difference
SMD: Standard mean difference
RR: Risk ratio
SD: Standard deviation
NOS: Newcastle-Ottawa Quality Assessment Scale
RH: Right lobe hepatectomy
LH: Left lobe hepatectomy
ALT: Alanine aminotransferase
AST: Aspartate aminotransferase
TB: Total bilirubin
LFT: Liver function test.

Authors' Contributions

Bin Zhang and Yu Pan wrote the paper and performed the research. Xiu-jun Cai and Ke Chen designed the study. Ming-Yu Chen and He-Pan Zhu collected the data. Hendi Maher and Yi-Bin Zhu performed the literature search and retrieved the data. Xiu-jun Cai, Jiang Chen, and Yi Dai analyzed the data and revised the manuscript.

Acknowledgments

This study was supported by Research Project of Zhejiang Provincial Education Department (no. N20140173).

References

[1] S. Raia, J. R. Nery, and S. Mies, "Liver transplantation from live donors," *The Lancet*, vol. 334, no. 8661, p. 497, 1989.

[2] D. G. Maluf, R. T. Stravitz, A. H. Cotterell et al., "Adult living donor versus deceased donor liver transplantation: A 6-year single center experience," *American Journal of Transplantation*, vol. 5, no. 1, pp. 149–156, 2005.

[3] D. Cherqui, O. Soubrane, E. Husson et al., "Laparoscopic living donor hepatectomy for liver transplantation in children," *The Lancet*, vol. 359, no. 9304, pp. 392–396, 2002.

[4] A. J. Koffron, R. Kung, T. Baker, J. Fryer, L. Clark, and M. Abecassis, "Laparoscopic-assisted right lobe donor hepatectomy," *American Journal of Transplantation*, vol. 6, no. 10, pp. 2522–2525, 2006.

[5] T. Kitajima, T. Kaido, T. Iida et al., "Short-term outcomes of laparoscopy-assisted hybrid living donor hepatectomy: a comparison with the conventional open procedure," *Surgical Endoscopy*, pp. 1–10, 2017.

[6] S. P. Hozo, B. Djulbegovic, and I. Hozo, "Estimating the mean and variance from the median, range, and the size of a sample," *BMC Medical Research Methodology*, vol. 5, article 13, 2005.

[7] J. P. T. Higgins, S. G. Thompson, J. J. Deeks, and D. G. Altman, "Measuring inconsistency in meta-analyses," *British Medical Journal*, vol. 327, no. 7414, pp. 557–560, 2003.

[8] T. B. Baker, C. L. Jay, D. P. Ladner et al., "Laparoscopy-assisted and open living donor right hepatectomy: A comparative study of outcomes," *Surgery*, vol. 146, no. 4, pp. 817–825, 2009.

[9] A. Thenappan, R. C. Jha, T. Fishbein et al., "Liver allograft outcomes after laparoscopic-assisted and minimal access live donor hepatectomy for transplantation," *The American Journal of Surgery*, vol. 201, no. 4, pp. 450–455, 2011.

[10] H. J. Choi, Y. K. You, G. H. Na, T. H. Hong, G. S. Shetty, and D. G. Kim, "Single-port laparoscopy-assisted donor right hepatectomy in living donor liver transplantation: Sensible approach or unnecessary hindrance?" *Transplantation Proceedings*, vol. 44, no. 2, pp. 347–352, 2012.

[11] S. Marubashi, H. Wada, K. Kawamoto et al., "Laparoscopy-assisted hybrid left-side donor hepatectomy," *World Journal of Surgery*, vol. 37, no. 9, pp. 2202–2210, 2013.

[12] K. Makki, V. K. Chorasiya, G. Sood, P. K. Srivastava, P. Dargan, and V. Vij, "Laparoscopy-assisted hepatectomy versus conventional (open) hepatectomy for living donors: When you know better, you do better," *Liver Transplantation*, vol. 20, no. 10, pp. 1229–1236, 2014.

[13] A. Soyama, M. Takatsuki, M. Hidaka et al., "Hybrid procedure in living donor liver transplantation," *Transplantation Proceedings*, vol. 47, no. 3, pp. 679–682, 2015.

[14] S.-W. Suh, K.-W. Lee, J.-M. Lee, Y. Choi, N.-J. Yi, and K.-S. Suh, "Clinical outcomes of and patient satisfaction with different incision methods for donor hepatectomy in living donor liver," *Liver Transplantation*, vol. 21, no. 1, pp. 72–78, 2015.

[15] S. Shen, W. Zhang, L. Jiang, L. Yan, and J. Yang, "Comparison of Upper Midline Incision With and Without Laparoscopic Assistance for Living-Donor Right Hepatectomy," *Transplantation Proceedings*, vol. 48, no. 8, pp. 2726–2731, 2016.

[16] A. Jain, P. Nemitz, R. Sharma et al., "Incidence of abdominal wall numbness post-liver transplantation and its complications," *Liver Transplantation*, vol. 15, no. 11, pp. 1488–1492, 2009.

[17] J. Xu, C. Hu, H.-L. Cao et al., "Meta-analysis of laparoscopic versus open hepatectomy for live liver donors," *PLoS ONE*, vol. 11, no. 10, Article ID e0165319, 2016.

[18] H.-S. Han, A. Shehta, S. Ahn, Y.-S. Yoon, J. Y. Cho, and Y. Choi, "Laparoscopic versus open liver resection for hepatocellular carcinoma: Case-matched study with propensity score matching," *Journal of Hepatology*, vol. 63, no. 3, article no. 5641, pp. 643–650, 2015.

[19] H. Moloo, F. Haggar, D. Coyle et al., "Hand assisted laparoscopic surgery versus conventional laparoscopy for colorectal surgery," *Cochrane Database of Systematic Reviews*, no. 10, Article ID CD006585, 2010.

[20] G. Berardi, F. Tomassini, and R. I. Troisi, "Comparison between minimally invasive and open living donor hepatectomy: A systematic review and meta-analysis," *Liver Transplantation*, vol. 21, no. 6, pp. 738–752, 2015.

[21] Y. L. Cheah, M. A. Simpson, J. J. Pomposelli, and E. A. Pomfret, "Incidence of death and potentially life-threatening near-miss events in living donor hepatic lobectomy: a world-wide survey," *Liver Transplantation*, vol. 19, no. 5, pp. 499–506, 2013.

[22] S. P. Cleary, H.-S. Han, M. Yamamoto, G. Wakabayashi, and H. J. Asbun, "The comparative costs of laparoscopic and open liver resection: a report for the 2nd International Consensus Conference on Laparoscopic Liver Resection," *Surgical Endoscopy*, vol. 30, no. 11, pp. 4691–4696, 2016.

25

Normal Uptake of ^{11}C-Acetate in Pancreas, Liver, Spleen, and Suprarenal Gland in PET

Bogdan Malkowski,[1,2] Pawel Wareluk,[3] Tomasz Gorycki,[4] Katarzyna Skrobisz,[4] and Michal Studniarek[3,4]

[1] *Department of Nuclear Medicine, Oncological Center of Bydgoszcz, Bydgoszcz, Poland*
[2] *Department of PET and Molecular Imaging, Collegium Medicum, University of Nicolaus Copernicus, Bydgoszcz, Poland*
[3] *Department of Diagnostic Imaging, Medical University of Warsaw, Warsaw, Poland*
[4] *Department of Radiology, Medical University of Gdańsk, Gdańsk, Poland*

Correspondence should be addressed to Katarzyna Skrobisz; kskrobisz@gumed.edu.pl

Academic Editor: Yousuke Nakai

Purpose. ^{11}C-Acetate is radiotracer being considered an alternative to ^{18}F-fluorodeoxyglucose. Evaluation of ^{11}C-acetate biodistribution in human parenchymal organs is described. *Methods and Materials.* 60 consecutive patients referred to ^{11}C-acetate PET CT suspected of renal or prostate cancer relapse with negative results (no recurrent tumor) were included in the study. Acquisition from the base of skull to upper thigh was made 20 min after i.v. injection of 720 MBq of ^{11}C-acetate. The distribution was evaluated by measuring the uptake in pancreas (uncinate process and body separately), liver, spleen, and left suprarenal gland. Clinical data of included patients showed no abnormalities in these organs. *Results.* Biodistributions of ^{11}C-acetate radiotracer were compared in different organs. Standardized uptake values of ^{11}C-acetate were significantly higher in pancreatic parenchyma (SUV mean 6,4) than in liver (SUV mean 3,3), spleen (SUV mean 4,5), or suprarenal gland (SUV mean 2,7) tissues. No significant difference was found between pancreatic head (SUV mean 6,4) and body (SUV mean 5,9) uptake. In case of all aforementioned organs, there were no differences either between both sexes or between formerly diagnosed tumors (renal and prostate). *Conclusions.* Evaluation of ^{11}C-acetate uptake differences in parenchymal organs will allow establishing normal patterns of distribution. High pancreatic uptake may be used in quantitative assessment of organ function in diffuse nonneoplastic pathology.

1. Introduction

^{11}C labelled acetate was a radiotracer first used for the assessment of myocardial viability over two decades ago [1]. Since then it has been evaluated as a promising tracer, mainly in oncological research, and also as a possible alternative to ^{18}F-fluorodeoxyglucose (FDG). However, ^{11}C-acetate is not as widely used in clinical practice and investigated as FDG. Relatively short half-life of approximately 20 minutes is one of the reasons for the above. Currently, positron emission tomography (PET) examinations with the use of ^{11}C-acetate are performed mostly in the fields of oncology, urology, and cardiology, with reports of unusual, rare tumor findings such as thymoma or cerebellopontine angle schwannoma [2].

The purpose of this study was to evaluate distribution of ^{11}C-acetate in human parenchymal organs during whole body PET examination combined with computed tomography (CT). Uptake of radiotracer was measured in pancreas (uncinate process and body separately), liver, spleen, and left suprarenal gland.

2. Methods and Materials

60 consecutive patients (22 women, 38 men) referred to ^{11}C-acetate PET CT suspected of renal or prostate cancer relapse with negative results (no recurrent tumor) were included in the study. 56 patients had kidney cancer and 7 patients had prostate cancer (three had both of them).

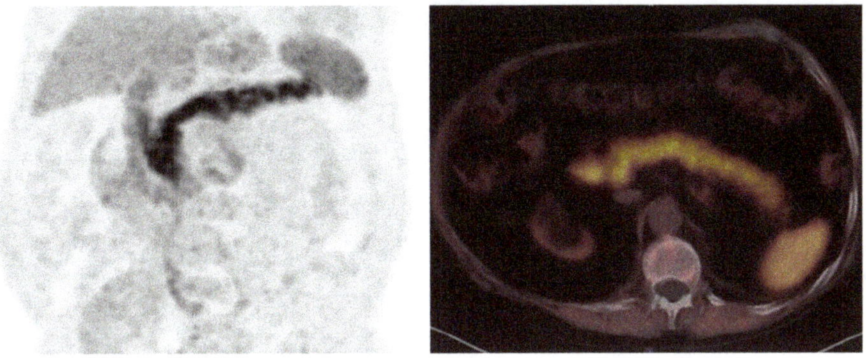

FIGURE 1: The dominant organ uptake of ^{11}C-acetate is seen in the pancreas.

PET/CT study were made using Biograph mCT 128. ^{11}C-Acetate was produced in our laboratory using Explora Acetate module according to the manufacturer instruction and GMP standards.

Acquisition was made 20 min after i.v. injection of 720 MBq of acetate. The acquisition from the base of skull to 1/3 upper thigh was performed. The parameters of the acquisition and reconstruction are presented in Table 1.

^{11}C-Acetate distribution was evaluated by placing the spherical 10 mm VOI and measuring the uptake values with isocontour tool. SUVs (max, peak, and mean) were recorded for pancreas (head and body separately), liver, spleen, and left suprarenal gland (Figure 1). The position of VOIs was the same for all patients and anatomical imagining (CT) was used to allocate them. Right suprarenals were not taken into account because of overlapping radioactivity from the liver. Clinical data of included patients showed no abnormalities in the all organs studied.

Statistical calculations were performed using STATISTICA (ver. 12.0, StatSoft Inc., 2014) statistical package and Excel (Microsoft) spreadsheet. Quantitative variables were characterized by the arithmetic mean, standard deviation, median, minimum and maximum values (range), and 95% CI (confidence interval). In contrast, the qualitative variables were presented using frequencies and percentages. To check whether a quantitative variable came from a normally distributed population, Shapiro-Wilk test was used. Leven (Brown-Forsythe) test was used to test the hypothesis of equal variances. The significance of differences between the two groups (unpaired model) was examined with the following tests: Student's t-test (or Welch t-test, in the absence of homogeneity of variance) or Mann–Whitney U test. The significance of differences between more than two groups was tested by an F test (ANOVA) or Kruskal-Wallis test (when ANOVA was inapplicable). If statistically significant differences between groups were present, post hoc tests (Tukey test for F, Dunn test for Kruskal-Wallis) were applied. In all the calculations the level of significance was set at $\alpha = 0.05$.

TABLE 1: The parameters of acquisition and reconstruction.

	^{11}C-Acetate
CT WB	
Topogram	Standard
Eff mAs	Care dose 4D
kV	120
Slice	5.0 mm
Acq	32 × 1.2 mm
Pitch	0.8
Direction	Craniocaudal
Kernel	B30f
FoV	780 mm
Increment	3.0 mm
PET WB	
Isotope	C-11
Pharm	Acetate
Scan range	Match CT range
Scan duration/bed	2.0 min
PET recon 1	
Output image	Corrected
Recon meth	TrueX + tof (UltraHD-PET)
Iteration	2
Subset	21
Image size	200
Filter	Gaussian
Zoom	1.0
FWHM	2.0
PET recon 2	
Output image	Uncorrected
Recon meth	Iterative + tof
Iteration	2
Subset	24
Image size	200
Filter	Gaussian
Zoom	1.0
FWHM	2.0
+	Standard AC recon

3. Results

Of all analyzed organs the head of the pancreas had highest SUVs values (SUV max 9.3, SUV peak 7.9, and SUV mean

Table 2: Comparison of ^{11}C-acetate uptake by organ.

	Pancreas head (N = 60)	Pancreas body (N = 60)	Liver (N = 60)	Spleen (N = 60)	Suprarenal gland (N = 60)	P value
SUV max						
Mean (SD)	9,3 (2,6)	9,0 (2,8)	5,2 (1,7)	6,4 (1,6)	4,2 (1,8)	
Range	4,6–15,9	4,0–16,1	2,6–9,1	3,5–10,6	2,2–15,3	0,001
Median	9,0	8,4	4,8	6,2	4,0	
95% CI	[8,6; 10,0]	[8,3; 9,7]	[4,7; 5,6]	[5,9; 6,8]	[3,8; 4,7]	
SUV peak						
Mean (SD)	7,9 (2,5)	7,2 (2,4)	4,2 (1,4)	5,4 (1,4)	3,5 (1,6)	
Range	3,9–15,0	2,7–13,3	2,1–7,4	2,6–9,2 1,5–13,3		0,001
Median	7,6	7,0	4,1	5,3	3,2	
95% CI	[7,3; 8,5]	[6,6; 7,8]	[3,9; 4,6]	[5,1; 5,8]	[3,0; 3,9]	
SUV mean						
Mean (SD)	6,4 (2,0)	5,9 (1,9)	3,3 (1,1)	4,5 (1,2)	2,7 (1,3)	
Range	3,0–12,3	2,3–10,8	1,6–5,7	2,1–7,7 1,4–10,8		0,001
Median	6,2	5,8	3,1	4,3	2,6	
95% CI	[5,9; 6,9]	[5,4; 6,3]	[3,0; 3,6]	[4,2; 4,8]	[2,4; 3,1]	

6.4). However no statistically significant difference was found between pancreatic head (SUV mean 6,4) and body (SUV mean 5,9) uptake (Table 1). Standardized uptake values of ^{11}C-acetate were significantly higher in pancreas (SUV mean of 6,4 for head and 5.9 for body) than in liver (SUV mean 3,3), spleen (SUV mean 4,5), or left suprarenal gland (SUV mean 2,7) (Table 2). In all organs there were no differences either between both sexes or between formerly diagnosed tumors (kidney and/or prostate cancer). The results were presented as an abstract and discussed at ECR 2016 Congress in Vienna [3].

4. Discussion

Acetate (CH_3COO^-) is an ion formed from acetic acid (CH_3COOH) by losing hydrogen ion. Physiologically, in human organism acetate is converted into acetyl-CoA and, depending on a cell type, involved in two main different metabolic pathways. The first is tricarboxylic acid cycle, resulting in energy, carbon dioxide, and water. The second, on the contrary, is anabolic pathway, leading to synthesis of cholesterol and fatty acids, which are later incorporated in the form of phospholipids into cell membranes [4]. Both pathways are also important in oncogenesis, as atypical, rapidly dividing cells are in need of energy and substrates for creating cell membranes. On this account the potential intracellular acetate utilization could be monitored in diagnostic and perhaps therapeutic applications in oncology [5]. Until now it was mainly used for imaging of renal, prostate, and bladder cancers.

For diagnostic purposes in nuclear medicine, acetate is labelled with ^{11}C carbon isotope produced from ^{14}N nitrogen by proton bombardment in a cyclotron. The labelling process requires considerable effort to convert gaseous precursors (radioactive CO_2 and methane) into more reactive molecules suitable for reaction with acetate [6]. After that, complete radiotracer is prepared for intravenous injection. Seltzer et al. evaluated ^{11}C-acetate estimated absorbed doses for healthy volunteers with pancreas, bowels, liver, kidneys, and spleen getting highest doses [7]. The radiotracer is not excreted in urine under normal circumstances. Few theories exist regarding distribution of ^{11}C-acetate, for example, its high concentration in pancreas which may correspond with increased lipid synthesis in acinar cells [7], incorporating into zymogens or generating hydrogen carbonate ions [8]. A recent study showed also potential of evaluating pancreatic exocrine function as ^{11}C-acetate activity increased in duodenum after secretin administration [9].

This study's purpose of evaluating ^{11}C-acetate uptake pattern in selected abdominal parenchymal organs has been undertaken only a few times before. The results are convergent with previous findings, stating the pancreas as an organ receiving highest absorbed doses [7]. Other organs (liver, spleen, and left suprarenal gland) showed significantly lower uptake of radiotracer, with spleen being second after pancreas. To our knowledge no study up to date tried to evaluate distribution of ^{11}C-acetate in different parts of pancreas, based on the fact that the uncinate process and the head have different embryological origins. No statistically significant differences were found in radiotracer uptake in body and uncinate process of pancreas in this study. Inclusion criteria in our study required no previous history of pancreas pathology and normal lab test results, but as other studies show [9, 10] it is possible to use ^{11}C-acetate in evaluating pancreas exocrine function.

In some forms of hereditary chronic pancreatitis, that is, coexisting with cystic fibrosis, there are no clinical symptoms of pancreatic exocrine or endocrine insufficiency [11]. The high risk of cancer development in these patients needs more radical treatment, but the patients usually do not accept the proposition until the pancreatic insufficiency is evident. Then ^{11}C-acetate PET/CT could be potentially decision-making tool. There is a need to develop more convenient tests to diagnose exocrine pancreatic insufficiency and monitor the disease progression.

The patients included had a history of kidney or/and prostate cancer but there was no difference in radiotracer distribution in both groups, as well as between male and female subjects.

^{11}C-Acetate uptake in suprarenal glands seems to be another interesting subject, as it was mentioned in only one study [12] regarding adrenal adenomas. Our results show that suprarenals had lowest uptake of examined organs. However it may be difficult to investigate right suprarenal glands due to problems with overlapping radioactivity from the liver.

5. Conclusions

The highest SUV max, SUV mean, and SUV peak values in pancreatic tissue in comparison to liver, spleen, and left suprarenal gland most probably indicate that specific organ function, that is, synthesis of hydrocarbonates or fatty acids, plays significant role in ^{11}C-acetate pancreatic uptake. It has to have a diagnostic potential in chronic pancreatic diseases. High pancreatic uptake may be used in the quantitative assessment of organ function in diffuse nonneoplastic pathology. Evaluation of ^{11}C- acetate uptake differences in parenchymal organs will allow establishing normal patterns of distribution and should lead to further studies of uptake changes in pancreatic disorders.

Authors' Contributions

B. Malkowski contributed to the idea and experimental organization. P. Wareluk contributed to the evaluation of the PET studies (1st evaluator). T. Gorycki contributed to the evaluation of the PET studies (2nd evaluator). K. Skrobisz contributed to the overwork of the results and preparing of the manuscript. M. Studniarek contributed to the overwork of the results and preparing of the manuscript and was the coordinator of the results.

References

[1] A. Luna, J. C. Vilanova, H. Da Cruz Jr., and S. E. LC Rossi, *Functional Imaging in Oncology*, Springer-Verlag, Berlin Heidelberg, 2014.

[2] I. Grassi, C. Nanni, V. Allegri et al., "The clinical use of PET with 11C-acetate," *American Journal of Nuclear Medicine and Molecular Imaging*, vol. 2, no. 1, pp. 33–47, 2012.

[3] B. Malkowski, P. Wareluk, K. Skrobisz, and M. Studniarek, "Normal uptake of 11C-acetate in pancreas, liver, spleen and suprarenal gland in PET," in *Proceedings of the Conference: ECR 2016*, 2016.

[4] J. V. Swinnen, P. P. Van Veldhoven, L. Timmermans et al., "Fatty acid synthase drives the synthesis of phospholipids partitioning into detergent-resistant membrane microdomains," *Biochemical and Biophysical Research Communications*, vol. 302, no. 4, pp. 898–903, 2003.

[5] L. M. Deford-Watts, A. Mintz, and S. J. Kridel, "The potential of 11C-acetate pet for monitoring the fatty acid synthesis pathway in tumors," *Current Pharmaceutical Biotechnology*, vol. 14, no. 3, pp. 300–312, 2013.

[6] N. Long, W. T. Wong, and E. H. Immergut, *The Chemistry of Molecular Imaging*, vol. 12, John Wiley and Sons, 2014.

[7] M. A. Seltzer, S. A. Jahan, R. Sparks et al., "Radiation dose estimates in humans for 11C-acetate whole-body PET," *Journal of Nuclear Medicine*, vol. 45, no. 7, pp. 1233–1236, 2004.

[8] P. D. Shreve and M. D. Gross, "Imaging of the pancreas and related diseases with PET carbon-11-acetate," *Journal of Nuclear Medicine*, vol. 38, no. 8, pp. 1305–1310, 1997.

[9] J. Hyun O, M. A. Lodge, S. Jagannath, J. M. Buscaglia, Y. Olagbemiro, and R. L. Wahl, "An exocrine pancreatic stress test with11C-acetate PET and secretin stimulation," *Journal of Nuclear Medicine*, vol. 55, no. 7, pp. 1128–1131, 2014.

[10] G. Karanikas and M. Beheshti, "11C-acetate PET/CT imaging: physiologic uptake, variants, and pitfalls," *PET Clinics*, vol. 9, no. 3, pp. 339–344, 2014.

[11] D. Lew, E. Afghani, and S. Pandol, "Chronic pancreatitis: current status and challenges for prevention and treatment," *Digestive Diseases and Sciences*, vol. 62, no. 7, pp. 1702–1712, 2017.

[12] D. Rubello, C. Bui, D. Casara, M. D. Gross, L. M. Fig, and B. Shapiro, "Functional scintigraphy of the adrenal gland," *European Journal of Endocrinology*, vol. 147, no. 1, pp. 13–28, 2002.

26

Bone Loss Prevention of Bisphosphonates in Patients with Inflammatory Bowel Disease

Yan Hu, Xiaoting Chen, Xiaojing Chen, Shuang Zhang, Tianyan Jiang, Jing Chang, and Yanhong Gao

Department of Geriatrics, Xinhua Hospital of Shanghai Jiaotong University, School of Medicine, Shanghai 2000092, China

Correspondence should be addressed to Jing Chang; changjingsh@163.com and Yanhong Gao; yhgao2010@yahoo.com

Academic Editor: Yvette Leung

Objective. The purpose of this study was to evaluate the effect of bisphosphonates in improving bone mineral density (BMD) and decreasing the occurrence rate of fractures and adverse events in patients with inflammatory bowel disease (IBD). *Methods.* Randomized controlled trials (RCTs) which use bisphosphonates in IBD patients were identified in PubMed, MEDLINE database, EMBASE database, Web of Knowledge, and the Cochrane Databases between 1990 and June 2016. People received bisphosphonate or placebos with a follow-up of at least one year were also considered. STATA 12.0 software was used for the meta-analysis. *Results.* Eleven randomized clinical trials were included in the meta-analysis. The data indicated that the percentage change in the increased BMD in the bisphosphonates groups was superior to that of the control groups at the lumbar spine and total hip. At the femoral neck, there was no significant difference between the two groups. The incidence of new fractures during follow-up showed significant reduction. The adverse event analysis revealed no significant difference between the two groups. *Conclusion.* Our results demonstrate that bisphosphonates therapy has an effect on bone loss in patients with IBD but show no evident efficiency at increasing the incidence of adverse events.

1. Introduction

Inflammatory bowel disease (IBD) includes Crohn's disease (CD), ulcerative colitis (UC), and indeterminate colitis and is characterized by chronic relapses and remitting inflammatory disorders of the gastrointestinal tract. Severe gastrointestinal symptoms including fatigue, abdominal pain, diarrhea, gastrointestinal bleeding, and damage to the structure and function of the gastrointestinal tract can occur due to this inflammation. The disease induces multisystem disorders, especially in the musculoskeletal system.

The disease itself, or chronic inflammation, smoking, glucocorticoid therapy, and so on, can cause skeletal system implications and bone disease [1, 2]. In recent years, the risk of low bone mineral density (BMD) and osteoporosis has increased in IBD patients at a prevalence between 22% and 77% compared with normal cases [3, 4]. The risk of fracture has likewise increased [5], and the risk of hip fracture has grown approximately 60% in patients with IBD [6]. The most relevant affecting factors are that patients always receive long-term corticosteroid therapy [7, 8]. Glucocorticoids increase the expression of the receptor activator for nuclear factor-kappa B ligand (RANKL) and decrease the expression of osteoprotegerin (OPG). Both of them play an important role in osteoclastogenesis to prolong the lifespan of osteoclasts [9]. Other factors such as nutritional interventions including dietary calcium and vitamin D intake and absorption, genetic factors, malabsorption, hypogonadism, bowel resection, and inflammatory cytokines such as TNF, IL-1beta, IL-2, and IL-17 may also have its impacts [10, 11].

Bisphosphonates are among the drugs most often used in the treatment of osteoporosis or osteopenia. They can be classified into two groups: nonnitrogen-containing bisphosphonates (e.g., etidronate and clodronate) and nitrogen-containing bisphosphonates (e.g., pamidronate, alendronate, risedronate, ibandronate, and zoledronate) [12]. Bisphosphonates have been found to prevent bone loss in patient with osteoporosis and corticosteroid-induced osteoporosis [13–15]. Alendronate has reported increased bone density in patients with glucocorticoid therapy. Cochrane systematic reviews have proved that alendronate and risedronate resulted in clinically important and statistically significant reductions in vertebral, nonvertebral, and hip fractures as a secondary form of prevention in postmenopausal women [16, 17]. The benefits of etidronate have also been demonstrated in the secondary prevention of vertebral fractures [17]. Moreover, calcium supplementation and vitamin D offer some benefits and somewhat prevent the development of osteoporosis or osteomalacia. Hormone replacement therapy (HRT), selective estrogen receptor modulators (SERMs), and sodium fluoride also have their effects [18, 19].

The number of people currently with IBD is increasing, and many have the potential to develop a bone disease. Focusing on early awareness in these individuals and defining the risk of fracture and adverse events in each patient to treat excessive bone loss and prevent osteoporotic fractures are important actions. According to the current limited data, bisphosphonates are the optimal choice for the therapy of both primary and glucocorticoid-induced osteoporosis in patients with IBD [20]. Several clinical trials have been conducted to analyse the effect of bisphosphonate on improving bone mineral density and decreasing fracture rates [21]. However, the effects of bisphosphonate used in patients with IBD have varied, and so have the experimental results [22]. In this meta-analysis, we unite and reanalyse previous clinical trials with the aim of developing further knowledge on the effect of bisphosphonates on bone loss and decreasing adverse events in patients with IBD.

2. Methods

2.1. Search Strategy. A literature search was performed from PubMed (1990–June 2016), MEDLINE database (1990–June 2016), EMBASE database (1990–June 2016), Web of Knowledge, and the Cochrane Controlled Trials Register in the Cochrane library. In the search, we used the terms: (inflammatory bowel disease OR ulcerative colitis OR Crohn's disease) and (osteoporosis or osteopenia or (bone and (density or mass or loss))) and (exp Diphosphonates/or (bisphosphonate* or alendron* or fosamax or etidron* or didronel or risedron* or actonel or ibandron* or bonivaor zolendron* or zometa or zomera or aclasta or reclastor pamidron* or aredia)). In addition, other relevant articles in hand were also searched. The language was restricted in English and the species was limited to humans in the search.

2.2. Study Selection. We included studies if they are randomized controlled trials (RCTs) which discussed the use of bisphosphonates in inflammatory bowel disease (IBD) patients, including the ones that only have Crohn's disease or only have ulcerative colitis. These recipients may be given calcium alone or vitamin D and calcium, while the control group received no treatment or placebo and may be given calcium alone or vitamin D and calcium. In addition, other inclusion criteria were as follows: (1) the participants' mean age being older than 18 years old; (2) the length of treatment being more than one year (including one year); (3) bisphosphonate in any dosage. There was no restriction about the gender of the participants. Duplications were excluded. BMDs were determined by dual-energy X-ray absorptiometry (DXA).

2.3. Statistical Analysis. In this meta-analysis, data analysis was conducted by the change in BMD values separately in the lumbar spine, total hip, and femoral neck. And the BMD values were expressed in percent change for both bisphosphonate and control groups. We used Stata/SE 12.0 program (Stata Corporation, College Station, TX, USA) for the total statistical analysis. Weighted mean differences (WMD) were calculated according to the percent change in BMD. Funnel plot was also drawn to assess the possible publication bias. The χ^2 test and I^2 statistic (represents the percentage of variability because of between-study variability) were applied to assess the heterogeneity among studies. If χ^2 p value < 0.1 or I > 50%, the statistic heterogeneity between studies was significant. Heterogeneity among studies was considered to be statistically significant when the p value was less than 0.1.

Moreover, subgroup analysis on the basis of treatment duration of studies (12 months and 24 months) was conducted for a further comparison. The incidence of new fractures and adverse events (AEs) was also conducted by using odds ratio (OR) between the bisphosphonate and control group.

3. Results

3.1. Literature Selection. According to the aforementioned search strategy and terms, 149 potentially relevant reports were found. Eleven random controlled trials (RCTs) [20, 22–31] met the inclusion criteria from these reports and others were found by additional articles that were considered eligible for this meta-analysis (Figure 1). The trials involved 785 participants. Three reports focused on participants with IBD [20, 26, 28], seven involved participants with Crohn's disease [22–25, 27, 29, 30], and one trial targeted patients with ulcerative colitis. All of the participants had osteopenia or osteoporosis. Only postmenopausal women were included in Palomba's [26] trial and excluded from Abitbol's [20] trial. Of all the eleven trials, two trials included adult patients with prolonged GC use [20, 31]. At baseline, there was generally a mild difference in the number of participants allocated to the intervention and control group except for von Tirpitz et al. [25]. There were three groups (two interventions and one placebo) in von Tirpitz et al. [25] and Klaus et al. [22]. Six studies [20, 23, 24, 26, 28, 31] were conducted in 12 months and the leaving papers were administered over the course of more than 1 year.

The characteristics of all of the trials are summarized in Table 1, including the number of patients, gender ratio, age, BMD, and duration. Table 2 compares the number of adverse events, nonvertebral and vertebral fractures between the two groups.

3.2. Effect of Bisphosphonates in Lumbar Spine BMD. Nine trials reported the percentage change of BMD in the lumbar

Table 1: Summary of the basic characteristics of the bisphosphonate and control groups.

Trial	Year	Intervention	Bisphosphonate administration	Control	Number of patients (intervention/ control)	Age (intervention/ control)	BMD (±SD g/cm^2) lumbar spine (intervention/ control)	BMD (±SD g/cm^2) Hip (intervention/ control)	BMD (±SD g/cm^2) T-score lumbar spine (intervention/ control)	BMD (±SD g/cm^2) T-score lumbar spine (intervention/ control)	Duration
Bartram et al.	2003	Pamidronate	30 mg/3 months i.v	No placebo	37/37	45.1 ± 11.4/ 43.5 ± 12.3	0.87 ± 0.09/0.86 ± 0.08	0.73 ± 0.01/0.78 ± 0.09	−1.84 ± 0.82/−1.91 ± 0.72	−2.34 ± 0.79/−1.92 ± 0.77	12
Haderslev et al.	2000	Alendronate	10 mg/day p.o	Placebo	15/17	44 ± 13/44 ± 12	0.74 ± 0.10/0.77 ± 0.09	0.74 ± 0.10/0.77 ± 0.09	−1.53/−1.21	−1.50/−1.70	12
Siffledeen et al.	2005	Etidronate	400 mg/14 days p.o	No placebo	71/72	40.0 ± 12.1/40.1 ± 14.1	0.94 ± 0.10/0.91 ± 0.11	0.86 ± 0.11/0.85 ± 0.11	−1.30 ± 0.85/−1.04 ± 0.75	−0.99 ± 0.72/−1.57 ± 0.97	24
Soo et al.	2012	risedronate	35 mg/day p.o	Placebo	45/43	39.8 ± 13.7/36.7 ± 12.7	0.936 ± 0.095/0.899 ± 0.075	0.886 ± 0.080/0.898 ± 0.097	−1.2 ± 0.9/−1.5 ± 0.7	−0.7 ± 0.6/−0.7 ± 0.6	24
Tirpitz et al.	2003	Ibandronate	1 mg/3 months i.v	No placebo	35/13	35.7 ± 1.8/37.15 ± 3.0	NA	NA	−2.29 ± 0.11/−1.57 ± 0.1	−2.29 ± 0.11/−1.57 ± 0.1	27
Klaus et al.	2011	Ibandronate	1 mg/3 months i.v	No placebo	54/32	33.8 ± 9.76/36.8 ± 13.1	0.90 ± 0.04/0.85 ± 0.08	0.90 ± 0.04/0.85 ± 0.08	−1.57 ± 0.31/−1.89 ± 0.71	−1.57 ± 0.31/−1.89 ± 0.71	42
Henderson et al.	2006	risedronate	5 mg/day p.o	Placebo	30/31	49.9 ± 12.8/47.2 ± 11.4	0.908 ± 0.082/0.898 ± 0.116	0.899 ± 0.127/0.867 ± 0.01	NA	NA	12
Palomba et al.	2005	risedronate	35 mg/week p.o	Placebo	45/45	52.3 ± 3.2/51.4 ± 3.0	0.561 ± 0.063/0.540 ± 0.062	0.561 ± 0.06/0.540 ± 0.062	NA	NA	12
van Bodegraven et al.	2014	risedronate	35 mg/week p.o	Placebo	64/67	43 ± 13/42 ± 13	0.94 ± 0.11/0.95 ± 0.11	0.81 ± 0.09/0.81 ± 0.11	−1.30 ± 0.61/−1.26 ± 0.78	−1.22 ± 0.63/−1.21 ± 0.51	24
Abitbol et al.	2007	Clodronate	900 mg/3 months i.v	Placebo	33/34	30/30	NA	NA	NA	NA	12
Kitazaki et al.	2009	alendronate	5 mg/day p.o	No placebo	19/20	41.2 ± 12.8/38.1 ± 15.5	0.926 ± 0.098/0.906 ± 0.125	NA	NA	NA	12

TABLE 2: Summary of the number of adverse events, nonvertebral and vertebral fractures between the bisphosphonate and control groups.

Trial	Year	Bisphosphonate group				Control group			
		Number of patients	Number of adverse events	Number of nonvertebral fractures	Number of vertebral fractures	Number of patients	Number of adverse events	Number of nonvertebral fractures	Number of vertebral fractures
Bartram et al.	2003	37	4			37	3		
Haderslev et al.	2000	15	12	0	1	17	13	1	2
Siffledeen et al.	2005	71	5		1	72	2		0
Soo et al.	2012	45	2			43	3		
Tirpitz et al.	2003	35	9			13	3		
Klaus et al.	2011	54	12		0	32	9		1
Henderson et al.	2006	30	18	1		31	19	1	
Palomba et al.	2005	45	5	0	5	45	2	4	14
van Bodegraven et al.	2014	64	0		0	67	1		1
Abitbol et al.	2007	33	26			34	24		
Kitazaki et al.	2009	19	3			20	1		

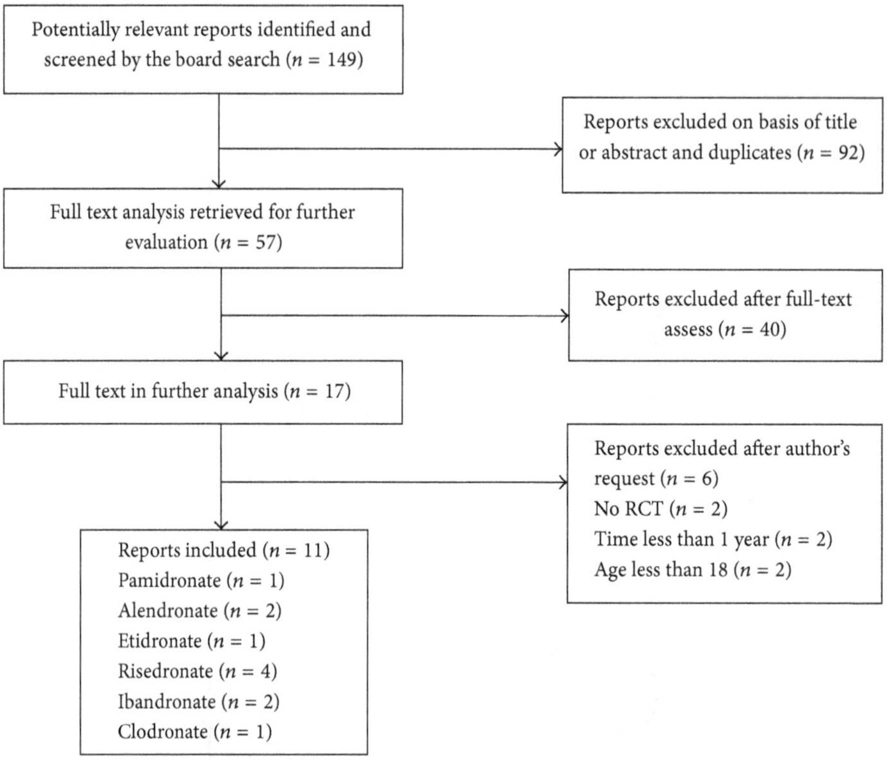

FIGURE 1: Flowchart of study selection in the meta-analysis.

spine in the bisphosphonate and control groups of IBD patients [20, 22–24, 26–30]. Tirpitz et al. [25] showed ΔT scores of spine BMD and found nonsignificant between groups. There was an increment of spine BMD values in the bisphosphonate group compared with the control group (WMD = 0.41, 95% CI: 0.18–0.64, p = 0.001) (Figure 2). The results of a fixed-effects model in the group were exactly the same as those of a random-effects model. Statistical moderate heterogeneity was found in this analysis (I^2 = 43.4%, p = 0.078). Moreover, the funnel plot also revealed some asymmetry (Figure 3) and Begg's and Egger's tests ruled out a trend toward publication bias (p = 0.466 and 0.281, resp.). Subgroup analysis targeting on treatment duration was established to determine this heterogeneity. For 12 months, the bisphosphonate group generated an increment in BMD values, and these trials were relatively homogeneous (I^2 = 39.4%, p = 0.143). The heterogeneity test for 24 months indicated that the statistical heterogeneity was large (I^2 = 65.8%, p = 0.054) (Figure 2).

3.3. Effect of Bisphosphonates in Total Hip BMD. Eight studies reported the percentage change in BMD at the total hip in the bisphosphonate groups and control groups [20, 23, 24, 26–30]. The BMD increased at the total hip in the group of IBD patients treated with bisphosphonate (WMD = 0.29, 95% CI: 0.11–0.46, p = 0.001) (Figure 4). The test for overall heterogeneity was small (p = 0.480). Either funnel plot or Begg's and Egger's tests showed no statistical evidence of publication bias. A further assessment included a subgroup analysis of the treatment duration. Seven trials conducted over 12 months revealed a superior effect in improving BMD of hip (WMD = 0.30, 95% CI: 0.08–0.53, p = 0.009). For the other two 24-month trials, the increase in BMD was not significant between the two groups (WMD = 0.27, 95% CI: −0.15–0.68, p = 0.206).

3.4. Effect of Bisphosphonates in Femoral Neck BMD. The four studies that examined the femoral neck BMD was assessed [20, 27–29]. A summary of the further treatment duration analysis conducted in the related studies is also given. It indicates that the bisphosphonate group was no different from the control group in terms of percentage change in BMD in femoral neck.

3.5. New Fractures Analysis. Six studies reported the incidences of new fractures during follow-up, including nonvertebral fractures and vertebral fractures [22, 23, 26–28, 30]. The pooled OR of total fractures was 0.30 (95% CI, 0.13–0.69, p = 0.005), indicating that bisphosphonate treatment was superior to control treatment in preventing vertebral fractures (OR = 0.38, 95% CI, 0.16–0.93, p = 0.035) instead of nonvertebral fractures (OR = 0.35, 95% CI, 0.06–1.95, p = 0.228) (Figure 5). Furthermore, pooled data showed significant effectiveness of bisphosphonates compared with controls at 12 months, with the ORs of 12 months and 24 months being 0.25 (95% CI, 0.10–0.64, p = 0.004) and 0.60 (95% CI, 0.09–3.84, p = 0.587) (Figure 5), respectively.

3.6. Adverse Event Analysis. All eleven of the studies showed the number of adverse events. No significant difference was

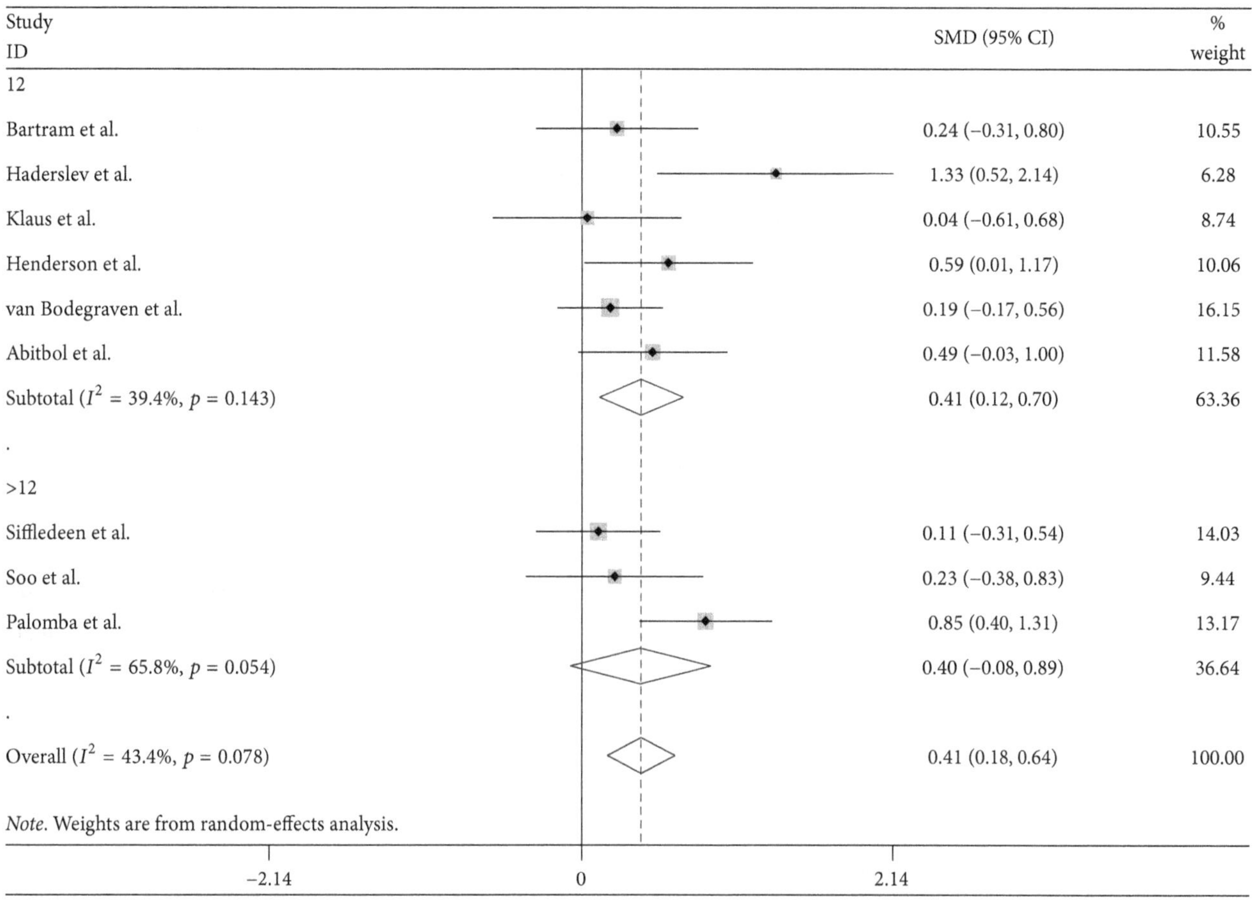
Study ID
SMD (95% CI)
% weight
12
Bartram et al. 0.24 (−0.31, 0.80) 10.55
Haderslev et al. 1.33 (0.52, 2.14) 6.28
Klaus et al. 0.04 (−0.61, 0.68) 8.74
Henderson et al. 0.59 (0.01, 1.17) 10.06
van Bodegraven et al. 0.19 (−0.17, 0.56) 16.15
Abitbol et al. 0.49 (−0.03, 1.00) 11.58
Subtotal (I^2 = 39.4%, p = 0.143) 0.41 (0.12, 0.70) 63.36
>12
Siffledeen et al. 0.11 (−0.31, 0.54) 14.03
Soo et al. 0.23 (−0.38, 0.83) 9.44
Palomba et al. 0.85 (0.40, 1.31) 13.17
Subtotal (I^2 = 65.8%, p = 0.054) 0.40 (−0.08, 0.89) 36.64
Overall (I^2 = 43.4%, p = 0.078) 0.41 (0.18, 0.64) 100.00
Note. Weights are from random-effects analysis.
−2.14
0
2.14

Figure 2: Randomized controlled trials of bisphosphonates in improving spinal BMD in IBD. Forest plot showing the weighted mean differences and 95% confidence interval of the percentage change in BMD in the lumbar spine in the bisphosphonate and control groups. A subgroup analysis of the treatment duration of the two groups is also shown.

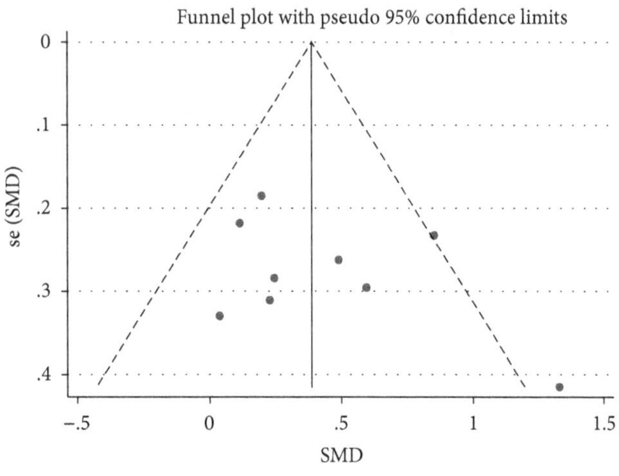

Figure 3: Funnel plot of studies included in Figure 2. Dots represent the results of each study. Funnel plots showing some asymmetry of nine trials reporting the efficacy of the bisphosphonates versus control groups in change of BMD in the lumbar spine in IBD patients.

found between the bisphosphonate and control groups (OR = 1.19, 95% CI, 0.77–1.85, $p = 0.426$) (Figure 6), demonstrating that bisphosphonate treatment was not associated with an increased incidence of adverse effects. Incidences of adverse effects were not increased with treatment duration. For 12 months and 24 months, the pooled ORs were 1.42 (95% CI, 0.80–2.53, $p = 0.227$) and 0.94 (95% CI, 0.48–1.84, $p = 0.848$), respectively. The shape of the funnel plot and the Egger's test ($p = 0.477$) (Figure 7) indicated no publication bias. Most of adverse events were gastric and intestinal

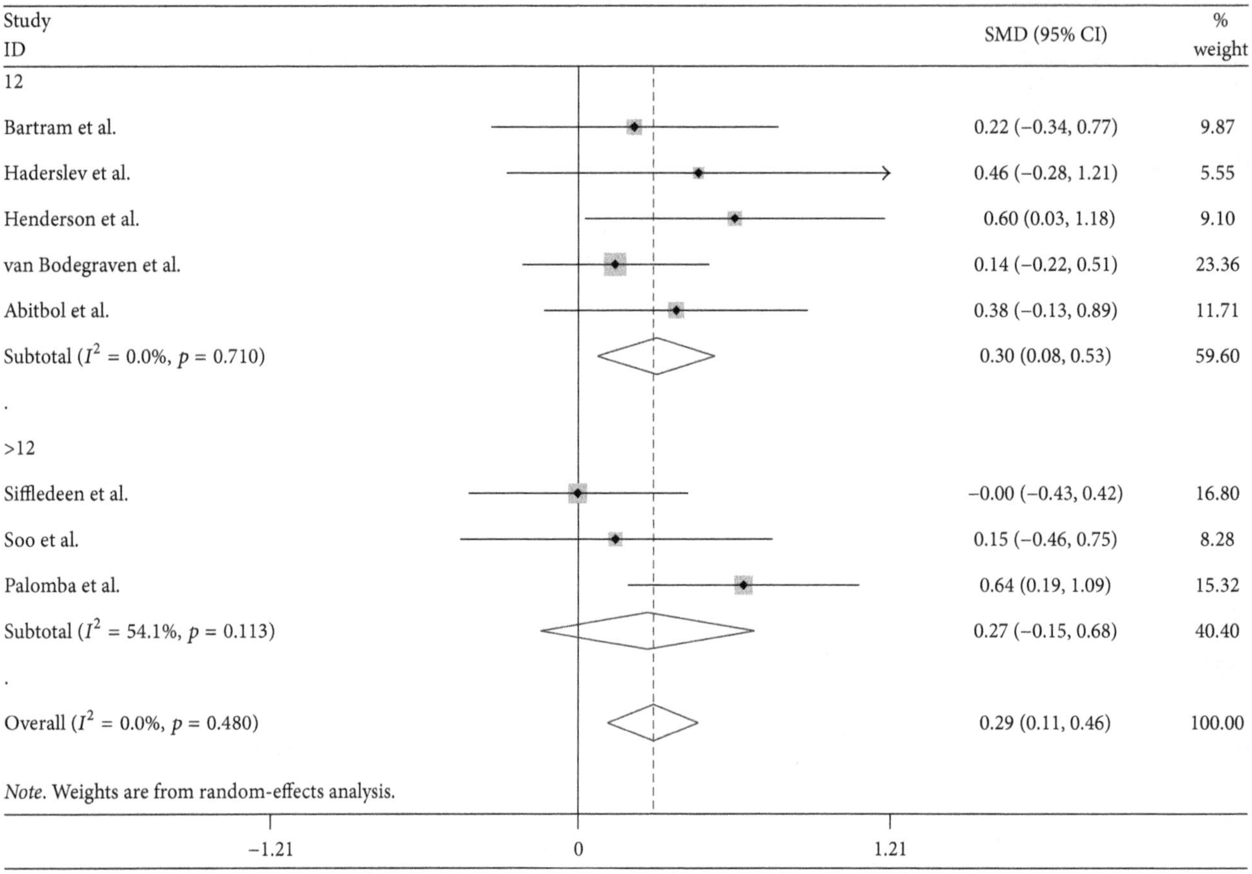
Study
ID
SMD (95% CI)
%
weight
12
Bartram et al.
0.22 (−0.34, 0.77)
9.87
Haderslev et al.
0.46 (−0.28, 1.21)
5.55
Henderson et al.
0.60 (0.03, 1.18)
9.10
van Bodegraven et al.
0.14 (−0.22, 0.51)
23.36
Abitbol et al.
0.38 (−0.13, 0.89)
11.71
Subtotal (I^2 = 0.0%, p = 0.710)
0.30 (0.08, 0.53)
59.60
>12
Siffledeen et al.
−0.00 (−0.43, 0.42)
16.80
Soo et al.
0.15 (−0.46, 0.75)
8.28
Palomba et al.
0.64 (0.19, 1.09)
15.32
Subtotal (I^2 = 54.1%, p = 0.113)
0.27 (−0.15, 0.68)
40.40
Overall (I^2 = 0.0%, p = 0.480)
0.29 (0.11, 0.46)
100.00
Note. Weights are from random-effects analysis.
−1.21
0
1.21

FIGURE 4: Randomized controlled trials of bisphosphonates in improving total hip BMD in IBD. Forest plot showing the weighted mean differences and 95% confidence interval of the percentage change in bone mineral density at the total hip in the bisphosphonate and control groups. A subgroup analysis of the treatment duration of the two groups is also shown.

diseases such as gaseous distention, bloating, and diarrhea. Three trials reported arthralgia [20, 26, 29] and two trials reported reversible bone pain [22, 27].

4. Discussion

IBD is a chronic and incurable disease, with increasing numbers of patients suffering from it. Among its complications, osteoporosis and fragility fracture are increasing common, especially in elderly patients. Long-term corticosteroid therapy has been considered one of the major causes of osteoporosis. Medications like bisphosphonates, vitamin D, calcitonin, teriparatide, parathyroid hormone, infliximab, and denosumab are effective for the prevention and treatment of osteoporosis [32]. Bisphosphonates can specifically bind to hydroxyl apatite in bone and inhibit osteoclast activity [14, 33] and is an effective treatment for GC-induced osteoporosis and postmenopausal osteoporosis. The studies enrolled in this meta-analysis showed that bisphosphonates can also reduce the risk of fractures in IBD patients. Only one clinical trial thus far showed that intranasal calcitonin is not able to increase BMD in young IBD patients [34]. Two prospective studies revealed the beneficial effect of infliximab on bone metabolism both in CD and in UC patients [35, 36]. For teriparatide, whether parathyroid hormone and denosumab can improve BMD or reduce the risk of fracture in IBD patients remains unknown.

This meta-analysis and systematic review was conducted to evaluate the effect of bisphosphonates in the prevention and treatment of bone loss in patients with IBD. The incidence of fractures and adverse events was also determined. Eleven RCTs were conducted in the analysis and contributed to some or all of the results of interest. The meta-analysis revealed that there was an increment in BMD at the lumbar spine and total hip in patients treated with bisphosphonates compared with the control group. Although the changes in lumbar spine and total hip BMD showed more significant improvement at 12 months, no difference was found at 24 months. No significant difference was found between the two groups in terms of BMD at the femoral neck, perhaps because the number of documents that noted the changes in the femoral neck BMD was small and the data we selected were taken from different trials. Also, there were six studies reporting the incidences of new fractures during follow-up, five of which reported vertebral fractures and three of which reported nonvertebral fractures, and significant difference between the treatment group and the control group can be seen, showing that bisphosphonates can reduce the risk of fractures, especially vertebral fractures. Similarly, short-term

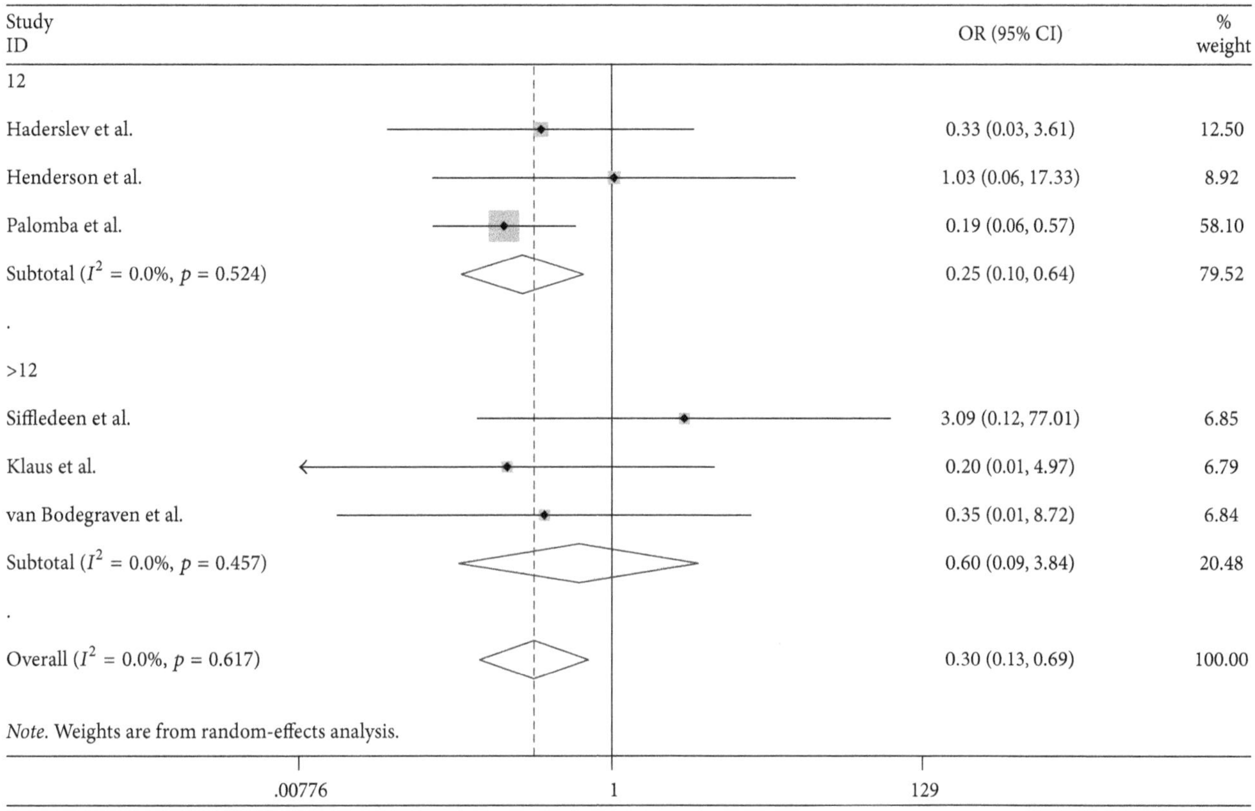

(a)

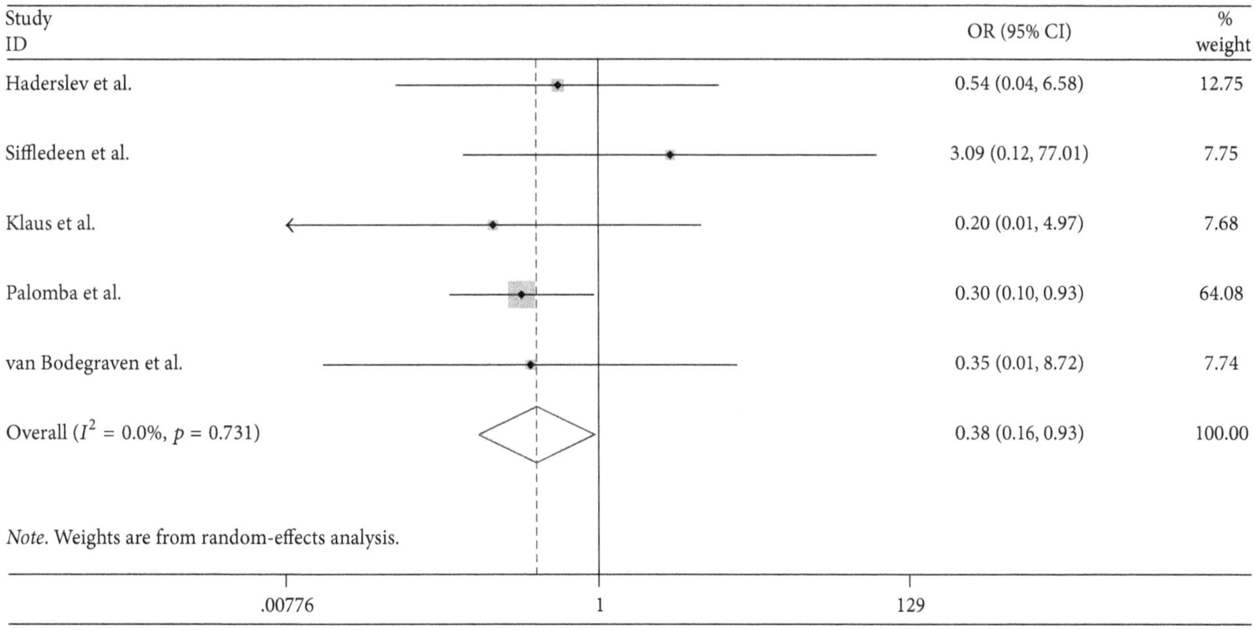

(b)

FIGURE 5: Randomized controlled trials of bisphosphonates in reducing new fractures and vertebrate fractures in IBD. (a) Forest plot showing the odds ratio and 95% confidence interval of the incidence of new fractures of the bisphosphonate and control groups. A subgroup analysis of the treatment duration of the two groups is also shown. (b) Forest plot showing the odds ratio and 95% confidence interval of the incidence of vertebrate fractures of the bisphosphonate and control groups.

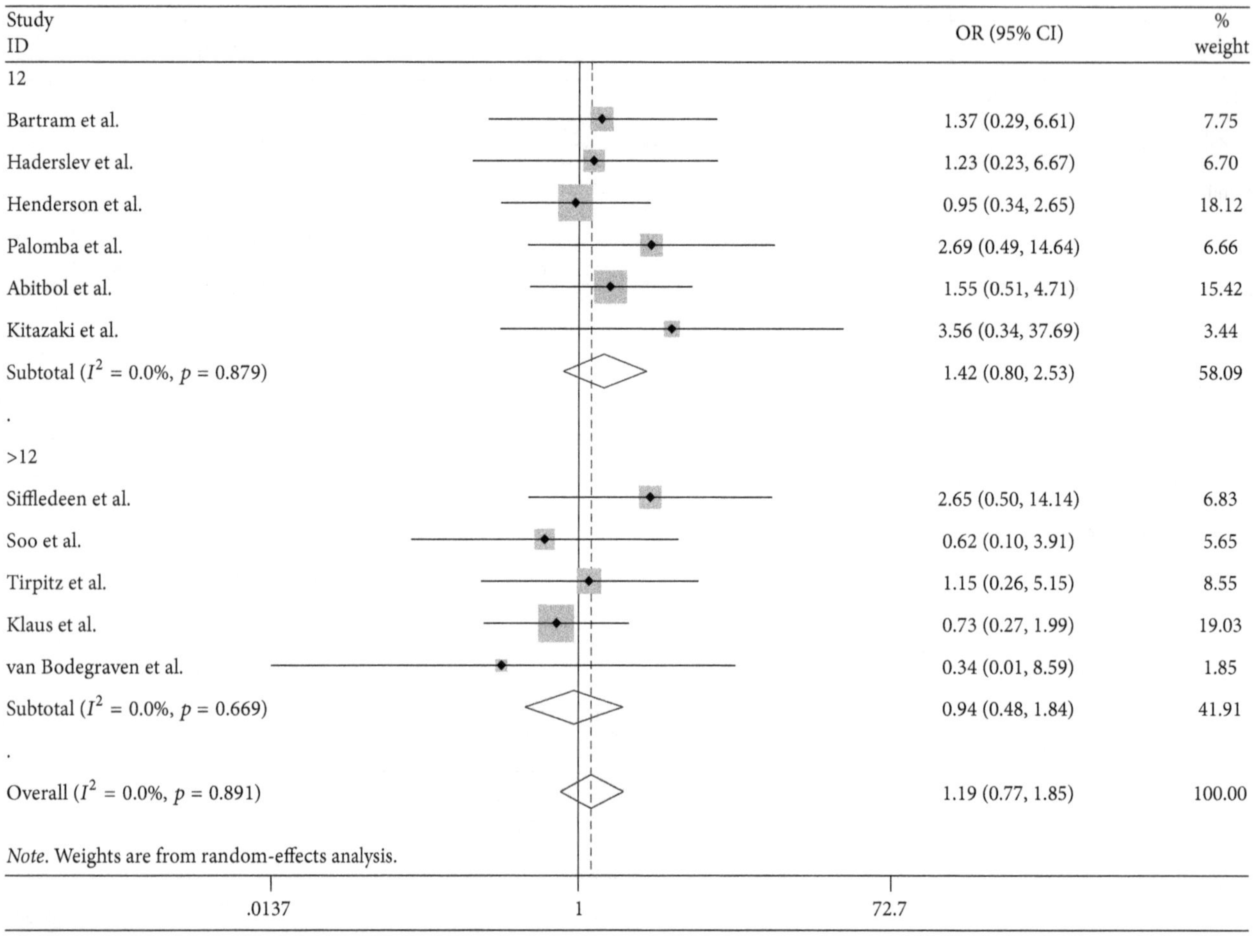

Study ID
OR (95% CI)
% weight
12
Bartram et al. 1.37 (0.29, 6.61) 7.75
Haderslev et al. 1.23 (0.23, 6.67) 6.70
Henderson et al. 0.95 (0.34, 2.65) 18.12
Palomba et al. 2.69 (0.49, 14.64) 6.66
Abitbol et al. 1.55 (0.51, 4.71) 15.42
Kitazaki et al. 3.56 (0.34, 37.69) 3.44
Subtotal (I^2 = 0.0%, p = 0.879) 1.42 (0.80, 2.53) 58.09
>12
Siffledeen et al. 2.65 (0.50, 14.14) 6.83
Soo et al. 0.62 (0.10, 3.91) 5.65
Tirpitz et al. 1.15 (0.26, 5.15) 8.55
Klaus et al. 0.73 (0.27, 1.99) 19.03
van Bodegraven et al. 0.34 (0.01, 8.59) 1.85
Subtotal (I^2 = 0.0%, p = 0.669) 0.94 (0.48, 1.84) 41.91
Overall (I^2 = 0.0%, p = 0.891) 1.19 (0.77, 1.85) 100.00
Note. Weights are from random-effects analysis.
.0137
1
72.7

FIGURE 6: Randomized controlled trials of bisphosphonates in adverse events. Forest plot showing the odds ratio and 95% confidence interval of the adverse event rates.

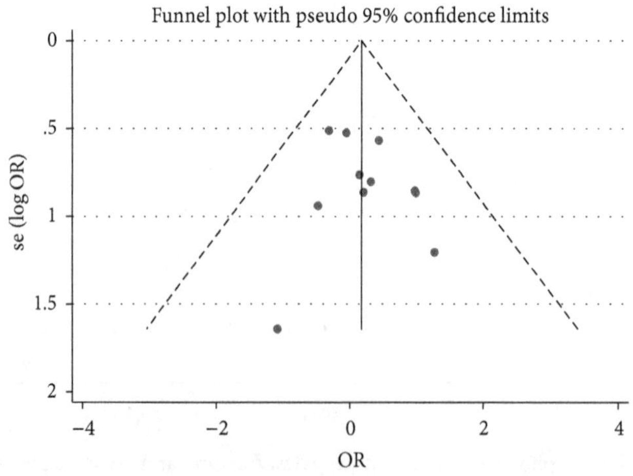

FIGURE 7: Funnel plot of studies included in Figure 6. Dots represent the results of each study. The funnel plot was visually examined, showing symmetrical characteristic of eleven trials reporting the adverse events. There was no asymmetry and statistical evidence of publication bias among the included studies.

treatment showed significant improvement while long-term treatment showed no difference. There are several explanations for these conflicted results. First, only three trials reported BMD change and the incidence of new fractures in the 24-month duration and therefore may not reflect the difference. Second, a longer duration and a high rate of withdrawal may have affected the results. Bisphosphonates had significant effect on the BMD in the lumbar spine and total hip compared with the placebo and no intervention groups as well as on the prevention of vertebral fractures.

From a bisphosphonate safety perspective, we could not find any statistically significant difference in the occurrence of adverse events between the bisphosphonate and control groups. Most of the adverse events were gastrointestinal reactions to the bisphosphonates in our review. At the same time, IBD itself also contributed to the adverse events. When the participants were aware of the treatment they were receiving, they might have been more or less likely to report adverse events. No other serious adverse events were described in the review. As such, no conclusions can be drawn in relation to the adverse events caused by bisphosphonates for patients with IBD.

We explored the presence of statistical heterogeneity using a chi-squared test and measured the quantity of heterogeneity by I^2. It showed a moderate heterogeneity at the lumbar spine ($I^2 = 43.4\%$, $p = 0.078$). To address our heterogeneity concerns, we used both fixed and random-effects models to make the chosen model more sensitive, and the results were coincident. There are several reasons for this heterogeneity. First, heterogeneity was brought into the meta-analysis by the study we included. In terms of the trials conducted by von Tirpitz et al. [25] and Klaus et al. [22], the number of participants was significantly different between the experiment and control groups when analysing the adverse event ratio. Postmenopausal women were excluded from Abitbol's [20] trial and exclusively included in Palomba's [26] trial suggesting that the result of this study should interpreted with caution. Second, the data related to the percentage change in BMD was limited because some citations only gave baseline and after-treatment T-scores [25] and the percentage change in the T-scores [22]. The primary statistics could not be found. In the femoral neck BMD, only four RCTs [20, 27–29] were reported. Third, our meta-analysis was based on published data; unpublished data was excluded, and heterogeneity was found. Finally, different bisphosphonate doses and administration regimen might have been potential sources of the observed heterogeneity.

Our meta-analysis was limited in several ways. All eleven of the included trials had small sample sizes, with an average of 78 participants with IBD. Small trials have less power, meaning that there was a lower chance of detecting a small but true effect as statistically significant. Another limitation was that seven RCTs focusing on Crohn's disease [22–25, 27, 29, 30] and three RCTs focusing on IBD were accepted [20, 26, 28] and one trial focusing on ulcerative colitis was accepted [31]. The number of trials focusing on IBD was relatively small. One trial assessed pamidronate versus no intervention, two trials assessed alendronate versus placebo and no intervention, respectively, two trials assessed ibandronate versus no intervention, one trial assessed etidronate versus no intervention, four trials assessed risedronate versus placebo, and one trial assessed clodronate versus placebo.

In summary, our integration of the available individual clinical trials indicated that some advantages were observed between the bisphosphonate and control treatments for BMD in the lumbar spine and total hip regions of patients with IBD. The bisphosphonates were found to be effective and safe. Clinicians should consider these results when choosing treatments for IBD patient with bone loss.

Authors' Contributions

Yan Hu and Xiaoting Chen are contributed equally to this article.

Acknowledgments

The reported work was supported in part by research grants from the Natural Science Foundation of China (81101360), Natural Science Foundation of Shanghai Technology Committee (no. 16ZR1422000), Medicine-Engineering Cross Project of Shanghai Jiao Tong University (no. YG2015MS67), and the Scientific Research Foundation for the Returned Overseas Chinese Scholars, State Education Ministry (no. 20134701) to Dr. Y. Gao.

References

[1] F. K. Ghishan and P. R. Kiela, "Advances in the understanding of mineral and bone metabolism in inflammatory bowel diseases," *American Journal of Physiology - Gastrointestinal and Liver Physiology*, vol. 300, no. 2, pp. G191–G201, 2011.

[2] C. A. Lima, "Risk factors for osteoporosis in inflammatory bowel disease patients," *World Journal of Gastrointestinal Pathophysiology*, vol. 6, no. 4, p. 210, 2015.

[3] M. Dinca, "Evolution of osteopenia in inflammatory bowel disease," *The American Journal of Gastroenterology*, vol. 94, no. 5, pp. 1292–1297.

[4] E. Miznerova, T. Hlavaty, T. Koller et al., "The prevalence and risk factors for osteoporosis in patients with inflammatory bowel disease," *Bratislava Medical Journal*, vol. 114, no. 08, pp. 439–445, 2013.

[5] C. N. Bernstein, J. F. Blanchard, W. Leslie, A. Wajda, and B. N. Yu, "The incidence of fracture among patients with inflammatory bowel disease: A population-based cohort study," *Annals of Internal Medicine*, vol. 133, no. 10, pp. 795–150, 2000.

[6] T. Card, J. West, R. Hubbard, and R. F. A. Logan, "Hip fractures in patients with inflammatory bowel disease and their relationship to corticosteroid use: A population based cohort study," *Gut*, vol. 53, no. 2, pp. 251–255, 2004.

[7] C. Schulte, A. U. Dignass, K. Mann, and H. Goebell, "Reduced bone mineral density and unbalanced bone metabolism in patients with inflammatory bowel disease," *Inflammatory Bowel Diseases*, vol. 4, no. 4, pp. 268–275, 1998.

[8] P. Miheller, K. Lorinczy, and P. L. Lakatos, "Clinical relevance of changes in bone metabolism in inflammatory bowel disease," *World Journal of Gastroenterology*, vol. 16, no. 44, pp. 5536–5542, 2010.

[9] T. Kondo, R. Kitazawa, A. Yamaguchi, and S. Kitazawa, "Dexamethasone promotes osteoclastogenesis by inhibiting osteoprotegerin through multiple levels," *Journal of Cellular Biochemistry*, vol. 103, no. 1, pp. 335–345, 2008.

[10] D. S. Amarasekara, J. Yu, and J. Rho, "Bone Loss Triggered by the Cytokine Network in Inflammatory Autoimmune Diseases," *Journal of Immunology Research*, vol. 2015, Article ID 832127, 2015.

[11] D. Q. Shih, S. R. Targan, and D. McGovern, "Recent advances in IBD pathogenesis: genetics and immunobiology," *Current Gastroenterology Reports*, vol. 10, no. 6, pp. 568–575, 2008.

[12] R. G. G. Russell, "Bisphosphonates: the first 40 years," *Bone*, vol. 49, no. 1, pp. 2–19, 2011.

[13] J. Y. Y. Leung, A. Y. Y. Ho, T. P. Ip, G. Lee, and A. W. C. Kung, "The efficacy and tolerability of risedronate on bone mineral density and bone turnover markers in osteoporotic Chinese women: A randomized placebo-controlled study," *Bone*, vol. 36, no. 2, pp. 358–364, 2005.

[14] S. A. Stoch, K. G. Saag, M. Greenwald et al., "Once-weekly oral alendronate 70 mg in patients with glucocorticoid-induced bone loss: A 12-month randomized, placebo-controlled clinical trial," *Journal of Rheumatology*, vol. 36, no. 8, pp. 1705–1714, 2009.

[15] D. M. Black, "Fracture Risk Reduction with Alendronate in Women with Osteoporosis: The Fracture Intervention Trial," *Journal of Clinical Endocrinology & Metabolism*, vol. 85, no. 11, pp. 4118–4124, 2000.

[16] G. A. Wells, A. Cranney, J. Peterson et al., "Alendronate for the primary and secondary prevention of osteoporotic fractures in postmenopausal women.," *Cochrane database of systematic reviews (Online)*, no. 1, p. CD001155, 2008.

[17] G. Wells, A. Cranney, J. Peterson et al., "Risedronate for the primary and secondary prevention of osteoporotic fractures in postmenopausal women," *Cochrane Database of Systematic Reviews*, vol. 23, no. 1, Article ID CD004523, 2008.

[18] C. v. Tirpitz, J. Klaus, J. Brückel et al., "Increase of bone mineral density with sodium fluoride in patients with Crohn's disease," *European Journal of Gastroenterology & Hepatology*, vol. 12, no. 1, pp. 19–24, 2000.

[19] H. N. de Souza, F. L. Lora, C. A. M. Kulak, N. C. P. Mañas, H. M. B. Amarante, and V. Z. C. Borba, "Low levels of 25-hydroxyvitamin D (25OHD) in patients with inflammatory bowel disease and its correlation with bone mineral density," *Arquivos Brasileiros de Endocrinologia e Metabologia*, vol. 52, no. 4, pp. 684–691, 2008.

[20] V. Abitbol, K. Briot, C. Roux et al., "A Double-Blind Placebo-Controlled Study of Intravenous Clodronate for Prevention of Steroid-Induced Bone Loss in Inflammatory Bowel Disease," *Clinical Gastroenterology and Hepatology*, vol. 5, no. 10, pp. 1184–1189, 2007.

[21] K. Saag, R. Emkey, and T. Schnitzer, "ALENDRONATE AND CORTICOSTEROID-INDUCED OSTEOPOROSIS," *Southern Medical Journal*, vol. 91, no. 11, p. 1084, 1998.

[22] J. Klaus, M. Reinshagen, K. Herdt et al., "Bones and Crohn's: No benefit of adding sodium fluoride or ibandronate to calcium and vitamin D," *World Journal of Gastroenterology*, vol. 17, no. 3, pp. 334–342, 2011.

[23] K. V. Haderslev, L. Tjellesen, H. A. Sorensen, and M. Staun, "Alendronate increases lumbar spine bone mineral density in patients with Crohn's disease," *Gastroenterology*, vol. 119, no. 3, pp. 639–646, 2000.

[24] S. A. Bartram, R. T. Peaston, D. J. Rawlings, R. M. Francis, and N. P. Thompson, "A randomized controlled trial of calcium with vitamin D, alone or in combination with intravenous pamidronate, for the treatment of low bone mineral density associated with Crohn's disease," *Alimentary Pharmacology and Therapeutics*, vol. 18, no. 11-12, pp. 1121–1127, 2003.

[25] C. Tirpitz, J. Klaus, and M. Steinkamp, "Therapy of osteoporosis in patients with Crohn's disease: a randomized study comparing sodium fluoride and ibandronate," *Alimentary pharmacology therapeutics*, vol. 17, pp. 807-16, 2003.

[26] S. Palomba, F. Orio Jr., F. Manguso et al., "Efficacy of risedronate administration in osteoporotic postmenopausal women affected by inflammatory bowel disease," *Osteoporosis International*, vol. 16, no. 9, pp. 1141–1149, 2005.

[27] J. S. Sifiledeen, R. N. Fedorak, K. Siminoski et al., "Randomized trial of etidronate plus calcium and vitamin D for treatment of low bone mineral density in Crohn's disease," *Clinical Gastroenterology and Hepatology*, vol. 3, no. 2, pp. 122–132, 2005.

[28] S. Henderson, N. Hoffman, and R. Prince, "A double-blind placebo-controlled study of the effects of the bisphosphonate risedronate on bone mass in patients with inflammatory bowel disease," *American Journal of Gastroenterology*, vol. 101, no. 1, pp. 119–123, 2006.

[29] I. Soo, J. Siffledeen, K. Siminoski, B. McQueen, and R. N. Fedorak, "Risedronate improves bone mineral density in Crohn's disease: A two year randomized controlled clinical trial," *Journal of Crohn's and Colitis*, vol. 6, no. 7, pp. 777–786, 2012.

[30] A. A. Van Bodegraven, N. Bravenboer, B. I. Witte et al., "Treatment of bone loss in osteopenic patients with Crohn's disease: A double-blind, randomised trial of oral risedronate 35 mg once weekly or placebo, concomitant with calcium and vitamin D supplementation," *Gut*, vol. 63, no. 9, pp. 1424–1430, 2014.

[31] S. Kitazaki, K. Mitsuyama, J. Masuda et al., "Clinical trial: Comparison of alendronate and alfacalcidol in glucocorticoid-associated osteoporosis in patients with ulcerative colitis," *Alimentary Pharmacology and Therapeutics*, vol. 29, no. 4, pp. 424–430, 2009.

[32] "Multiple choice in the management of the menopause: Weighted scores for the answers," *Climacteric*, vol. 14, no. 6, pp. 703-704, 2011.

[33] Y. Okada, M. Nawata, S. Nakayamada, K. Saito, and Y. Tanaka, "Alendronate protects premenopausal women from bone loss and fracture associated with high-dose glucocorticoid therapy," *Journal of Rheumatology*, vol. 35, no. 11, pp. 2249–2254, 2008.

[34] H. M. Pappa, T. M. Saslowsky, R. Filip-Dhima et al., "Efficacy and harms of nasal calcitonin in improving bone density in young patients with inflammatory bowel disease: A randomized, placebo-controlled, double-blind trial," *American Journal of Gastroenterology*, vol. 106, no. 8, pp. 1527–1543, 2011.

[35] S. G. Veerappan, M. Healy, B. Walsh, C. A. O'Morain, J. S. Daly, and B. M. Ryan, "A 1-year prospective study of the effect of infliximab on bone metabolism in inflammatory bowel disease patients," *European Journal of Gastroenterology and Hepatology*, vol. 28, no. 11, pp. 1335–1344, 2016.

[36] B. M. Ryan, M. G. V. M. Russel, L. Schurgers et al., "Effect of antitumour necrosis factor-α therapy on bone turnover in patients with active Crohn's disease: A prospective study," *Alimentary Pharmacology and Therapeutics*, vol. 20, no. 8, pp. 851–857, 2004.

27

New Insights in Genetic Cholestasis: From Molecular Mechanisms to Clinical Implications

Eva Sticova,[1,2] **Milan Jirsa**,[3] **and Joanna Pawłowska**[4]

[1] *Clinical and Transplant Pathology Centre, Institute for Clinical and Experimental Medicine, Prague 4, 140 21, Czech Republic*
[2] *Department of Pathology, Third Faculty of Medicine, Charles University, Prague 10, 100 00, Czech Republic*
[3] *Laboratory of Experimental Hepatology, Experimental Medicine Centre, Institute for Clinical and Experimental Medicine, Prague 4, 140 21, Czech Republic*
[4] *Department of Gastroenterology, Hepatology, Nutritional Disorders and Pediatrics, The Children's Memorial Health Institute (CMHI), Warsaw 04-730, Poland*

Correspondence should be addressed to Eva Sticova; eva.sticova@ikem.cz

Academic Editor: Emmanuel Tsochatzis

Cholestasis is characterised by impaired bile secretion and accumulation of bile salts in the organism. Hereditary cholestasis is a heterogeneous group of rare autosomal recessive liver disorders, which are characterised by intrahepatic cholestasis, pruritus, and jaundice and caused by defects in genes related to the secretion and transport of bile salts and lipids. Phenotypic manifestation is highly variable, ranging from progressive familial intrahepatic cholestasis (PFIC)—with onset in early infancy and progression to end-stage liver disease—to a milder intermittent mostly nonprogressive form known as benign recurrent intrahepatic cholestasis (BRIC). Cases have been reported of initially benign episodic cholestasis that subsequently transitions to a persistent progressive form of the disease. Therefore, BRIC and PFIC seem to represent two extremes of a continuous spectrum of phenotypes that comprise one disease. Thus far, five representatives of PFIC (named PFIC1-5) caused by pathogenic mutations present in both alleles of *ATP8B1*, *ABCB11*, *ABCB4*, *TJP2*, and *NR1H4* have been described. In addition to familial intrahepatic cholestasis, partial defects in *ATP8B1*, *ABCB11*, and *ABCB4* predispose patients to drug-induced cholestasis and intrahepatic cholestasis in pregnancy. This review summarises the current knowledge of the clinical manifestations, genetics, and molecular mechanisms of these diseases and briefly outlines the therapeutic options, both conservative and invasive, with an outlook for future personalised therapeutic strategies.

1. Introduction

Cholestasis is characterised by an impairment of bile secretion and transport, leading to the subsequent accumulation of toxic bile components in the organism. Bile salts (BS), the main organic solutes in bile, are physiological detergents that facilitate the absorption and transport of lipids, vitamins, and nutrients. BS also play an important role in cell signalling as part of key metabolic processes.

2. Bile Salt Synthesis

BS are synthesised from cholesterol in the liver. The size of the total BS pool in human adults is 3-4 g [1, 2]. There are two main pathways of BS synthesis. The classic (neutral) biosynthesis pathway, localised exclusively in the liver and accounting for at least 75% of the total BS pool, starts with modification of the sterol ring, followed by side chain cleavage reactions to synthesise cholic and chenodeoxycholic acid, constituting the primary BS in humans. The first and rate-limiting enzyme in this pathway is microsomal cholesterol 7 alpha-hydroxylase (CYP7A1). In the alternative (acidic) pathway of BS synthesis, side chain oxidation precedes modification of the sterol ring. The first enzyme in the alternative pathway is mitochondrial sterol-27 hydroxylase (encoded by *CYP27A1*). Primary BS are conjugated at the side chain either with taurine or glycine, while water soluble conjugates are excreted into bile where they are rapidly incorporated in mixed micelles containing phospholipids (predominantly phosphatidylcholine) and cholesterol. Thereafter, they are

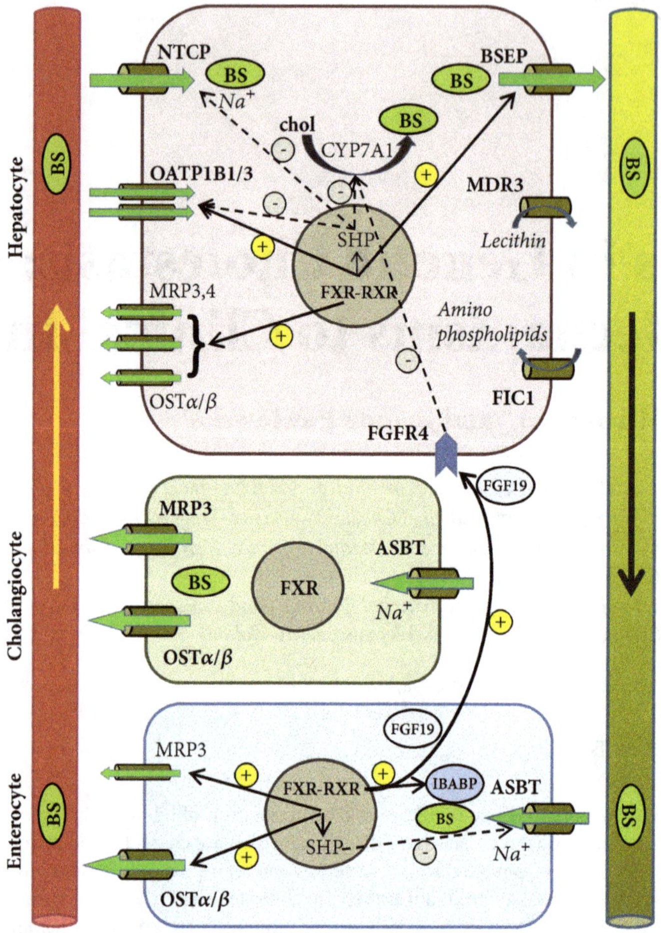

FIGURE 1: Bile salt and lipid transporters and their regulatory pathways.

transported into the intestinal tract where they are deconjugated, oxidised, and dehydroxylated to form 7-deoxycholic and lithocholic acid as part of a reaction catalysed by bacterial 7 alpha-dehydroxylases. Finally, most intestinal BS (95%) are reabsorbed in the distal part of the small intestine and transported to the liver via the portal blood and, to a lesser extent, via the hepatic artery in a process known as enterohepatic circulation. The BS pool is recycled 4-12 times a day. BS lost in the faeces (0.2-0.6 g/day) are replenished by *de novo* synthesis in the liver [1–3].

3. Bile Salt and Lipid Transporters

Bile acids form dissociated sodium or potassium salts in body fluids with neutral pH. Therefore, BS transporters are designed as anion transporters. Enterohepatic circulation of BS is driven by several specific transport systems expressed predominantly in hepatocytes and biliary and intestinal epithelia (Figure 1).

In hepatocytes, Na+-dependent taurocholate cotransporting peptide (NTCP, also known as the sodium/bile acid cotransporter), encoded by *SLC10A1* (solute carrier family 10 member 1), represents the major conjugated BS uptake system from the blood, contributing 80% of the transport capacity. NTCP is localised in the basolateral (sinusoidal) membrane, and its driving force, the Na^+ concentration gradient, is maintained by Na^+/K^+-ATPase [4, 5]. NTCP deficiency has recently been shown to cause severe familial predominantly conjugated hypercholanemia with no cholestatic jaundice, pruritus, and liver disease [6].

Unconjugated BS are transported by the multispecific ATP- and Na^+-independent basolateral uptake transporters, organic anion-transporting polypeptide 1B1 (OATP1B1, also termed OATP-C, OATP2, SLC21A6, or LST-1, encoded by *SLCO1B1*), and 1B3 (OATP1B3, synonyms OATP8, SLC21A8, or LST3, encoded by *SLCO1B3*) [4, 7, 8]. They play a secondary role in liver uptake of conjugated BS since the presence of both OATP1Bs only partly compensates for NTCP deficiency [6].

The basolateral domain of hepatocytes also possesses several ATP-dependent efflux pumps, which constitute the multidrug resistance protein (MRP) subfamily (ABCC). ABCC proteins transport organic anions including BS [9, 10].

MRP3 (encoded by *ABCC3*) is a basolateral transporter of BS, glucuronide, and anionic conjugates, including glutathione [11–13]. In the liver, MRP3 is expressed predominantly in the centrilobular hepatocytes, and its expression is low under physiological conditions. MRP3 expression rate is upregulated during cholestasis and independently of any cholestatic manifestation, in individuals with Dubin-Johnson syndrome or after repeated administration of ethinylestradiol [11, 14, 15]. As well as in hepatocytes, Northern blotting of various human tissues indicates the presence of MRP3 in the bile duct epithelium, gallbladder, intestine, pancreas, and kidney [16].

MRP4 (gene *ABCC4*) is an inducible basolateral transporter that cotransports taurine and glycine conjugates of cholic acid with glutathione. It is also a high-affinity transporter of sulphated BS, dehydroepiandrosterone sulphate, eicosanoids, and uric acid, as well as signalling molecules such as cAMP and cGMP [17]. Although MRP4 expression in the liver is low, it can be induced by BS in cholestasis [18, 19]. Strong upregulation of human MRP4 has been demonstrated in patients with BS export pump (BSEP) deficiency [20].

The heterodimeric organic solute transporter OSTα-OSTβ, initially identified as a basolateral BS efflux system in enterocytes (see below), is also localised in the sinusoidal membrane of hepatocytes [21]. Hepatic OSTα-OSTβ expression increases in patients with primary biliary cirrhosis and in bile duct-ligated rodents [22]. Thus, during cholestasis, MRP3, MRP4, and OSTα-OSTβ may provide effective protection against hepatocellular BS overload.

The transfer of BS from the liver to the bile canaliculus is determined by several transport proteins in the canalicular (apical) membrane of hepatocytes, mainly ATP-dependent BSEP and MRPs.

BSEP, encoded by *ABCB11*, is responsible for the ATP-dependent transport of predominantly monovalent conjugated BS across the hepatocyte canalicular membrane. It is exclusively expressed in the liver and localised predominantly in the canalicular microvillar (but not the intermicrovillar) membrane and to a lesser extent in subcanalicular (subapical) vesicles [23]. Expression of BSEP is sensitive to the flux of BS through hepatocytes. The BSEP promoter contains an inverted repeat DNA element (IR-1), a binding site for the farnesoid X receptor (FXR), which plays an important role in maintaining BS homeostasis (see below).

Multidrug resistance protein 3 (MDR3, gene *ABCB4*) is understood to act as a floppase, which translocates phospholipids from the inner to the outer leaflet of the lipid bilayer of the canalicular membrane [24]. Mutations in *ABCB4* cause cholestasis, which is characterised by the decreased biliary lecithin output, impaired formation of mixed micelles, and the production of more hydrophilic bile with potent detergent properties, resulting in membrane damage [25, 26].

Familial intrahepatic cholestasis type 1 transporter (FIC1, gene *ATP8B1*), a member of the type 4 subfamily of P-type ATPases (P4 ATPase), is a flippase that mediates the translocation of aminophospholipids from the outer (exoplasmic) to the inner (cytoplasmic) leaflet of the plasma membrane [27]. In most eukaryotic cells, phosphatidylcholine and sphingolipids are concentrated in the exoplasmic leaflet, whereas the aminophospholipids (phosphatidylserine and phosphatidylethanolamine) are largely confined to the cytoplasmic leaflet. FIC1 thus helps in maintaining asymmetry and fluidity characteristics of plasma membranes, the essential prerequisites for proper function of transmembrane embedded pumps [27].

Cholangiocytes are important modifiers of bile composition. Conjugated BS need to be actively transported into cholangiocytes via apical sodium-dependent bile acid transporter (ASBT, gene *SLC10A2*) and are exported into the peribiliary capillary plexus via the heterodimeric transporter OSTα-OSTβ and via MRP3 [28, 29]. Under physiological conditions, BS transporters in cholangiocytes can play a major role in the regulation of intracellular concentrations of BS as signalling molecules. In obstructive cholestasis, cholangiocellular BS receptors may facilitate the removal of BS from stagnant bile [3, 28, 29].

An important step in maintaining BS homeostasis is the reabsorption of BS in the intestinal lumen, predominantly in the ileum. Intestinal epithelial cells reabsorb the majority of secreted BS through ASBT, localised in the brush border membrane of enterocytes. Human ASBT, also called ileal bile acid transporter or ileal sodium-dependent bile acid transporter, consists of 348 amino acids. It transports conjugated and unconjugated BS with a higher affinity for chenodeoxycholic and deoxycholic acid than for taurocholate [30]. After uptake into the enterocyte, the transcellular movement of BS is mediated by cytosolic ileal bile acid-binding protein, also known as fatty acid-binding protein 6 or gastrotropin (IBABP, FABP6, gene *FABP6*), that is cytoplasmically attached to ASBT [30].

The heterodimeric organic solute transporter OSTα-OSTβ (OSTα, gene *SLC51A*; OSTβ, gene *SLC51B*) is expressed in the basolateral membrane of enterocytes and effluxes BS to the portal blood. In humans, OSTα-OSTβ is expressed at high levels in a variety of tissues and is the primary transporter of BS into the systemic circulation [21, 22, 30].

Furthermore, MRP3 may also participate in the basolateral transport of BS in human enterocytes, although its overall contribution is small [10].

4. Regulation of Bile Salt Synthesis and Trafficking

The BS biosynthesis and enterohepatic circulation are tightly regulated at many levels but particularly by transcriptional and posttranscriptional mechanisms [2, 3]. A key regulator of BS synthesis and enterohepatic flow is the nuclear farnesoid X receptor (FXR), a major BS-responsive ligand-activated transcription factor with a high affinity for several major endogenous BS [2, 31, 32]. Expression levels of the FXR gene (also known as the *NR1H4* gene—nuclear receptor subfamily 1, group H, member 4) are highest in the intestine, predominantly in the ileal epithelium, liver, and kidneys [31, 32].

FXR acts as an agonist-dependent transcriptional activator of its direct target genes. The preferred DNA-binding sequence for FXR within its target promoters is a variant of inverted repeat-1 motif (IR-1) to which FXR binds as a heterodimer with the retinoid X receptor (RXR). FXR can also downregulate the transcription of specific target genes indirectly via another nuclear receptor, the small heterodimer partner (SHP, the *NR0B2* gene). SHP is an atypical orphan nuclear receptor without a DNA-binding domain. It acts as a repressor of nuclear receptors, as well as of transcription factors belonging to other protein families [2, 31, 33].

FXR plays a key role in controlling the enterohepatic circulation of BS, largely by directly regulating the expression of several hepatobiliary transporters (Figure 1). In the liver, the heterodimer FXR-RXR induces the expression of BSEP by binding to an IR-1 element at the promoter [34, 35]. Likewise, FXR can directly transactivate the *ABCC2, ABCB4,* and *SLCO1B3* genes [36, 37].

The FXR-RXR complex directly induces the expression of OSTα-OSTβ (in ileal enterocytes and in the basolateral membrane of hepatocytes) as well as intestinal expression of the intestinal bile acid-binding protein (IBABP) [22, 37].

In addition to directly activating the main BS efflux systems, under cholestatic conditions, FXR concurrently downregulates the main BS uptake systems, primarily NTCP in the basolateral membrane of hepatocytes and ASBT in the ileal epithelium. OATP1B1 is also suppressed by an FXR-dependent pathway during cholestasis. FXR-mediated repression of target genes is indirect and mainly effected via SHP [2, 33, 37].

As well as regulating transport systems involved in the enterohepatic flow of BS, FXR represses the transcription of genes that encode regulatory enzymes in both classical and alternative BS biosynthetic pathways, predominantly *CYP7A1* and *CYP27A1* [2, 33].

There are two important FXR-dependent mechanisms for BS-induced inhibition of *CYP7A1* gene transcription: the FXR/SHP pathway in the liver and the FXR/FGF19/FGFR4 pathway in the intestine [2, 37].

In the liver, the heterodimer FXR/RXR, after binding retinoic acid and BS, induces the expression of SHP. The interaction of SHP with liver receptor homologue-1 (LRH-1, also NR5A2, gene *NR5A2*) and hepatocyte nuclear factor-4α (HNF4α, also NR2A1, gene *HNF4A*) inhibits *CYP7A1* transcription [2, 32, 33]. In the *CYP27A1* gene, the BS response element contains a DNA-binding site for HNF4α only, not for LRH-1 [2, 31].

In the intestine, FXR induces an intestinal hormone, fibroblast growth factor 19 (FGF19, gene *FGF19*), which activates hepatic FGF receptor 4 (FGFR4, gene *FGFR4*) and downregulates BS synthesis by inhibiting *CYP71A* expression. The FXR/FGF19/FGFR4 pathway seems to be the physiological mechanism for feedback regulation of BS biosynthesis. Furthermore, the FGF19 autocrine pathway exists in the human liver [2, 31, 37, 38].

Along with FXR-related regulation of BS biosynthesis, there are several FXR-independent mechanisms of *CYP7A1* inhibition mediated by pregnane X receptor (PXR), vitamin D receptor (VDR), the cytokines tumour necrosis factor α (TNFα) and interleukin 1β (IL-1β), transforming growth factor β1 (TGFβ1), epidermal growth factor receptor (EGFR), and others. These factors activate signalling pathways, which play roles in protecting against BS toxicity during cholestatic liver injury [2, 31, 32, 37].

Finally, FXR also directly transactivates genes encoding enzymes that metabolise BS, such as human uridine 5'-diphosphate-glucuronosyltransferase 2B4 (UGT2B4, encoded by *UGT2B4*). Interestingly, FXR binds the *UGT2B4* promoter as a monomer without previous heterodimerisation with RXR [32].

Several nuclear receptors such as FXR, RXR, LXR, and SHP are also expressed in cholangiocytes, but their role in bile duct biology remains to be elucidated [29].

5. Familial Intrahepatic Cholestasis

Up- and downregulation of transport systems involved in bile formation can explain the impaired liver uptake and excretion of biliary constituents, which result in cholestasis and jaundice in some hereditary and many common acquired liver disorders. Hereditary diseases characterised by hepatocanalicular cholestasis, which is caused by defects in hepatobiliary transporters, their regulator FXR, and in tightness of the liver epithelium, include progressive familial intrahepatic cholestasis (PFIC) types 1 to 5, benign recurrent intrahepatic cholestasis (BRIC) 1 and 2, familial cholelithiasis caused by a lack of biliary secretion of phospholipids (Low Phospholipid-Associated Cholelithiasis or Gallbladder Disease-1), intrahepatic cholestasis of pregnancy (ICP), and several other rare disorders. Hereditary predisposition also plays an important role in drug-induced intrahepatic cholestasis, including cholestasis induced by hormonal contraceptives [39, 40].

5.1. Progressive Familial Intrahepatic Cholestasis. PFIC, first described in 1969 [41], is a genetically heterogeneous group of autosomal recessive disorders caused by mutations in genes that encode hepatocanalicular transporters of BS and phospholipids, their regulator FXR, and TJP2 which is essential for tightness of cell junctions between the epithelial cells lining the bile ducts. The exact incidence of PFIC is not known, but it is estimated to be in the region of 1/50000 to 1/100000 births. Both genders are equally affected [42]. Clinically, PFIC usually manifests in the first year of life and is characterised by jaundice, severe pruritus, hepatosplenomegaly, steatorrhoea, and retardation of growth and mental development. Further symptoms caused by a deficit of fat-soluble vitamins include coagulopathy, osteopaenia, and neuromuscular disorders. Without adequate treatment, the disease progresses to liver fibrosis and cirrhosis and usually ends in death due to liver failure in the first or, more rarely, in the second decade of life [40, 42].

The PFIC group consists of five representatives (PFIC 1-5), which are classified into two main categories according to levels of serum γ-glutamyl transferase (GGT) activity. GGT is considered a cholestatic enzyme and, when elevated, is associated with damage to the apical membranes of bile ducts and the disruption of intercellular connections due to high concentrations of BS in bile. However, in some cholestatic diseases, synthesis or canalicular secretion of BS is virtually absent and there are no conditions that predispose either to the release of membrane GGT from damaged cholangiocytes or to leakage of bile into the extracellular space and subsequently the blood. This explains why, in hereditary

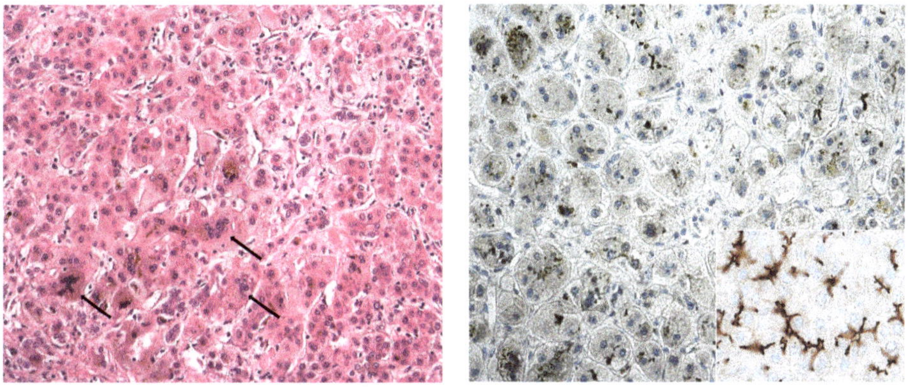

(a) (b)

FIGURE 2: *Histopathology of ABCB11 disease.* (a) Giant-cell hepatitis (arrows) with hepatocanalicular cholestasis and (b) complete absence of ABCB11/BSEP protein are typical findings in PFIC2 patients. Inset: immunohistochemical positivity of BSEP in the apical (canalicular) domain of hepatocytes in a healthy control. (a) Hematoxylin and eosin, original magnification x200. (b, inset) Immunohistochemical staining with ABCB11 Rabbit Polyclonal Antibody (NBP1-89319, Novus Biologicals, USA), original magnification x200 (b), x400 (inset).

cholestasis, GGT activity is increased only in disorders of phospholipid secretion (PFIC3).

5.1.1. Progressive Familial Intrahepatic Cholestasis Type 1 (PFIC1). PFIC1 (*ATP8B1* disease, OMIM #211600), formerly Byler's disease [41], is the consequence of a severe defect in the gene encoding ATPase, *ATP8B1/FIC1* (familial intrahepatic cholestasis 1), localised in the long arm of the 18th chromosome (18q21) [43, 44]. ATP8B1 deficiency, which causes membrane phospholipid asymmetry of the canalicular membrane, reduces the capacity of the liver to secrete bile [45, 46]. In addition to the previously described common symptoms of PFIC, clinical manifestation of PFIC1 also includes a wide range of extrahepatic symptoms. Extrahepatic manifestations of *ATP8B1* disease include elevated sweat chloride concentrations, delayed pubescence and growth, and watery diarrhoea as well as impaired hearing and/or pancreatitis [47]. These symptoms often persist, while diarrhoea even tends to worsen after liver transplantation (LTX). Liver allografts in PFIC1 patients may display diffuse steatosis with a variable necroinflammatory component, with subsequent fibrosis [48]. Both diarrhoea and steatosis/steatohepatitis may improve after biliary diversion [49].

Laboratory findings with regard to PFIC1 have reported cholestasis with low serum levels of GGT, increased serum concentrations of primary BS, and normal levels of cholesterol. Aminotransferases are initially within the reference range, but during disease progression they gradually increase by up to tenfold [41]. Histopathological changes predominantly involve canalicular cholestasis accentuated around the central veins. The interlobular ducts can be hypoplastic due to subnormal bile flow. Giant-cell changes of hepatocytes are generally not observed in biopsies. Liver fibrosis progression corresponds with the respective stage of the disease and can terminate in cirrhosis. A typical ultrastructural finding is the presence of Byler-type coarsely granular bile in the bile canaliculi [50]. Molecular diagnosis is based on the detection of pathogenic mutations in both alleles of the *ATP8B1* gene. The milder intermittent nonprogressive form of *ATP8B1* deficiency is called BRIC1 (see below).

5.1.2. Progressive Familial Intrahepatic Cholestasis Type 2 (PFIC2). PFIC2 (*ABCB11* disease, OMIM #601847) is caused by mutations in *ABCB11*, which is located on the long arm of the second chromosome (2q24) and encodes the canalicular transport protein ABCB11/BSEP [51]. Clinical and laboratory findings with regard to PFIC2 are similar to PFIC1 but extrahepatic symptoms are not present. Additionally, in PFIC2 the formation of gallstones and the early elevation of serum aminotransferase activity can occur. The development of hepatobiliary malignancies, both hepatocellular carcinoma and cholangiocarcinoma, can be a serious complication of PFIC2, which is not observed in PFIC1 [52, 53]. Screening for liver tumours is recommended from the first year of life in PFIC2 patients.

Except for PFIC2, mutations in *ABCB11* may result in a milder nonprogressive form of PFIC2 known as BRIC2 as well as other forms of cholestasis such as ICP and/or drug-induced cholestasis (see below).

Histologically, the typical findings in the liver biopsies of PFIC2 patients are giant-cell (syncycial) hepatitis with hepatocanalicular cholestasis, while extramedullary haemopoiesis is frequently discernible within lobules. Interlobular bile ducts can be hypoplastic, and ductular proliferation at the peripheries of portal triads is commonly observed. The ABCB11/BSEP protein is usually undetectable immunohistochemically (Figure 2). Ultrastructurally, canalicular bile can be either amorphous or filamentous but is not coarsely granular [51].

Untreated PFIC2 usually leads to progressive liver fibrosis and cirrhosis, the development of which is more rapid than in PFIC1. One curative method for patients with PFIC2 is LTX. Unlike in PFIC1, steatosis and steatohepatitis are not present in liver allografts in the case of PFIC2. However, in some patients, a recurrence of the PFIC2 phenotype, accompanied by elevated serum levels of BS and bilirubin with almost normal GGT activity, has been observed after LTX [54, 55]. It has been shown that canalicular immunostaining of the BSEP, MDR3, and MRP2 proteins is preserved in the liver graft biopsies and no discernible changes in BSEP immunoreactivity distribution between the apical membrane and the cytoplasm have been reported; nonetheless, *de novo* polyclonal inhibitory antibodies directed against the first extracellular loop of BSEP have been observed in the posttransplant serum of patients, a condition known as Autoimmune BSEP Disease (AIBD) [56, 57]. The exact mechanism by which BS transport is inhibited by anti-BSEP antibodies is still unknown. It is supposed that the cross-linking of BSEP molecules, which in turn disrupts the structure and function of canalicular membranes, and/or the direct mechanical occlusion of the BSEP pore, might explain the inhibitory effects of the antibodies [56, 57]. It is estimated that up to 8% of transplanted PFIC2 patients develop anti-BSEP antibodies [56]. This may be explained by the insufficient autotolerance against BSEP exhibited in some patients with severe *ABCB11* mutations, resulting in the complete absence of the BSEP protein. The causal relationship between recurrent cholestasis in the liver grafts of PFIC2 patients and the occurrence of *de novo* antibodies directed against BSEP is further supported by observations that plasmapheresis and the administration of anti-CD20 antibodies (rituximab) may alleviate symptoms of cholestasis [54–57].

Interestingly, posttransplant development of inhibitory autoantibodies directed against FIC1 and MDR3 transporters with corresponding phenotypes has not yet been documented in patients with PFIC1 and PFIC3, respectively [44].

5.1.3. Progressive Familial Intrahepatic Cholestasis Type 3 (PFIC3). PFIC3 (*ABCB4* disease, OMIM #602347) is caused by mutations in both alleles of the *ABCB4/MDR3* gene that encode phospholipid transporter MDR3, expressed in the canalicular (apical) membrane of hepatocytes [26]. As well as PFIC3, there is evidence that either biallelic or monoallelic *ABCB4* defects may cause or predispose patients to a wide spectrum of human liver diseases, such as Low Phospholipid-Associated Cholelithiasis Syndrome (LPAC, OMIM #600803), Intrahepatic Cholestasis of Pregnancy (ICP, OMIM #147480), drug-induced liver injury, transient neonatal cholestasis, small duct sclerosing cholangitis, and adult biliary fibrosis or cirrhosis [58–61]. Moreover, hepatocellular carcinoma and intrahepatic cholangiocarcinoma have been documented in patients with *ABCB4/MDR3* mutations [61].

Clinical and laboratory findings associated with PFIC3 correspond to the other two forms of PFIC, but are characterised by the absence of extrahepatic symptoms (except for cholelithiasis). Unlike PFIC1 and PFIC2, elevated serum GGT activity and normal cholesterol levels are typically observed, as exhibited by the MDR3 deficit [26, 62].

Histopathological findings in connection with *ABCB4* disease are variable. Syncytial (giant-cell) changes, cholestasis, portal inflammatory infiltrate, and periportal ductular proliferation accompanied by various stages of fibrosis have been observed in liver tissue. Lipid crystals within bile ducts and fibroobliterative bile duct lesions can be seen. Immunohistochemistry has indicated the absence of the canalicular MDR3 protein, predominantly in early onset forms; however, its use is limited compared to PFIC2. Ultrastructurally, bile is dense and amorphous in PFIC3 [26, 61].

Prolonged cholestasis in PFIC3 is associated with significant accumulation of copper in liver tissue and with increased urine copper excretion, i.e., findings that overlap with the diagnostic criteria for Wilson's disease [63, 64].

5.1.4. Progressive Familial Intrahepatic Cholestasis Type 4 (PFIC4). The fourth form of PFIC (PFIC4, *TJP2* deficiency, OMIM #615878), first described in 2014 [65], is clinically similar to PFIC2 and caused by homozygous or compound heterozygous mutations in the *TJP2* gene, located in the 9q12 chromosome. Tight junction protein 2 (TJP2, also zona occludens-2) is a cytoplasmic component of cell-cell junctional complexes expressed in most epithelia and creates a link between transmembrane tight junction proteins and the actin cytoskeleton. Complete TJP2 deficiency is associated with a significant reduction in an integral tight junction protein, claudin-1, predominantly in the canalicular membranes of liver cells, which subsequently leads to the disruption of intercellular connections and the leakage of bile through the paracellular space into the liver parenchyma [65, 66].

Patients with *TJP2* deficiency display severe progressive cholestatic liver disease in early childhood, which puts them at increased risk of developing hepatocellular carcinoma [67]. Serum GGT activity is normal or, at most, slightly increased, while expression of the canalicular proteins BSEP and MDR3 is maintained. In addition to liver impairment, extrahepatic features have been identified in PFIC4 patients, including neurological and respiratory disorders [66]. A single homozygous missense mutation in *TJP2* has been previously described as causing benign familial hypercholanemia, a rare disorder of oligogenic inheritance, which usually manifests in elevated serum BS concentrations, pruritus, and fat malabsorption, but which does not lead to the development of liver disease [68].

5.1.5. Progressive Familial Intrahepatic Cholestasis Type 5 (PFIC5). PFIC5 (OMIM #617049), first described in 2016 [69], is a cholestatic disorder caused by mutations in *NR1H4*, a gene located at 12q23.1, which encodes FXR, the key regulator of BS metabolism (see above). Homozygous loss of FXR function is associated with severe neonatal cholestasis and early onset vitamin K-independent coagulopathy, which rapidly progresses to end-stage liver disease. The nonresponsiveness of coagulopathy to vitamin K treatment is likely a direct consequence of the loss of FXR function, representing an important distinguishing diagnostic feature of *NR1H4*-related cholestasis. In addition to low (or normal) GGT activity, serum levels of alpha-fetoprotein are typically elevated [69].

Liver biopsies have shown diffuse giant-cell transformation of hepatocytes with hepatocellular cholestasis and ductular proliferation. Progressive fibrosis and even micronodular cirrhosis are evident at later stages. BSEP is undetectable in the apical domains of hepatocytes, which is consistent with low activity of GGT; MDR3 expression, on the other hand, is maintained [69].

Since FXR affects several metabolic pathways, some *NR1H4* variations may be associated with susceptibility to various human diseases. *NR1H4* single-nucleotide polymorphisms seem to be correlated with differences in glucose homeostasis, gallstone formation, ICP, inflammatory bowel disease, and several other disorders [70, 71].

5.2. Benign Recurrent Intrahepatic Cholestasis (BRIC). BRIC is a group of genetically heterogeneous autosomal recessive diseases, characterised by intermittent episodes of cholestasis. They are caused by mutations in the *ATP8B1* and *ABCB11* genes (the same as in PFIC1 and PFIC2) and probably in at least one other as yet unidentified gene [72]. There are two genetically characterised forms of BRIC: BRIC1 (Summerskill-Walshe-Tygstrup syndrome, OMIM #243300) and BRIC2 (OMIM #605479), caused by partial deficiency in ATP8B1 [39, 73] and ABCB11 [74], respectively. The disease typically manifests before the second decade of life, but the age of the first manifestation can vary greatly. The same variability has been documented in the duration of cholestatic episodes (several days to several months) and their intensity. Infection or pregnancy may act as a triggering factor. The clinical manifestations include jaundice, pruritus, fatigue, anorexia, and steatorrhoea. Increase of bilirubin and BS levels in serum has been observed during cholestatic attacks, but GGT activity and serum cholesterol levels tend to be normal. Aminotransferase activity is usually normal or only slightly elevated, while biochemical parameters fall within normal ranges. Liver biopsies performed during cholestatic attacks have demonstrated hepatocanalicular cholestasis without fibrosis. During the asymptomatic period, the histological picture is completely normal. Since canalicular expression of BSEP protein in hepatocytes is mostly maintained, immunohistology is of limited significance in these cases. Diagnosis of BRIC1 and BRIC2 is based on demonstrating evidence of mutations in both alleles of the corresponding genes, *ATP8B1* and *ABCB11*.

While mutations causing PFIC are often located in the conserved regions of the genes that encode conserved functional domains of the corresponding proteins, mutations in BRIC only partially impact protein function and expression. However, several cases of initially benign episodic cholestasis that have subsequently transitioned to a persistent progressive form of the disease have been reported [75]. Thus, BRIC and PFIC seem to represent two extremes of a continuous spectrum of phenotypes of the one disease.

The administration of statins, corticosteroids, cholestyramine, or ursodeoxycholic acid (UDCA) is usually not very effective in BRIC patients. Improvement of pruritus and shortening of symptomatic phase has been described in BRIC patients treated with the antibiotic rifampicin, a potent human activator of PXR [76, 77]. However, severe hepatotoxicity after long-term administration of rifampicin has been reported in patients with cholestatic disorders [77, 78]. Nasobiliary drainage seems to have a prompt effect during cholestatic episodes, but the mechanism of action remains unclear [79].

5.3. Intrahepatic Cholestasis of Pregnancy (ICP). ICP (OMIM #147480), also known as obstetric cholestasis, is characterised by cholestasis and pruritus with onset in pregnancy, usually in the third trimester. It is associated with abnormal liver function in the absence of other liver diseases and resolves completely after delivery [80, 81]. The incidence of ICP varies with geographical location and ethnicity. Seasonal variations indicate higher incidence in winter months, as reported in some countries, and it more commonly occurs in association with multiple pregnancies and following in vitro fertilisation. In Europe, ICP affects about 1% of all pregnancies [81]. A typical symptom is intense pruritus, commonly localised in the palms and the soles, which progresses during pregnancy. Elevated levels of serum BS and increased liver aminotransferase activity are typical laboratory findings in such cases. Increased serum bilirubin levels have been observed in a small proportion of cases, while jaundice only rarely occurs in affected women [81].

ICP usually resolves soon after delivery. Although the disease is considered relatively benign for the mother, there is an increased rate of adverse foetal outcomes, including foetal distress, foetal asphyxia, stillbirth, or even intrauterine death: all known complications of ICP [81, 82]. ICP may also be associated with an abnormal metabolic profile in afflicted women, especially higher prevalence of dyslipidaemia, impaired glucose tolerance, and maternal comorbidities, e.g., gestational diabetes and preeclampsia [82, 83]. Administration of UDCA improves clinical symptoms, predominantly pruritus, and may even reduce the risk of premature birth [84–86].

Mutations in *ABCB4, ABCB11,* and *ATP8B1* have been identified in some patients suffering from ICP [87–90]. Additionally, variations in *NR1H4* may be implicated in ICP, possibly via downregulation of BSEP expression [71].

6. Conclusions and Perspectives

Identification of the genes involved in hereditary cholestasis has advanced our understanding of the molecular mechanisms behind bile formation and transport.

Recently, mutations in *TJP2* and *NR1H4* have been found in patients with apparent BSEP deficiency, normal serum GGT activity, and no mutations in *ABCB11*. However, there are rare cases of genetic cholestasis causes of which have yet to be identified. Therefore it seems likely that other yet unidentified genes involved in secretion and/or transport of cholephiles may be responsible for FIC-like phenotypes.

Current therapeutic regimens in FIC patients comprise both nonsurgical and surgical approaches. Nonsurgical therapy includes drugs, predominantly UDCA and rifampicin, and nasobiliary drainage, the latter being predominantly used in BRIC patients with intractable pruritus during long-lasting cholestatic episodes [76, 77, 79]. However, the mechanism responsible for the instant and complete relief from pruritus is still unclear.

In addition to cholestyramine, phenobarbital, S-adenosylmethionine, opiate antagonists, UDCA, rifampicin, and serotonin antagonists and its reuptake inhibitors seem to be beneficial in managing refractory pruritus in patients with PFIC [77, 91, 92]. Furthermore, clinical and biochemical improvements have been observed in BRIC patients with intractable pruritus after using the molecular adsorbent recirculating system (MARS) and the Prometheus system, an extracorporeal liver support therapy based on fractionated plasma separation and adsorption [93].

Surgical therapies include partial biliary diversion, i.e., mechanical interruption of BS enterohepatic circulation in order to prevent reabsorption of pruritogens (unidentified thus far) and their precursors, which is primarily useful in noncirrhotic children with low-GGT PFIC, permanent cholestasis and/or intense refractory pruritus, and orthotopic LTX, which is still the ultimate treatment modality for many PFIC patients [91]. However, as well as the risks associated with these invasive procedures, other serious postoperative-related complications have been reported, particularly in PFIC1 patients with extradigestive symptoms, which can persist or even worsen, most likely due to extrahepatic expression of FIC1 [47]. Moreover, the development of steatosis and steatohepatitis leading to progressive liver allograft fibrosis in PFIC1 patients [48] and recurrence of the PFIC2 phenotype in *ABCB11* deficiency may represent other serious complications after LTX, and for some patients may even necessitate retransplantation [54–57].

Importantly, because of the shortage of cadaveric donors, parental living-related LTX is often considered in PFIC patients. As heterozygous conditions can cause mild-to-moderate disease expression under certain circumstances, the use of blood relatives as donors is seen as controversial. In such cases, it is likely that the heterozygous status of the donor allograft could pose a risk of complications during the late posttransplant period, such as lithiasis or cholestasis, which can be precipitated by infections or by drugs administered to the patient. However, the results of a recent study indicate that the PFIC heterozygote status of the organ donor does not increase the risk of liver dysfunction [94].

The limited effectiveness of current conservative procedures along with the complications of invasive methods, particularly LTX, stress the need for the development and introduction of new treatment options. Total biliary diversion, pharmacological diversion of BS, and hepatocyte transplantation as well as gene- and mutation-targeted pharmacotherapies represent promising future therapeutic approaches. The latter two methods provide the basis for personalised treatment strategies in FIC patients. Pharmacological chaperones (e.g., 4-phenylbutyrate), agonists of nuclear receptors (e.g., statins, fibrates, 6-ethyl chenodeoxycholic acid), endoplasmic reticulum-associated degradation inhibitors (MG132), and several other mutation-specific drugs can be used to increase the expression of functional proteins and mitigate or even eliminate deficient phenotypes [95–97].

Nevertheless, despite the indisputable progress in the therapy of FIC patients, the increased risks of hepatobiliary malignancies, particularly in relation to *ABCB11* deficiency, still remain serious life-threatening complications. Further studies are required in order to elucidate the complex pathogenesis of cholestasis, unlock the mechanism of cholestatic pruritus, and improve the clinical management of both hereditary and acquired cholestatic liver diseases.

Abbreviations

ABC: ATP-binding cassette subfamily
ABCB4: ATP-binding cassette, subfamily B, member 4
ABCB11: ATP-binding cassette, subfamily B, member 11
AIBD: Autoimmune BSEP Disease
ASBT: Apical sodium-dependent bile acid transporter
ATP8B1: ATPase, aminophospholipid transporter, class I, type 8B, member 1
BRIC: Benign Recurrent Intrahepatic Cholestasis
BS: Bile salts
BSEP: Bile salt export pump
CYP7A1: Cholesterol 7 alpha-hydroxylase
CYP27A1: Sterol-27 hydroxylase
FGF19: Fibroblast growth factor 19
FGFR4: Fibroblast growth factor receptor 4
FIC: Familial intrahepatic cholestasis
FXR: Farnesoid X-activated receptor
GGT: γ-Glutamyl transferase
HNF4α: Hepatocyte nuclear factor 4α
IBABP: Intestinal bile acid-binding protein
ICP: Intrahepatic cholestasis of pregnancy
IR-1: Inverted repeat DNA element with 1 nucleotide spacing
LPAC: Low Phospholipid-Associated Cholelithiasis Syndrome
LTX: Liver allograft transplantation
LXR: Liver X receptor
MDR3: Multidrug resistance protein 3
MRP: Multidrug resistance-associated protein
NR1H4: Nuclear receptor subfamily 1, group H, member 4
NTCP: Na+-taurocholate cotransporting polypeptide/solute carrier family 10 member 1
OATP: Organic anion-transporting polypeptide
OMIM: Electronic database Online Mendelian Inheritance in ManTM
OST: Organic solute transporter
PFIC: Progressive Familial Intrahepatic Cholestasis
PXR: Pregnane X receptor
RXR: Retinoid X receptor
SHP: Small heterodimer partner
SLC22A: Solute carrier family 22 (organic cation transporter), member 1
SLCO: Solute carrier organic anion transporter family
TJP2: Tight junction protein 2; zona occludens-2
UDCA: Ursodeoxycholic acid
UGT2B4: Uridine 5′-diphosphate-glucuronosyltransferase 2B4.

Acknowledgments

Milan Jirsa was supported by Ministry of Health, Czech Republic—Conceptual Development of Research Organization ("Institute for Clinical and Experimental Medicine-IKEM, IN 00023001").

References

[1] N. B. Javitt, "Bile acid synthesis from cholesterol: regulatory and auxiliary pathways.," *The FASEB Journal*, vol. 8, no. 15, pp. 1308–1311, 1994.

[2] J. Y. L. Chiang, "Bile acids: regulation of synthesis," *Journal of Lipid Research*, vol. 50, no. 10, pp. 1955–1966, 2009.

[3] J. L. Boyer, "Bile formation and secretion," *Comprehensive Physiology*, vol. 3, no. 3, pp. 1035–1078, 2013.

[4] B. Hagenbuch and P. J. Meier, "Sinusoidal (basolateral) bile salt uptake systems of hepatocytes," *Seminars in Liver Disease*, vol. 16, no. 2, pp. 129–136, 1996.

[5] B. Hagenbuch, B. Stieger, M. Foguet, H. Lübbert, and P. J. Meier, "Functional expression cloning and characterization of the hepatocyte Na+/bile acid cotransport system," *Proceedings of the National Acadamy of Sciences of the United States of America*, vol. 88, no. 23, pp. 10629–10633, 1991.

[6] F. M. Vaz, C. C. Paulusma, H. Huidekoper et al., "Sodium taurocholate cotransporting polypeptide (SLC10A1) deficiency: Conjugated hypercholanemia without a clear clinical phenotype," *Hepatology*, vol. 61, no. 1, pp. 260–267, 2015.

[7] B. Hagenbuch and P. J. Meier, "Organic anion transporting polypeptides of the OATP/SLC21 family: Phylogenetic classification as OATP/SLCO super-family, new nomenclature and molecular/functional properties," *Pflügers Archiv - European Journal of Physiology*, vol. 447, no. 5, pp. 653–665, 2004.

[8] B. Hagenbuch and B. Stieger, "The SLCO (former SLC21) superfamily of transporters," *Molecular Aspects of Medicine*, vol. 34, no. 2-3, pp. 396–412, 2013.

[9] M. Müller and P. L. M. Jansen, "The secretory function of the liver: New aspects of hepatobiliary transport," *Journal of Hepatology*, vol. 28, no. 2, pp. 344–354, 1998.

[10] G. J. E. J. Hooiveld, J. E. Van Montfoort, D. K. F. Meijer, and M. Müller, "Function and regulation of ATP-binding cassette transport proteins involved in hepatobiliary transport," *European Journal of Pharmaceutical Sciences*, vol. 12, no. 4, pp. 525–543, 2001.

[11] J. König, D. Rost, Y. Cui, and D. Keppler, "Characterization of the human multidrug resistance protein isoform MRP3 localized to the basolateral hepatocyte membrane," *Hepatology*, vol. 29, no. 4, pp. 1156–1163, 1999.

[12] H. Zeng, G. Liu, P. A. Rea, and G. D. Kruh, "Transport of amphipathic anions by human multidrug resistance protein 3," *Cancer Research*, vol. 60, pp. 4779–4784, 2000.

[13] Y.-M. A. Lee, Y. Cui, J. König et al., "Identification and functional characterization of the natural variant MRP3-Arg1297His of human multidrug resistance protein 3 (MRP3/ABCC3)," *Pharmacogenetics*, vol. 14, no. 4, pp. 213–223, 2004.

[14] M. Donner, "Up-regulation of basolateral multidrug resistance protein 3 (Mrp3) in cholestatic rat liver," *Hepatology*, vol. 34, no. 2, pp. 351–359, 2001.

[15] M. L. Ruiz, J. P. Rigalli, A. Arias et al., "Induction of hepatic multidrug resistance-associated protein 3 by ethynylestradiol is independent of cholestasis and mediated by estrogen receptor," *Drug Metabolism and Disposition*, vol. 41, no. 2, pp. 275–280, 2013.

[16] N. J. Cherrington, D. P. Hartley, N. Li, D. R. Johnson, and C. D. Klaassen, "Organ distribution of multidrug resistance proteins 1, 2, and 3 (Mrp1, 2, and 3) mRNA and hepatic induction of Mrp3 by constitutive androstane receptor activators in rats," *The Journal of Pharmacology and Experimental Therapeutics*, vol. 300, no. 1, pp. 97–104, 2002.

[17] C. A. Ritter, G. Jedlitschky, H. Meyer Zu Schwabedissen, M. Grube, K. Köck, and H. K. Kroemer, "Cellular export of drugs and signaling molecules by the ATP-binding cassette transporters MRP4 (ABCC4) and MRP5 (ABCC5)," *Drug Metabolism Reviews*, vol. 37, no. 1, pp. 253–278, 2005.

[18] F. G. M. Russel, J. B. Koenderink, and R. Masereeuw, "Multidrug resistance protein 4 (MRP4/ABCC4): a versatile efflux transporter for drugs and signalling molecules," *Trends in Pharmacological Sciences*, vol. 29, no. 4, pp. 200–207, 2008.

[19] D. Keppler, "Progress in the molecular characterization of hepatobiliary transporters," *Digestive Diseases*, vol. 35, no. 3, pp. 197–202, 2017.

[20] V. Keitel, M. Burdelski, U. Warskulat et al., "Expression and localization of hepatobiliary transport proteins in progressive familial intrahepatic cholestasis," *Hepatology*, vol. 41, no. 5, pp. 1160–1172, 2005.

[21] N. Ballatori, F. Fang, W. V. Christian, N. Li, and C. L. Hammond, "Ostα-Ostβ is required for bile acid and conjugated steroid disposition in the intestine, kidney, and liver," *American Journal of Physiology-Gastrointestinal and Liver Physiology*, vol. 295, no. 1, pp. G179–G186, 2008.

[22] J. L. Boyer, M. Trauner, A. Mennone et al., "Upregulation of a basolateral FXR-dependent bile acid efflux transporter OSTalpha-OSTbeta in cholestasis in humans and rodents," *American Journal of Physiology-Gastrointestinal and Liver Physiology*, vol. 290, no. 6, pp. G1124–G1130, 2006.

[23] T. Gerloff, B. Stieger, B. Hagenbuch et al., "The sister of P-glycoprotein represents the canalicular bile salt export pump of mammalian liver," *The Journal of Biological Chemistry*, vol. 273, no. 16, pp. 10046–10050, 1998.

[24] A. M. van der Bliek, F. Baas, T. Ten Houte de Lange, P. M. Kooiman, T. van der Velde-Koerts, and P. Borst, "The human mdr3 gene encodes a novel P-glycoprotein homologue and gives rise to alternatively spliced mRNAs in liver," *EMBO Journal*, vol. 6, no. 11, pp. 3325–3331, 1987.

[25] A. J. Smith, J. L. Timmermans-Hereijgers, and B. Roelofsen, "The human MDR3 P-glycoprotein promotes translocation of phosphatidylcholine through the plasma membrane of fibroblasts from transgenic mice," *FEBS Letters*, vol. 354, no. 3, pp. 263–266, 1994.

[26] J. M. L. de Vree, E. Jacquemin, E. Sturm et al., "Mutations in the MDR3 gene cause progressive familial intrahepatic cholestasis," *Proceedings of the National Acadamy of Sciences of the United States of America*, vol. 95, no. 1, pp. 282–287, 1998.

[27] A. Groen, M. R. Romero, C. Kunne et al., "Complementary functions of the flippase ATP8B1 and the floppase ABCB4 in maintaining canalicular membrane integrity," *Gastroenterology*, vol. 141, no. 5, pp. 1927–1937, 2011.

[28] P. A. Dawson, T. Lan, and A. Rao, "Thematic review series: Bile acids. Bile acid transporters," *Journal of Lipid Research*, vol. 50, no. 12, pp. 2340–2357, 2009.

[29] E. Halilbasic, T. Claudel, and M. Trauner, "Bile acid transporters

and regulatory nuclear receptors in the liver and beyond," *Journal of Hepatology*, vol. 58, no. 1, pp. 155–168, 2013.

[30] B. L. Shneider, "Intestinal bile acid transport: Biology, physiology, and pathophysiology," *Journal of Pediatric Gastroenterology and Nutrition*, vol. 32, no. 4, pp. 407–417, 2001.

[31] T. Claudel, G. Zollner, M. Wagner, and M. Trauner, "Role of nuclear receptors for bile acid metabolism, bile secretion, cholestasis, and gallstone disease," *Biochimica et Biophysica Acta (BBA) - Molecular Basis of Disease*, vol. 1812, no. 8, pp. 867–878, 2011.

[32] J. J. Eloranta and G. A. Kullak-Ublick, "The role of FXR in disorders of bile acid homeostasis," *Physiology Journal*, vol. 23, no. 5, pp. 286–295, 2008.

[33] B. Goodwin, S. A. Jones, R. R. Price et al., "A regulatory cascade of the nuclear receptors FXR, SHP-1, and LRH-1 represses bile acid biosynthesis," *Molecular Cell*, vol. 6, no. 3, pp. 517–526, 2000.

[34] M. Müller, P. L. M. Jansen, K. N. Faber et al., "Farnesoid X receptor and bile salts are involved in transcriptional regulation of the gene encoding the human bile salt export pump," *Hepatology*, vol. 35, no. 3, pp. 589–596, 2002.

[35] M. Ananthanarayanan, N. Balasubramanian, M. Makishima, D. J. Mangelsdorf, and F. J. Suchy, "Human bile salt export pump promoter is transactivated by the farnesoid X receptor/bile acid receptor," *The Journal of Biological Chemistry*, vol. 276, no. 31, pp. 28857–28865, 2001.

[36] L. Huang, A. Zhao, J. L. Lew et al., "Farnesoid X receptor activates transcription of the phospholipid pump MDR3," *The Journal of Biological Chemistry*, vol. 278, no. 51, pp. 51085–51090, 2003.

[37] M. Wagner, G. Zollner, and M. Trauner, "Nuclear receptor regulation of the adaptive response of bile acid transporters in cholestasis," *Seminars in Liver Disease*, vol. 30, no. 2, pp. 160–177, 2010.

[38] Y. Zhang, H. R. Kast-Woelbern, and P. A. Edwards, "Natural structural variants of the nuclear receptor farnesoid X receptor affect transcriptional activation," *The Journal of Biological Chemistry*, vol. 278, no. 1, pp. 104–110, 2003.

[39] S. W. C. Van Mil, R. H. J. Houwen, and L. W. J. Klomp, "Genetics of familial intrahepatic cholestasis syndromes," *Journal of Medical Genetics*, vol. 42, no. 6, pp. 449–463, 2005.

[40] V. E. H. Carlton, L. Pawlikowska, and L. N. Bull, "Molecular basis of intrahepatic cholestasis," *Annals of Medicine*, vol. 36, no. 8, pp. 606–617, 2004.

[41] R. J. Clayton, F. L. Iber, B. H. Ruebner, and V. A. Mckusick, "Byler Disease: Fatal Familial Intrahepatic Cholestasis in an Amish Kindred," *American Journal of Diseases of Children*, vol. 117, no. 1, pp. 112–124, 1969.

[42] E. Jacquemin, "Progressive familial intrahepatic cholestasis," *Clinics and Research in Hepatology and Gastroenterology*, vol. 36, supplement 1, pp. S26–S35, 2012.

[43] L. N. Bull, M. J. T. Van Eijk, L. Pawlikowska et al., "A gene encoding a P-type ATPase mutated in two forms of hereditary cholestasis," *Nature Genetics*, vol. 18, no. 3, pp. 219–224, 1998.

[44] L. W. J. Klomp, J. C. Vargas, S. W. C. Van Mil et al., "Characterization of mutations in ATP8B1 associated with hereditary cholestasis," *Hepatology*, vol. 40, no. 1, pp. 27–38, 2004.

[45] P. Ujhazy, D. Ortiz, S. Misra et al., "Familial intrahepatic cholestasis 1: Studies of localization and function," *Hepatology* vol. 34, no. 4 I, pp. 768–775, 2001.

[46] C. C. Paulusma, A. Groen, C. Kunne et al., "Atp8b1 deficiency in mice reduces resistance of the canalicular membrane to hydrophobic bile salts and impairs bile salt transport," *Hepatology*, vol. 44, no. 1, pp. 195–204, 2006.

[47] S. W. C. Van Mil, L. W. J. Klomp, L. N. Bull, and R. H. J. Houwen, "FIC1 disease: A spectrum of intrahepatic cholestatic disorders," *Seminars in Liver Disease*, vol. 21, no. 4, pp. 535–544, 2001.

[48] A. Miyahawa-Hayashino, H. Egawa, T. Yorifuji et al., "Allograft steatohepatitis in progressive familial intrahepatic cholestasis type 1 after living donor liver transplantation," *Liver Transplantation*, vol. 15, no. 6, pp. 610–618, 2009.

[49] E. Nicastro, X. Stephenne, F. Smets et al., "Recovery of graft steatosis and protein-losing enteropathy after biliary diversion in a PFIC 1 liver transplanted child," *Pediatric Transplantation*, vol. 16, no. 5, pp. E177–E182, 2012.

[50] K. Evason, K. E. Bove, M. J. Finegold et al., "Morphologic findings in progressive familial intrahepatic cholestasis 2 (PFIC2): Correlation with genetic and immunohistochemical studies," *The American Journal of Surgical Pathology*, vol. 35, no. 5, pp. 687–696, 2011.

[51] S. S. Strautnieks, L. N. Bull, A. S. Knisely et al., "A gene encoding a liver-specific ABC transporter is mutated in progressive familial intrahepatic cholestasis," *Nature Genetics*, vol. 20, no. 3, pp. 233–238, 1998.

[52] A. S. Knisely, S. S. Strautnieks, Y. Meier et al., "Hepatocellular carcinoma in ten children under five years of age with bile salt export pump deficiency," *Hepatology*, vol. 44, no. 2, pp. 478–486, 2006.

[53] A. O. Scheimann, S. S. Strautnieks, A. S. Knisely, J. A. Byrne, R. J. Thompson, and M. J. Finegold, "Mutations in Bile Salt Export Pump (ABCB11) in Two Children with Progressive Familial Intrahepatic Cholestasis and Cholangiocarcinoma," *Journal of Pediatrics*, vol. 150, no. 5, pp. 556–559, 2007.

[54] V. Keitel, M. Burdelski, Z. Vojnisek, L. Schmitt, D. Häussinger, and R. Kubitz, "De novo bile salt transporter antibodies as a possible cause of recurrent graft failure after liver transplantation: A novel mechanism of cholestasis," *Hepatology*, vol. 50, no. 2, pp. 510–517, 2009.

[55] P. Jara, L. Hierro, P. Martínez-Fernández et al., "Recurrence of bile salt export pump deficiency after liver transplantation," *The New England Journal of Medicine*, vol. 361, no. 14, pp. 1359–1367, 2009.

[56] R. Kubitz, C. Dröge, S. Kluge et al., "Autoimmune BSEP Disease: Disease Recurrence After Liver Transplantation for Progressive Familial Intrahepatic Cholestasis," *Clinical Reviews in Allergy & Immunology*, vol. 48, no. 2-3, pp. 273–284, 2015.

[57] J. Stindt, S. Kluge, C. Dröge et al., "Bile salt export pump-reactive antibodies form a polyclonal, multi-inhibitory response in antibody-induced bile salt export pump deficiency," *Hepatology*, vol. 63, no. 2, pp. 524–537, 2016.

[58] E. Jacquemin, J. M. DeVree, D. Cresteil et al., "The wide spectrum of multidrug resistance 3 deficiency: from neonatal cholestasis to cirrhosis of adulthood," *Gastroenterology*, vol. 120, no. 6, pp. 1448–1458, 2001.

[59] O. Rosmorduc and R. Poupon, "Low phospholipid associated cholelithiasis: association with mutation in the *MDR3/ABCB4* gene," *Orphanet Journal of Rare Diseases*, vol. 2, article 29, 2007.

[60] A. Davit-Spraul, E. Gonzales, C. Baussan, and E. Jacquemin, "The spectrum of liver diseases related to ABCB4 gene mutations: Pathophysiology and clinical aspects," *Seminars in Liver Disease*, vol. 30, no. 2, pp. 134–146, 2010.

[61] D. Wendum, V. Barbu, O. Rosmorduc, L. Arrivé, J.-F. Fléjou, and R. Poupon, "Aspects of liver pathology in adult patients with MDR3/ABCB4 gene mutations," *Virchows Archiv*, vol. 460, no. 3, pp. 291–298, 2012.

[62] R. P. J. Oude Elferink and C. C. Paulusma, "Function and pathophysiological importance of ABCB4 (MDR3 P-glycoprotein)," *Pflügers Archiv - European Journal of Physiology*, vol. 453, no. 5, pp. 601–610, 2007.

[63] A. Davit-Spraul, E. Gonzales, C. Baussan, and E. Jacquemin, "Progressive familial intrahepatic cholestasis," *Clinical Pediatrics*, vol. 51, pp. 689–691, 2012.

[64] S. Boga, D. Jain, and M. L. Schilsky, "Presentation of progressive familial intrahepatic cholestasis type 3 mimicking wilson disease: molecular genetic diagnosis and response to treatment," *Pediatric Gastroenterology, Hepatology & Nutrition*, vol. 18, no. 3, p. 202, 2015.

[65] M. Sambrotta, S. Strautnieks, E. Papouli et al., "Mutations in TJP2 cause progressive cholestatic liver disease," *Nature Genetics*, vol. 46, no. 4, pp. 326–328, 2014.

[66] M. Sambrotta and R. J. Thompson, "Mutations in TJP2, encoding zona occludens 2, and liver disease," *Tissue Barriers*, vol. 3, no. 3, Article ID e1026537, 2015.

[67] S. Zhou, P. M. Hertel, M. J. Finegold et al., "Hepatocellular carcinoma associated with tight-junction protein 2 deficiency," *Hepatology*, vol. 62, no. 6, pp. 1914–1916, 2015.

[68] V. E. H. Carlton, B. Z. Harris, E. G. Puffenberger et al., "Complex inheritance of familial hypercholanemia with associated mutations in TJP2 and BAAT," *Nature Genetics*, vol. 34, no. 1, pp. 91–96, 2003.

[69] N. Gomez-Ospina, C. J. Potter, R. Xiao et al., "Mutations in the nuclear bile acid receptor FXR cause progressive familial intrahepatic cholestasis," *Nature Communications*, vol. 7, Article ID 10713, 2016.

[70] I. Koutsounas, S. Theocharis, I. Delladetsima, E. Patsouris, and C. Giaginis, "Farnesoid x receptor in human metabolism and disease: the interplay between gene polymorphisms, clinical phenotypes and disease susceptibility," *Expert Opinion on Drug Metabolism & Toxicology*, vol. 11, no. 4, pp. 523–532, 2015.

[71] S. W. C. van Mil, A. Milona, P. H. Dixon et al., "Functional Variants of the Central Bile Acid Sensor FXR Identified in Intrahepatic Cholestasis of Pregnancy," *Gastroenterology*, vol. 133, no. 2, pp. 507–516, 2007.

[72] C. Dröge, M. Bonus, U. Baumann et al., "Sequencing of FIC1, BSEP and MDR3 in a large cohort of patients with cholestasis revealed a high number of different genetic variants," *Journal of Hepatology*, vol. 67, no. 6, pp. 1253–1264, 2017.

[73] L. N. Bull, V. E. H. Carlton, N. L. Stricker et al., "Genetic and morphological findings in progressive familial intrahepatic cholestasis (Byler disease [PFIC-1] and Byler syndrome): Evidence for heterogeneity," *Hepatology*, vol. 26, no. 1, pp. 155–164, 1997.

[74] S. W. C. Van Mil, W. L. Van Der Woerd, G. Van Der Brugge et al., "Benign recurrent intrahepatic cholestasis type 2 is caused by mutations in ABCB11," *Gastroenterology*, vol. 127, no. 2, pp. 379–384, 2004.

[75] N. A. M. Van Ooteghem, L. W. J. Klomp, G. P. Van Berge-Henegouwen, and R. H. J. Houwen, "Benign recurrent intrahepatic cholestasis progressing to progressive familial intrahepatic cholestasis: Low GGT cholestasis is a clinical continuum," *Journal of Hepatology*, vol. 36, no. 3, pp. 439–443, 2002.

[76] F. Balsells, R. Wyllie, R. Steffen, and M. Kay, "Benign recurrent intrahepatic cholestasis: Improvement of pruritus and shortening of the symptomatic phase with rifampin therapy: A case report," *Clinical Pediatrics*, vol. 36, no. 8, pp. 483–485, 1997.

[77] U. Beuers, M. Trauner, P. Jansen, and R. Poupon, "New paradigms in the treatment of hepatic cholestasis: From UDCA to FXR, PXR and beyond," *Journal of Hepatology*, vol. 62, no. 1, pp. S25–S37, 2015.

[78] L. Bachs, A. Parés, M. Elena, C. Piera, and J. Rodés, "Effects of long-term rifampicin administration in primary biliary cirrhosis," *Gastroenterology*, vol. 102, no. 6, pp. 2077–2080, 1992.

[79] J. M. Stapelbroek, K. J. Van Erpecum, L. W. J. Klomp et al., "Nasobiliary drainage induces long-lasting remission in benign recurrent intrahepatic cholestasis," *Hepatology*, vol. 43, no. 1, pp. 51–53, 2006.

[80] F. Lammert, H.-U. Marschall, A. Glantz, and S. Matern, "Intrahepatic cholestasis of pregnancy: molecular pathogenesis, diagnosis and management," *Journal of Hepatology*, vol. 33, no. 6, pp. 1012–1021, 2000.

[81] P. H. Dixon and C. Williamson, "The pathophysiology of intrahepatic cholestasis of pregnancy," *Clinics and Research in Hepatology and Gastroenterology*, vol. 40, no. 2, pp. 141–153, 2016.

[82] M. G. Martineau, C. Raker, P. H. Dixon et al., "The metabolic profile of intrahepatic cholestasis of pregnancy is associated with impaired glucose tolerance, dyslipidemia, and increased fetal growth," *Diabetes Care*, vol. 38, no. 2, pp. 243–248, 2015.

[83] D. G. Goulis, I. A. L. Walker, M. De Swiet, C. W. G. Redman, and C. Williamson, "Preeclampsia with Abnormal Liver Function Tests Is Associated with Cholestasis in a Subgroup of Cases," *Hypertension in Pregnancy*, vol. 23, no. 1, pp. 19–27, 2004.

[84] A. Glantz, H.-U. Marschall, F. Lammert, and L.-Å. Mattsson, "Intrahepatic cholestasis of pregnancy: A randomized controlled trial comparing dexamethasone and ursodeoxycholic acid," *Hepatology*, vol. 42, no. 6, pp. 1399–1405, 2005.

[85] R. Zapata, L. Sandoval, J. Palma et al., "Ursodeoxycholic acid in the treatment of intrahepatic cholestasis of pregnancy. A 12-year experience," *Liver International*, vol. 25, no. 3, pp. 548–554, 2005.

[86] T. Binder, P. Salaj, T. Zima, and L. Vítek, "Randomized prospective comparative study of ursodeoxycholic acid and S-adenosyl-L-methionine in the treatment of intrahepatic cholestasis of pregnancy," *Journal of Perinatal Medicine*, vol. 34, no. 5, pp. 383–391, 2006.

[87] P. H. Dixon, N. Weerasekera, K. J. Linton et al., "Heterozygous MDR3 missense mutation associated with intrahepatic cholestasis of pregnancy: Evidence for a defect in protein trafficking," *Human Molecular Genetics*, vol. 9, no. 8, pp. 1209–1217, 2000.

[88] C. Gendrot, Y. Bacq, M.-C. Brechot, J. Lansac, and C. Andres, "A second heterozygous MDR3 nonsense mutation associated with intrahepatic cholestasis of pregnancy," *Journal of Medical Genetics*, vol. 40, no. 3, article e32, 2003.

[89] A. Floreani, I. Carderi, D. Paternoster et al., "Intrahepatic cholestasis of pregnancy: Three novel MDR3 gene mutations," *Alimentary Pharmacology & Therapeutics*, vol. 23, no. 11, pp. 1649–1653, 2006.

[90] J. N. Painter, M. Savander, A. Ropponen et al., "Sequence variation in the ATP8B1 gene and intrahepatic cholestasis of

pregnancy," *European Journal of Human Genetics*, vol. 13, no. 4, pp. 435–439, 2005.

[91] W. L. Van Der Woerd, R. H. J. Houwen, and S. F. J. Van De Graaf, "Current and future therapies for inherited cholestatic liver diseases," *World Journal of Gastroenterology*, vol. 23, no. 5, pp. 763–775, 2017.

[92] A. Thébaut, D. Habes, F. Gottrand et al., "Sertraline as an additional treatment for cholestatic pruritus in children," *Journal of Pediatric Gastroenterology and Nutrition*, vol. 64, no. 3, pp. 431–435, 2017.

[93] U. Ołdakowska-Jedynak, I. Jankowska, M. Hartleb et al., "Treatment of pruritus with Prometheus dialysis and absorption system in a patient with benign recurrent intrahepatic cholestasis," *Hepatology Research*, vol. 44, no. 10, pp. E304–E308, 2014.

[94] L. Cutillo, M. Najimi, F. Smets et al., "Safety of living-related liver transplantation for progressive familial intrahepatic cholestasis," *Pediatric Transplantation*, vol. 10, no. 5, pp. 570–574, 2006.

[95] E. Gonzales, B. Grosse, B. Schuller et al., "Targeted pharmacotherapy in progressive familial intrahepatic cholestasis type 2: Evidence for improvement of cholestasis with 4-phenylbutyrate," *Hepatology*, vol. 62, no. 2, pp. 558–566, 2015.

[96] E. Gonzales and E. Jacquemin, "Mutation specific drug therapy for progressive familial or benign recurrent intrahepatic cholestasis: A new tool in a near future?" *Journal of Hepatology*, vol. 53, no. 2, pp. 385–387, 2010.

[97] M. Trauner, C. D. Fuchs, E. Halilbasic, and G. Paumgartner, "New therapeutic concepts in bile acid transport and signaling for management of cholestasis," *Hepatology*, vol. 65, no. 4, pp. 1393–1404, 2017.

28

"Fatal Gastrointestinal and Peritoneal Ischemic Disease" of Unknown Cause at Arba Minch Hospital, Southern Ethiopia

Jilcha Diribi Feyisa[1] **Melka Kenea,**[2] **Efrem Gashaw,**[2] **Eskezyiaw Agedew Getahun**[3] **Barry Leon Hicks,**[4] **and Hailemichael Desalegn**[1]

[1]*Department of Internal Medicine, Saint Paul's Hospital Millennium Medical College, Ethiopia*
[2]*Department of Surgery, Arba Minch General Hospital, Ethiopia*
[3]*Department of Public Health, College of Health Sciences, Arba Minch University, Ethiopia*
[4]*Department of Surgery, Arba Minch University, Ethiopia*

Correspondence should be addressed to Jilcha Diribi Feyisa; jilcha.diribi@sphmmc.edu.et

Academic Editor: Maikel P. Peppelenbosch

Gastrointestinal and peritoneal ischemic disease due to unknown etiology present with intestinal obstruction and/or peritonitis otherwise in healthy patient emerged as fatal disease at Arba Minch General Hospital. This disorder was diagnosed based on intraoperative finding. Clinical presentation and natural history of disease progression were similar. It is estimated that about 6–10 lives are being claimed each year at Arba Minch Hospital with this disease of unidentified cause accounting for the largest figure of surgical department. Here we report case analysis and literature review illustrating clinical presentation, workup, preoperative diagnosis, intraoperative diagnosis, and final outcome of fatal gastrointestinal and peritoneal ischemic disease.

1. Introduction

Fatal gastrointestinal and peritoneal ischemic disease (FGPID) is a pathology which describes ischemic changes to intraperitoneal organs including bowel, peritoneum, omentum, gallbladder, mesentery, and mesenteric lymph nodes. Although this disease is acknowledged as emerging problem at Arba Minch General Hospital (AMGH) years ago, there was no study so far in this hospital to identify cause and possible factors behind, whereas the mortality is high and continuing. This is clearly reflected by outnumbered death reports during surgical morning session and monthly reports. Besides, there are no in depth clinical evaluation, investigation, and recorded data of those patients apart from having the routines. Therefore, the definite pathology, possible cause, natural history, and immediate cause of death remain obscure. The blindly tried options of managements are unsuccessful so far.

We could not identify similar case reports, but entire and localized bowel ischemia can occur due to vascular and nonvascular causes identified due to eosinophilic gastroenteritis and mesenteric vascular disorders [1, 2]. Ischemia of intraperitoneal organs with obstruction feature are identified in these reports specifically with eosinophilic gastroenteritis (EGE) and ischemic bowel disease/mesenteric ischemia (MI) [3–5].

2. Case Presentation and Analysis

In this report we analyzed medical records of 8 consecutive patients who were operated and found to have ischemia of peritoneum and the whole bowel from April 1/2015 to December 1/2016 in AMGH, southern Ethiopia. A retrospective analysis of cases and literature review have been done. Data was collected using structured data sheet. The results were annualized manually and descriptive statics were used.

Among 8 patients analyzed with gastrointestinal and peritoneal ischemic disease of unknown cause in Arba Minch General Hospital, 6 were females and 2 males, with mean age of 26 years ±12.54 and SD range of 11-45 years. 4

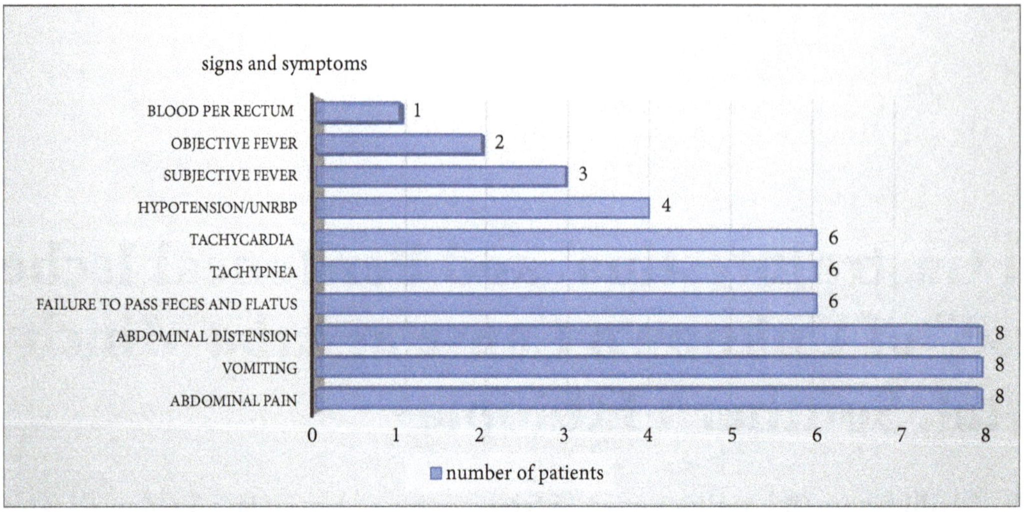

FIGURE 1: Clinical symptoms and signs on presentation of patients with fatal gastrointestinal and peritoneal ischemic disease discussed in this case report. UNRBP: unrecordable blood pressure.

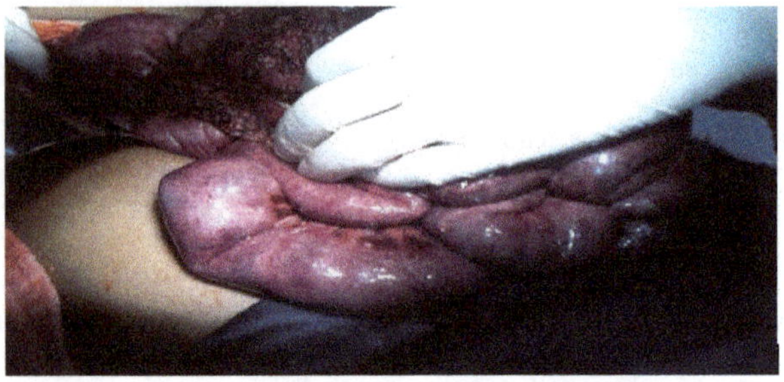

FIGURE 2: Gross specimen showing patchy ischemia of small intestine, peritoneum, and omentum from patient having gastrointestinal and peritoneal ischemic disease.

of the patients are from Chencha woreda while the rest are from Bonke woreda. All patients were presented as acute abdomen. Abdominal pain, vomiting, and abdominal distension were presenting symptoms in all cases (Figure 1). Six of patients had failure to pass feces and flatus. Three of the cases presented with hypovolemic shock. Six of them had tachycardia and all were tachypneic, with average pulse rate of 119 ±25.83 bit/minute and average respiratory rate of 36± 8.25 breath/minute. Only two of the cases had objective fever with axillary temperature of >38°C and average temperature of 37.47°C±1.2 SD on presentation.

The preoperative clinical diagnosis in six of the cases was small bowel obstruction with generalized peritonitis. Three of them were presumed to have generalized peritonitis, one acute pancreatitis, and one suspected to have mesenteric ischemia. Two of the cases were consulted to obstetric side for possible ruptured ovarian cyst. The intraoperative finding in all eight cases, however, confirmed gastrointestinal and peritoneal ischemic disease with no cause identified. All patients had ischemic changes which involved the whole bowel (stomach, small bowel, large bowel to rectum), peritoneum, and omentum (Figure 2). Pancreas condition was normal except one case which got edematous. In addition all cases have hemorrhagic ascites. Six patients were found to have abdominal wall involvement while gallbladder was involved in one case. Mesenteric lymphadenopathy (LAP) was observed only in 2 cases. Mesenteric arteries are found pulsating in all of the cases.

Regarding outcome after operation, five of the cases died in hospital within 2 hours up to eighth postoperative day's intervals. One patient was self-discharged against medical advice as she was getting deteriorated. She did not revisited hospital and hence her final outcome was not traced. One patient was improved and discharged on 21st postoperative day. She was appointed to surgical referral clinic but she did not appear on her appointment date. Her case was so not confirmed as she was not traced for her final outcome (Table 1).

3. Discussion

The present report addressed ischemic changes to entire bowel, peritoneum, and other intraperitoneal viscera's with ileus as remarking presentation. There have been reports on intestinal and/or peritoneal ischemic changes with different clinical presentation from different corners of the world specifically from far east countries even if hardly available with similar presentation [1–6]. There is a paucity of literature in our country, Ethiopia, regarding ischemic disease involving intraperitoneal viscera. Oral based discussion made among surgical seniors from Black Lion, Jimma, Gondar, Hawassa, and Arba Minch University Hospitals however indicated that a number of patients were seen in Jimma hospital Having ischemia of the whole bowel (personal communication, Seifu, MD, 2015, AMGH). Interpersonal communication made with medical practitioner from Mizan Tepi Hospital also revealed the presence of similar cases diagnosed on the basis of intraoperative finding (personal communication, Ruth Shimelis, MD, November 2016, SPHMMC).

The result of the analysis showed invariable ischemic changes of stomach, small bowel, large bowel, peritoneum, and omentum. Matsushita M et al. reported eosinophilic

TABLE 1: Postoperative outcome of patients diagnosed with FGPD of unknown cause.

Patient	Outcome	Date of death/discharge (post-operative)	Condition on discharge (if discharged)	Condition after discharge (if discharged)
Patient 1	Death	4th		
Patient 2	Death	8.5 hours		
Patient 3	Discharge	21st	Improved, appointed to SRC	Not revisited, not traced
Patient 4	Death	2 hours		
Patient 5	Self-discharge	8th	Deteriorated	Not revisited, not traced
Patient 6	Death	6th		
Patient 7	Death	In Recovery Room		
Patient 8	Death	3rd		

SRC: surgical referral clinic.

gastroenteritis involving the entire digestive tract [1]. The result of our study indicated that six of the patients were presumed to have intestinal obstruction. A case series report from Mangalore, South India, of four patients who presented with intestinal obstruction showed a similar clinical presentation to our cases. Histopathological report of those cases confirmed EGE in all cases [3]. All presented with abdominal pain, vomiting, weight loss, diarrhea, and abdominal distension which are the major presenting symptoms of EGE in descending order as per a study done in USA by Talley on clinicopathological aspect of EGE [3, 7]. Hemorrhagic ascites were found in all of the case. As per Klein classification of EGE, the muscular layer involvement was found to be present with intestinal obstruction while serosal type is studied as the cause for ascites [8]. Female predominance is found in the same report (three females and one male) though other reports on EGE showed male predominance [3, 7]. EGE commonly occurs in children. Mean age at diagnosis is third to fifth decade, commonly in fifth decade which is closely parallel age group of our case [7]. Clinical misdiagnosis is common in EGE especially when it is present with obstructive feature. In the case report from India, patients are clinically misdiagnosed as Intestinal Tuberculosis, volvulus, neoplasm, and other uncertainty for obstruction [3]. This is because diagnosis of EGE is challenging and one of the exclusion pathologies [8]. This might be similar to our cases where there is clinical misdiagnosis though the actual pathology is yet not confirmed. EGE was repeatedly reported as allergic condition in more than half of the cases [9]. The seasonality and area specific nature of our cases may so suggest its possibility. It is also reported in connection with parasitic infection [10]. Beside Ascariasis found intraoperatively in one of our cases, the burden of infectious disease in the region which can have systemic presentation involving those anatomical parts needs high consideration in this regard raising the possibility.

The other reasonable pathology mentioned in literature resulting in ischemic change to bowel is obstruction of mesenteric arteries or systemic hypoperfusion termed as mesenteric ischemia [2, 6, 11]. Consistent with our case, it is repeatedly reported as fatal condition necessitating immediate medical and surgical intervention. A clinical series done over the last 15 years summarizing the possible outcome of acute type mesenteric ischemia showed a mortality rate of 70% with a range of 59%-93%. Clinical analysis done 70 years earlier than this report also showed similar figure [11]. It is comparable to 75% fatality of our case. Mesenteric ischemia is reported to affect every segment of gastrointestinal tract. Many of case reports are however on isolated small bowel or colonic ischemia since multiple collateral vessels are available in upper segment. Ischemic colitis is commonly reported in association with mesenteric vascular disease [1, 2, 12]. A case report from Staten Island University Hospital, Staten Island, NY, USA, explains an ischemic bowel injury which occurred following angiography [6]. It needs obstruction of abdominal aorta, small mesenteric arterial occlusion, or nonocclusive type mesenteric ischemia to result in involvement of the whole bowel and other intraperitoneal viscera [13]. This contradicts our finding of whole bowel involvement in all cases. Intraoperatively identified pulsatile mesenteric arteries of patients in our case also question the possibility of mesenteric ischemia. Still it cannot be ruled out with the possibility of small penetrating arterial occlusion or nonocclusive type of mesenteric ischemia. Similar to our cases abdominal pain is the usual manifestation of mesenteric ischemia mimicking peritonitis. It outranges abdominal finding raising high clinical suspicion of the case. According to a study done in series of 58 cases, abdominal pain was present in 95% of cases while metabolic acidosis (44%), nausea (44%), vomiting (35%), diarrhea (35%), tachycardia (33%), blood per rectum (16%), and constipation (7%) were also present [11, 14]. Except diarrhea and unconfirmed metabolic acidosis, all were the presenting features of our cases.

We could not find literature which explains the involvement of gall bladder, omentum, and abdominal wall with this listed clinical presentation found in our case.

4. Limitations

Incomplete recording of medical records, limited laboratory investigations done, unavailability of imaging modalities, failure to collect histopathological result sent as the fatal nature of disease resulting in death before bringing to hospital, difficulty of tracing family back due to lack of precise address on cards were the limitations faced.

5. Conclusion

The involvement of the whole bowel with peritoneum, omentum, abdominal wall, and gall bladder in some cases without selection of arteries, presence of mesenteric pulse intraoperatively, evidences high possibility of nonvascular disease. Absence of cardiac and renal comorbidities also makes nonocclusive disease unlikely. Higher incidence observed among third to fifth decade (25.75 years ±12.54 SD) having age range of 11-45 years with inclusion of children as well, higher incidence in female, patchy nature of ischemia, presence of hemorrhagic fluid, acute onset of disease, nonmechanical nature of intestinal obstruction, and area and season specific nature of the disease suggest the possibility of exposure to food allergens or nutritional poisoning, environmental toxins, or allergens. The presence of tachypnea in all of patients might also strengthen the possibility of allergen induced hypersensitivity. The possibility of infectious cause and autoimmune or neoplastic causes is still not ruled out.

Additional Points

Recommendation. We recommend the need for further research to identify the possible cause of this fatal illness. Based on different literature sources and experience, the nature of intraoperative features affecting specific communities in a seasonal pattern needs to have urgent multidisciplinary approach from clinicians, epidemiologists, and pathologists to identify the cause of this fatal disease and recommend effective measures.

Acknowledgments

We are very grateful to the staff of the Department of Surgery at Arba Minch University and all Ethiopian patients who were willing to provide us with necessary information to the extent of exposing their body in uncomfortable setup so as to bring knowledge transformation in medical practice.

References

[1] M. Matsushita, K. Hajiro, Y. Morita, H. Takakuwa, and T. Suzaki, "Eosinophilic Gastroenteritis Involving the Entire Digestive Tract," *American Journal of Gastroenterology*, vol. 90, no. 10, pp. 1868–1870, 1995.

[2] S. K. Gandhi, M. M. Hanson, A. M. Vernava, D. L. Kaminski, and W. E. Longo, "Ischemic colitis," *Diseases of the Colon & Rectum*, vol. 39, no. 1, pp. 88–100, 1996.

[3] A. Krishnappa, S. A. Shariff, and A. D. Kumar, "Eosinophilic gastroenteritis presenting as Intestinal Obstruction – a case series" MVJ Medical college and Research Hospital, Bangalore," *India online journal of Health and allied Science*, vol. 10, no. 2, 2011.

[4] T. Miyamoto, T. Shibata, S. Matsuura, M. Kagesawa, Y. Ishizawa, and K. Tamiya, "Eosinophilic gastroenteritis with ileus and ascites," *Internal Medicine*, vol. 35, no. 10, pp. 779–782, 1996.

[5] E. Shweiki, J. C. West, J. W. Klena et al., "Eosinophilic gastroenteritis presenting as an obstructing cecal mass - A case report and review of the literature," *American Journal of Gastroenterology*, vol. 94, no. 12, pp. 3644-3645, 1999.

[6] S. Kedia, V. Raj Bhatt, A. Koirala et al., "Acute mesenteric ischemia: a sequela of abdominal aortography," *Journal of Community Hospital Internal Medicine Perspectives (JCHIMP)*, vol. 4, no. 1, p. 22894, 2014.

[7] N. J. Talley, R. G. Shorter, S. F. Phillips, and A. R. Zinsmeister, "Eosinophilic gastroenteritis: a clinicopathological study of patients with disease of the mucosa, muscle layer, and subserosal tissues," *Gut*, vol. 31, no. 1, pp. 54–58, 1992.

[8] N. C. Klein, R. L. Hargrove, M. H. Sleisenger, and G. H. Jeffries, "Eosinophilic gastroenteritis," *Medicine*, vol. 49, no. 4, pp. 299–319, 1970.

[9] C. Prussin, "Eosinophilic gastroenteritis and related eosinophilic disorders," *Gastroenterology Clinics of North America*, vol. 43, no. 2, pp. 317–327, 2014.

[10] J. K. Triantafillidis, A. Parasi, P. Cherakakis, and M. Sklavaina, "Eosinophilic gastroenteritis: Current aspects on etiology, pathogenesis, diagnosis and treatment," *Annals of Gastroenterology*, vol. 15, no. 2, pp. 106–115, 2002.

[11] "American Gastroenterological Association medical position statement: Guidelines on osteoporosis in gastrointestinal diseases, This document presents the official recommendations of the American Gastroenterological Association (AGA) Committee on Osteoporosis in Gastrointestinal Disease. It was approved by the Clinical Practice Committee on September 21, 2002, and by the AGA Governing Board on November 1, 2002.," *Gastroenterology*, vol. 124, no. 3, pp. 791–794, 2003.

[12] J. D. Rosenblum, C. M. Boyle, and L. B. Schwartz, "The mesenteric circulation: Anatomy and physiology," *Surgical Clinics of North America*, vol. 77, no. 2, pp. 289–306, 1997.

[13] http://www.mayoclinic.org/diseases-conditions/mesenteric-ischemia/basics/definition/CON-20035882.

[14] W. M. Park, P. Gloviczki, K. J. Cherry Jr. et al., "Contemporary management of acute mesenteric ischemia: Factors associated with survival," *Journal of Vascular Surgery*, vol. 35, no. 3, pp. 445–452, 2002.

29

Nonalcoholic Fatty Liver Disease Cirrhosis: A Review of Its Epidemiology, Risk Factors, Clinical Presentation, Diagnosis, Management, and Prognosis

Bei Li, Chuan Zhang, and Yu-Tao Zhan

Department of Gastroenterology, Beijing Tongren Hospital, Capital Medical University, Beijing 100730, China

Correspondence should be addressed to Yu-Tao Zhan; yutaozhan@263.net

Academic Editor: Pascal Lapierre

Cirrhosis is the common end stage of a number of chronic liver conditions and a significant cause of morbidity and mortality. With the growing epidemic of obesity and metabolic syndrome, nonalcoholic fatty liver disease (NAFLD) has become the most common cause of chronic liver disease worldwide and will become one of the leading causes of cirrhosis. Increased awareness and understanding of NAFLD cirrhosis are essential. To date, there has been no published systematic review on NAFLD cirrhosis. Thus, this article reviews recent studies on the epidemiology, risk factors, clinical presentation, diagnosis, management, and prognosis of NAFLD cirrhosis.

1. Introduction

Cirrhosis is the end stage of a wide number of chronic liver conditions that share common features of necroinflammation, fibrosis, and regenerative nodules, which modify the normal liver structure to reduce its functional mass and alter the vascular architecture [1]. Cirrhosis has become a major public health problem and a significant cause of morbidity and mortality [2]. It is the 13th most common cause of mortality worldwide [3]. Global cirrhosis deaths have increased from 1.54% of all deaths in 1980 to 1.95% in 2010 [4], causing more than one million deaths each year [5]. The most common primary etiologies for cirrhosis are chronic hepatitis B, alcoholic liver disease, chronic hepatitis C, and nonalcoholic fatty liver disease (NAFLD) [2]. Chronic hepatitis B is the most common cause of cirrhosis in most parts of Asia and sub-Saharan Africa [4], whereas alcoholic liver disease and chronic hepatitis C are the main causes in most developed countries. In recent years, with the rising incidence of obesity, NAFLD has become one of the leading causes of cirrhosis in some countries [6]. By 2020, the number of individuals with NAFLD cirrhosis is predicted to exceed that of those with hepatitis B- and C-related cirrhosis, and NAFLD cirrhosis will become the leading indication for liver transplantation [7].

2. Epidemiology

With the ongoing epidemic of obesity and metabolic syndrome, NAFLD has become the most common cause of chronic liver disease worldwide [8]. The global prevalence of NAFLD was estimated to be about 24% [9]. Cirrhosis is an important factor for liver-related morbidity and mortality in patients with NAFLD [10]. However, we still do not have a detailed understanding on how often NAFLD cirrhosis occurs. Existing studies with different study objects, diagnostic methods, and other variable parameters showed the inconsistent epidemiological results of NAFLD cirrhosis.

2.1. General Population Study. Kabbany et al. analyzed the National Health and Nutrition Examination Survey (USA) data between 2009 and 2012. Cirrhosis was diagnosed by an AST to platelet ratio index >2 and abnormal liver function tests. NAFLD cirrhosis was defined as cirrhosis that presented with at least one of the following: obesity, diabetes, insulin resistance, and metabolic syndrome. They reported that the prevalence of NAFLD cirrhosis was 0.178% [11]. Fung et al. performed a prospective cross-sectional study of 2493 volunteers recruited from the general population and the Red Cross Transfusion Center in Hong Kong (China). Cirrhosis was diagnosed by transient elastography (TE). They found that the incidence of NAFLD cirrhosis was 0.17 % [12].

2.2. Diseases or Morbidity Patients Study. A study on 1799 patients with type 2 diabetes (T2DM) showed that the prevalence of NAFLD cirrhosis diagnosed by TE was 11.2% [13]. A review of 16 individual studies of 2,956 patients with severe obesity revealed that 5.8% of patients have NAFLD cirrhosis [8]. Those studies suggested that patients with T2DM or severe obesity have high incidence of NAFLD cirrhosis [14].

2.3. Hospitalized Patients with Cirrhosis Study. Xiong et al. performed a retrospective study of 1,582 patients with cirrhosis at Daping Hospital (China). Cirrhosis was diagnosed based on clinical symptoms, imaging data, and/or histological findings. This study found that the prevalence of NAFLD cirrhosis was 1.9% [15]. Michitaka et al. analyzed data from 33,379 patients with cirrhosis at 58 hospitals including all university and other major hospitals in Japan. Cirrhosis was diagnosed by autopsy, laparoscopy or abdominal imaging, laboratory findings, and clinical findings compatible with cirrhosis. This analysis showed that NAFLD cirrhosis constituted 2.1% of all cases of cirrhosis [16]. Karageorgos et al. studied 812 cases of cirrhosis from a liver disease center (Greece). The diagnosis of cirrhosis was confirmed by liver biopsy in compensated cirrhosis and clinical evidence in decompensated cirrhosis. They found that NAFLD cirrhosis constituted 15.5% of all cases of cirrhosis [17]. Hsiang et al. reported a retrospective study from a secondary care hospital in South Auckland (New Zealand). The diagnosis of cirrhosis was based on clinical, biochemical, histological, transient elastography, or radiological evidence accompanied by clinical signs of cirrhosis. The author found that NAFLD cirrhosis was prevalent in 16.4% of cirrhotic patients [18]. Those studies suggested that the prevalence of NAFLD cirrhosis is relatively lower in hospitalized patients with cirrhosis.

2.4. Liver Transplant Patient Studies. One study from the Nordic Liver Transplant between 2011 and 2015 reported that NASH cirrhosis was about 6.1% of adult patients (91/1476) listed for liver transplantation [19]. Another study from United Network for Organ Sharing database showed that NASH cirrhosis accounts for 5% of all young US patients listed for liver transplantation [20], and NASH cirrhosis increased from 1% to 16% from 2002 to 2016. The analysis of data from the Organ Procurement and Transplantation Network (OPTN) database from 2000 to 2014 also supported the increased tendency of NASH cirrhosis over time with an increase of 55.4% between 2016 and 2030 [21].

3. Risk Factor

3.1. Histological Subtype. Histological subtype is the greatest risk factor for the progression of NAFLD to cirrhosis. NAFLD has been divided into two main histological subtypes: nonalcoholic fatty liver (NAFL) and nonalcoholic steatohepatitis (NASH) [22]. The incidence of progression to cirrhosis is higher in NASH than in NAFL. A longitudinal study with a mean of 15.6 years of follow-up showed that only 1% of patients with NAFL developed cirrhosis, whereas 11% of those with NASH developed cirrhosis [23]. Moreover, NASH progressed more rapidly to cirrhosis. The annual fibrosis progression rate in patients with NASH was 0.14 stages, compared with 0.07 stages in patients with NAFL [24].

3.2. Metabolic Factors. Many studies suggested that diabetes is the strongest metabolic factor of progression of NAFLD to cirrhosis [25]. Porepa et al. used administrative health databases in Ontario (Canada) (1994–2006) to perform a population-based matched retrospective cohort study. 438,069 individuals with newly diagnosed diabetes were matched to 2,059,708 individuals without diabetes. After a median follow-up duration of 6.4 years, 1,119 (3.71%) patients with diabetes developed cirrhosis and 1,896 (1.34%) individuals without diabetes developed cirrhosis [26]. Nderitu et al. examined 509,436 participants from the Swedish Apolipoprotein Mortality Risk (AMORIS) cohort between 1985 and 1996 and found that 2,775 participants developed cirrhosis; diabetes and high blood glucose were associated with cirrhosis independent of obesity [27]. Other metabolic factors, including hyperlipidemia, obesity, and hypertension, were also important risk factors for NAFLD cirrhosis.

3.3. Genetic Polymorphisms. Genetic factors are believed to contribute to 30%–50% of the risk for high-prevalence diseases, such as obesity, T2DM, cardiovascular disease (CVD), and cirrhosis [28]. Genome-wide association studies (GWAS) and candidate gene studies have contributed greatly to our understanding of the genetic contribution to NAFLD progression. GWAS studies have identified some of the genetic variants associated with NAFLD progression. Among the loci identified, the nonsynonymous single-nucleotide polymorphism (SNP) in PNPLA3 (rs738409 c.444 C4G, p.Ile148Met), patatin-like phospholipase domain containing 3, has been validated across multiple patient cohorts. Notably, presence of this SNP has been robustly associated with the development of NAFLD cirrhosis [29]. One study of over 1000 individuals with biopsy-proven NAFLD demonstrated that the SNP in transmembrane 6 superfamily member 2 (rs58542926 c.449 C>T, p.Glu167Lys) was associated with increased risk for advanced fibrosis independent of gender, age at biopsy, BMI, T2DM, and PNPLA3 rs738409 genotype [30].

3.4. Age. In a retrospective cohort study from the United Kingdom, 351 patients with biopsy-proven NAFLD were divided into an older (≥60), a middle-aged (50 to 60), and a younger (≤50) group. Cirrhotic patients were significantly older than noncirrhotic patients. Older patients had significantly more risk factors, including hypertension, obesity, diabetes, and hyperlipidemia [31]. In a cross-sectional multicenter study from the United States, 796 patients with biopsy-proven NAFLD were classified into the elderly patients group (≥65) and the nonelderly patients group (18 to 65). Elderly patients with NAFLD had significantly higher rates of advanced fibrosis than nonelderly patients with NAFLD. Moreover, the elderly patients did not have more risk factors such as diabetes or insulin resistance [32]. However, the association between age and cirrhosis in NAFLD may be related to the duration of disease rather than the age itself [33].

3.5. Other Factors. Other risk factors for progression to cirrhosis in patients with NAFLD include gender, ethnicity, and family history of metabolic traits. Data on gender differences in the development of cirrhosis in patients with NAFLD are discordant [34]. A longitudinal study of patients with NAFLD found that gender was not an independent risk factor for the progression of fibrosis. A few studies suggested that male gender is a strong independent risk factor for fibrosis. Some studies showed that the risk of advanced fibrosis is higher in females than in males. Although the risk of NASH was higher in Hispanics and lower in Blacks than Whites, the proportion of patients with significant fibrosis did not significantly differ among racial or ethnic groups in United States. Thus, ethnicity is not a risk factor for the development of cirrhosis in patients with NAFLD [35]. A recent study showed that 68.8% (779/1133) of patients with NASH cirrhosis have the family history of metabolic traits, and those patients have increased risk of cirrhosis diagnosis at an early age of <45 years. Those results suggested that the family history of metabolic traits is a risk factor for cirrhosis and associated with early age at diagnosis of NAFLD cirrhosis [36].

4. Clinical and Liver Function Features

The clinical presentations of NAFLD cirrhosis were analyzed from several early studies [37–39]. The majority of patients with NAFLD cirrhosis are female, older than 50 years, and frequently with obesity and/or T2DM. Patients with NAFLD cirrhosis are at risk of the same complications of cirrhosis as with any other etiology of liver disease [40]. Ascites is the first and most common clinical feature of decompensation, but occurs at a slower rate in patients with NAFLD cirrhosis than in patients with HCV cirrhosis [23]. Once ascites develops, the rate of hepatorenal syndrome in patients with NAFLD cirrhosis is similar to that in patients with HCV cirrhosis [41]. The incidences of variceal hemorrhage, hepatic encephalopathy, and hepatocellular carcinoma (HCC) were similar in NAFLD cirrhosis and HCV cirrhosis patients. Liver enzyme abnormalities are found in patients with NAFLD cirrhosis, but the degrees of liver enzyme abnormality are mild. The mean values of serum ALT, AST, AKP, and GGT are usually no more than three times of the upper limit of normal values.

5. Diagnosis

The diagnosis of decompensated cirrhosis is relatively easy for patients with NAFLD and is mainly based on (1) having risk factors for progression to cirrhosis, (2) excluding the other causes of cirrhosis, and (3) having cirrhosis complications. However, the diagnosis of compensated cirrhosis is difficult in patients with NAFLD due to absence of symptoms. Liver biopsy, imaging, and scoring systems for fibrosis are important methods for the diagnosis of compensated cirrhosis in patients with NAFLD.

5.1. Liver Biopsy. Liver biopsy represents the gold standard for diagnosis of cirrhosis. Key features of NASH, such as steatosis, ballooning, and Mallory-Denk bodies, are important histological features for the diagnosis of NAFLD cirrhosis. Steatosis is the histological feature that ties together all of the various forms of NAFLD. Steatosis may become inconspicuous in cirrhosis. However, a diagnosis of NAFLD cirrhosis can still be made if the critical features of ballooning and Mallory-Denk bodies are observed [42]. All histologic features of NASH may not be evident once it progresses to cirrhosis. Therefore, cirrhosis without features of NASH may be diagnosed as "cryptogenic cirrhosis". T2DM and obesity are important factors for the development of NAFLD cirrhosis. In addition to excluding other known causes of cirrhosis, T2DM, obesity, and other comorbidities may help diagnose NAFLD cirrhosis without key NASH features in liver histology. Although liver biopsy is considered as the gold standard for the diagnosis of NAFLD cirrhosis, it is invasive and has several limitations, including sampling bias and complications (transient pain, anxiety and discomfort, hemorrhage, and rarely death) [43, 44].

5.2. Imaging Methods. In recent years, noninvasive alternative diagnostic imaging methods have been validated in comparison with liver biopsy and demonstrated good diagnostic accuracy for the diagnosis of cirrhosis. One of these techniques is TE, which produces a 'liver stiffness measurement' (LSM) using pulsed-echo ultrasound as a surrogate marker of fibrosis. A LSM >13.0 kPa is taken as the cut-off for clinically relevant cirrhosis [45]. A meta-analysis study of 7 articles showed that the sensitivity and the specificity of TE for the diagnosis of NAFLD cirrhosis were 96.2 % and 92.2%, respectively [46]. However, the failure rate of the M probe of TE is high in patients with BMI >30 kg/m^2 or T2DM [47]. The diagnostic accuracy for the liver fibrosis of XL probe of TE is similar to that of M probe [48]. As a result, in clinical practice, if the M probe is unreliable, the XL probe could be used [49]. Another noninvasive imaging technique for the diagnosis of cirrhosis is magnetic resonance elastography (MRE). Recent study showed that MRE has higher diagnostic accuracy in detecting liver fibrosis in patients with NAFLD compared to TE [50]. MRE may be a promising noninvasive technique for the diagnosis of NAFLD cirrhosis. The important limitation of TE and MRE is that they are not widely available.

5.3. Score Systems for Fibrosis. Based on demographic factors and blood tests, several scoring systems for the assessment of fibrosis or cirrhosis in NAFLD have been proposed: NAFLD fibrosis score (NFS), fibrosis-4-score (FIB-4), BARD (BMI-AST/ALT-Diabetes), enhanced liver fibrosis panel (ELF), Hepascore, Fibro Meter™, Fibro Test™, and so on [51]. NFS and FIB-4 are better than scoring systems in predicting advanced fibrosis in patients with NAFLD. NFS and FIB-4 have been recommended as screening tools to identify NAFLD patients with higher likelihoods of advanced fibrosis and/or cirrhosis in the NAFLD practice guideline from the American Association for the Study of Liver Diseases (AASLD) [52]. NFS is characterized by two cut-off values: lower cut-off value and higher cut-off value. The lower cut-off

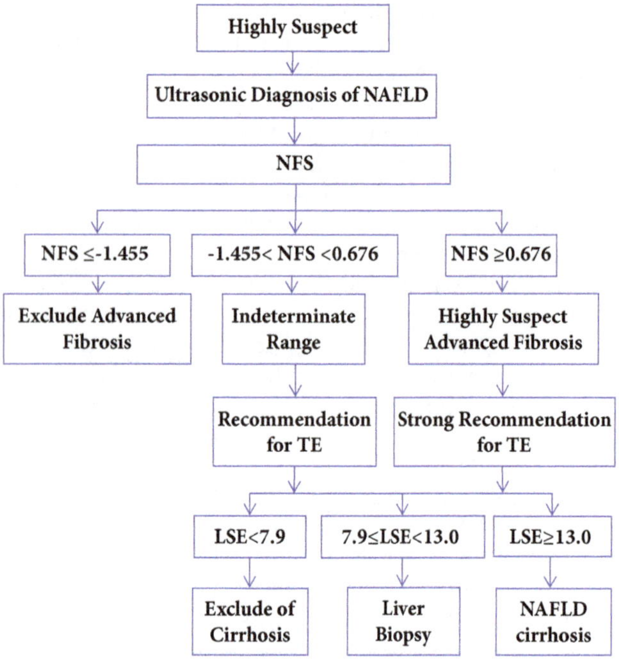

FIGURE 1: Proposal of diagnostic algorithm for classification of patients affected by NAFLD. NAFLD: nonalcoholic fatty liver disease; NFS: NAFLD fibrosis score; TE: transient elastography; LSE: liver stiffness measurement; kPa: kilopascal.

value has the highest negative predictive value to exclude advanced fibrosis. The higher cut-off value has the highest positive predictive value to identify patients with advanced fibrosis. The "gray area" between the two cut-off values is the indeterminate range [53]. FIB-4 also offers dual cut-off values as NFS: patients with score <1.45 are unlikely whereas patients with score >3.25 are likely to have advanced fibrosis.

Considering the different accuracy, cost, and availability of these diagnosis methods for cirrhosis, the selection of diagnostic approach for patients with suspected NAFLD cirrhosis could be suggested as follows: (1) NFS (or FIB-4) is first used for patients with diagnosed NAFLD. (2) Cirrhosis in patients with a NFS below the lower cut-off level can be excluded. Patients with a NFS above the indeterminate range or higher cut-off level require further diagnostic testing with TE. (3) Cirrhosis in patients with a TE < 7.9 kPa can be excluded. Patients with a TE 7.9~13.0 kPa should consider liver biopsy. Patients with a TE >13.0 kPa are diagnosed as cirrhosis. A proposal of diagnostic algorithm is illustrated in Figure 1 (modified according to [45, 53]).

6. Management

Obesity is of great prognostic relevance to patients with cirrhosis, and weight loss is important in patients with NAFLD cirrhosis. However, weight loss should not be recommended in patients with decompensated end-stage liver disease due to the risk of protein calorie malnutrition [54]. Antifibrotic therapy is an important strategy for the prevention and reversion of NAFLD cirrhosis. Emerging drugs including activator of farnesoid X receptor (Obeticholic acid), antagonist of C-C chemokine receptors type 2 and 5 (Cenicriviroc), and inhibitor of apoptosis signaling kinase-1 (Selonsertib) have been confirmed to have antifibrotic effect and will be expected to be developed as potential therapy for NAFLD cirrhosis [55]. Alcohol is a confirmed factor for liver injury. Alcohol should be prohibited in patients with NAFLD cirrhosis. Other conditions enhancing the development of cirrhosis in patients with NAFLD include diabetes, hyperlipidemia, and hypertension, which should be screened for and treated. The prevention, screening, and treatment of CVD and cirrhosis complications are critical for the prognosis of NAFLD cirrhosis. Liver transplant is an effective treatment for end-stage liver disease in patients with NAFLD cirrhosis.

6.1. Surveillance and Prevention of Cardiovascular Disease. Patients with NAFLD cirrhosis have a high prevalence of CVD. Careful attention should be paid to the surveillance of CVD. Noninvasive functional cardiac testing is recommended in patients with NASH cirrhosis, with progression to invasive tests when noninvasive testing is abnormal or inconclusive [54]. Hyperlipidemia is an important factor for the development of CVD. Statins, as drugs for lipid-reduction, are recommended for the prevention of CVD in patients with NAFLD cirrhosis who meet criteria based on current recommendations, but they should be avoided in patients with decompensated cirrhosis [52].

6.2. Screening and Management of Gastroesophageal Varices. Gastroesophageal variceal hemorrhage is a severe fatal complication of cirrhosis. Patients with NAFLD cirrhosis should be screened and managed for gastroesophageal varices according to AASLD practice guidelines [56]: (1) Patients with compensated cirrhosis (CC) without varices on screening endoscopy should have endoscopy repeated every 2 years; patients with CC with small varices on screening endoscopy should have endoscopy repeated every year; patients with CC without varices or with small varices who develop decompensation should have a repeat endoscopy when this occurs. (2) Traditional nonselective beta-blockers (NSBBs) (propranolol, nadolol, and carvedilol) or endoscopic variceal ligation (EVL) is recommended for the prevention of first variceal hemorrhage in patients with medium or large varices; NSBB is the recommended therapy for patients with high-risk small esophageal varices; the combination of NSBB and EVL is first-line therapy in the prevention of rebleeding.

6.3. Surveillance and Management of Hepatocellular Carcinoma. There is substantial evidence that cirrhosis is a common cause for the development of HCC [57]. Patients with NAFLD cirrhosis are at higher risk for HCC [58]. The cumulative incidence of HCC from NAFLD cirrhosis has been reported as 2.4% and 12.8% over a median follow-up of 3.2 to 7.2 years [59]. International societies recommend HCC surveillance in selected target populations, including patients with cirrhosis of any cause [60]. AASLD recommends that patients with NAFLD cirrhosis should be considered for HCC screening with ultrasound testing and with or without measurement of blood alpha-fetoprotein (AFP) levels, every 6 months [52, 61]. The treatment of HCC in patients with

NAFLD cirrhosis may be referred to the AASLD practice guidelines [61]. T2DM significantly increases the risk of developing HCC [62]. Metformin and statins significantly reduce the risk of HCC among patients with diabetes [63]. Statins and metformin have been suggested as potential strategies for the primary prevention of HCC in patients with NAFLD and diabetes [60, 62].

6.4. Liver Transplantation. Liver transplant is an effective treatment for end-stage liver disease, with an overall one-year survival of around 91% and a three-year survival of around 80%. Survival rates up to ten years are similar for patients receiving transplants for NAFLD cirrhosis and those receiving transplants for other indications, such as HCV cirrhosis and alcoholic cirrhosis. Guidelines for liver transplantation for patients with nonalcoholic steatohepatitis recommend that the indications for liver transplantation include NASH cirrhosis or HCC [54]. Studies of post-transplant survival outcomes suggested that NASH cirrhosis is associated with higher 30-day mortality, predominantly from an increase in CVD, and that severe obesity is likely to increase postoperative and long term mortality [64]. Thus, patients should undergo preoperative assessment and management of CVD and optimization of nutritional status. Following liver transplantation for patients with NAFLD cirrhosis, NAFLD recurs in at least 1/3 of patients [65]. Reduced mobility and commonly used immunosuppression regimens place those patients at higher risks of developing obesity, diabetes, and hypertension or exacerbating these conditions if previously present. As a result, body weight, hypertension, diabetes, and hyperlipidemia should continue to be monitored and managed in posttransplant patients.

7. Prognosis

Studies on the prognosis of NAFLD cirrhosis were reported mostly several years ago. The 5-year survival rate of 68 patients with NASH cirrhosis was 75.2% [48]. The death of patients with NAFLD cirrhosis is caused by complications. Once cirrhosis develops, prognosis is negatively impacted, with potential development of cirrhosis complications. The 5-year occurrence rates of ascites, varices, encephalopathy, and HCC of 68 patients with NASH cirrhosis were 19.1%, 28.2%, 16.1%, and 11.3%, respectively [38]. The 10-year occurrence rates of ascites, variceal hemorrhage, encephalopathy, and HCC of 152 patients with NASH cirrhosis were 14%, 12%, 15%, and 7%, respectively [66]. Bhala compared the natural history of NAFLD cirrhosis to HCV cirrhosis and found that patients with NAFLD cirrhosis appeared to have lower rates of liver-related complications and lower rates of HCC than patients with HCV infection of a similar disease stage, cardiovascular mortality was greater in patients with NAFLD related cirrhosis, and these two groups of patients had similar overall mortality [39]. NAFLD cirrhosis is the larger proportion of cryptogenic cirrhosis. The studies on the natural history of cryptogenic cirrhosis showed that the cumulated incidence of HCC in patients with cryptogenic cirrhosis was similar to that in patients with HCV cirrhosis, and patients with cryptogenic cirrhosis have a higher risk of developing severe liver complications [67, 68]. These existing data strongly suggested that NAFLD cirrhosis has a poor prognosis.

8. Conclusions

NAFLD is becoming one of the leading causes of cirrhosis. Risk factors for the progression to cirrhosis in patients with NAFLD include NASH, metabolic factors, genetic polymorphisms, and older age. The clinical presentations of NAFLD cirrhosis are similar to those of cirrhosis caused by other etiology. The diagnosis of decompensated cirrhosis is relatively easy for patients with NAFLD. Liver biopsy, imaging, and scoring systems for fibrosis are important methods for the diagnosis of compensated cirrhosis in patients with NAFLD. Reducing weight, prohibiting drinking, managing other risk factors for progressing to cirrhosis, and antifibrosis are fundamental treatments. Screening, treatment, and prevention of cirrhosis complications and CVD are crucial for the management of NAFLD cirrhosis. Liver transplant is an effective treatment for end-stage liver disease in patients with NAFLD cirrhosis. The prognosis of NAFLD cirrhosis is poor. The prevention and treatment of NAFLD cirrhosis should be emphasized.

Acknowledgments

This research was supported by the National Natural Science Foundation of China (Grant no. 8157040055).

References

[1] R. G. de la Garza, L. A. Morales-Garza, I. Martin-Estal, and I. Castilla-Cortazar, "Insulin-like growth factor-1 deficiency and cirrhosis establishment," *Journal of Clinical Medicine Research*, vol. 9, no. 4, pp. G233–G247, 2017.

[2] C. Stasi, C. Silvestri, F. Voller, and F. Cipriani, "Epidemiology of liver cirrhosis," *Journal of Clinical and Experimental Hepatology*, vol. 5, no. 3, p. 272, 2015.

[3] N. Abbas, J. Makker, H. Abbas, and B. Balar, "Perioperative care of patients with liver cirrhosis: a review," *Health Services Insights*, pp. G1–G12, 2017.

[4] A. A. Mokdad, A. D. Lopez, and S. Shahraz, "Liver cirrhosis mortality in 187 countries between 1980 and 2010: a systematic analysis," *BMC Medicine*, vol. 12, article 145, 2014.

[5] A. Safaei, A. A. Oskouie, S. R. Mohebbi et al., "Metabolomic analysis of human cirrhosis, hepatocellular carcinoma, non-alcoholic fatty liver disease and non-alcoholic steatohepatitis diseases," *Gastroenterol Hepatol Bed Bench*, vol. 9, no. 3, pp. G158–G173, 2016.

[6] A. Kadayifci, V. Tan, P. C. Ursell, R. B. Merriman, and N. M. Bass, "Clinical and pathologic risk factors for atherosclerosis in cirrhosis: A comparison between NASH-related cirrhosis and cirrhosis due to other aetiologies," *Journal of Hepatology*, vol. 49, no. 4, pp. 595–599, 2008.

[7] E. H. van den Berg, R. M. Douwes, V. E. de Meijer, T. C. Schreuder, and H. Blokzijl, "Liver transplantation for NASH cirrhosis is not performed at the expense of major post-operative morbidity," *Digestive and Liver Disease*, vol. 50, no. 1, pp. G68–G75, 2018.

[8] A. Wree, L. Broderick, A. Canbay, H. M. Hoffman, and A. E. Feldstein, "From NAFLD to NASH to cirrhosis-new insights into disease mechanisms," *Nature Reviews Gastroenterology & Hepatology*, vol. 10, no. 11, pp. G627–G636, 2013.

[9] Z. M. Younossi, A. B. Koenig, D. Abdelatif, Y. Fazel, L. Henry, and M. Wymer, "Global epidemiology of nonalcoholic fatty liver disease—meta-analytic assessment of prevalence, incidence, and outcomes," *Hepatology*, vol. 64, no. 1, pp. G73–G84, 2016.

[10] P. Angulo, "Long-term mortality in nonalcoholic fatty liver disease: is liver histology of any prognostic significance?" *Hepatology*, vol. 51, no. 2, pp. G373–G375, 2010.

[11] M. N. Kabbany, P. K. C. Selvakumar, K. Watt et al., "Prevalence of nonalcoholic steatohepatitis-associated cirrhosis in the United States: an analysis of national health and nutrition examination survey data," *American Journal of Gastroenterology*, vol. 112, no. 4, pp. G581–G587, 2017.

[12] J. Fung, C.-K. Lee, M. Chan, W.-K. Seto, C.-L. Lai, and M.-F. Yuen, "High prevalence of non-alcoholic fatty liver disease in the Chinese—results from the Hong Kong liver health census," *Liver International*, vol. 35, no. 2, pp. G542–G549, 2015.

[13] R. Kwok, K. C. Choi, G. L.-H. Wong et al., "Screening diabetic patients for non-alcoholic fatty liver disease with controlled attenuation parameter and liver stiffness measurements: a prospective cohort study," *Gut*, vol. 65, pp. G1359–G1368, 2016.

[14] A. Lonardo, F. Nascimbeni, A. Mantovani, and G. Targher, "Hypertension, diabetes, atherosclerosis and NASH: cause or consequence?" *Journal of Hepatology*, vol. 68, no. 2, pp. G335–G352, 2018.

[15] J. Xiong, J. Wang, J. Huang, W. Sun, J. Wang, and D. Chen, "Non-alcoholic steatohepatitis-related liver cirrhosis is increasing in China: a ten-year retrospective study," *Clinics*, vol. 70, no. 8, pp. G563–G568, 2015.

[16] K. Michitaka, S. Nishiguchi, Y. Aoyagi, Y. Hiasa, Y. Tokumoto, and M. Onji, "Etiology of liver cirrhosis in Japan: a nationwide survey," *Journal of Gastroenterology*, vol. 45, no. 1, pp. G86–G94, 2010.

[17] S. A. Karageorgos, S. Stratakou, M. Koulentaki et al., "Long-term change in incidence and risk factors of cirrhosis and hepatocellular carcinoma in crete, Greece: a 25-year study," *Annals of Gastroenterology*, vol. 30, no. 3, pp. G357–G363, 2017.

[18] J. C. Hsiang, W. W. Bai, Z. Raos et al., "Epidemiology, disease burden and outcomes of cirrhosis in a large secondary care hospital in South Auckland, New Zealand," *Internal Medicine Journal*, vol. 45, no. 2, pp. G160–G169, 2015.

[19] M. Holmer, E. Melum, H. Isoniemi et al., "Nonalcoholic fatty liver disease is an increasing indication for liver transplantation in the Nordic countries," *Liver International*, pp. G1–G9, 2018.

[20] I. Doycheva, D. Issa, K. D. Watt, R. Lopez, G. Rifai, and N. Alkhouri, "Nonalcoholic steatohepatitis is the most rapidly increasing indication for liver transplantation in young adults in the United States," *Journal of Clinical Gastroenterology*, vol. 52, no. 4, pp. G339–G346, 2018.

[21] N. D. Parikh, W. J. Marrero, J. Wang et al., "Projected increase in obesity and non-alcoholic-steatohepatitis-related liver transplantation waitlist additions in the United States," *Hepatology*, 2017.

[22] M. S. Siddiqui, M. Fuchs, M. O. Idowu et al., "Severity of nonalcoholic fatty liver disease and progression to cirrhosis are associated with atherogenic lipoprotein profile," *Clinical Gastroenterology and Hepatology*, vol. 13, no. 5, pp. G1000–G1008.e3, 2015.

[23] A. Marengo, R. I. K. Jouness, and E. Bugianesi, "Progression and natural history of nonalcoholic fatty liver disease in adults," *Clinics in Liver Disease*, vol. 20, no. 2, pp. G313–G324, 2016.

[24] S. Singh, A. M. Allen, Z. Wang, L. J. Prokop, M. H. Murad, and R. Loomba, "Sa1052 fibrosis progression in nonalcoholic fatty liver versus nonalcoholic steatohepatitis: a systematic review and meta-analysis of paired-biopsy studies," *Gastroenterology*, vol. 146, no. 5, pp. G947–G948, 2014.

[25] L. Valenti, E. Bugianesi, U. Pajvani, and G. Targher, "Non-alcoholic fatty liver disease: cause or consequence of type 2 diabetes?" *Liver International*, vol. 36, no. 11, pp. G1563–G1579, 2016.

[26] L. Porepa, J. G. Ray, P. Sanchez-Romeu, and G. L. Booth, "Newly diagnosed diabetes mellitus as a risk factor for serious liver disease," *Canadian Medical Association Journal*, vol. 182, no. 11, pp. E526–E531, 2010.

[27] P. Nderitu, C. Bosco, H. Garmo et al., "The association between individual metabolic syndrome components, primary liver cancer and cirrhosis: a study in the Swedish AMORIS cohort," *International Journal of Cancer*, vol. 141, no. 6, pp. G1148–G1160, 2017.

[28] Q. M. Anstee, D. Seth, and C. P. Day, "Genetic factors that affect risk of alcoholic and nonalcoholic fatty liver disease," *Gastroenterology*, vol. 150, no. 8, pp. G1728–G1744, 2016.

[29] L. Valenti, A. Al-Serri, A. K. Daly et al., "Homozygosity for the patatin-like phospholipase-3/adiponutrin i148m polymorphism influences liver fibrosis in patients with nonalcoholic fatty liver disease," *Hepatology*, vol. 51, no. 4, pp. G1209–G1217, 2010.

[30] Y. L. Liu, H. L. Reeves, A. D. Burt et al., "TM6SF2 rs58542926 influences hepatic fibrosis progression in patients with non-alcoholic fatty liver disease," *Nature Communications*, vol. 5, p. G4309, 2014.

[31] J. Frith, C. P. Day, E. Henderson, A. D. Burt, and J. L. Newton, "Non-alcoholic fatty liver disease in older people," *Gerontology*, vol. 55, no. 6, pp. G607–G613, 2009.

[32] M. Noureddin, K. P. Yates, I. A. Vaughn et al., "Clinical and histological determinants of nonalcoholic steatohepatitis and advanced fibrosis in elderly patients," *Hepatology*, vol. 58, no. 5, pp. G1644–G1654, 2013.

[33] G. Vernon, A. Baranova, and Z. M. Younossi, "Systematic review: the epidemiology and natural history of non-alcoholic fatty liver disease and non-alcoholic steatohepatitis in adults," *Alimentary Pharmacology & Therapeutics*, vol. 34, no. 3, pp. G274–G285, 2011.

[34] S. Ballestri, F. Nascimbeni, E. Baldelli, A. Marrazzo, D. Romagnoli, and A. Lonardo, "NAFLD as a sexual dimorphic disease: role of gender and reproductive status in the development and progression of nonalcoholic fatty liver disease and inherent cardiovascular risk," *Advances in Therapy*, vol. 36, pp. G1291–G1326, 2017.

[35] N. E. Rich, S. Oji, A. R. Mufti et al., "Racial and ethnic disparities in nonalcoholic fatty liver disease prevalence, severity, and outcomes in the United States: a systematic review and meta-analysis," *Clinical Gastroenterology and Hepatology*, vol. 16, no. 2, pp. 198–210.e2, 2018.

[36] A. S. Bhadoria, C. K. Kedarisetty, C. Bihari et al., "Impact of family history of metabolic traits on severity of non-alcoholic steatohepatitis related cirrhosis: a cross-sectional study," *Liver International*, vol. 37, no. 9, pp. G1397–G1404, 2017.

[37] J. M. Hui, J. G. Kench, S. Chitturi et al., "Long-term outcomes of cirrhosis in nonalcoholic steatohepatitis compared with hepatitis C," *Hepatology*, vol. 38, no. 2, pp. G420–G427, 2003.

[38] S. Yatsuji, E. Hashimoto, M. Tobari, M. Taniai, K. Tokushige, and K. Shiratori, "Clinical features and outcomes of cirrhosis due to non-alcoholic steatohepatitis compared with cirrhosis caused by chronic hepatitis C," *Journal of Gastroenterology and Hepatology*, vol. 24, no. 2, pp. G248–G254, 2009.

[39] N. Bhala, P. Angulo, D. van der Poorten et al., "The natural history of nonalcoholic fatty liver disease with advanced fibrosis or cirrhosis: an international collaborative study," *Hepatology*, vol. 54, no. 4, pp. G1208–G1216, 2011.

[40] J. K. Dyson, Q. M. Anstee, and S. McPherson, "Non-alcoholic fatty liver disease: a practical approach to treatment," *Frontline Gastroenterol*, vol. 5, pp. G277–G286, 2014.

[41] S. Caldwell and C. Argo, "The natural history of non-alcoholic fatty liver disease," *Digestive Diseases*, vol. 28, no. 1, pp. G162–G168, 2010.

[42] G. T. Brown and D. E. Kleiner, "Histopathology of nonalcoholic fatty liver disease and nonalcoholic steatohepatitis," *Metabolism—Clinical and Experimental*, vol. 65, no. 8, pp. G1080–G1086, 2016.

[43] F. Shen, R. D. Zheng, Y. Q. Mi et al., "Controlled attenuation parameter for non-invasive assessment of hepatic steatosis in Chinese patients," *World Journal of Gastroenterology*, vol. 20, no. 16, pp. G4702–G4711, 2014.

[44] C. Laurent, "Diagnosis of non-alcoholic fatty liver disease/non-alcoholic steatohepatitis: non-invasive tests are enough," *Liver International*, vol. 38, pp. G67–G70, 2018.

[45] E. M. Koehler, E. P. C. Plompen, J. N. L. Schouten et al., "Presence of diabetes mellitus and steatosis is associated with liver stiffness in a general population: the Rotterdam study," *Hepatology*, vol. 63, no. 1, pp. G138–G147, 2016.

[46] S.-A. Hashemi, S.-M. Alavian, and M. Gholami-Fesharaki, "Assessment of transient elastography (FibroScan) for diagnosis of fibrosis in non-alcoholic fatty liver disease: a systematic review and meta-analysis," *Caspian Journal of Internal Medicine*, vol. 7, no. 4, pp. G242–G252, 2016.

[47] J. K. Dyson, Q. M. Anstee, and S. McPherson, "Non-alcoholic fatty liver disease: a practical approach to diagnosis and staging," *Frontline Gastroenterology*, vol. 5, no. 3, pp. G211–G218, 2014.

[48] D. Festi, R. Schiumerini, G. Marasco, E. Scaioli, F. Pasqui, and A. Colecchia, "Non-invasive diagnostic approach to non-alcoholic fatty liver disease: current evidence and future perspectives," *Expert Review of Gastroenterology & Hepatology*, vol. 9, no. 8, pp. G1039–1053, 2015.

[49] V. De Lédinghen, V. W.-S. Wong, J. Vergniol et al., "Diagnosis of liver fibrosis and cirrhosis using liver stiffness measurement: comparison between M and XL probe of FibroScan," *Journal of Hepatology*, vol. 56, no. 4, pp. G833–G839, 2012.

[50] K. Imajo, T. Kessoku, Y. Honda et al., "Magnetic resonance imaging more accurately classifies steatosis and fibrosis in patients with nonalcoholic fatty liver disease than transient elastography," *Gastroenterology*, vol. 150, no. 3, pp. 626–637.e7, 2016.

[51] P. Stål, "Liver fibrosis in non-alcoholic fatty liver disease— diagnostic challenge with prognostic significance," *World Journal of Gastroenterology*, vol. 21, no. 39, pp. G11077–G11087, 2015.

[52] N. Chalasani, Z. Younossi, J. E. Lavine et al., "The diagnosis and management of nonalcoholic fatty liver disease: practice guidance from the American Association for the study of liver diseases," *Hepatology*, vol. 67, no. 1, pp. G328–G357, 2018.

[53] D. Festi, R. Schiumerini, G. Marasco, E. Scaioli, F. Pasqui, and A. Colecchia, "Non-invasive diagnostic approach to non-alcoholic fatty liver disease: current evidence and future perspectives," *Expert Review of Gastroenterology & Hepatology*, vol. 9, no. 8, pp. G1039–G1053, 2015.

[54] P. N. Newsome, M. E. Allison, P. A. Andrews et al., "Guidelines for liver transplantation for patients with alcoholic steatohepatitis," *Gut*, vol. 61, no. 4, pp. G484–G500, 2012.

[55] J. Wattacheril, D. Issa, and A. Sanyal, "Nonalcoholic Steatohepatitis (NASH) and hepatic fibrosis: emerging therapies," *Annual Review of Pharmacology and Toxicology*, vol. 58, no. 1, pp. G649–G662, 2018.

[56] G. Garcia-Tsao, J. G. Abraldes, A. Berzigotti, and J. Bosch, "Portal hypertensive bleeding in cirrhosis: risk stratification, diagnosis, and management: 2016 practice guidance by the American Association for the study of liver diseases," *Hepatology*, vol. 65, no. 1, pp. G310–G335, 2017.

[57] N. N. Than, A. Ghazanfar, J. Hodson et al., "Comparing clinical presentations, treatments and outcomes of hepatocellular carcinoma due to hepatitis C and non-alcoholic fatty liver disease," *QJM*, vol. 110, no. 2, pp. G73–G81, 2017.

[58] K. Shetty, J. Chen, J. Shin, W. Jogunoori, and L. Mishra, "Pathogenesis of hepatocellular carcinoma development in non-alcoholic fatty liver disease," *Current Hepatology Reports*, vol. 14, no. 2, pp. G119–G127, 2015.

[59] G. Baffy, E. M. Brunt, and S. H. Caldwell, "Hepatocellular carcinoma in non-alcoholic fatty liver disease: an emerging menace," *Journal of Hepatology*, vol. 56, no. 6, pp. 1384–1391, 2012.

[60] E. Degasperi and M. Colombo, "Distinctive features of hepatocellular carcinoma in non-alcoholic fatty liver disease," *The Lancet Gastroenterology & Hepatology*, vol. 1, no. 2, pp. G156–G164, 2016.

[61] J. K. Heimbach, L. M. Kulik, R. S. Finn et al., "AASLD guidelines for the treatment of hepatocellular carcinoma," *Hepatology*, vol. 67, no. 1, pp. 358–380, 2018.

[62] P. Wainwright, E. Scorletti, and C. D. Byrne, "Type 2 diabetes and hepatocellular carcinoma: risk factors and pathogenesis," *Current Diabetes Reports*, vol. 17, no. 4, article 20, 2017.

[63] H. B. El-Serag, M. L. Johnson, C. Hachem, and R. O. Morgana, "Statins are associated with a reduced risk of hepatocellular carcinoma in a large cohort of patients with diabetes," *Gastroenterology*, vol. 136, no. 5, pp. G1601–G1608, 2009.

[64] R. S. Khan and P. N. Newsome, "Non-alcoholic fatty liver disease and liver transplantation," *Metabolism*, vol. 65, no. 8, pp. G1208–G1223, 2016.

[65] P. Zezos and E. L. Renner, "Liver transplantation and non-alcoholic fatty liver disease," *World Journal of Gastroenterology*, vol. 20, no. 42, pp. G15532–G15538, 2014.

[66] A. J. Sanyal, C. Banas, C. Sargeant et al., "Similarities and differences in outcomes of cirrhosis due to nonalcoholic steatohepatitis and hepatitis C," *Hepatology*, vol. 43, no. 4, pp. G682–G689, 2006.

30

The Prevalence of Hjortsjo Crook Sign of Right Posterior Sectional Bile Duct and Bile Duct Anatomy in ERCP

Hanan M. Alghamdi,[1] Afnan F. Almuhanna,[2] Bander F. Aldhafery,[2] Raed M. AlSulaiman,[3] Ahmed Almarhabi,[3] and Abdulaziz AlQurain[3]

[1]*Department of Surgery, King Fahd Hospital of the University, University of Imam Abdulrahman Bin Faisal College of Medicine, Dammam, Saudi Arabia*
[2]*Department of Radiology, King Fahd Hospital of the University, University of Imam Abdulrahman Bin Faisal College of Medicine, Dammam, Saudi Arabia*
[3]*Department of Internal Medicine, King Fahd Hospital of the University, University of Imam Abdulrahman Bin Faisal College of Medicine, Dammam, Saudi Arabia*

Correspondence should be addressed to Hanan M. Alghamdi; hmalghamdi@uod.edu.sa

Academic Editor: Kevork M. Peltekian

Aim. The frequency of the Right Posterior Sectional Bile Duct (RPSBD) hump sign in cholangiogram when it crosses over the right portal vein known as Hjortsjo Crook Sign and the bile duct anatomy are studied. Knowledge of the implication of positive sign can facilitate safe resection for both bile duct and portal vein. *Methods.* Prospectively, we included 237 patients with indicated ERCP during a period from March 2010 to January 2015. *Results.* The mean age (±SD) and male to female ratio were 38.8 (±19.20) and 1 : 1.28, respectively. All patients are Arab from Middle Eastern origin, had biliary stone disease, and underwent diagnostic and therapeutic ERCP. Positive Hjortsjo Crook Sign was found in 17.7% (42) of patients. The sign was found to be equally more frequent in Nakamura's RPSBD anatomical variant types I, II, and IV in 8.4% (20), 6.8% (16), and 2.1% (5), respectively, while rare anatomical variant type III showed no positive sign. *Conclusion.* Hjortsjo Crook Sign frequently presents in RPSBD variation types I, II, and IV in our patients.

1. Introduction

The anatomy of the bile duct (BD) is resembling that of the portal system and liver segments. Based on the literature, the proportion of biliary anatomical variations varies between 28% and 43%. Most of hilar bile ducts anatomical variations stem from different Right Posterior Sectional Bile Duct (RPSBD) origin [1, 2].

Shimizu's operative series showed that the RPSBD is most commonly supraportal in 84%, infraportal in 13%, and rarely a combination of both in 3% (the segment VII duct being supraportal and segment VI being infraportal) [3]. Furthermore, Nakamura's operative series report the supraportal RPSBD to be most common in BD variant type I (65%, the classic form where the RPSBD and the anterior sectional BD join to form a single right hepatic duct), type II (9.2%, the RPSBD joins the confluence, forming trifurcation), and type IV (15.8%, the RPSBD joins the left hepatic duct), whereas the infraportal RPSBD is reported to be most common in type III (8.3%) and that of the combination in type V (1.7%) [4].

The recognition of the hump appearance in animal cholangiogram being due to supraportal upward course of the RPSBD was first reported by Hjortsjo Crooks in 1951 [5]. The sign can be positive for the supraportal type BD in the classic Nakamura type I, II, or IV. Recognition of Hjortsjo Crook Sign (HCS) in ERCP can enrich our preoperative knowledge of biliary anatomical variation; their precise delineation and anticipation for technical modifications are vital to achieving safe curative liver resection [3] and liver transplantation [4, 6–8] and to avoiding biliary injury in common general surgical procedure like cholecystectomy [9–11].

TABLE 1: Patient demographic data.

	N = 237
Age:	
(i) Mean (±SD)	38.8 (19.20)
(ii) Median (range)	34.033 (18–97)
Gender	
Male	104
Female	133
M : F ratio	1 : 1.28
Nationality	
Saudi	199
Others (Middle Eastern)	37
Total	237

N: number.

TABLE 2: Biochemical profile of all patients.

Variables	Normal ranges	N = 237 Mean ± SD
T Bili	(0.1–1.0)	8.7655 ± 21.78339
D Bili	0.0–0.4	6.9978 ± 17.24988
Alkaline phosphatase	50–140	254.0222 ± 224.22206
PT	11–14	12.6705 ± 2.45859
GGTP	5–85	269.8923 ± 325.76886
Albumin	3.5–4.8	3.7143 ± 3.64814
WBC	4–11	8.4414 ± 3.75207
Platelet	140–440	285.0127 ± 138.17845
Amylase	25–125	218.7683 ± 484.17567
Lipase	4–24	1348.9000 ± 4559.71331

T Bili: total bilirubin; D Bili: direct bilirubin; PT: prothrombin time; N: number.

Our study describes the characteristics of HCS of the RPSBD anatomy in relation to the right portal vein (RPV) among Middle Eastern population using ERCP cholangiogram. To date, the relation of the different anatomical variation of the RPSBD to the RPV based on HCS has never been examined before in humans.

2. Materials and Methods

2.1. Patients and Methods. This prospective study was carried out during the period from March 2010 to January 2015. We prospectively included 237 consecutive patients who have undergone ERCPs fulfilling the inclusion criteria of being from adult age group (above 18 years old), being from Middle Eastern origin, and having the underlying condition of biliary disease only. Furthermore, patients with complete imaging study and without any prior history of liver resection or biliary instrumentation were considered also as inclusion criteria, while criteria like incomplete study, previous liver surgery, and previous liver transplantation were considered as exclusion criteria. Relevant demographic and laboratory data are obtained and depicted in Tables 1 and 2. The ERCP cholangiogram was reviewed by two radiologists separately. Further filling and focused image in ERCP were done if needed during the procedure (with standard ERCP technique using semiprone position); then the biliary anatomy and the HCS are interpreted by two different radiologists.

This research is supported by the University of Imam Abdulrahman Bin Faisal (formerly known as University of Dammam) (Institutional Research Board: 201054); accordingly, the ethics approval was obtained and informed consent was weaved.

2.2. Statistical Analysis. Data analyses included descriptive statistics computed for continuous variables, including means, standard deviations (SD), and minimum and maximum values as well as 95% CI. Frequencies were used for categorical variables. In this study, there was no attempt at imputation for missing data. For all tests, significance is defined as $p < 0.05$ (95% confidence interval). All statistical analyses were done using SPSS 12 (Chicago, Illinois, USA).

3. Result

Most of our patients are from youthful age groups due to general young population with mean age (±SD) of 38.8 (±19.20). The predominance of female gender (male to female ratio was 1 : 1.28) reflects the prevalence of the biliary disease in females (Table 1). All patients are Arab from Middle Eastern origin, had biliary stone disease, and underwent diagnostic and therapeutic ERCP. Biochemical data for all patients is in line with biliary stone complications (Table 2).

Anatomical variation of RPSBD based on Nakamura's classification is depicted in Table 3 and showed predominance of types I, II, and IV to be 61.1%, 17.8%, and 16%. Type III RPSBD variant was rare in our population (3.4%) while type V is not detected. Only four patients (1.7%) had undetermined RPSBD anatomical variation.

Most importantly, positive HCS was detected more frequently among patients with type I RPSBD anatomy, in 20 patients (8.4%). The second commonest occurrence of positive HCS was found in type II RPSBD variant, in 13 patients (6.8%). On the other hand, a rare type III RPSBD anatomy was found in only 8 patients and all were found to have negative HCS. One more positive HCS was found in undermined type of RPSBD (0.4%). The presence of positive HCS is depicted in Table 3.

4. Discussion

Knowledge of details of hepatobiliary anatomy is vital while performing complex surgical procedures such as hepatobiliary surgeries or liver transplant. This is particularly essential when it comes to anatomic areas with high rates of variations. Multiple biliary orifices in hilar transection plane requiring complex reconstruction are as common as 26% in Ohkubo's and 39.6% in Kasahara's operative series, requiring complex hilar dissection [1, 6]. Hence, the extensive preoperative imaging studies to determine the bile ducat anatomical variant are of paramount importance.

In typical biliary duct course, the lateral hepatic bile duct supplying segments VI and VII and the paramedian hepatic bile duct supplying segments V and VIII reunite to form

TABLE 3: Comparative evaluation of different types of Hjortsjo Crook Sign.

RPSBD anatomical variant[§]	Positive HCS N (%)	Negative HCS N (%)	Total
Type I 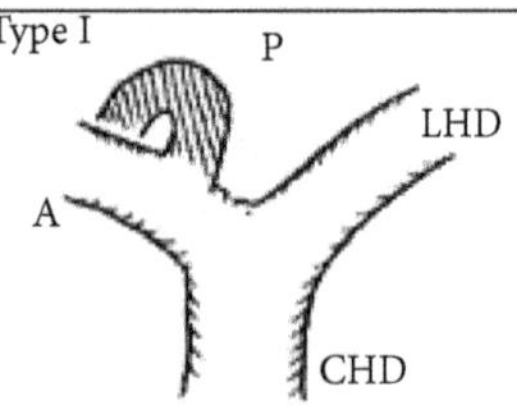	20 (8.4)	125 (52.7)	*145 (61.1)*
Type II 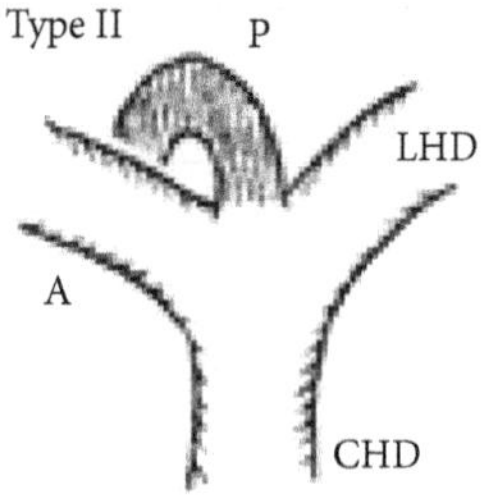	16 (6.8)	26 (11)	*42 (17.8)*
Type III 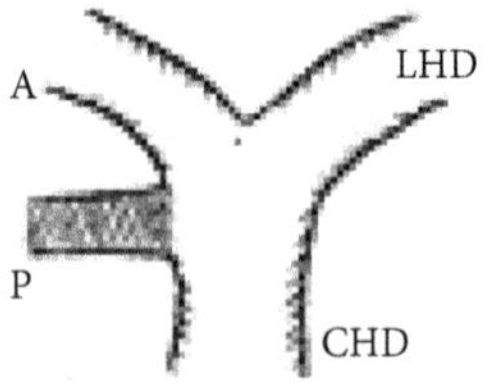	0	8 (3.4)	*8 (3.4)*
Type IV 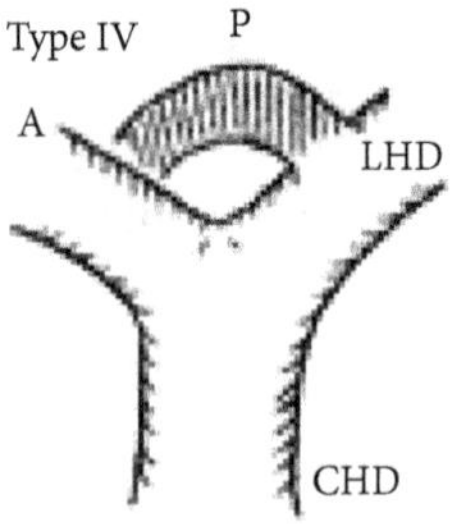	5 (2.1)	33 (13.9)	*38 (16)*
Type V Mixed type	0	0	*0*
Undetermined	1 (0.4)	3 (1.3)	*4 (1.7)*
Total	*42 (17.7)*	*195 (82.3)*	

RPSBD: Right Posterior Sectional Bile Duct. [§]Nakamura's classification of RPSBD. LHD: left hepatic duct. CHD: common hepatic duct. A: Right Anterior Sectional Bile Duct. P: Right Posterior Sectional Bile Duct. N: number. HCS: Hjortsjo Crook Sign. Data are frequency counts (percentage of total).

the right hepatic bile duct (RHD). However, it has been reported that this kind of modal disposition is only associated with 57% of the cases [12]. Many anatomic variations of the convergence of biliary ducts are reported, where the RHD may join the main hepatic duct below the normal confluence level (anterior region in 9% of cases and posterior region in 16% of cases). However, there are situations where the right anterior and posterior segmental bile ducts do not form the right hepatic duct and in 6% to 9% of the cases the right anterior segmental duct joins the left hepatic duct while in 7% to 14% of the cases the anterior segmental duct joins the hilar confluence and forms and three-branch type hilar confluence (c); similarly, in 9% to 27% cases, the posterior segmental duct joins the left hepatic duct [12–14].

To determine the specific anatomical variations, several studies have been conducted using different modalities like cadaveric research [15], intraoperative cholangiogram [16, 17], or imaging such as ultrasonography [18] and magnetic resonance cholangiography [19, 20]. On the other hand, ERCP is the standard technique in this field and provides, if done properly, a detailed anatomy of the extrahepatic and the intrahepatic biliary anatomy as well [21].

Due to expansion and advancement in surgical intervention in hepatobiliary conditions and transplant, this area has moved from anatomy books and being an area of clinical research to fulfilling practical needs [22]. Previous studies based on West or Far East patient population have reported anatomic variants of hepatobiliary system detected by intraoperative cholangiography, MRCP (magnetic resonance cholangiography), or ERCP [23–26].

The ERCP procedure was used in this study to document the variant biliary anatomy of the RPSBD and to investigate the usefulness of positive HCS in delineation of the RPSBD in relation to right postal vein as demonstrated in cholangiogram obtained through ERCP.

To our knowledge, this is the first study to examine the relationship between HCS and the various patterns of the RPSBD variable anatomy in humans and the reported data can be better representative database for our population.

The anatomical variations of RPSBD are similar to the international published data with predominance of types I and II (61.1% and 17.8%, resp.). However, we found more frequently type IV (16%) than type III (3.4%) (Table 3). Low incidence of type III in which the RPSBD drains into the common bile duct was recognized as "cysticohepatic ducts" and its prevalence is very low (1-2%). Our findings are consistent with other studies that reported only 2% of the cases where the RPSBD drained into the cystic duct. Prior information on HCS will help in dealing with the anatomical abnormality especially in the context of RPSBD, where the cystic duct can be ligated between the gallbladder and the point at which the duct joins [27, 28].

We found HCS to be positive in 17.7% of the patients and more frequently positive in types I, II, and IV RPSBD anatomy in 8.4%, 6.8%, and 2.1%, respectively. On the other hand, in a rare type III RPSBD anatomy, all were found to have negative HCS. One more positive HCS was found in undermined type of RPSBD (0.4%) (Table 3).

A possible limitation of this study was that it did not evaluate the patterns of HCS in a healthy population [29]. Irrespective of that, our data may be more representative of the general population than data from other populations.

In conclusion, our study reveals that types I, II, and IV RPSBD anatomical variation is more commonly showing positive HCS than any other type. Prior knowledge of this sign is essential to achieve curative resection in some cases with an abnormal pattern of the RPSBD. Since elusive knowledge of the biliary anatomy at hepatic hilum in hepatobiliary surgery may easily lead to postoperative biliary complication

[4, 8], preoperative recognition as well as intraoperative understanding of the RPSBD is apparently important for safe and curative resection in patients with aberrant biliary system. Likewise, avoiding biliary complications for both donor and recipient in living donor liver transplantation (LDLT) is critical to achieving safety for both. One of the major biliary complications in patients undergoing LDLT is the anatomical limitations contributed by multiple tiny bile ducts and the differential blood supplies. Recognizing these anomalies with the aid of HCS preoperatively, this may result in dramatic drop in the incidence of biliary complications and improve outcome and selection of donors in LDLT in our populations. Although in LDLT the donor will not undergo ERCP as standard evaluation test, the knowledge of the importance of HCS can be useful for comparison of data obtained from less sensitive modalities like magnetic resonance cholangiopancreatography (MRCP).

References

[1] M. Ohkubo, M. Nagino, J. Kamiya et al., "Surgical anatomy of the bile ducts at the hepatic hilum as applied to living donor liver transplantation," *Annals of Surgery*, vol. 239, no. 1, pp. 82–86, 2004.

[2] S. G. Puente and G. C. Bannura, "Radiological anatomy of the biliary tract: variations and congenital abnormalities," *World Journal of Surgery*, vol. 7, no. 2, pp. 271–276, 1983.

[3] H. Shimizu, S. Sawada, F. Kimura et al., "Clinical significance of biliary vascular anatomy of the right liver for hilar cholangiocarcinoma applied to left hemihepatectomy," *Annals of Surgery* vol. 249, no. 3, pp. 435–439, 2009.

[4] T. Nakamura, K. Tanaka, T. Kiuchi et al., "Anatomical variations and surgical strategies in right lobe living donor liver transplantation: lessons from 120 cases," *Transplantation*, vol. 73, no. 12; pp. 1896–1903, 2002.

[5] C. H. Hjortsjo, "The topography of the intrahepatic duct systems," *Acta anatomica*, vol. 11, no. 4, pp. 599–615, 1951.

[6] M. Kasahara, H. Egawa, K. Tanaka et al., "Variations in biliary anatomy associated with trifurcated portal vein in right-lobe living-donor liver transplantation," *Transplantation*, vol. 79, no. 5, pp. 626-627, 2005.

[7] T. L. Huang, Y. F. Cheng, C. L. Chen, T. Y. Chen, and T. Y. Lee, "Variants of the bile ducts: clinical application in the potential donor of living-related hepatic transplantation," *Transplantation Proceedings*, vol. 28, no. 3, pp. 1669-1670, 1996.

[8] Y. F. Cheng, T. L. Huang, C. L. Chen, Y. S. Chen, and T. Y. Lee, "Variations of the intrahepatic bile ducts: application in living related liver transplantation and splitting liver transplantation," *Clinical Transplantation*, vol. 11, no. 4, pp. 337–340, 1997.

[9] R. A. Christensen, E. VanSonnenberg, A. A. Nemcek Jr., and H. B. D'Agostino, "Inadvertent ligation of the aberrant right hepatic duct at cholecystectomy: radiologic diagnosis and therapy," *Radiology*, vol. 183, no. 2, pp. 549–553, 1992.

[10] K. D. Lillemoe, J. A. Petrofski, M. A. Choti, A. C. Venbrux, and J. L. Cameron, "Isolated right segmental hepatic duct injury: a diagnostic and therapeutic challenge," *Journal of Gastrointestinal Surgery*, vol. 4, no. 2, pp. 168–177, 2000.

[11] M. A. Turner and A. S. Fulcher, "The cystic duct: normal anatomy and disease processes," *Radiographics*, vol. 21, no. 1, pp. 3–22, 2001.

[12] C. Couinaud, *Le Foie. Etudes Anatomiquesetchirurgicales*, Edition Masson, 1957.

[13] J. E. Healey and P. C. Schroy, "Anatomy of the biliary ducts within the human liver: analysis of the prevailing pattern of branchings and the major variations of the biliary ducts," *Archives of Surgery*, vol. 66, no. 5, pp. 599–616, 1953.

[14] G. S. Gazelle, M. J. Lee, and P. R. Mueller, "Cholangiographic segmental anatomy of the liver.," *RadioGraphics*, vol. 14, no. 5, pp. 1005–1013, 1994.

[15] G. A. Kune, "The influence of structure and function in the surgery of the biliary tract," *Annals of the Royal College of Surgeons of England*, vol. 47, pp. 78–91, 1970.

[16] J. A. Hamlin, "Biliary ductal anomalies," in *Operative Biliary Radiology*, G. Berci and J. A. Hamlin, Eds., pp. 110-16, Williams and Wilkins, Philadelphia, Pa, USA, 1st edition, 1981.

[17] J. W. Choi, T. K. Kim, K. W. Kim et al., "Anatomic variation in intrahepatic bile ducts: an analysis of intraoperative cholangiograms in 300 consecutive donors for living donor liver transplantation," *Korean Journal of Radiology*, vol. 4, no. 2, pp. 85–90, 2003.

[18] R.-Q. Zheng, G.-H. Chen, E.-J. Xu et al., "Evaluating biliary anatomy and variations in living liver donors by a new technique: three-dimensional contrast-enhanced ultrasonic cholangiography," *Ultrasound in Medicine and Biology*, vol. 36, no. 8, pp. 1282–1287, 2010.

[19] K. J. Mortelé and P. R. Ros, "Anatomicvariants of the biliary tree: MR cholangiographic findings and clinical applications," *American Journal of Roentgenology*, vol. 177, no. 2, pp. 389–394, 2001.

[20] C. Aube, J.-J. Tuech, B. Delorme et al., "Contribution of magnetic resonance cholangiography to the anatomic study of bile ducts," *Hepato-Gastroenterology*, vol. 51, pp. 1600–1604, 2004.

[21] D. J. Gulliver, P. B. Cotton, and J. Baillie, "Anatomic variants and artifacts in ERCP interpretation," *American Journal of Roentgenology*, vol. 156, no. 5, pp. 975–980, 1991.

[22] T. Kiuchi and H. Okajima, "Anatomical variants and anomalies," in *Living-Donor Liver Transplantation: Surgical Technique and Innovations*, K. Tanaka, Y. Inomata, and S. Kaihara, Eds., p. 17, Prous Science, Barcelona, Spain, 2003.

[23] H. Kida, M. Uchimura, and K. Okamoto, "Intrahepatic architecture of bile and portal vein," *Journal of Biliary Tract and Pancreas*, vol. 8, pp. 1–7, 1987 (Japanese).

[24] S. Ishiyama, Y. Yamada, Y. Narishima, T. Yamaki, Y. Kunii, and H. Yamauchi, "Surgical anatomy of the hilar bile duct carcinoma," *Journal of Biliary Tract and Pancreas*, vol. 20, pp. 811–829, 1999 (Japanese).

[25] C. M. Lee, H. C. Chen, T. K. Leung, and Y. Y. Chen, "Magnetic resonance cholangiopancreatography of anatomical variants of the biliary tree in Taiwanese," *Journal of the Formosan Medical Association*, vol. 103, pp. 155–159, 2004.

[26] H.-J. Kim, M.-H. Kim, S.-K. Lee et al., "Nomal structure, variations, and anomalies of the pancreaticobiliary ducts of Koreans: A nationwide cooperative prospective study," *Gastrointestinal Endoscopy*, vol. 55, no. 7, pp. 889–896, 2002.

[27] J. Champetier, C. Létoublon, I. Alnaasan, and B. Charvin, "The cystohepatic ducts: surgical implications," *Surgical and Radiologic Anatomy*, vol. 13, no. 3, pp. 203–211, 1991.

[28] S. H. Reid, S.-R. Cho, C.-I. Shaw, and M. A. Turner, "Anomalous hepatic duct inserting into the cystic duct," *American Journal of Roentgenology*, vol. 147, no. 6, pp. 1181-1182, 1986.

[29] M. L. Freeman, D. B. Nelson, S. Sherman et al., "Complications of endoscopic biliary sphincterotomy," *The New England Journal of Medicine*, vol. 335, no. 13, pp. 909–918, 1996.

31

Current Perspectives Regarding Stem Cell-Based Therapy for Liver Cirrhosis

Kyeong-Ah Kwak,[1] Hyun-Jae Cho,[2] Jin-Young Yang,[3] and Young-Seok Park[1]

[1]*Department of Oral Anatomy, School of Dentistry, Seoul National University and Dental Research Institute, Seoul, Republic of Korea*
[2]*Department of Preventive and Social Dentistry, School of Dentistry, Seoul National University and Dental Research Institute, Seoul, Republic of Korea*
[3]*Department of Dental Hygiene, Daejeon Institute of Science and Technology, Daejeon, Republic of Korea*

Correspondence should be addressed to Young-Seok Park; ayoayo7@snu.ac.kr

Academic Editor: Emmanuel Tsochatzis

Liver cirrhosis is a major cause of mortality and a common end of various progressive liver diseases. Since the effective treatment is currently limited to liver transplantation, stem cell-based therapy as an alternative has attracted interest due to promising results from preclinical and clinical studies. However, there is still much to be understood regarding the precise mechanisms of action. A number of stem cells from different origins have been employed for hepatic regeneration with different degrees of success. The present review presents a synopsis of stem cell research for the treatment of patients with liver cirrhosis according to the stem cell type. Clinical trials to date are summarized briefly. Finally, issues to be resolved and future perspectives are discussed with regard to clinical applications.

1. Introduction

Liver fibrosis results from sustained injury, which can be inflicted by various factors such as viruses, drugs, alcohol, metabolic diseases, and autoimmune attacks [1]. Prolonged exposure to these harmful factors causes hepatocyte apoptosis, inflammatory cell recruitment, endothelial cell impairment, and, lastly, activation of hepatic stellate cells, the major cells involved in liver fibrosis. Liver fibrosis is a kind of scar tissue formation in response to liver damage [2–9]. Histologically, it is caused by an imbalance between extracellular matrix synthesis and degradation [10–12].

Liver cirrhosis is a condition where scar tissue replaces the healthy tissue of the liver and regenerative nodules with surrounding fibrous bands develop as a result of the injury [13]. Cirrhosis is the common end of progressive liver disease of various causes, resulting in chronic liver failure entailing complications such as hepatic encephalopathy, spontaneous bacterial peritonitis, ascites, and esophageal varices [14]. Unfortunately, the majority of cases are usually in an irreversible state when diagnosed. Despite current advancements in its management [15, 16], cirrhosis was the 14th leading cause of death worldwide in 2012 [17]. Orthotopic liver transplantation is known to be the only definite solution to end-stage cirrhosis.

However, several problems preclude the prevalent application of the procedure, including immunological rejection and the scarcity of donor sources [18].

In fact, the liver has an inherent regenerative capacity to a substantial degree [19], and, thus, the cessation of those harmful factors may prevent further progression of fibrosis and reverse the situation in some cases [20]. In cases where hepatocyte proliferation is insufficient for recovery from liver injury, bipotent resident liver progenitor cells (LPC) are activated and participate in liver regeneration by differentiating into hepatocytes and biliary epithelial cells [19, 21–23]. However, fibrosis is inevitable when regeneration is exceeded by destruction. Clinical signs of liver failure usually appear after about 80 to 90% of the parenchyma has been destroyed.

Hepatocyte transplantation has been proposed as an alternative approach to transplantation, since hepatocytes have been proven to be strongly associated with liver repair [24–28]. While hepatocyte transplantation is safe in humans, its applicability remains limited due to organ availability, failure of donor engraftment, weak viability in cell culture, and vulnerability to cryopreservation damage [25, 26, 29–32].

Instead of hepatocytes, the transplantation of stem cells has shown therapeutic potential for liver function improvement according to recent experimental studies and human studies [20, 26, 33–40]. Although they remain unclear, the major potential mechanisms have been proposed as a twofold; one is the improvement of the microenvironments through paracrine effects, and the other is the replacement of functional hepatocytes [20].

To date, several kinds of stem cells have been investigated for their therapeutic feasibility and clinical potential in liver cirrhosis [41–43]. The present article briefly reviews the current literature according to the types of stem cells and discusses the future perspectives of stem cell-based therapy in liver cirrhosis.

2. Sources of Stem Cells

Hepatocytes obtained via autopsy of patients who received bone marrow transplantation suggested that they are pluripotent cells in bone marrow [44, 45]. Currently, at least three types of bone marrow-derived cells are known to differentiate into hepatocyte-like cells (HLCs): hematopoietic stem cells (HSCs), mesenchymal stem cells (MSCs), and endothelial progenitor cells (EPCs), though early infusion trials did not discriminate the origins of those cells from bone marrow-derived stromal cells with some improvement [32, 46–52]. A large number of preclinical studies have proven the feasibility of HSCs, MSCs, and EPCs to restore hepatic function in models of liver injury [53–57]. In addition, other stem cells including embryonic stem cells (ESCs) and induced pluripotent stem cells (iPSCs) can also be differentiated into HLCs [58–60]. HLCs can contribute to the remodeling of cirrhotic liver [20, 61–68].

2.1. Hematopoietic Stem Cells. HSCs are the predominant population of stem cells within bone marrow and express CD34 as the cell surface marker. They can renew themselves and differentiate into progenitor cells [69, 70]. HSCs can easily be made to leave the bone marrow and circulate into the blood. The mobilization of HSCs resident in bone marrow can be brought about at a low magnitude through tissue injury [71, 72] or in high amounts after artificial priming [73, 74]. Granulocyte-colony stimulating factor is the most widely studied and widely used mobilizing agent [75–80].

HLCs derived from HSCs have been demonstrated to contribute to liver regeneration [65, 81–83]. In general, two mechanisms were proposed with substantial support. One was the de novo generation of hepatocytes through transdifferentiation, and the other was the genetic reprogramming of resident hepatocytes through cell fusion [45, 46, 84]. However, the infused HSCs do not seem to be a primary source of newly generated hepatocytes [85, 86]. Rather, their roles are likely to be associated with macrophages, which produce collagenases, phagocytose dead cells, and facilitate liver regeneration [87–89]. Therefore, the clinical benefit of HSC therapy occurs through paracrine signaling interactions involving various cytokines and growth factors [86, 90, 91]. Furthermore, HSCs likely stimulate neoangiogenesis [92].

2.2. Endothelial Progenitor Cells. EPCs are immature endothelial cells that can be found in both peripheral blood vessels and bone marrow. They arise from hemangioblasts and participate in the neovascularization of damaged tissue throughout the whole body [93–99]. Due to their common expression of CD34, EPCs and HSCs are assumed to have a common precursor [94, 100–106]. However, EPCs are likely to be differentiated from various cell lineages, as evidenced by their diverse surface markers [102, 104, 107–113].

The transplantation of EPCs led to the suspension of liver fibrosis by suppressing activating HSCs, according to an animal study [55]. They also promoted hepatocyte proliferation and increased matrix metalloproteinase activity [114]. These effects were associated with increased secretion of growth factors [115–117].

2.3. Mesenchymal Stem Cells. MSCs are a rarer population in bone marrow compared to HSCs, which are capable of self-renewal and differentiation into HLCs as well as cell types of mesenchymal origin [68, 118–128]. Traditionally, MSCs have frequently been isolated from bone marrow [129], but, recently, they have been obtained from many other tissues including umbilical cord blood, adipose tissue, and placenta [130–142]. There seems to be source-dependent differences among MSCs [143].

As a therapeutic advantage, MSCs can easily be expanded ex vivo without losing their differentiation potential, and they can also be migrated to the injured areas in response to homing signals [1]. Furthermore, the MSCs have immunomodulatory properties [144–156], through both adaptive and innate immune systems [157, 158], and secrete a variety of trophic factors such as growth factors and cytokines beneficial for liver regeneration [159–164]. Some of these trophic factors are known to revive hepatocytes reaching their replicative senescence [38, 165, 166]. With these advantages as a cell therapy source, the MSCs are the most widely studied stem cells, both experimentally and clinically [59, 167–174].

The precise therapeutic mechanisms of MSCs in liver regeneration have yet to be sufficiently elucidated. Accumulating evidence strongly supports the inference that the effects of MSCs are mediated mostly via paracrine mechanisms rather than transdifferentiation [175–179], although the infused bone marrow-derived MSCs (BM-MSCs) have been shown to engraft into host livers and ameliorate fibrosis in experimental animal models of liver fibrosis [54, 180–183]. MSC transplantation has also demonstrated preclinical efficacy in mitigating liver fibrosis as in other organs [53, 54, 181, 184–187]. Strategies to enhance the effects of MSC in cirrhosis have been investigated, including the facilitation of transdifferentiation into functional hepatocytes [59, 68, 120, 168, 188]. Interestingly, however, the in vivo transdifferentiation of MSCs into hepatocytes has been rarely observed in animal models [54, 189–192].

Rather, the MSCs downregulate proinflammatory and fibrogenic cytokine activity, stimulate hepatocellular proliferation, and promote collagen degradation by matrix metalloproteinase [53, 54, 181, 190–193]. The paracrine effects modulate the functioning of activated hepatic stellated cells [56, 194, 195]. Evidence from treatment with MSC-conditioned medium reconfirmed the paracrine effects of MSCs such as the increased proliferation and reduced apoptosis of hepatocytes subsequent to the upregulation of several anti-inflammatory and antifibrotic cytokines [196, 197]. How each of these signaling molecules individually contributes to hepatic regeneration, however, remains to be further elucidated [46].

2.4. Embryogenic Stem Cells. Thomson et al. derived and characterized human ESCs from the inner mass of a blastocyst for the first time in 1998 [198]. ESCs have pluripotency and can differentiate into hepatocyte-like cells, which possess some properties of mature hepatocytes [199–205]. Hepatocytes generated from ESCs in vitro and hepatocytes differentiated from ESCs have been demonstrated to express a number of hepatocyte-related genes and mimic hepatic functions. ESC-derived hepatocytes bear the typical morphology of mature hepatocyte and colonized liver tissue upon transplantation. The cardinal pathways associated with activin A and Wnt3a and FGF signaling are essential for ESC to differentiate into hepatic lineage [200, 206–217]. ESC-derived hepatocyte-like cells promoted the cell recovery of injured liver by cell replacement [201, 210, 218, 219] and paracrine mechanism to stimulate endogenous regeneration. However, it still remains unclear whether ESCs-derived hepatocytes have the origin of definitive endoderm or primitive endoderm. The recent study using ESCs combined with MSCs showed promising results [201, 220]. Human ESCs are likely resistant to cryopreservation, which mature hepatocytes can hardly endure. Studies using ESCs have provided the molecular basis of hepatocyte differentiation. Despite the promising results, the application of human ESCs has always been precluded by practical and ethical barriers.

2.5. Induced Pluripotent Stem Cells. The iPSCs were first developed by Dr. Yamanaka from mouse fibroblasts in 2006, which were reprogrammed into a state of pluripotency like that of ESCs [98]. These iPSCs have been reported to be differentiated to neuron cells [221], neurospheres [222], cardiomyocytes [223–225], hematopoietic and endothelial cells [226], and insulin-secreting islet-like clusters [227]. A number of protocols to differentiate iPSCs into HLCs have been described [60, 228–242]. Unfortunately, the iPSC-derived HLCs showed minimal activity, reaching around 0.3 to 10% of the activity of primary hepatocytes [231].

In animal experiments, the iPSC-derived HLC transplantation halted lethal fulminant hepatic failure, promoted regeneration, and improved function [234, 235, 243–245]. Due to immunosuppression and possible unlimited supply, the patient-corrected human iPSCs have great potential to be utilized in personalized cell therapy [230, 246, 247]. However, several issues regarding iPSC usage should be properly addressed prior to clinical application, including teratoma formation and tumorigenicity, controversy about immunogenicity, long-term safety and efficacy, and optimal reprogramming and manufacturing processes [248–250].

2.6. Other Cells. Fetal hepatic progenitor cells have been of interest due to their ease of isolation, high proliferation rate, superior repopulation capacity, lower immunogenicity, and resistance to cryopreservation in contrast to adult counterparts [251–256]. Annex stem cells derived from umbilical cord, placenta, and amniotic fluid have easily accessible sources, but they can be categorized as MSCs with respective differences according to their origin [257–261].

3. Clinical Trials Using Stem Cell-Based Therapy

Early autologous bone marrow-derived stem cell transplantation resulted in amelioration of liver injury and functional improvements, and they probably included a mixed cell population of HSCs, MSCs, and EPCs [53, 55, 82, 124, 262, 263]. A number of single-arm, phase I clinical studies with small samples have been performed and have shown some promise in patients with liver cirrhosis [31, 48, 49, 123, 264–270]. The infusion of bone marrow-derived stem cells has sometimes been used as a supportive measure for patients with partial hepatectomy [271–273]. Although the precise mechanisms are still unresolved, the findings from those studies with small sample sizes have provided assurance that no critical complications occurred after the procedures. Furthermore, the posttransplantation incidence of hepatocellular carcinoma was not increased despite the enduring concern [68, 274, 275].

A trial using human fetal liver-derived stem cells enrolling 25 patients with cirrhosis demonstrated improved mean model for end-stage liver disease (MELD) scores [276], although long-term outcomes were not properly reported [277]. There have been several clinical studies using HSCs with promising results [278–281] since Pai et al. [37] reported that the autologous infusion of CD34+ cells improved the serum albumin level and the Child-Pugh score. However, most results have shown only temporary effects and there still remains many questions yet to be answered [280].

The most frequently studied stem cells are the MSCs; thus, their mechanisms of actions are also better understood. In particular, BM-MSCs have been prevalently utilized. In two early pilot studies, autologous injections of BM-MSCs in a few patients were reported to result in improvement of liver function [35, 267]. The safety and short-term efficacy of BM-MSCs were evidenced in two groups of 20 patients each, which showed significantly improved Child-Pugh and MELD scores [47]. Subsequent studies continued to confirm the efficacy of BM-MSC transplantation in varying sizes of samples [282–285]. Notably, one randomized controlled trial using autologous MSCs in cirrhotic patients failed to demonstrate beneficial effects, in contrast to the prior reports [286].

The transplanted cells were mostly infused intravenously, except in three studies using the hepatic artery [284, 285] and one featuring direct injection into the spleen [282]. Not a small variation existed in the numbers of infused cells and the administration frequencies. Although the overall study qualities did not surpass the level of moderate or poor, the results seemed promising in terms of MELD scores and liver function improvements [1]. Specifically, most studies did not include histologic evaluations [287].

As other kinds of MSCs, umbilical cord-derived MSCs (UC-MSCs) were evaluated in clinical trials. UC-MSC infusion was well tolerated and resulted in significant functional improvement and increased survival rates [288–290].

To summarize, stem cell trials in patients with liver cirrhosis have demonstrated generalized functional improvements. In addition, improvements were also found in the MELD and Child-Pugh scores. Unfortunately, these beneficial effects were attenuated with time or were not measured. Therefore, it can be temporarily concluded that treatment using stem cells might be slightly superior to current conventional treatment according to two systematic reviews [1, 42] (Table 1).

4. Discussion

Liver cirrhosis is a major cause of mortality and incurs great healthcare burdens across the world [291–294]. Liver transplantation is the only effective treatment. The survival rate after liver transplantation has progressively increased and the rate of survival after one year of surgery is currently 83% after one year. However, the shortage of organs is a serious problem contributing to the increasing mortality rate of patients on the waiting list [295, 296]. Allogeneic hepatocyte transplantation [297, 298] also entails limited availability with only modest benefits reported [26, 299, 300].

Efforts have been made to develop antifibrotic therapies. Unfortunately, there are no antifibrotic drugs available in a current clinical setting [301–303] even if several reports have been published from preclinical and clinical studies [304–306]. The targets of the drug are primarily associated with the activities of hepatic stellate cells: the downregulation of cell activation [307–310], neutralization of fibrogenic and proliferative cell responses [311–313], promotion of cell apoptosis [314], and promotion of matrix degradation [315, 316]. Clinical studies have, however, failed to yield meaningful results compared with preclinical studies [287, 317–319].

In this regard, stem cell-based therapy is considered a promising therapeutic alternative based on the discrepancy between the demand and supply of donor livers for transplantation. Stem cell clinical trials have resulted in promising outcomes [20, 209, 230, 246, 277, 320–325]. There are advantages and disadvantages depending on which source of stem cells is used in the cell-based therapies. For example, ethical issues and behavioral uncertainties in vivo are major problems of ESCs or iPSCs to be used clinically although they are the most capability of producing HLCs [20]. Teratoma formation and the use of immunomodulatory drugs are other concerns of stem cell uses. For all kinds of stem cell-based therapies, the progressive liver fibrosis and hepatocellular carcinoma are still the fearful medium- or long-term adverse effects. Prior to clinical use, the in vivo safety should be confirmed including toxicity and tumorigenicity. Regulatory challenges and financial burden cast somewhat different kinds of translational barrier.

Among stem cells of various origins, MSCs have attracted attention due to their advantages and have been extensively investigated in experimental studies and in clinical trials. Nevertheless, there are still a number of issues to be addressed. First, the ideal delivery route of MSCs has not been elucidated, and it is unstandardized in clinical trials to date. MSCs differentiate into myofibroblasts instead of hepatocytes depending on the injection route [326, 327]. The optimal dose and number of injections are another practical issue when comparing the results from clinical trials. In addition, sophisticated methods of tracking engrafted MSCs are still lacking. Therefore, it is impossible to predict the fate of transplanted cells, although the survival duration is important for sustained efficacy [328–330]. Recently, labeling cells with superparamagnetic iron oxide nanoparticles and reporter genes have been suggested with advanced imaging technologies [331–336]. Finally, the quality of the clinical studies reported to date is far from sufficient to reach a definite conclusion. Patient enrollment must differentiate clearly between patients with compensated cirrhosis and patients with impaired function. Only randomized controlled designs can assess the reliable clinical benefit. Long-term follow-up and histologic evidence should be recommended in cases where they are available [42, 250, 337].

With advances in novel biotechnology, strategies have been devised to enhance the effects of stem cell-based therapy. For example, the microencapsulation of MSCs in microspheres was proposed to evade unwanted differentiation into myoblasts [338]. To promote the homing of MSCs, the use of MSCs modified by liver-specific receptors has been suggested [339]. Genome editing using CRISPR/Cas9 is a very promising technology widely used in current functional genomics [18, 340, 341]. The three-dimensional culture technique is another example for providing an expansion and differentiation platform for hepatocytes [342, 343].

Rapidly developing iPSC technologies provide an unprecedented opportunity for researchers and clinicians [344]. Recent studies have shown that iPSC-derived hepatocytes can be used for the investigation of the genetic and molecular mechanisms of liver disorders [240, 242, 244, 345–356]. They can be utilized for multiple applications, including drug safety screening of new drugs [214, 357–359] and disease modeling [240, 360]. Disease-specific iPSCs could provide invaluable opportunities to elucidate the pathologic mechanism of disease and develop curative treatment options.

5. Conclusion

Liver fibrosis progresses to cirrhosis, which is the result of the extracellular matrix deposition in the parenchyma. Curative treatment for cirrhosis is currently limited to orthotopic liver transplantation, and a worldwide shortage of donor organs results in the deaths of patients waiting for organs. Stem cell-based therapy has emerged as a promising alternative with accumulating evidence from experimental and clinical

Table 1: Main clinical trials of stem cell therapy for liver cirrhosis.

Trial number	Study phase (type)	Cell source	#	Eligibility criteria	Primary outcome measure	Secondary outcome measure	Time frame	Start date	End date	Location
NCT01875081	Phase II (randomized open)	BM-MSC	72	Histologically or clinically diagnosed as alcoholic liver cirrhosis Classified as Child-Pugh grade B or C	Histopathological evaluation	Histopathological evaluation score, MELD score, Child-Pugh grade, and so on	6 months	2012.11	2016.03 (completed)	Korea
NCT02943889	Phase I/II (non-randomized open)	BM-MSC	40	Decompensated liver cirrhosis Child class b or c	Improvement of liver function in form of improvement in Child score	Postpone or overcome liver transplantation complications	6, 24 months	2016.10	2017.08 (not yet recruiting)	None
NCT02786017	Phase I/II (randomized double-blinded controlled)	UC-MSC	40	Subjects who are decompensated cirrhosis of any cause Child-pugh score ≥7	Change in the model for end-stage liver disease (MELD) score	Change in Child-Pugh score, clinical laboratory parameters of liver function	1 and 3 days 1 and 2 weeks 1, 3, 6, 12, and 24 months	2016.05	2018.12 (recruiting)	China
NCT01591200	Phase II (randomized open)	AlloMSC	40	Child class B or C, Child-Pugh scores of ≥7 and <14 MELD scores of at least 10	Safety	Liver function improvement, Child-Pugh score, MELD score, SF36-QOL, and so on	24 months	2012.06	2016.04 (completed)	India
NCT01120925	Phase I/II (randomized quadruple blind controlled)	BM-MSC	30	MELD score of 12 or Child score B or C Serum ALT 1/5 times more than normal	Liver function test	Cirrhosis mortality	6 months	2010.05	2013.07 (completed)	Iran
NCT00420134	Phase I/II (randomized single-blinded)	MSC	30	MELD score of at least 10 Patent portal vein on color Doppler examination of the live Normal alpha-feto protein serum levels	Liver function test MELD score	Cirrhosis mortality	6 months	2006.02	2009.06 (completed)	Iran

TABLE 1: Continued.

Trial number	Study phase (type)	Cell source	#	Eligibility criteria	Primary outcome measure	Secondary outcome measure	Time frame	Start date	End date	Location
NCT01013194	Phase I/II (non-randomized open)	FLC	25	A score ≥ B8 based on the Child-Pugh-Turcotte classification and/or MELD score ≥ 14	Survival	Analysis of Child-Pugh score, meld score from baseline to 1-year follow-up	6 and 12 months	2007.02	2011.07 (completed)	Italy
NCT01342250	Phase I/II (randomized open)	UC-MSC	20	Decompensated liver cirrhosis, Child-Pugh B/C (7–12 points) or Meld score ≦ 21.	Survival	Liver function improvement, Child-Pugh score, MELD score, SF36-QOL, and so on	24 months	2010.10	2011.10 (completed)	China
NCT02652351	Phase I (open)	UC-MSC	20	Clinical, radiological, or biochemical evidence of liver cirrhosis	Severity of adverse events	Hepatic function, liver fibrosis index	1, 3, 6, and 12 months	2016.03	2016.10 (recruiting)	China
NCT01147380	Phase I (non-randomized open)	NK	18	Subjects who need to meet the liver transplant eligibility criteria Cardiac and pulmonary function	Side effect of cadaveric donor liver NK cell infusion	NK cell infusion-related toxicity, anti-HCC, HCV effect	12 and 24 months	2010.06	2014.12 (completed)	USA
NCT03254758	Phase I/II (open)	AD-MSC	15	Chronic hepatitis C or nonalcoholic steatohepatitis (NASH) Child-Pugh grade B liver cirrhosis	Child-Pugh score, safety profile	Child-Pugh score, safety profile	6 months	2017.07	2018.12 (recruiting)	Japan
NCT01333228	Phase I/II (open)	BM-EPC	14	Liver cirrhosis (Child-Pugh 8 or above)	Safety and tolerability	Effect on liver function, portal hypertension, complications of liver cirrhosis	12 months	2012.06	2015.03 (completed)	Spain
NCT01503749	Phase I (randomized open)	PB-MNC (G-CSF)	9	Advanced liver cirrhosis with Child-Pugh score 8 or 9	Severe adverse events	Change in Child-Pugh score and MELD score	1–4 weeks 2–6 months	2012.01	2014.08 (completed)	-
NCT00713934	Phase I/II (randomized single-blinded)	BMMNC BMHSC	7	Liver biopsy showing histological cirrhosis, grade B or C (Child-Pugh score) liver cirrhosis in sonography study Liver crrhosis in sonography study	Liver function test MELD score	Cirrhosis mortality	6 months	2008.01	2009.02 (completed)	Iran

Table 1: Continued.

Trial number	Study phase (type)	Cell source	#	Eligibility criteria	Primary outcome measure	Secondary outcome measure	Time frame	Start date	End date	Location
NCT02297867	Phase I (open)	ADSC	6	Investigators without HBV, HCV, HIV, syphilis, and so on	MELD	None	1–6 months	2015.07	2018.01 (active, not recruiting)	Taiwan
NCT02705742	Phase I/II (open)	AD-MSC	5	Clinical, radiologic, and pathologically proven liver cirrhosis due to HCV hepatitis	All cause mortality	-	12 months	2016.01	2017.12 (recruiting)	Turkey
NCT01454336	Phase I (open)	BM-MSC	3	Approved cirrhosis by elastography, biopsy, sonography	ALT, AST, serum albumin, liver fibrosis	Progression of fibrosis	12 months	2010.06	2013.07 (completed)	Iran

#Number of enrollments; MELD, model for end-stage liver disease; UC-MSC, umbilical cord mesenchymal stem cell; AlloMSC, allogeneic MSC; FLC, fetal liver cell; BM-EPC, bone marrow-derived endothelial progenitor cells; PB-MNC, peripheral blood mononucleated cells; BMHSC, bone marrow CD133+ hematopoietic stem cell.

studies. Varieties of stem cells including MSCs, HSCs, EPCs, ESCs, and iPSCs have been investigated for their feasibility and/or clinical potentials. Among them, MSCs have been most studied and are relatively well understood. A primary mechanism of action has been proposed as paracrine effects rather than transdifferentiation. The results from clinical trials seem very promising from the perspectives of functional improvement and clinical parameters. However, long-term efficacy has not yet been proven, and standardized trial protocols are needed. Novel technologies are expected to overcome the current hurdles related to clinical application of stem cell-based therapy.

Authors' Contributions

Kyeong-Ah Kwak and Hyun-Jae Cho contributed equally to this work.

Acknowledgments

This research was supported by Ministry of Food and Drug Safety of Korea (Grant 17172MFDS202).

References

[1] Y. W. Eom, K. Y. Shim, and S. K. Baik, "Mesenchymal stem cell therapy for liver fibrosis," *Korean Journal of Internal Medicine*, vol. 30, no. 5, pp. 580–589, 2015.

[2] R. Bataller and D. A. Brenner, "Liver fibrosis," *The Journal of Clinical Investigation*, vol. 115, no. 2, pp. 209–218, 2005.

[3] R. Domitrović and H. Jakovac, "Effects of standardized bilberry fruit extract (Mirtoselect®) on resolution of CCl4-induced liver fibrosis in mice," *Food and Chemical Toxicology*, vol. 49, no. 4, pp. 848–854, 2011.

[4] S. Ghatak, A. Biswas, G. K. Dhali, A. Chowdhury, J. L. Boyer, and A. Santra, "Oxidative stress and hepatic stellate cell activation are key events in arsenic induced liver fibrosis in mice," *Toxicology and Applied Pharmacology*, vol. 251, no. 1, pp. 59–69, 2011.

[5] W. K. Hong, M. Y. Kim, S. K. Baik et al., "The usefulness of non-invasive liver stiffness measurements in predicting clinically significant portal hypertension in cirrhotic patients: Korean data.," *Clinical and Molecular Hepatology*, vol. 19, no. 4, pp. 370–375, 2013.

[6] T. Kisseleva and D. A. Brenner, "Mechanisms of fibrogenesis," *Experimental Biology and Medicine*, vol. 233, no. 2, pp. 109–122, 2008.

[7] H. Malhi and G. J. Gores, "Cellular and molecular mechanisms of liver injury," *Gastroenterology*, vol. 134, no. 6, pp. 1641–1654, 2008.

[8] K. M. Moon, G. Kim, S. K. Baik et al., "Ultrasonographic scoring system score versus liver stiffness measurement in prediction of cirrhosis.," *Clinical and Molecular Hepatology*, vol. 19, no. 4, pp. 389–398, 2013.

[9] V. K. Snowdon and J. A. Fallowfield, "Models and Mechanisms of Fibrosis Resolution," *Alcoholism: Clinical and Experimental Research*, vol. 35, no. 5, pp. 794–799, 2011.

[10] R. Lichtinghagen, D. Michels, C. I. Haberkorn et al., "Matrix metalloproteinase (MMP)-2, MMP-7, and tissue inhibitor of metalloproteinase-1 are closely related to the fibroproliferative process in the liver during chronic hepatitis C," *Journal of Hepatology*, vol. 34, no. 2, pp. 239–247, 2001.

[11] A. El Taghdouini and L. A. van Grunsven, "Epigenetic regulation of hepatic stellate cell activation and liver fibrosis," *Expert Review of Gastroenterology & Hepatology*, vol. 10, no. 12, pp. 1397–1408, 2016.

[12] A. El Taghdouini, A. L. Sørensen, A. H. Reiner et al., "Genome-wide analysis of DNA methylation and gene expression patterns in purified, uncultured human liver cells and activated hepatic stellate cells," *Oncotarget* , vol. 6, no. 29, pp. 26729–26745, 2015.

[13] D. Schuppan and N. H. Afdhal, "Liver cirrhosis," *The Lancet*, vol. 371, no. 9615, pp. 838–851, 2008.

[14] H. R. Perez and J. H. Stoeckle, "Stuttering: clinical and research update," *Can Fam Physician*, vol. 62, pp. 479–484, 2016.

[15] N. Carbonell, A. Pauwels, L. Serfaty, O. Fourdan, V. G. Lévy, and R. Poupon, "Improved survival after variceal bleeding in patients with cirrhosis over the past two decades," *Hepatology*, vol. 40, no. 3, pp. 652–659, 2004.

[16] K. Stokkeland, L. Brandt, A. Ekbom, and R. Hultcrantz, "Improved prognosis for patients hospitalized with esophageal varices in Sweden 1969–2002," *Hepatology*, vol. 43, no. 3, pp. 500–505, 2006.

[17] R. Lozano, M. Naghavi, K. Foreman et al., "Global and regional mortality from 235 causes of death for 20 age groups in 1990 and 2010: A systematic analysis for the Global Burden of Disease Study 2010," *The Lancet*, vol. 380, no. 9859, pp. 2095–2128, 2012.

[18] Y. Guo, B. Chen, L.-J. Chen, C.-F. Zhang, and C. Xiang, "Current status and future prospects of mesenchymal stem cell therapy for liver fibrosis," *Journal of Zhejiang University SCIENCE B*, vol. 17, no. 11, pp. 831–841, 2016.

[19] J. W. Kung and S. J. Forbes, "Stem cells and liver repair," *Current Opinion in Biotechnology*, vol. 20, no. 5, pp. 568–574, 2009.

[20] Z. Zhang and F.-S. Wang, "Stem cell therapies for liver failure and cirrhosis," *Journal of Hepatology*, vol. 59, no. 1, pp. 183–185, 2013.

[21] T. G. Bird, S. Lorenzini, and S. J. Forbes, "Activation of stem cells in hepatic diseases," *Cell and Tissue Research*, vol. 331, no. 1, pp. 283–300, 2008.

[22] Y. Y. Dan and G. C. Yeoh, "Liver stem cells: A scientific and clinical perspective," *Journal of Gastroenterology and Hepatology*, vol. 23, no. 5, pp. 687–698, 2008.

[23] V. Papp, A. Rókusz, K. Dezso et al., "Expansion of hepatic stem cell compartment boosts liver regeneration," *Stem Cells and Development*, vol. 23, no. 1, pp. 56–65, 2014.

[24] N. Fausto, J. S. Campbell, and K. J. Riehle, "Liver regeneration," *Hepatology*, vol. 43, no. 2, pp. S45–S53, 2006.

[25] G. K. Michalopoulos and M. C. DeFrances, "Liver regeneration," *Science*, vol. 276, no. 5309, pp. 60–65, 1997.

[26] R. Gramignoli, M. Vosough, K. Kannisto, R. C. Srinivasan, and S. C. Strom, "Clinical hepatocyte transplantation: practical limits and possible solutions," *European Surgical Research*, vol. 54, no. 3-4, pp. 162–177, 2015.

[27] M. Najimi and E. Sokal, "Liver cell transplantation," *Minerva Pediatrica*, vol. 57, no. 5, pp. 243–257, 2005.

[28] S. C. Strom, J. R. Chowdhury, and I. J. Fox, "Hepatocyte transplantation for the treatment of human disease," *Seminars in Liver Disease*, vol. 19, no. 1, pp. 39–48, 1999.

[29] J. Puppi, S. C. Strom, R. D. Hughes et al., "Improving the techniques for human hepatocyte transplantation: Report from a consensus meeting in London," *Cell Transplantation*, vol. 21, no. 1, pp. 1–10, 2012.

[30] K. A. Soltys, A. Soto-Gutiérrez, M. Nagaya et al., "Barriers to the successful treatment of liver disease by hepatocyte transplantation," *Journal of Hepatology*, vol. 53, no. 4, pp. 769–774, 2010.

[31] S. Terai, T. Ishikawa, K. Omori et al., "Improved liver function in patients with liver cirrhosis after autologous bone marrow cell infusion therapy," *Stem Cells*, vol. 24, no. 10, pp. 2292–2298, 2006.

[32] S. Terai, H. Tanimoto, M. Maeda et al., "Timeline for development of autologous bone marrow infusion (ABMi) therapy and perspective for future stem cell therapy," *Journal of Gastroenterology*, vol. 47, no. 5, pp. 491–497, 2012.

[33] K.-A. Cho, G.-W. Lim, S.-Y. Joo et al., "Transplantation of bone marrow cells reduces CCl 4-induced liver fibrosis in mice," *Liver International*, vol. 31, no. 7, pp. 932–939, 2011.

[34] A. Gasbarrini, G. L. Rapaccini, S. Rutella et al., "Rescue therapy by portal infusion of autologous stem cells in a case of drug-induced hepatitis," *Digestive and Liver Disease*, vol. 39, no. 9, pp. 878–882, 2007.

[35] P. Kharaziha, P. M. Hellström, B. Noorinayer et al., "Improvement of liver function in liver cirrhosis patients after autologous mesenchymal stem cell injection: a phase I-II clinical trial," *European Journal of Gastroenterology & Hepatology*, vol. 21, no. 10, pp. 1199–1205, 2009.

[36] N. Levičar, M. Pai, N. A. Habib et al., "Long-term clinical results of autologous infusion of mobilized adult bone marrow derived CD34 + cells in patients with chronic liver disease," *Cell Proliferation*, vol. 41, no. 1, pp. 115–125, 2008.

[37] M. Pai, D. Zacharoulis, M. N. Milicevic et al., "Autologous infusion of expanded mobilized adult bone marrow-derived CD34+ cells into patients with alcoholic liver cirrhosis," *American Journal of Gastroenterology*, vol. 103, no. 8, pp. 1952–1958, 2008.

[38] I. Sakaida, S. Terai, N. Yamamoto et al., "Transplantation of bone marrow cells reduces CCl_4-induced liver fibrosis in mice," *Hepatology*, vol. 40, no. 6, pp. 1304–1311, 2004.

[39] M. R. Alison, S. Islam, and S. M. L. Lim, "Cell therapy for liver disease," *Current Opinion in Molecular Therapeutics*, vol. 11, no. 4, pp. 364–374, 2009.

[40] A. G. Bonavita, K. Quaresma, V. Cotta-De-Almeida, M. A. Pinto, R. M. Saraiva, and L. A. Alves, "Hepatocyte xenotransplantation for treating liver disease: Review Article," *Xenotransplantation*, vol. 17, no. 3, pp. 181–187, 2010.

[41] S. M. Park, "Stem cell research in gastroenterology," *The Korean journal of gastroenterology = Taehan Sohwagi Hakhoe chi*, vol. 43, no. 4, pp. 221–225, 2004.

[42] X. Qi, X. Guo, and C. Su, "Clinical outcomes of the transplantation of stem cells from various human tissue sources in the management of Liver Cirrhosis: A systematic review and meta-analysis," *Current Stem Cell Research & Therapy*, vol. 10, no. 2, pp. 166–180, 2015.

[43] E. Y. Shevela, N. M. Starostina, A. I. Pal'tsev et al., "Efficiency of Cell Therapy in Liver Cirrhosis," *Bulletin of Experimental Biology and Medicine*, vol. 160, no. 4, pp. 542–547, 2016.

[44] M. R. Alison, R. Poulsom, R. Jeffery et al., "Hepatocytes from non-hepatic adult stem cells," *Nature*, vol. 406, no. 6793, p. 257, 2000.

[45] N. D. Theise, M. Nimmakayalu, R. Gardner et al., "Liver from bone marrow in humans," *Hepatology*, vol. 32, no. 1, pp. 11–16, 2000.

[46] J. M. Vainshtein, R. Kabarriti, K. J. Mehta, J. Roy-Chowdhury, and C. Guha, "Bone marrow-derived stromal cell therapy in cirrhosis: Clinical evidence, cellular mechanisms, and implications for the treatment of Hepatocellular carcinoma," *International Journal of Radiation Oncology • Biology • Physics*, vol. 89, no. 4, pp. 786–803, 2014.

[47] M.-E. M. Amer, S. Z. El-Sayed, W. A. El-Kheir et al., "Clinical and laboratory evaluation of patients with end-stage liver cell failure injected with bone marrow-derived hepatocyte-like cells," *European Journal of Gastroenterology & Hepatology*, vol. 23, no. 10, pp. 936–941, 2011.

[48] A. C. Lyra, M. B. P. Soares, L. F. M. da Silva et al., "Infusion of autologous bone marrow mononuclear cells through hepatic artery results in a short-term improvement of liver function in patients with chronic liver disease: a pilot randomized controlled study," *European Journal of Gastroenterology & Hepatology*, vol. 22, no. 1, pp. 33–42, 2010.

[49] A. C. Lyra, M. B. Pereira Soares, L. F. Maia da Silva et al., "Feasiblity and safety of autologous bone marrow mononuclear cell transplantation in patients with advanced chronic liver disease," *World Journal of Gastroenterology*, vol. 13, no. 7, pp. 1067–1073, 2007.

[50] T. Saito, K. Okumoto, H. Haga et al., "Potential therapeutic application of intravenous autologous bone marrow infusion in patients with alcoholic liver cirrhosis," *Stem Cells and Development*, vol. 20, no. 9, pp. 1503–1510, 2011.

[51] T. Takami, S. Terai, and I. Sakaida, "Stem cell therapy in chronic liver disease," *Current Opinion in Gastroenterology*, vol. 28, no. 3, pp. 203–208, 2012.

[52] S. Terai, T. Takami, N. Yamamoto et al., "Status and prospects of liver cirrhosis treatment by using bone marrow-derived cells and mesenchymal cells," *Tissue Engineering - Part B: Reviews*, vol. 20, no. 3, pp. 206–210, 2014.

[53] M. T. Abdel Aziz, H. M. Atta, S. Mahfouz et al., "Therapeutic potential of bone marrow-derived mesenchymal stem cells on experimental liver fibrosis," *Clinical Biochemistry*, vol. 40, no. 12, pp. 893–899, 2007.

[54] B. Fang, M. Shi, L. Liao, S. Yang, Y. Liu, and R. C. Zhao, "Systemic infusion of FLK1+ mesenchymal stem cells ameliorate carbon tetrachloride-induced liver fibrosis in mice," *Transplantation*, vol. 78, no. 1, pp. 83–88, 2004.

[55] T. Nakamura, T. Torimura, M. Sakamoto et al., "Significance and Therapeutic Potential of Endothelial Progenitor Cell Transplantation in a Cirrhotic Liver Rat Model," *Gastroenterology*, vol. 133, no. 1, pp. 91–e1, 2007.

[56] S. Oyagi, M. Hirose, M. Kojima et al., "Therapeutic effect of transplanting HGF-treated bone marrow mesenchymal cells into CCl4-injured rats," *Journal of Hepatology*, vol. 44, no. 4, pp. 742–748, 2006.

[57] Y. Zhan, Y. Wang, L. Wei et al., "Differentiation of Hematopoietic Stem Cells into Hepatocytes in Liver Fibrosis in Rats," *Transplantation Proceedings*, vol. 38, no. 9, pp. 3082–3085, 2006.

[58] R. Kia, R. L. C. Sison, J. Heslop et al., "Stem cell-derived hepatocytes as a predictive model for drug-induced liver injury: are we there yet?" *British Journal of Clinical Pharmacology*, vol. 75, no. 4, pp. 885–896, 2013.

[59] S.-N. Shu, L. Wei, J.-H. Wang, Y.-T. Zhan, H.-S. Chen, and Y. Wang, "Hepatic differentiation capability of rat bone marrow-derived mesenchymal stem cells and hematopoietic stem cells," *World Journal of Gastroenterology*, vol. 10, no. 19, pp. 2818–2822, 2004.

[60] K. Si-Tayeb, F. K. Noto, M. Nagaoka et al., "Highly efficient generation of human hepatocyte-like cells from induced pluripotent stem cells," *Hepatology*, vol. 51, no. 1, pp. 297–305, 2010.

[61] Y. W. Eom, G. Kim, and S. K. Baik, "Mesenchymal stem cell therapy for cirrhosis: Present and future perspectives," *World Journal of Gastroenterology*, vol. 21, no. 36, pp. 10253–10261, 2015.

[62] T. R. Brazelton, F. M. V. Rossi, G. I. Keshet, and H. M. Blau, "From marrow to brain: expression of neuronal phenotypes in adult mice," *Science*, vol. 290, no. 5497, pp. 1775–1779, 2000.

[63] G. Ferrari, G. Cusella-De Angelis, M. Coletta et al., "Muscle regeneration by bone marrow-derived myogenic progenitors," *Science*, vol. 279, no. 5356, pp. 1528–1530, 1998.

[64] A. Ianus, G. G. Holz, N. D. Theise, and M. A. Hussain, "In vivo derivation of glucose-competent pancreatic endocrine cells from bone marrow without evidence of cell fusion," *The Journal of Clinical Investigation*, vol. 111, no. 6, pp. 843–850, 2003.

[65] E. Lagasse, H. Connors, M. Al-Dhalimy et al., "Purified hematopoietic stem cells can differentiate into hepatocytes *in vivo*," *Nature Medicine*, vol. 6, no. 11, pp. 1229–1234, 2000.

[66] D. Orlic, J. Kajstura, S. Chimenti et al., "Bone marrow cells regenerate infarcted myocardium," *Nature*, vol. 410, no. 6829, pp. 701–705, 2001.

[67] B. E. Petersen, W. C. Bowen, K. D. Patrene et al., "Bone marrow as a potential source of hepatic oval cells," *Science*, vol. 284, no. 5417, pp. 1168–1170, 1999.

[68] R. E. Schwartz, M. Reyes, L. Koodie et al., "Multipotent adult progenitor cells from bone marrow differentiate into functional hepatocyte-like cells," *The Journal of Clinical Investigation*, vol. 109, no. 10, pp. 1291–1302, 2002.

[69] S. Hombach-Klonisch, S. Panigrahi, I. Rashedi et al., "Adult stem cells and their trans-differentiation potential - Perspectives and therapeutic applications," *Journal of Molecular Medicine*, vol. 86, no. 12, pp. 1301–1314, 2008.

[70] G. Menichella, M. Lai, R. Serafini et al., "Large volume leukapheresis for collecting hemopoietic progenitors: Role of CD 34+ precount in predicting successful collection," *The International Journal of Artificial Organs*, vol. 22, no. 5, pp. 334–341, 1999.

[71] G. De Silvestro, M. Vicarioto, C. Donadel, M. Menegazzo, P. Marson, and A. Corsini, "Mobilization of peripheral blood hematopoietic stem cells following liver resection surgery," *Hepato-Gastroenterology*, vol. 51, no. 57, pp. 805–810, 2004.

[72] R. M. Lemoli, L. Catani, S. Talarico et al., "Mobilization of bone marrow-derived hematopoietic and endothelial stem cells after orthotopic liver transplantation and liver resection," *Stem Cells*, vol. 24, no. 12, pp. 2817–2825, 2006.

[73] M. Mohty and A. D. Ho, "In and out of the niche: perspectives in mobilization of hematopoietic stem cells," *Experimental Hematology*, vol. 39, no. 7, pp. 723–729, 2011.

[74] L. B. To, D. N. Haylock, P. J. Simmons, and C. A. Juttner, "The biology and clinical uses of blood stem cells," *Blood*, vol. 89, no. 7, pp. 2233–2258, 1997.

[75] D. Metcalf, "The molecular control of cell division, differentiation commitment and maturation in haemopoietic cells," *Nature*, vol. 339, no. 6219, pp. 27–30, 1989.

[76] A. C. Piscaglia, T. D. Shupe, S.-H. Oh, A. Gasbarrini, and B. E. Petersen, "Granulocyte-Colony Stimulating Factor Promotes Liver Repair and Induces Oval Cell Migration and Proliferation in Rats," *Gastroenterology*, vol. 133, no. 2, pp. 619–631, 2007.

[77] O. Quintana-Bustamante, A. Alvarez-Barrientos, A. V. Kofman et al., "Hematopoietic mobilization in mice increases the presence of bone marrow-derived hepatocytes via in vivo cell fusion," *Hepatology*, vol. 43, no. 1, pp. 108–116, 2006.

[78] E. Tsolaki, E. Athanasiou, E. Gounari et al., "Hematopoietic stem cells and liver regeneration: Differentially acting hematopoietic stem cell mobilization agents reverse induced chronic liver injury," *Blood Cells, Molecules, and Diseases*, vol. 53, no. 3, pp. 124–132, 2014.

[79] E. Yannaki, E. Athanasiou, A. Xagorari et al., "G-CSF-primed hematopoietic stem cells or G-CSF per se accelerate recovery and improve survival after liver injury, predominantly by promoting endogenous repair programs," *Experimental Hematology*, vol. 33, no. 1, pp. 108–119, 2005.

[80] E. Tsolaki and E. Yannaki, "Stem cell-based regenerative opportunities for the liver: State of the art and beyond," *World Journal of Gastroenterology*, vol. 21, no. 43, pp. 12334–12350, 2015.

[81] Y.-Y. Jang, M. I. Collector, S. B. Baylin, A. M. Diehl, and S. J. Sharkis, "Hematopoietic stem cells convert into liver cells within days without fusion," *Nature Cell Biology*, vol. 6, no. 6, pp. 532–539, 2004.

[82] S. Khurana and A. Mukhopadhyay, "Characterization of the potential subpopulation of bone marrow cells involved in the repair of injured liver tissue," *Stem Cells*, vol. 25, no. 6, pp. 1439–1447, 2007.

[83] N. D. Theise, S. Badve, R. Saxena et al., "Derivation of hepatocytes from bone marrow cells in mice after radiation-induced myeloablation," *Hepatology*, vol. 31, no. 1, pp. 235–240, 2000.

[84] T. W. Austin and E. Lagasse, "Hepatic regeneration from hematopoietic stem cells," *Mechanisms of Development*, vol. 120, no. 1, pp. 131–135, 2003.

[85] T. Kisseleva and D. A. Brenner, "The phenotypic fate and functional role for bone marrow-derived stem cells in liver fibrosis," *Journal of Hepatology*, vol. 56, no. 4, pp. 965–972, 2012.

[86] S. S. Thorgeirsson and J. W. Grisham, "Hematopoietic cells as hepatocyte stem cells: a critical review of the evidence," *Hepatology*, vol. 43, no. 1, pp. 2–8, 2006.

[87] J. A. Thomas, C. Pope, D. Wojtacha et al., "Macrophage therapy for murine liver fibrosis recruits host effector cells improving fibrosis, regeneration, and function," *Hepatology*, vol. 53, no. 6, pp. 2003–2015, 2011.

[88] L. Boulter, O. Govaere, T. G. Bird et al., "Macrophage-derived Wnt opposes Notch signaling to specify hepatic progenitor cell fate in chronic liver disease," *Nature Medicine*, vol. 18, no. 4, pp. 572–579, 2012.

[89] X. Aldeguer, F. Debonera, A. Shaked et al., "Interleukin-6 from intrahepatic cells of bone marrow origin is required for normal murine liver regeneration," *Hepatology*, vol. 35, no. 1, pp. 40–48, 2002.

[90] F. S. Loffredo, M. L. Steinhauser, J. Gannon, and R. T. Lee, "Bone marrow-derived cell therapy stimulates endogenous cardiomyocyte progenitors and promotes cardiac repair," *Cell Stem Cell*, vol. 8, no. 4, pp. 389–398, 2011.

[91] X. L. Tang, G. Rokosh, S. K. Sanganalmath et al., "Intracoronary administration of cardiac progenitor cells alleviates left ventricular dysfunction in rats with a 30-day-old infarction," *Circulation*, vol. 121, no. 2, pp. 293–305, 2010.

[92] B. Larrivee and A. Karsan, "Involvement of marrow-derived endothelial cells in vascularization," *Handbook of Experimental Pharmacology*, pp. 89–114, 2007.

[93] T. Asahara, H. Masuda, T. Takahashi et al., "Bone marrow origin of endothelial progenitor cells responsible for postnatal vasculogenesis in physiological and pathological neovascularization," *Circulation Research*, vol. 85, no. 3, pp. 221–228, 1999.

[94] T. Asahara, T. Murohara, A. Sullivan et al., "Isolation of putative progenitor endothelial cells for angiogenesis," *Science*, vol. 275, no. 5302, pp. 964–967, 1997.

[95] T. Asahara, T. Takahashi, H. Masuda et al., "VEGF contributes to postnatal neovascularization by mobilizing bone marrow-derived endothelial progenitor cells," *EMBO Journal*, vol. 18, no. 14, pp. 3964–3972, 1999.

[96] C. Kalka, H. Masuda, T. Takahashi et al., "Transplantation of ex vivo expanded endothelial progenitor cells for therapeutic neovascularization," *Proceedings of the National Acadamy of Sciences of the United States of America*, vol. 97, no. 7, pp. 3422–3427, 2000.

[97] A. Kawamoto, H.-C. Gwon, H. Iwaguro et al., "Therapeutic potential of ex vivo expanded endothelial progenitor cells for myocardial ischemia," *Circulation*, vol. 103, no. 5, pp. 634–637, 2001.

[98] T. Takahashi, C. Kalka, H. Masuda et al., "Ischemia- and cytokine-induced mobilization of bone marrow-derived endothelial progenitor cells for neovascularization," *Nature Medicine*, vol. 5, no. 4, pp. 434–438, 1999.

[99] J.-I. Yamaguchi, K. F. Kusano, O. Masuo et al., "Stromal cell-derived factor-1 effects on *ex vivo* expanded endothelial progenitor cell recruitment for ischemic neovascularization," *Circulation*, vol. 107, no. 9, pp. 1322–1328, 2003.

[100] T. Asahara and A. Kawamoto, "Endothelial progenitor cells for postnatal vasculogenesis," *American Journal of Physiology-Cell Physiology*, vol. 287, no. 3, pp. C572–C579, 2004.

[101] A. S. Bailey, S. Jiang, M. Afentoulis et al., "Transplanted adult hematopoietic stems cells differentiate into functional endothelial cells," *Blood*, vol. 103, no. 1, pp. 13–19, 2004.

[102] K. Choi, M. Kennedy, A. Kazarov, J. C. Papadimitriou, and G. Keller, "A common precursor for hematopoietic and endothelial cells," *Development*, vol. 125, no. 4, pp. 725–732, 1998.

[103] E. Pelosi, M. Valtieri, S. Coppola et al., "Identification of the hemangioblast in postnatal life," *Blood*, vol. 100, no. 9, pp. 3203–3208, 2002.

[104] D. Ribatti, "The discovery of endothelial progenitor cells. An historical review," *Leukemia Research*, vol. 31, no. 4, pp. 439–444, 2007.

[105] Q. Shi, S. Rafii, M. Wu Hong-De et al., "Evidence for circulating bone marrow-derived endothelial cells," *Blood*, vol. 92, no. 2, pp. 362–367, 1998.

[106] C. Urbich and S. Dimmeler, "Endothelial progenitor cells: functional characterization," *Trends in Cardiovascular Medicine*, vol. 14, no. 8, pp. 318–322, 2004.

[107] A. Al-Khaldi, N. Eliopoulos, D. Martineau, L. Lejeune, K. Lachapelle, and J. Galipeau, "Postnatal bone marrow stromal cells elicit a potent VEGF-dependent neoangiogenic response in vivo," *Gene Therapy*, vol. 10, no. 8, pp. 621–629, 2003.

[108] A. P. Beltrami, L. Barlucchi, D. Torella et al., "Adult cardiac stem cells are multipotent and support myocardial regeneration," *Cell*, vol. 114, no. 6, pp. 763–776, 2003.

[109] B. Dome, J. Dobos, J. Tovari et al., "Circulating bone marrow-derived endothelial progenitor cells: characterization, mobilization, and therapeutic considerations in malignant disease," *Cytometry Part A*, vol. 73, no. 3, pp. 186–193, 2008.

[110] N. Kubis, Y. Tomita, A. Tran-Dinh et al., "Vascular fate of adipose tissue-derived adult stromal cells in the ischemic murine brain: A combined imaging-histological study," *NeuroImage*, vol. 34, no. 1, pp. 1–11, 2007.

[111] A. Miranville, C. Heeschen, C. Sengenès, C. A. Curat, R. Busse, and A. Bouloumié, "Improvement of postnatal neovascularization by human adipose tissue-derived stem cells," *Circulation*, vol. 110, no. 3, pp. 349–355, 2004.

[112] V. Planat-Benard, J.-S. Silvestre, B. Cousin et al., "Plasticity of human adipose lineage cells toward endothelial cells: physiological and therapeutic perspectives," *Circulation*, vol. 109, no. 5, pp. 656–663, 2004.

[113] A. E. Wurmser, K. Nakashima, R. G. Summers et al., "Cell fusion-independent differentiation of neural stem cells to the endothelial lineage," *Nature*, vol. 430, no. 6997, pp. 350–356, 2004.

[114] L. Wang, X. Wang, G. Xie, L. Wang, C. K. Hill, and L. D. DeLeve, "Liver sinusoidal endothelial cell progenitor cells promote liver regeneration in rats," *The Journal of Clinical Investigation*, vol. 122, no. 4, pp. 1567–1573, 2012.

[115] P. Beaudry, Y. Hida, T. Udagawa et al., "Endothelial progenitor cells contribute to accelerated liver regeneration," *Journal of Pediatric Surgery*, vol. 42, no. 7, pp. 1190–1198, 2007.

[116] E. Taniguchi, M. Kin, T. Torimura et al., "Endothelial progenitor cell transplantation improves the survival following liver injury in mice," *Gastroenterology*, vol. 130, no. 2, pp. 521–531, 2006.

[117] T. Ueno, T. Nakamura, T. Torimura, and M. Sata, "Angiogenic cell therapy for hepatic fibrosis," *Medical Molecular Morphology*, vol. 39, no. 1, pp. 16–21, 2006.

[118] K. Fukuda and J. Fujita, "Mesenchymal, but not hematopoietic, stem cells can be mobilized and differentiate into cardiomyocytes after myocardial infarction in mice," *Kidney International*, vol. 68, no. 5, pp. 1940–1943, 2005.

[119] K. K. Hirschi and M. A. Goodell, "Hematopoietic, vascular and cardiac fates of bone marrow-derived stem cells," *Gene Therapy*, vol. 9, no. 10, pp. 648–652, 2002.

[120] Y. Jiang, B. N. Jahagirdar, R. L. Reinhardt et al., "Pluripotency of mesenchymal stem cells derived from adult marrow," *Nature*, vol. 418, no. 6893, pp. 41–49, 2002.

[121] Y. N. Kallis, M. R. Alison, and S. J. Forbes, "Bone marrow stem cells and liver disease," *Gut*, vol. 56, no. 5, pp. 716–724, 2007.

[122] G. Keilhoff, A. Goihl, K. Langnäse, H. Fansa, and G. Wolf, "Transdifferentiation of mesenchymal stem cells into Schwann cell-like myelinating cells," *European Journal of Cell Biology*, vol. 85, no. 1, pp. 11–24, 2006.

[123] C. Krabbe, J. Zimmer, and M. Meyer, "Neural transdifferentiation of mesenchymal stem cells - A critical review," *APMIS-Acta Pathologica, Microbiologica et Immunologica Scandinavica*, vol. 113, no. 11-12, pp. 831–844, 2005.

[124] S. Masson, D. J. Harrison, J. N. Plevris, and P. N. Newsome, "Potential of hematopoietic stem cell therapy in hepatology: A critical review," *Stem Cells*, vol. 22, no. 6, pp. 897–907, 2004.

[125] M. F. Pittenger, J. D. Mosca, and K. R. McIntosh, "Human Mesenchymal Stem Cells: Progenitor Cells for Cartilage, Bone, Fat and Stroma," in *Lymphoid Organogenesis*, vol. 251 of *Current Topics in Microbiology and Immunology*, pp. 3–11, Springer Berlin Heidelberg, Berlin, Heidelberg, 2000.

[126] W. S. N. Shim, S. Jiang, P. Wong et al., "Ex vivo differentiation of human adult bone marrow stem cells into cardiomyocyte-like cells," *Biochemical and Biophysical Research Communications*, vol. 324, no. 2, pp. 481–488, 2004.

[127] L. Song and R. S. Tuan, "Transdifferentiation potential of human mesenchymal stem cells derived from bone marrow," *The FASEB Journal*, vol. 18, no. 9, pp. 980–982, 2004.

[128] C. Toma, M. F. Pittenger, K. S. Cahill, B. J. Byrne, and P. D. Kessler, "Human mesenchymal stem cells differentiate to a cardiomyocyte phenotype in the adult murine heart," *Circulation*, vol. 105, no. 1, pp. 93–98, 2002.

[129] M. F. Pittenger, A. M. Mackay, S. C. Beck et al., "Multilineage potential of adult human mesenchymal stem cells," *Science*, vol. 284, no. 5411, pp. 143–147, 1999.

[130] C. De Bari, F. Dell'Accio, P. Tylzanowski, and F. P. Luyten, "Multipotent mesenchymal stem cells from adult human synovial membrane," *Arthritis & Rheumatology*, vol. 44, no. 8, pp. 1928–1942, 2001.

[131] P. S. In't Anker, S. A. Scherjon, C. Kleijburg-van der Keur et al., "Isolation of mesenchymal stem cells of fetal or maternal origin from human placenta," *Stem Cells*, vol. 22, no. 7, pp. 1338–1345, 2004.

[132] P. S. In 't Anker, W. A. Noort, S. A. Scherjon et al., "Mesenchymal stem cells in human second-trimester bone marrow, liver, lung, and spleen exhibit a similar immunophenotype but a heterogeneous multilineage differentiation potential," *Haematologica*, vol. 88, no. 8, pp. 845–852, 2003.

[133] P. S. In 't Anker, S. A. Scherjon, C. Kleijburg-van der Keur et al., "Amniotic fluid as a novel source of mesenchymal stem cells for therapeutic transplantation," *Blood*, vol. 102, no. 4, pp. 1548-1549, 2003.

[134] Y. Jiang, B. Vaessen, T. Lenvik, M. Blackstad, M. Reyes, and C. M. Verfaillie, "Multipotent progenitor cells can be isolated from postnatal murine bone marrow, muscle, and brain," *Experimental Hematology*, vol. 30, no. 8, pp. 896–904, 2002.

[135] V. Sottile, C. Halleux, F. Bassilana, H. Keller, and K. Seuwen, "Stem cell characteristics of human trabecular bone-derived cells," *Bone*, vol. 30, no. 5, pp. 699–704, 2002.

[136] O. K. Lee, T. K. Kuo, W. M. Chen, K. D. Lee, S. L. Hsieh, and T. H. Chen, "Isolation of multipotent mesenchymal stem cells from umbilical cord blood," *Blood*, vol. 103, no. 5, pp. 1669–1675, 2004.

[137] P. A. Zuk, M. Zhu, P. Ashjian et al., "Human adipose tissue is a source of multipotent stem cells," *Molecular Biology of the Cell (MBoC)*, vol. 13, no. 12, pp. 4279–4295, 2002.

[138] C. Campagnoli, I. A. G. Roberts, S. Kumar, P. R. Bennett, I. Bellantuono, and N. M. Fisk, "Identification of mesenchymal stem/progenitor cells in human first-trimester fetal blood, liver, and bone marrow," *Blood*, vol. 98, no. 8, pp. 2396–2402, 2001.

[139] D. A. de Ugarte, K. Morizono, A. Elbarbary et al., "Comparison of multi-lineage cells from human adipose tissue and bone marrow," *Cells Tissues Organs*, vol. 174, no. 3, pp. 101–109, 2003.

[140] A. Erices, P. Conget, and J. J. Minguell, "Mesenchymal progenitor cells in human umbilical cord blood," *British Journal of Haematology*, vol. 109, no. 1, pp. 235–242, 2000.

[141] N. J. Zvaifler, L. Marinova-Mutafchieva, G. Adams et al., "Mesenchymal precursor cells in the blood of normal individuals," *Arthritis Research & Therapy*, vol. 2, no. 6, pp. 477–488, 2000.

[142] M. D. Kim, S. S. Kim, H. Y. Cha et al., "Therapeutic effect of hepatocyte growth factor-secreting mesenchymal stem cells in a rat model of liver fibrosis," *Experimental & molecular medicine*, vol. 46, p. e110, 2014.

[143] B. M. Manzini, A. da Silva Santos Duarte, S. Sankaramanivel et al., "Useful properties of undifferentiated mesenchymal stromal cells and adipose tissue as the source in liver-regenerative therapy studied in an animal model of severe acute fulminant hepatitis," *Cytotherapy*, vol. 17, no. 8, pp. 1052–1065, 2015.

[144] M. Sundin, O. Ringdén, B. Sundberg, S. Nava, C. Götherström, and K. Le Blanc, "No alloantibodies against mesenchymal stromal cells, but presence of anti-fetal calf serum antibodies, after transplantation in allogeneic hematopoietic stem cell recipients," *Haematologica*, vol. 92, no. 9, pp. 1208–1215, 2007.

[145] S. Asari, S. Itakura, K. Ferreri et al., "Mesenchymal stem cells suppress B-cell terminal differentiation," *Experimental Hematology*, vol. 37, no. 5, pp. 604–615, 2009.

[146] A. Corcione, F. Benvenuto, E. Ferretti et al., "Human mesenchymal stem cells modulate B-cell functions," *Blood*, vol. 107, no. 1, pp. 367–372, 2006.

[147] W. Zhang, W. Ge, C. Li et al., "Effects of mesenchymal stem cells on differentiation, maturation, and function of human monocyte-derived dendritic cells," *Stem Cells and Development*, vol. 13, no. 3, pp. 263–271, 2004.

[148] B. Zhang, R. Liu, D. Shi et al., "Mesenchymal stem cells induce mature dendritic cells into a novel Jagged-2 dependent regulatory dendritic cell population," *Blood*, vol. 113, no. 1, pp. 46–57, 2009.

[149] G. M. Spaggiari, A. Capobianco, S. Becchetti, M. C. Mingari, and L. Moretta, "Mesenchymal stem cell-natural killer cell interactions: evidence that activated NK cells are capable of killing MSCs, whereas MSCs can inhibit IL-2-induced NK-cell proliferation," *Blood*, vol. 107, no. 4, pp. 1484–1490, 2006.

[150] S. Aggarwal and M. F. Pittenger, "Human mesenchymal stem cells modulate allogeneic immune cell responses," *Blood*, vol. 105, no. 4, pp. 1815–1822, 2005.

[151] H. Cao, J. Yang, J. Yu et al., "Therapeutic potential of transplanted placental mesenchymal stem cells in treating Chinese miniature pigs with acute liver failure," *BMC Medicine*, vol. 10, article 56, 2012.

[152] K. English, J. M. Ryan, L. Tobin, M. J. Murphy, F. P. Barry, and B. P. Mahon, "Cell contact, prostaglandin E2 and transforming growth factor beta 1 play non-redundant roles in human mesenchymal stem cell induction of CD4+CD25Highforkhead box P3+ regulatory T cells," *Clinical & Experimental Immunology*, vol. 156, no. 1, pp. 149–160, 2009.

[153] K.-A. Cho, S.-Y. Ju, S. J. Cho et al., "Mesenchymal stem cells showed the highest potential for the regeneration of injured liver tissue compared with other subpopulations of the bone marrow," *Cell Biology International*, vol. 33, no. 7, pp. 772–777, 2009.

[154] I. Pascual-Miguelañez, J. Salinas-Gomez, D. Fernandez-Luengas et al., "Systemic treatment of acute liver failure with adipose derived stem cells," *Journal of Investigative Surgery*, vol. 28, no. 2, pp. 120–126, 2015.

[155] F. Salomone, I. Barbagallo, L. Puzzo, C. Piazza, and G. Li Volti, "Efficacy of adipose tissue-mesenchymal stem cell transplantation in rats with acetaminophen liver injury," *Stem Cell Research*, vol. 11, no. 3, pp. 1037–1044, 2013.

[156] X. Zhu, B. He, X. Zhou, and J. Ren, "Effects of transplanted bone-marrow-derived mesenchymal stem cells in animal models of acute hepatitis," *Cell and Tissue Research*, vol. 351, no. 3, pp. 477–486, 2013.

[157] G. Chamberlain, J. Fox, B. Ashton, and J. Middleton, "Concise review: mesenchymal stem cells: their phenotype, differentiation capacity, immunological features, and potential for homing," *Stem Cells*, vol. 25, no. 11, pp. 2739–2749, 2007.

[158] A. Gebler, O. Zabel, and B. Seliger, "The immunomodulatory capacity of mesenchymal stem cells," *Trends in Molecular Medicine*, vol. 18, no. 2, pp. 128–134, 2012.

[159] K.-A. Cho, S.-Y. Woo, J.-Y. Seoh, H.-S. Han, and K.-H. Ryu, "Mesenchymal stem cells restore CCl_4-induced liver injury by an antioxidative process," *Cell Biology International*, vol. 36, no. 12, pp. 1267–1274, 2012.

[160] L. F. Quintanilha, T. Takami, Y. Hirose et al., "Canine mesenchymal stem cells show antioxidant properties against thioacetamide-induced liver injury in vitro and in vivo," *Hepatology Research*, vol. 44, no. 10, pp. E206–E217, 2014.

[161] E. R. Marsden, Z. Hu, K. Fujio, H. Nakatsukasa, S. S. Thorgeirsson, and R. P. Evarts, "Expression of acidic fibroblast growth factor in regenerating liver and during hepatic differentiation," *Laboratory Investigation*, vol. 67, no. 4, pp. 427–433, 1992.

[162] G. K. Michalopoulos, "Liver regeneration after partial hepatectomy: critical analysis of mechanistic dilemmas," *The American Journal of Pathology*, vol. 176, no. 1, pp. 2–13, 2010.

[163] K. Nozawa, Y. Kurumiya, A. Yamamoto, Y. Isobe, M. Suzuki, and S. Yoshida, "Up-regulation of telomerase in primary cultured rat hepatocytes," *The Journal of Biochemistry*, vol. 126, no. 2, pp. 361–367, 1999.

[164] E. M. Webber, P. J. Godowski, and N. Fausto, "In vivo response of hepatocytes to growth factors requires an initial priming stimulus," *Hepatology*, vol. 19, no. 2, pp. 489–497, 1994.

[165] S. U. Kim, H. J. Oh, I. R. Wanless, S. Lee, K.-H. Han, and Y. N. Park, "The Laennec staging system for histological subclassification of cirrhosis is useful for stratification of prognosis in patients with liver cirrhosis," *Journal of Hepatology*, vol. 57, no. 3, pp. 556–563, 2012.

[166] L. Wang, X. Wang, L. Wang et al., "Hepatic vascular endothelial growth factor regulates recruitment of rat liver sinusoidal endothelial cell progenitor cells," *Gastroenterology*, vol. 143, no. 6, pp. 1555–e2, 2012.

[167] C. Lange, P. Bassler, M. V. Lioznov et al., "Liver-specific gene expression in mesenchymal stem cells is induced by liver cells," *World Journal of Gastroenterology*, vol. 11, no. 29, pp. 4497–4504, 2005.

[168] J. M. Luk, P. P. Wang, C. K. Lee, J. H. Wang, and S. T. Fan, "Hepatic potential of bone marrow stromal cells: development of in vitro co-culture and intra-portal transplantation models," *Journal of Immunological Methods*, vol. 305, no. 1, pp. 39–47, 2005.

[169] A. Banas, T. Teratani, Y. Yamamoto et al., "Rapid hepatic fate specification of adipose-derived stem cells and their therapeutic potential for liver failure," *Journal of Gastroenterology and Hepatology*, vol. 24, no. 1, pp. 70–77, 2009.

[170] N. Ishkitiev, K. Yaegaki, B. Calenic et al., "Deciduous and permanent dental pulp mesenchymal cells acquire hepatic morphologic and functional features in vitro," *Journal of Endodontics*, vol. 36, no. 3, pp. 469–474, 2010.

[171] K.-D. Lee, T. K.-C. Kuo, J. Whang-Peng et al., "In vitro hepatic differentiation of human mesenchymal stem cells," *Hepatology*, vol. 40, no. 6, pp. 1275–1284, 2004.

[172] L. Ling, Y. Ni, Q. Wang et al., "Transdifferentiation of mesenchymal stem cells derived from human fetal lung to hepatocyte-like cells," *Cell Biology International*, vol. 32, no. 9, pp. 1091–1098, 2008.

[173] M. J. Seo, S. Y. Suh, Y. C. Bae, and J. S. Jung, "Differentiation of human adipose stromal cells into hepatic lineage *in vitro* and *in vivo*," *Biochemical and Biophysical Research Communications*, vol. 328, no. 1, pp. 258–264, 2005.

[174] Y.-B. Zheng, Z.-L. Gao, C. Xie et al., "Characterization and hepatogenic differentiation of mesenchymal stem cells from human amniotic fluid and human bone marrow: a comparative study," *Cell Biology International*, vol. 32, no. 11, pp. 1439–1448, 2008.

[175] A. Xagorari, E. Siotou, M. Yiangou et al., "Protective effect of mesenchymal stem cell-conditioned medium on hepatic cell apoptosis after acute liver injury," *International Journal of Clinical and Experimental Pathology*, vol. 6, no. 5, pp. 831–840, 2013.

[176] D. van Poll, B. Parekkadan, C. H. Cho et al., "Mesenchymal stem cell-derived molecules directly modulate hepatocellular death and regeneration *in vitro* and *in vivo*," *Hepatology*, vol. 47, no. 5, pp. 1634–1643, 2008.

[177] B. Parekkadan, D. van Poll, K. Suganuma et al., "Mesenchymal stem cell-derived molecules reverse fulminant hepatic failure," *PLoS ONE*, vol. 2, no. 9, article e941, 2007.

[178] S. Yuan, T. Jiang, R. Zheng, L. Sun, G. Cao, and Y. Zhang, "Effect of bone marrow mesenchymal stem cell transplantation on acute hepatic failure in rats," *Experimental and Therapeutic Medicine*, vol. 8, no. 4, pp. 1150–1158, 2014.

[179] S. Zhang, L. Chen, T. Liu et al., "Human umbilical cord matrix stem cells efficiently rescue acute liver failure through paracrine effects rather than hepatic differentiation," *Tissue Engineering Part A*, vol. 18, no. 13-14, pp. 1352–1364, 2012.

[180] Y. O. Jang, M. Y. Kim, M. Y. Cho, S. K. Baik, Y. Z. Cho, and S. O. Kwon, "Effect of bone marrow-derived mesenchymal stem cells on hepatic fibrosis in a thioacetamide-induced cirrhotic rat model," *BMC Gastroenterology*, vol. 14, no. 1, article 198, 2014.

[181] D. C. Zhao, J. X. Lei, R. Chen et al., "Bone marrow-derived mesenchymal stem cells protect against experimental liver fibrosis in rats," *World Journal of Gastroenterology*, vol. 11, no. 22, pp. 3431–3440, 2005.

[182] Y. Wang, F. Lian, J. Li et al., "Adipose derived mesenchymal stem cells transplantation via portal vein improves microcirculation and ameliorates liver fibrosis induced by CCl4 in rats," *Journal of Translational Medicine*, vol. 10, no. 1, article 133, 2012.

[183] F. Yu, S. Ji, L. Su et al., "Adipose-derived mesenchymal stem cells inhibit activation of hepatic stellate cells invitro and ameliorate rat liver fibrosis invivo," *Journal of the Formosan Medical Association*, vol. 114, no. 2, pp. 130–138, 2015.

[184] V. Ninichuk, O. Gross, S. Segerer et al., "Multipotent mesenchymal stem cells reduce interstitial fibrosis but do not delay progression of chronic kidney disease in collagen4A3-deficient mice," *Kidney International*, vol. 70, no. 1, pp. 121–129, 2006.

[185] S. Ohnishi, H. Sumiyoshi, S. Kitamura, and N. Nagaya, "Mesenchymal stem cells attenuate cardiac fibroblast proliferation and collagen synthesis through paracrine actions," *FEBS Letters*, vol. 581, no. 21, pp. 3961–3966, 2007.

[186] L. A. Ortiz, F. Gambelli, C. McBride et al., "Mesenchymal stem cell engraftment in lung is enhanced in response to bleomycin exposure and ameliorates its fibrotic effects," *Proceedings of the National Acadamy of Sciences of the United States of America*, vol. 100, no. 14, pp. 8407–8411, 2003.

[187] M. Rojas, J. Xu, C. R. Woods et al., "Bone marrow-derived mesenchymal stem cells in repair of the injured lung," *American Journal of Respiratory Cell and Molecular Biology*, vol. 33, no. 2, pp. 145–152, 2005.

[188] I. Aurich, L. P. Mueller, H. Aurich et al., "Functional integration of hepatocytes derived from human mesenchymal stem cells into mouse livers," *Gut*, vol. 56, no. 3, pp. 405–415, 2007.

[189] L.-J. Dai, H. Y. Li, L.-X. Guan, G. Ritchie, and J. X. Zhou, "The therapeutic potential of bone marrow-derived mesenchymal stem cells on hepatic cirrhosis," *Stem Cell Research*, vol. 2, no. 1, pp. 16–25, 2009.

[190] T. K. Kuo, S.-P. Hung, C.-H. Chuang et al., "Stem cell therapy for liver disease: parameters governing the success of using bone marrow mesenchymal stem cells," *Gastroenterology*, vol. 134, no. 7, pp. 2111.e3–2121.e3, 2008.

[191] V. Rabani, M. Shahsavani, M. Gharavi, A. Piryaei, Z. Azhdari, and H. Baharvand, "Mesenchymal stem cell infusion therapy in a carbon tetrachloride-induced liver fibrosis model affects matrix metalloproteinase expression," *Cell Biology International*, vol. 34, no. 6, pp. 601–605, 2010.

[192] Y. Sato, H. Araki, J. Kato et al., "Human mesenchymal stem cells xenografted directly to rat liver are differentiated into human hepatocytes without fusion," *Blood*, vol. 106, no. 2, pp. 756–763, 2005.

[193] S. Pulavendran, J. Vignesh, and C. Rose, "Differential anti-inflammatory and anti-fibrotic activity of transplanted mesenchymal vs. Hematopoietic stem cells in carbon tetrachloride-induced liver injury in mice," *International Immunopharmacology*, vol. 10, no. 4, pp. 513–519, 2010.

[194] N. Lin, K. Hu, S. Chen et al., "Nerve growth factor-mediated paracrine regulation of hepatic stellate cells by multipotent mesenchymal stromal cells," *Life Sciences*, vol. 85, no. 7-8, pp. 291–295, 2009.

[195] B. Parekkadan, D. van Poll, Z. Megeed et al., "Immunomodulation of activated hepatic stellate cells by mesenchymal stem cells," *Biochemical and Biophysical Research Communications*, vol. 363, no. 2, pp. 247–252, 2007.

[196] T. Kinnaird, E. S. Burnett, M. Shou et al., "Local delivery of marrow-derived stromal cells augments collateral perfusion through paracrine mechanisms," *Circulation*, vol. 109, no. 12, pp. 1543–1549, 2004.

[197] M. F. Pittenger, "Mesenchymal stem cells from adult bone marrow," *Methods in Molecular Biology*, vol. 449, pp. 27–44, 2008.

[198] J. A. Thomson, J. Itskovitz-Eldor, S. S. Shapiro et al., "Embryonic stem cell lines derived from human blastocysts," *Science*, vol. 282, no. 5391, pp. 1145–1147, 1998.

[199] G. Brolén, L. Sivertsson, P. Björquist et al., "Hepatocyte-like cells derived from human embryonic stem cells specifically via definitive endoderm and a progenitor stage," *Journal of Biotechnology*, vol. 145, no. 3, pp. 284–294, 2010.

[200] D. C. Hay, J. Fletcher, C. Payne et al., "Highly efficient differentiation of hESCs to functional hepatic endoderm requires ActivinA and Wnt3a signaling," *Proceedings of the National Acadamy of Sciences of the United States of America*, vol. 105, no. 34, pp. 12301–12306, 2008.

[201] D.-H. Woo, S.-K. Kim, H.-J. Lim et al., "Direct and indirect contribution of human embryonic stem cellderived hepatocyte-like cells to liver repair in mice," *Gastroenterology*, vol. 142, no. 3, pp. 602–611, 2012.

[202] K. Cameron, R. Tan, W. Schmidt-Heck et al., "Recombinant Laminins Drive the Differentiation and Self-Organization of hESC-Derived Hepatocytes," *Stem Cell Reports*, vol. 5, no. 6, pp. 1250–1262, 2015.

[203] Y. Duan, A. Catana, Y. Meng et al., "Differentiation and enrichment of hepatocyte-like cells from human embryonic stem cells in vitro and in vivo," *Stem Cells*, vol. 25, no. 12, pp. 3058–3068, 2007.

[204] N. Lavon, O. Yanuka, and N. Benvenisty, "Differentiation and isolation of hepatic-like cells from human embryonic stem cells," *Differentiation*, vol. 72, no. 5, pp. 230–238, 2004.

[205] H. Rashidi, S. Alhaque, D. Szkolnicka, O. Flint, and D. C. Hay, "Fluid shear stress modulation of hepatocyte-like cell function," *Archives of Toxicology*, vol. 90, no. 7, pp. 1757–1761, 2016.

[206] G. M. Morrison, I. Oikonomopoulou, R. P. Migueles et al., "Anterior definitive endoderm from ESCs reveals a role for FGF signaling," *Cell Stem Cell*, vol. 3, no. 4, pp. 402–415, 2008.

[207] S. Agarwal, K. L. Holton, and R. Lanza, "Efficient differentiation of functional hepatocytes from human embryonic stem cells," *Stem Cells*, vol. 26, no. 5, pp. 1117–1127, 2008.

[208] J. Cai, Y. Zhao, Y. Liu et al., "Directed differentiation of human embryonic stem cells into functional hepatic cells," *Hepatology*, vol. 45, no. 5, pp. 1229–1239, 2007.

[209] S. J. Forbes, S. Gupta, and A. Dhawan, "Cell therapy for liver disease: from liver transplantation to cell factory," *Journal of Hepatology*, vol. 62, no. 1, supplement, pp. S157–S169, 2015.

[210] H. Basma, A. Soto-Gutiérrez, G. R. Yannam et al., "Differentiation and transplantation of human embryonic stem cell-derived hepatocytes," *Gastroenterology*, vol. 136, no. 3, pp. 990.e4–999.e4, 2009.

[211] Y. Duan, X. Ma, W. E. I. Zou et al., "Differentiation and characterization of metabolically functioning hepatocytes from human embryonic stem cells," *Stem Cells*, vol. 28, no. 4, pp. 674–686, 2010.

[212] T. N. Bukong, T. Lo, G. Szabo, and A. Dolganiuc, "Novel developmental biology-based protocol of embryonic stem cell differentiation to morphologically sound and functional yet immature hepatocytes," *Liver International*, vol. 32, no. 5, pp. 732–741, 2012.

[213] D. C. Hay, D. Zhao, J. Fletcher et al., "Efficient differentiation of hepatocytes from human embryonic stem cells exhibiting markers recapitulating liver development in vivo," *Stem Cells*, vol. 26, no. 4, pp. 894–902, 2008.

[214] C. N. Medine, B. Lucendo-Villarin, C. Storck et al., "Developing high-fidelity hepatotoxicity models from pluripotent stem cells," *Stem Cells Translational Medicine*, vol. 2, no. 7, pp. 505–509, 2013.

[215] N. S. Sharma, E. J. Wallenstein, E. Novik, T. Maguire, R. Schloss, and M. L. Yarmush, "Enrichment of hepatocyte-like cells with upregulated metabolic and differentiated function derived from embryonic stem cells using s-nitrosoacetylpenicillamine," *Tissue Engineering - Part C: Methods*, vol. 15, no. 2, pp. 297–306, 2009.

[216] T. Touboul, N. R. F. Hannan, S. Corbineau et al., "Generation of functional hepatocytes from human embryonic stem cells under chemically defined conditions that recapitulate liver development," *Hepatology*, vol. 51, no. 5, pp. 1754–1765, 2010.

[217] N. Tuleuova, J. Y. Lee, J. Lee, E. Ramanculov, M. A. Zern, and A. Revzin, "Using growth factor arrays and micropatterned co-cultures to induce hepatic differentiation of embryonic stem cells," *Biomaterials*, vol. 31, no. 35, pp. 9221–9231, 2010.

[218] H. Yamamoto, G. Quinn, A. Asari et al., "Differentiation of embryonic stem cells into hepatocytes: Biological functions and therapeutic application," *Hepatology*, vol. 37, no. 5, pp. 983–993, 2003.

[219] L. Tolosa, J. Caron, Z. Hannoun et al., "Transplantation of hESC-derived hepatocytes protects mice from liver injury," *Stem Cell Research & Therapy*, vol. 6, article 246, 2015.

[220] K. Moriya, M. Yoshikawa, K. Saito et al., "Embryonic stem cells develop into hepatocytes after intrasplenic transplantation in CCl_4-treated mice," *World Journal of Gastroenterology*, vol. 13, no. 6, pp. 866–873, 2007.

[221] O. Cooper, G. Hargus, M. Deleidi et al., "Differentiation of human ES and Parkinson's disease iPS cells into ventral midbrain dopaminergic neurons requires a high activity form of SHH, FGF8a and specific regionalization by retinoic acid," *Molecular and Cellular Neuroscience*, vol. 45, no. 3, pp. 258–266, 2010.

[222] S. Nori, Y. Okada, A. Yasuda et al., "Grafted human-induced pluripotent stem-cell-derived neurospheres promote motor functional recovery after spinal cord injury in mice," *Proceedings of the National Acadamy of Sciences of the United States of America*, vol. 108, no. 40, pp. 16825–16830, 2011.

[223] T. Tanaka, S. Tohyama, M. Murata et al., "*In vitro* pharmacologic testing using human induced pluripotent stem cell-derived cardiomyocytes," *Biochemical and Biophysical Research Communications*, vol. 385, no. 4, pp. 497–502, 2009.

[224] N. Yokoo, S. Baba, S. Kaichi et al., "The effects of cardioactive drugs on cardiomyocytes derived from human induced pluripotent stem cells," *Biochemical and Biophysical Research Communications*, vol. 387, no. 3, pp. 482–488, 2009.

[225] J. Zhang, G. F. Wilson, A. G. Soerens et al., "Functional cardiomyocytes derived from human induced pluripotent stem cells," *Circulation Research*, vol. 104, no. 4, pp. e30–e41, 2009.

[226] K.-D. Choi, J. Yu, K. Smuga-Otto et al., "Hematopoietic and endothelial differentiation of human induced pluripotent stem cells," *Stem Cells*, vol. 27, no. 3, pp. 559–567, 2009.

[227] K. Tateishi, J. He, O. Taranova, G. Liang, A. C. D'Alessio, and Y. Zhang, "Generation of insulin-secreting islet-like clusters from human skin fibroblasts," *The Journal of Biological Chemistry*, vol. 283, no. 46, pp. 31601–31607, 2008.

[228] S. Gerbal-Chaloin, N. Funakoshi, A. Caillaud, C. Gondeau, B. Champon, and K. Si-Tayeb, "Human induced pluripotent stem cells in hepatology: beyond the proof of concept," *The American Journal of Pathology*, vol. 184, no. 2, pp. 332–347, 2014.

[229] Y. Kondo, T. Iwao, K. Nakamura et al., "An efficient method for differentiation of human induced pluripotent stem cells into hepatocyte-like cells retaining drug metabolizing activity," *Drug Metabolism and Pharmacokinetics*, vol. 29, no. 3, pp. 237–243, 2014.

[230] H. Okano, M. Nakamura, K. Yoshida et al., "Steps toward safe cell therapy using induced pluripotent stem cells," *Circulation Research*, vol. 112, no. 3, pp. 523–533, 2013.

[231] Z. Song, J. Cai, Y. Liu et al., "Efficient generation of hepatocyte-like cells from human induced pluripotent stem cells," *Cell Research*, vol. 19, no. 11, pp. 1233–1242, 2009.

[232] M. Baxter, S. Withey, S. Harrison et al., "Phenotypic and functional analyses show stem cell-derived hepatocyte-like cells better mimic fetal rather than adult hepatocytes," *Journal of Hepatology*, vol. 62, no. 3, pp. 581–589, 2015.

[233] G. J. Sullivan, D. C. Hay, I.-H. Park et al., "Generation of functional human hepatic endoderm from human induced pluripotent stem cells," *Hepatology*, vol. 51, no. 1, pp. 329–335, 2010.

[234] Y.-F. Chen, C.-Y. Tseng, H.-W. Wang, H.-C. Kuo, V. W. Yang, and O. K. Lee, "Rapid generation of mature hepatocyte-like cells from human induced pluripotent stem cells by an efficient three-step protocol," *Hepatology*, vol. 55, no. 4, pp. 1193–1203, 2012.

[235] S. Asgari, M. Moslem, K. Bagheri-Lankarani, B. Pournasr, M. Miryounesi, and H. Baharvand, "Differentiation and Transplantation of Human Induced Pluripotent Stem Cell-derived Hepatocyte-like Cells," *Stem Cell Reviews and Reports*, vol. 9, no. 4, pp. 493–504, 2013.

[236] K. Takayama, M. Inamura, K. Kawabata et al., "Generation of metabolically functioning hepatocytes from human pluripotent stem cells by FOXA2 and HNF1α transduction," *Journal of Hepatology*, vol. 57, no. 3, pp. 628–636, 2012.

[237] K. Takayama, M. Inamura, K. Kawabata et al., "Efficient generation of functional hepatocytes from human embryonic stem cells and induced pluripotent stem cells by HNF4α transduction," *Molecular Therapy*, vol. 20, no. 1, pp. 127–137, 2012.

[238] Q. Zhang, Y. Yang, J. Zhang et al., "Efficient derivation of functional hepatocytes from mouse induced pluripotent stem cells by a combination of cytokines and sodium butyrate," *Chinese Medical Journal*, vol. 124, no. 22, pp. 3786–3793, 2011.

[239] A. Ghodsizadeh, A. Taei, M. Totonchi et al., "Generation of liver disease-specific induced pluripotent stem cells along with efficient differentiation to functional hepatocyte-like cells," *Stem Cell Reviews and Reports*, vol. 6, no. 4, pp. 622–632, 2010.

[240] S. T. Rashid, S. Corbineau, N. Hannan et al., "Modeling inherited metabolic disorders of the liver using human induced pluripotent stem cells," *The Journal of Clinical Investigation*, vol. 120, no. 9, pp. 3127–3136, 2010.

[241] P. Sancho-Bru, P. Roelandt, N. Narain et al., "Directed differentiation of murine-induced pluripotent stem cells to functional hepatocyte-like cells," *Journal of Hepatology*, vol. 54, no. 1, pp. 98–107, 2011.

[242] S. Zhang, S. Chen, W. Li et al., "Rescue of ATP7B function in hepatocyte-like cells from Wilson's disease induced pluripotent stem cells using gene therapy or the chaperone drug curcumin," *Human Molecular Genetics*, vol. 20, no. 16, Article ID ddr223, pp. 3176–3187, 2011.

[243] S. Espejel, G. R. Roll, and K. J. McLaughlin, "Induced pluripotent stem cell-derived hepatocytes have the functional and proliferative capabilities needed for liver regeneration in mice," *The Journal of Clinical Investigation*, vol. 120, no. 9, pp. 3120–3126, 2010.

[244] K. Yusa, S. T. Rashid, H. Strick-Marchand et al., "Targeted gene correction of alpha1-antitrypsin deficiency in induced pluripotent stem cells," *Nature*, vol. 478, no. 7369, pp. 391–394, 2011.

[245] J. Harding and O. Mirochnitchenko, "Preclinical studies for induced pluripotent stem cell-based therapeutics," *The Journal of Biological Chemistry*, vol. 289, no. 8, pp. 4585–4593, 2014.

[246] V. K. Singh, M. Kalsan, N. Kumar, A. Saini, and R. Chandra, "Induced pluripotent stem cells: applications in regenerative medicine, disease modeling, and drug discovery," *Frontiers in Cell and Developmental Biology*, vol. 3, no. 2, 2015.

[247] S. J. Yu, J.-H. Yoon, W. Kim et al., "Ultrasound-guided percutaneous portal transplantation of peripheral blood monocytes in patients with liver cirrhosis," *Korean Journal of Internal Medicine*, vol. 32, no. 2, pp. 261–268, 2017.

[248] T. Zhao, Z.-N. Zhang, Z. Rong, and Y. Xu, "Immunogenicity of induced pluripotent stem cells," *Nature*, vol. 474, no. 7350, pp. 212–215, 2011.

[249] R. Araki, M. Uda, Y. Hoki et al., "Negligible immunogenicity of terminally differentiated cells derived from induced pluripotent or embryonic stem cells," *Nature*, vol. 494, no. 7435, pp. 100–104, 2013.

[250] L. Tolosa, E. Pareja, and M. J. Gómez-Lechón, "Clinical Application of Pluripotent Stem Cells: An Alternative Cell-Based Therapy for Treating Liver Diseases?" *Transplantation*, vol. 100, no. 12, pp. 2548–2557, 2016.

[251] Y. Haruna, K. Saito, S. Spaulding, M. A. Nalesnik, and M. A. Gerber, "Identification of bipotential progenitor cells in human liver development," *Hepatology*, vol. 23, no. 3, pp. 476–481, 1996.

[252] E. Schmelzer, L. Zhang, A. Bruce et al., "Human hepatic stem cells from fetal and postnatal donors," *The Journal of Experimental Medicine*, vol. 204, no. 8, pp. 1973–1987, 2007.

[253] N. Shiojiri and T. Mizuno, "Differentiation of functional hepatocytes and biliary epithelial cells from immature hepatocytes of the fetal mouse in vitro," *Anatomy and Embryology*, vol. 187, no. 3, pp. 221–229, 1993.

[254] T. Cantz, D. M. Zuckerman, M. R. Burda et al., "Quantitative gene expression analysis reveals transition of fetal liver progenitor cells to mature hepatocytes after transplantation in uPA/RAG-2 mice," *The American Journal of Pathology*, vol. 162, no. 1, pp. 37–45, 2003.

[255] M. Oertel, A. Menthena, Y.-Q. Chen, B. Teisner, C. H. Jensen, and D. A. Shafritz, "Purification of fetal liver stem/progenitor cells containing all the repopulation potential for normal adult rat liver," *Gastroenterology*, vol. 134, no. 3, pp. 823–832, 2008.

[256] J. S. Sandhu, P. M. Petkov, M. D. Dabeva, and D. A. Shafritz, "Stem cell properties and repopulation of the rat liver by fetal liver epithelial progenitor cells," *The American Journal of Pathology*, vol. 159, no. 4, pp. 1323–1334, 2001.

[257] C. van de Ven, D. Collins, M. B. Bradley, E. Morris, and M. S. Cairo, "The potential of umbilical cord blood multipotent stem cells for nonhematopoietic tissue and cell regeneration," *Experimental Hematology*, vol. 35, no. 12, pp. 1753–1765, 2007.

[258] D. Campard, P. A. Lysy, M. Najimi, and E. M. Sokal, "Native umbilical cord matrix stem cells express hepatic markers and differentiate into hepatocyte-like cells," *Gastroenterology*, vol. 134, no. 3, pp. 833–848, 2008.

[259] K. Teramoto, K. Asahina, Y. Kumashiro et al., "Hepatocyte differentiation from embryonic stem cells and umbilical cord blood cells," *Journal of Hepato-Biliary-Pancreatic Sciences*, vol. 12, no. 3, pp. 196–202, 2005.

[260] C.-C. Chien, B. L. Yen, F.-K. Lee et al., "*In vitro* differentiation of human placenta-derived multipotent cells into hepatocyte-like cells," *Stem Cells*, vol. 24, no. 7, pp. 1759–1768, 2006.

[261] M. Bhatia, A. G. Elefanty, S. J. Fisher, R. Patient, T. Schlaeger, and E. Y. Snyder, *Current Protocols in Stem Cell Biology*, John Wiley & Sons, Inc., Hoboken, NJ, USA, 2007.

[262] S. Lorenzini and P. Andreone, "Stem cell therapy for human liver cirrhosis: A cautious analysis of the results," *Stem Cells*, vol. 25, no. 9, pp. 2383-2384, 2007.

[263] Y. Q. Xu and Z. C. Liu, "Therapeutic Potential of Adult Bone Marrow Stem Cells in Liver Disease and Delivery Approaches," *Stem Cell Reviews and Reports*, vol. 4, no. 2, pp. 101–112, 2008.

[264] M. Y. Gordon, N. Levičar, M. Pai et al., "Characterization and clinical application of human $CD34^+$ stem/progenitor cell populations mobilized into the blood by granulocyte colony-stimulating factor," *Stem Cells*, vol. 24, no. 7, pp. 1822–1830, 2006.

[265] A. A. Khan, N. Parveen, V. S. Mahaboob et al., "Safety and Efficacy of Autologous Bone Marrow Stem Cell Transplantation Through Hepatic Artery for the Treatment of Chronic Liver Failure: A Preliminary Study," *Transplantation Proceedings*, vol. 40, no. 4, pp. 1140–1144, 2008.

[266] J. K. Kim, Y. N. Park, J. S. Kim et al., "Autologous bone marrow infusion activates the progenitor cell compartment in patients with advanced liver cirrhosis," *Cell Transplantation*, vol. 19, no. 10, pp. 1237–1246, 2010.

[267] M. Mohamadnejad, K. Alimoghaddam, M. Mohyeddin-Bonab et al., "Phase 1 trial of autologous bone marrow mesenchymal stem cell transplantation in patients with decompensated liver cirrhosis," *Archives of Iranian Medicine*, vol. 10, no. 4, pp. 459–466, 2007.

[268] M. Mohamadnejad, M. Namiri, M. Bagheri et al., "Phase 1 human trial of autologous bone marrow-hematopoietic stem cell transplantation in patients with decompensated cirrhosis," *World Journal of Gastroenterology*, vol. 13, no. 24, pp. 3359–3363, 2007.

[269] H. Salama, A.-R. Zekri, M. Zern et al., "Autologous hematopoietic stem cell transplantation in 48 patients with end-stage chronic liver diseases," *Cell Transplantation*, vol. 19, no. 11, pp. 1475–1486, 2010.

[270] E. Yannaki, A. Anagnostopoulos, D. Kapetanos et al., "Lasting amelioration in the clinical course of decompensated alcoholic cirrhosis with boost infusions of mobilized peripheral blood stem cells," *Experimental Hematology*, vol. 34, no. 11, pp. 1583–1587, 2006.

[271] J. Schulte Am Esch II, W. T. Knoefel, M. Klein et al., "Portal application of autologous $CD133^+$ bone marrow cells to the liver: a novel concept to support hepatic regeneration," *Stem Cells*, vol. 23, no. 4, pp. 463–470, 2005.

[272] G. Fürst, J. Schulte Am Esch, L. W. Poll et al., "Portal vein embolization and autologous CD133+ bone marrow stem cells for liver regeneration: Initial experience," *Radiology*, vol. 243, no. 1, pp. 171–179, 2007.

[273] A. Ismail, A. Aldorry, M. Shaker et al., "Simultaneous injection of autologous mononuclear cells with TACE in HCC patients; Preliminary study," *Journal of Gastrointestinal Cancer*, vol. 42, no. 1, pp. 11–19, 2011.

[274] A. E. Karnoub, A. B. Dash, A. P. Vo et al., "Mesenchymal stem cells within tumour stroma promote breast cancer metastasis," *Nature*, vol. 449, no. 7162, pp. 557–563, 2007.

[275] I. Matushansky, E. Hernando, N. D. Socci et al., "Derivation of sarcomas from mesenchymal stem cells via inactivation of the Wnt pathway," *The Journal of Clinical Investigation*, vol. 117, no. 11, pp. 3248–3257, 2007.

[276] A. A. Khan, M. V. Shaik, N. Parveen et al., "Human fetal liver-derived stem cell transplantation as supportive modality in the management of end-stage decompensated liver cirrhosis," *Cell Transplantation*, vol. 19, no. 4, pp. 409–418, 2010.

[277] G. Lanzoni, T. Oikawa, Y. Wang et al., "Concise review: clinical programs of stem cell therapies for liver and pancreas," *Stem Cells*, vol. 31, no. 10, pp. 2047–2060, 2013.

[278] G. R. Burganova, "Effectiveness of autologous hematopoietic stem cells transplantation in patients with liver cirrhosis," *Experimental & Clinical Gastroenterology*, vol. no. 4, pp. 91–97, 2012.

[279] A. King, D. Barton, H. A. Beard et al., "REpeated AutoLogous Infusions of STem cells in Cirrhosis (REALISTIC): a multicentre, phase II, open-label, randomised controlled trial of repeated autologous infusions of granulocyte colony-stimulating factor (GCSF) mobilised CD133+ bone marrow stem cells in patients with cirrhosis. A study protocol for a randomised controlled trial," *BMJ Open*, vol. 5, no. 3, Article ID e007700, 2015.

[280] C. Margini, R. Vukotic, L. Brodosi, M. Bernardi, and P. Andreone, "Bone marrow derived stem cells for the treatment of

end-stage liver disease," *World Journal of Gastroenterology*, no. 27, pp. 9098–9105, 2014.

[281] A. R. Zekri, H. Salama, and E. Medhat, "The impact of repeated autologous infusion of haematopoietic stem cells in patients with liver insufficiency," *Stem Cell Research & Therapy*, vol. 6, no. 1, p. 118, 2015.

[282] M. A. Amin, D. Sabry, L. A. Rashed et al., "Short-term evaluation of autologous transplantation of bone marrow-derived mesenchymal stem cells in patients with cirrhosis: Egyptian study," *Clinical Transplantation*, vol. 27, no. 4, pp. 607–612, 2013.

[283] M. El-Ansary, I. Abdel-Aziz, S. Mogawer et al., "Phase II trial: undifferentiated versus differentiated autologous mesenchymal stem cells transplantation in Egyptian patients with HCV induced liver cirrhosis," *Stem Cell Reviews and Reports*, vol. 8, no. 3, pp. 972–981, 2012.

[284] Y. O. Jang, Y. J. Kim, S. K. Baik et al., "Histological improvement following administration of autologous bone marrow-derived mesenchymal stem cells for alcoholic cirrhosis: a pilot study," *Liver International*, vol. 34, no. 1, pp. 33–41, 2014.

[285] L. Peng, D.-Y. Xie, B.-L. Lin et al., "Autologous bone marrow mesenchymal stem cell transplantation in liver failure patients caused by hepatitis B: short-term and long-term outcomes," *Hepatology*, vol. 54, no. 3, pp. 820–828, 2011.

[286] M. Mohamadnejad, K. Alimoghaddam, M. Bagheri et al., "Randomized placebo-controlled trial of mesenchymal stem cell transplantation in decompensated cirrhosis," *Liver International*, vol. 33, no. 10, pp. 1490–1496, 2013.

[287] S. Berardis, P. D. Sattwika, M. Najimi, and E. M. Sokal, "Use of mesenchymal stem cells to treat liver fibrosis: current situation and future prospects," *World Journal of Gastroenterology*, vol. 21, no. 3, pp. 742–758, 2015.

[288] M. Shi, Z. Zhang, and R. Xu, "Human mesenchymal stem cell transfusion is safe and improves liver function in acute-on-chronic liver failure patients," *Stem Cells Translational Medicine*, vol. 1, no. 10, pp. 725–731, 2012.

[289] L. Wang, J. Li, H. Liu et al., "A pilot study of umbilical cord-derived mesenchymal stem cell transfusion in patients with primary biliary cirrhosis," *Journal of Gastroenterology and Hepatology*, vol. 28, no. 1, pp. 85–92, 2013.

[290] Z. Zhang, H. Lin, M. Shi et al., "Human umbilical cord mesenchymal stem cells improve liver function and ascites in decompensated liver cirrhosis patients," *Journal of Gastroenterology and Hepatology*, vol. 27, supplement 2, pp. 112–120, 2012.

[291] M. Blachier, H. Leleu, M. Peck-Radosavljevic, D.-C. Valla, and F. Roudot-Thoraval, "The burden of liver disease in Europe: a review of available epidemiological data," *Journal of Hepatology*, vol. 58, no. 3, pp. 593–608, 2013.

[292] J. Polson and W. M. Lee, "AASLD position paper: The management of acute liver failure," *Hepatology*, vol. 41, no. 5, pp. 1179–1197, 2005.

[293] R. Jalan, P. Gines, J. C. Olson et al., "Acute-on chronic liver failure," *Journal of Hepatology*, vol. 57, no. 6, pp. 1336–1348, 2012.

[294] R. Williams, "Global challenges in liver disease," *Hepatology*, vol. 44, no. 3, pp. 521–526, 2006.

[295] N. Kemmer, A. Alsina, and G. W. Neff, "Orthotopic liver transplantation in a multiethnic population: Role of spatial accessibility," *Transplantation Proceedings*, vol. 43, no. 10, pp. 3780–3782, 2011.

[296] S. J. Kim, C. W. Choi, D. H. Kang et al., "Emergency endoscopic variceal ligation in cirrhotic patients with blood clots in the stomach but no active bleeding or stigmata increases the risk of rebleeding," *Clinical and Molecular Hepatology*, vol. 22, no. 4, pp. 466–476, 2016.

[297] I. J. Fox and J. Roy-Chowdhury, "Hepatocyte transplantation," *Journal of Hepatology*, vol. 40, no. 6, pp. 878–886, 2004.

[298] S. C. Strom, R. A. Fisher, M. T. Thompson et al., "Hepatocyte transplantation as a bridge to orthotopic liver transplantation in terminal liver failure," *Transplantation*, vol. 63, no. 4, pp. 559–569, 1997.

[299] A. Dhawan, "Clinical human hepatocyte transplantation: Current status and challenges," *Liver Transplantation*, vol. 21, pp. S39–S44, 2015.

[300] M. C. Hansel, R. Gramignoli, K. J. Skvorak et al., "The history and use of human hepatocytes for the treatment of liver diseases: the first 100 patients," *Current Protocols in Toxicology*, vol. 62, pp. 14-12, 2014.

[301] S. L. Friedman, "Liver fibrosis—from bench to bedside," *Journal of Hepatology*, vol. 38, supplement 1, pp. 38–53, 2003.

[302] J.-T. Li, Z.-X. Liao, J. Ping, D. Xu, and H. Wang, "Molecular mechanism of hepatic stellate cell activation and antifibrotic therapeutic strategies," *Journal of Gastroenterology*, vol. 43, no. 6, pp. 419–428, 2008.

[303] E. Mormone, J. George, and N. Nieto, "Molecular pathogenesis of hepatic fibrosis and current therapeutic approaches," *Chemico-Biological Interactions*, vol. 193, no. 3, pp. 225–231, 2011.

[304] E. Albanis and S. L. Friedman, "Antifibrotic agents for liver disease," *American Journal of Transplantation*, vol. 6, no. 1, pp. 12–19, 2006.

[305] M. Ismail and M. Pinzani, "Reversal of hepatic fibrosis: pathophysiological basis of antifibrotic therapies," *Hepatic Medicine: Evidence and Research*, pp. 69–80, 2011.

[306] D. C. Rockey, "Current and future anti-fibrotic therapies for chronic liver disease," *Clinics in Liver Disease*, vol. 12, no. 4, pp. 939–962, 2008.

[307] R. Belfort, S. A. Harrison, K. Brown et al., "A placebo-controlled trial of pioglitazone in subjects with nonalcoholic steatohepatitis," *The New England Journal of Medicine*, vol. 355, no. 22, pp. 2297–2307, 2006.

[308] P. J. Pockros, L. Jeffers, N. Afdhal et al., "Final results of a double-blind, placebo-controlled trial of the antifibrotic efficacy of interferon-γ1b in chronic hepatitis C patients with advanced fibrosis or cirrhosis," *Hepatology*, vol. 45, no. 3, pp. 569–578, 2007.

[309] A. J. Sanyal, N. Chalasani, K. V. Kowdley et al., "Pioglitazone, vitamin E, or placebo for nonalcoholic steatohepatitis," *The New England Journal of Medicine*, vol. 362, no. 18, pp. 1675–1685, 2010.

[310] H.-L. Weng, B.-E. Wang, J.-D. Jia et al., "Effect of interferon-gamma on hepatic fibrosis in chronic hepatitis B virus infection: A randomized controlled study," *Clinical Gastroenterology and Hepatology*, vol. 3, no. 8, pp. 819–828, 2005.

[311] B. K. A. Dayyeh, M. Yang, J. L. Dienstag, and R. T. Chung, "The effects of angiotensin blocking agents on the progression of liver fibrosis in the HALT-C Trial cohort," *Digestive Diseases and Sciences*, vol. 56, no. 2, pp. 564–568, 2011.

[312] Q. Lang, Q. Liu, N. Xu et al., "The antifibrotic effects of TGF-β1 siRNA on hepatic fibrosis in rats," *Biochemical and Biophysical Research Communications*, vol. 409, no. 3, pp. 448–453, 2011.

[313] T. Nakamura, R. Sakata, T. Ueno, M. Sata, and H. Ueno, "Inhibition of transforming growth factor β prevents progression of liver fibrosis and enhances hepatocyte regeneration in dimethylnitrosamine- treated rats," *Hepatology*, vol. 32, no. 2, pp. 247–255, 2000.

[314] M. C. Wright, R. Issa, D. E. Smart et al., "Gliotoxin stimulates the apoptosis of human and rat hepatic stellate cells and enhances the resolution of liver fibrosis in rats," *Gastroenterology*, vol. 121, no. 3, pp. 685–698, 2001.

[315] S. Salgado, J. Garcia, J. Vera et al., "Liver cirrhosis is reverted by urokinase-type plasminogen activator gene therapy," *Molecular Therapy*, vol. 2, no. 6, pp. 545–551, 2000.

[316] H. Sugino, N. Kumagai, S. Watanabe et al., "Polaprezinc attenuates liver fibrosis in a mouse model of non-alcoholic steatohepatitis," *Journal of Gastroenterology and Hepatology*, vol. 23, no. 12, pp. 1909–1916, 2008.

[317] E. Mezey, J. J. Potter, L. Rennie-Tankersley, J. Caballeria, and A. Pares, "A randomized placebo controlled trial of vitamin E for alcoholic hepatitis," *Journal of Hepatology*, vol. 40, no. 1, pp. 40–46, 2004.

[318] D. R. Nelson, Z. Tu, C. Soldevila-Pico et al., "Long-term interleukin 10 therapy in chronic hepatitis C patients has a proviral and anti-inflammatory effect," *Hepatology*, vol. 38, no. 4, pp. 859–868, 2003.

[319] N. Nikolaidis, J. Kountouras, O. Giouleme et al., "Colchicine treatment of liver fibrosis," *Hepato-Gastroenterology*, vol. 53, no. 68, pp. 281–285, 2006.

[320] M. Esrefoglu, "Role of stem cells in repair of liver injury: Experimental and clinical benefit of transferred stem cells on liver failure," *World Journal of Gastroenterology*, vol. 19, no. 40, pp. 6757–6773, 2013.

[321] M. A. Habeeb, "Hepatic stem cells: A viable approach for the treatment of liver cirrhosis," *World Journal of Stem Cells*, vol. 7, no. 5, p. 859, 2015.

[322] C. Hu and L. Li, "In Vitro and in Vivo Hepatic Differentiation of Adult Somatic Stem Cells and Extraembryonic Stem Cells for Treating End Stage Liver Diseases," *Stem Cells International*, vol. 2015, Article ID 871972, 2015.

[323] P. A. Lysy, D. Campard, F. Smets et al., "Persistence of a chimerical phenotype after hepatocyte differentiation of human bone marrow mesenchymal stem cells," *Cell Proliferation*, vol. 41, no. 1, pp. 36–58, 2008.

[324] C. Nicolas, Y. Wang, J. Luebke-Wheeler, and S. Nyberg, "Stem Cell Therapies for Treatment of Liver Disease," *Biomedicines*, vol. 4, no. 1, p. 2, 2016.

[325] Y. Yu, X. Wang, and S. Nyberg, "Potential and Challenges of Induced Pluripotent Stem Cells in Liver Diseases Treatment," *Journal of Clinical Medicine*, vol. 3, no. 3, pp. 997–1017, 2014.

[326] R. M. Baertschiger, V. Serre-Beinier, P. Morel et al., "Fibrogenic potential of human multipotent mesenchymal stromal cells in injured liver," *PLoS ONE*, vol. 4, no. 8, Article ID e6657, 2009.

[327] L. V. di Bonzo, I. Ferrero, C. Cravanzola et al., "Human mesenchymal stem cells as a two-edged sword in hepatic regenerative medicine: engraftment and hepatocyte differentiation versus profibrogenic potential," *Gut*, vol. 57, no. 2, pp. 223–231, 2008.

[328] B. Raore, T. Federici, J. Taub et al., "Cervical multilevel intraspinal stem cell therapy: Assessment of surgical risks in gottingen minipigs," *The Spine Journal*, vol. 36, no. 3, pp. E164–E171, 2011.

[329] L. Xu, D. K. Ryugo, T. Pongstaporn, K. Johe, and V. E. Koliatsos, "Human neural stem cell grafts in the spinal cord of SOD1 transgenic rats: Differentiation and structural integration into the segmental motor circuitry," *Journal of Comparative Neurology*, vol. 514, no. 4, pp. 297–309, 2009.

[330] J. Yan, L. Xu, A. M. Welsh et al., "Extensive neuronal differentiation of human neural stem cell grafts in adult rat spinal cord," *PLoS Medicine*, vol. 4, no. 2, article e39, 2007.

[331] J. Chen, F. Wang, Y. Zhang et al., "In vivo tracking of superparamagnetic iron oxide nanoparticle labeled chondrocytes in large animal model.," *Annals of Biomedical Engineering*, vol. 40, no. 12, pp. 2568–2578, 2012.

[332] S.-L. Hu, J.-Q. Zhang, X. Hu et al., "In vitro labeling of human umbilical cord mesenchymal stem cells with superparamagnetic iron oxide nanoparticles," *Journal of Cellular Biochemistry*, vol. 108, no. 2, pp. 529–535, 2009.

[333] M. Neri, C. Maderna, C. Cavazzin et al., "Efficient in vitro labeling of human neural precursor cells with superparamagnetic iron oxide particles: Relevance for in vivo cell tracking," *Stem Cells*, vol. 26, no. 2, pp. 505–516, 2008.

[334] S. S. Yaghoubi, D. O. Campbell, C. G. Radu, and J. Czernin, "Positron emission tomography reporter genes and reporter probes: gene and cell therapy applications," *Theranostics*, vol. 2, no. 4, pp. 374–391, 2012.

[335] F. Wang, J. E. Dennis, A. Awadallah et al., "Transcriptional profiling of human mesenchymal stem cells transduced with reporter genes for imaging," *Physiological Genomics*, vol. 37, no. 1, pp. 23–34, 2009.

[336] S. J. Zhang and J. C. Wu, "Comparison of imaging techniques for tracking cardiac stem cell therapy," *Journal of Nuclear Medicine*, vol. 48, no. 12, pp. 1916–1919, 2007.

[337] K. T. Suk, J.-H. Yoon, M. Y. Kim et al., "Transplantation with autologous bone marrow-derived mesenchymal stem cells for alcoholic cirrhosis: Phase 2 trial," *Hepatology*, vol. 64, no. 6, pp. 2185–2197, 2016.

[338] R. P. H. Meier, R. Mahou, P. Morel et al., "Microencapsulated human mesenchymal stem cells decrease liver fibrosis in mice," *Journal of Hepatology*, vol. 62, no. 3, pp. 634–641, 2015.

[339] Y. Wang, X. Yu, E. Chen, and L. Li, "Liver-derived human mesenchymal stem cells: A novel therapeutic source for liver diseases," *Stem Cell Research & Therapy*, vol. 7, no. 1, article no. 71, 2016.

[340] F. Zhang, Y. Wen, and X. Guo, "CRISPR/Cas9 for genome editing: Progress, implications and challenges," *Human Molecular Genetics*, vol. 23, no. 1, pp. R40–R46, 2014.

[341] C. Smith, L. Abalde-Atristain, C. He et al., "Efficient and allele-specific genome editing of disease loci in human iPSCs," *Molecular Therapy*, vol. 23, no. 3, pp. 570–577, 2015.

[342] M. Vosough, E. Omidinia, M. Kadivar et al., "Generation of functional hepatocyte-like cells from human pluripotent stem cells in a scalable suspension culture," *Stem Cells and Development*, vol. 22, no. 20, pp. 2693–2705, 2013.

[343] S. Ogawa, J. Surapisitchat, C. Virtanen et al., "Three-dimensional culture and cAMP signaling promote the maturation of human pluripotent stem cell-derived hepatocytes," *Development*, vol. 140, no. 15, pp. 3285–3296, 2013.

[344] M. C. Hansel, J. C. Davila, M. Vosough et al., "The Use of Induced Pluripotent Stem Cells for the Study and Treatment of Liver Diseases," *Current Protocols in Toxicology*, vol. 67, pp. 14-13, 2016.

[345] S. M. Choi, Y. Kim, J. S. Shim et al., "Efficient drug screening and gene correction for treating liver disease using patient-specific stem cells," *Hepatology*, vol. 57, no. 6, pp. 2458–2468, 2013.

[346] N. Dianat, C. Steichen, L. Vallier, A. Weber, and A. Dubart-Kupperschmitt, "Human pluripotent stem cells for modelling human liver diseases and cell therapy," *Current Gene Therapy*, vol. 13, no. 2, pp. 120–132, 2013.

[347] K. Hussain, B. Challis, N. Rocha et al., "An activating mutation of *AKT2* and human hypoglycemia," *Science*, vol. 334, no. 6055, p. 474, 2011.

[348] M. Li, K. Suzuki, N. Y. Kim, G.-H. Liu, and J. C. I. Belmonte, "A cut above the rest: targeted genome editing technologies in human pluripotent stem cells," *The Journal of Biological Chemistry*, vol. 289, no. 8, pp. 4594–4599, 2014.

[349] T. Egashira, S. Yuasa, and K. Fukuda, "Novel insights into disease modeling using induced pluripotent stem cells," *Biological & Pharmaceutical Bulletin*, vol. 36, no. 2, pp. 182–188, 2013.

[350] R. Eggenschwiler, K. Loya, and G. Wu, "Sustained knockdown of a disease-causing gene in patient-specific induced pluripotent stem cells using lentiviral vector-based gene therapy," *Stem Cells Translational Medicine*, vol. 2, no. 9, pp. 641–654, 2013.

[351] U. Grieshammer and K. A. Shepard, "Proceedings: consideration of genetics in the design of induced pluripotent stem cell-based models of complex disease," *Stem Cells Translational Medicine*, vol. 3, no. 11, pp. 1253–1258, 2014.

[352] H. Inoue, N. Nagata, H. Kurokawa, and S. Yamanaka, "IPS cells: a game changer for future medicine," *EMBO Journal*, vol. 33, no. 5, pp. 409–417, 2014.

[353] F. T. Merkle and K. Eggan, "Modeling human disease with pluripotent stem cells: From genome association to function," *Cell Stem Cell*, vol. 12, no. 6, pp. 656–668, 2013.

[354] K. Moriya, M. Yoshikawa, Y. Ouji et al., "Embryonic stem cells reduce liver fibrosis in CCl4-treated mice," *International Journal of Clinical and Experimental Pathology*, vol. 89, no. 6, pp. 401–409, 2008.

[355] R. Schwartz, K. Trehan, L. Andrus et al., "Su1581 Modeling Hepatitis C Virus Infection Using Human Induced Pluripotent Stem Cells," *Gastroenterology*, vol. 142, no. 5, p. S-971, 2012.

[356] F. Soldner and R. Jaenisch, "iPSC disease modeling," *Science*, vol. 338, no. 6111, pp. 1155-1156, 2012.

[357] G. Holmgren, A.-K. Sjögren, I. Barragan et al., "Long-term chronic toxicity testing using human pluripotent stem cell-derived hepatocytes," *Drug Metabolism and Disposition*, vol. 42, no. 9, pp. 1401–1406, 2014.

[358] D. Szkolnicka, S. L. Farnworth, B. Lucendo-Villarin et al., "Accurate prediction of drug-induced liver injury using stem cell-derived populations," *Stem Cells Translational Medicine*, vol. 3, no. 2, pp. 141–148, 2014.

[359] D. Szkolnicka, B. Lucendo-Villarin, J. K. Moore, K. J. Simpson, S. J. Forbes, and D. C. Hay, "Reducing hepatocyte injury and necrosis in response to paracetamol using noncoding RNAs," *Stem Cells Translational Medicine*, vol. 5, no. 6, pp. 764–772, 2016.

[360] M. A. Cayo, J. Cai, A. Delaforest et al., "JD induced pluripotent stem cell-derived hepatocytes faithfully recapitulate the pathophysiology of familial hypercholesterolemia," *Hepatology*, vol. 56, no. 6, pp. 2163–2171, 2012.

32

The Effect of Prucalopride on Small Bowel Transit Time in Hospitalized Patients Undergoing Capsule Endoscopy

Majid Alsahafi,[1,2] Paula Cramer,[1] Nazira Chatur,[1] and Fergal Donnellan[1]

[1]*Division of Gastroenterology, Vancouver General Hospital, University of British Columbia, Vancouver, BC, Canada*
[2]*Department of Medicine, King Abdulaziz University, Jeddah, Saudi Arabia*

Correspondence should be addressed to Fergal Donnellan; fergal.donnellan@vch.ca

Academic Editor: Salvatore Cucchiara

Background. The inpatient status is a well-known risk factor for incomplete video capsule endoscopy (VCE) examinations due to prolonged transit time. We aimed to evaluate the effect of prucalopride on small bowel transit time for hospitalized patients undergoing VCE. *Methods.* We included all hospitalized patients who underwent VCE at a tertiary academic center from October 2011 through September 2016. A single 2 mg dose of prucalopride was given exclusively for all patients who underwent VCE between March 2014 and December 2015. VCE studies were excluded if the capsule was retained or endoscopically placed, if other prokinetic agents were given, in cases with technical failure, or if patients had prior gastric or small bowel resection. *Results.* 442 VCE were identified, of which 68 were performed in hospitalized patients. 54 inpatients were included, of which 29 consecutive patients received prucalopride. The prucalopride group had a significantly shorter small bowel transit time compared to the control group (92 versus 275.5, $p < 0.001$). There was a trend for a higher completion rate in the prucalopride group (93.1% versus 76%, $p = 0.12$). *Conclusions.* Our results suggest that the administration of prucalopride prior to VCE is a simple and effective intervention to decrease small bowel transit time.

1. Introduction

Small bowel video capsule endoscopy (VCE) has revolutionized the management of small bowel disorders and is considered now the first line to investigate for obscure gastrointestinal bleeding [1–5]. Optimal diagnostic utility depends not only on adequate small bowel visualization, but also on the completion of small bowel examination. Because of the limited battery time, 16.5% of VCE studies are incomplete [6]. Prolongation of the small bowel transit may result in lower completion rates, which limits the diagnostic utility of VCE and increases the cost associated with further diagnostic testing.

Inpatient VCE is commonly performed to investigate the source of obscure gastrointestinal bleeding. The inpatient status is a well-known risk factor for incomplete small bowel examination with a reported completion rate as low as 64%, limiting the diagnostic utility of VCE [7–11]. The performance of VCE after hospital discharge is potentially associated with a decrease in the diagnostic yield, delays therapeutic interventions, and is not always possible. Several studies have shown that VCE performed during or early after the bleeding event is associated with a higher diagnostic yield [10, 12–15]. Therefore, interventions to shorten small bowel transit time are particularly needed for hospitalized patients to increase the completion rates. The experience with purgatives and prokinetic agents revealed mixed results with no conclusive benefit [16–18].

Prucalopride is a 5-HT4 receptor agonist that has been shown to improve colonic motility. It has been approved in Canada and Europe for treatment of chronic idiopathic constipation in women who fail to respond to laxatives. In addition to improving colonic motility, animal and human studies suggest that prucalopride stimulates motility in the stomach and small intestine, and as a result it has the potential to decrease the transit times in the stomach and the small bowel [19–24]. The effect of prucalopride on small bowel transit time (SBTT) in patients undergoing VCE has not been previously investigated. We therefore aimed to determine the effect of prucalopride on SBTT for hospitalized patients who are particularly at risk for prolongation of SBTT.

2. Methods

2.1. Patients. The study was approved by the University of British Columbia Clinical Research Ethics Board and the Vancouver Coastal Health Research Institute. We included all hospitalized patients who underwent VCE at Vancouver General Hospital from October 2011 through September 2016. Vancouver General Hospital is a tertiary, academic center and the largest hospital in British Columbia, Canada. Inpatient VCE were identified through a prospective capsule endoscopy database that includes data related to all patients who underwent VCE at our center. The database includes information related to patients' demographics, indication for VCE, use of prokinetics, and completeness of small bowel examination. VCE studies were excluded if the capsule was retained or endoscopically placed, if other prokinetic agents were given, or if the patient had prior gastric or small bowel resection. Capsule retention is defined as the presence of the capsule endoscope in the digestive tract for a minimum of 2 weeks or more, or when the capsule is retained indefinitely in the small bowel unless a targeted medical or surgical intervention is initiated. VCE studies with technical failure, including accidental removal of the sensor/recorder, were also excluded. In addition to the data recorded in the database, we retrospectively reviewed the hospital electronic medical records, pre-VCE clinical assessment forms, and the VCE reports to collect data on medical comorbidities and the use of the following medications: narcotics, antiplatelet drugs, nonsteroidal anti-inflammatory drugs, warfarin, and other anticoagulants.

2.2. VCE Procedure. Prior to January 2015, all small bowel VCE studies were performed using Endocapsule EC1 (Olympus, Tokyo, Japan). After this date, all VCE studies were performed using Pillcam SB3 (Given Imaging, Yokneam, Israel). Patients were given standard instructions as per our usual practice including a clear liquid diet after lunch the day prior to VCE, followed by an overnight fast. They were permitted to resume a clear fluid diet and to have a light meal two and four hours after the beginning of recording, respectively. Patients received 2 L of polyethylene glycol starting at 4 pm the day before the procedure. Between March 2014 and December 2015, all hospitalized patients were given a 2 mg single dose of prucalopride orally at the time of VCE as per our protocol during this period. No patient received prucalopride outside this period. Apart from the bowel preparation, no other mucosal cleansing or antibubbles agents were given. All patients had the VCE recorders disconnected after 8 hours of recording.

2.3. VCE Interpretation. Data related to VCE interpretation was collected from the VCE reports. One of two gastroenterologists with experience in VCE reviewed and interpreted the VCE images at a maximum rate of 15 images per second as per our usual practice. The reviewers were not blinded to clinical data but they were unaware of the study hypothesis as the study hypothesis was conceived after all VCE were done. We collected data on gastric transit time (GTT), SBTT, small bowel completion rate, and the diagnostic yield. SBTT was defined as the time from the first duodenal image to the first cecal image. GTT was defined as the time from the first gastric image to the first duodenal image.

Small bowel completion rate and the diagnostic yield were defined as the proportion of VCE in which the cecum was reached and the proportion of VCE with positive findings, respectively. The findings on VCE were categorized as positive or negative using a modified version of a previously reported P0–P2 system [25]. The VCE study was considered positive if a significant lesion (P2) was reported. The presence of fresh blood of unclear source was considered a positive finding as this suggests the site of bleeding and helps with further management. Alternatively, the VCE study was considered negative if no abnormality was found (P0) or an abnormality of uncertain significance was reported (P1). Abnormalities of uncertain significance included minor isolated erosions and small nonspecific red spots.

2.4. Statistical Analysis. The mean and standard deviation and/or the median with range were used for continuous variables as appropriate. The percentage and count were used for categorical variables. Statistical analysis was performed with the Chi-square test or Fisher exact test for categorical variables as appropriate. The SBTT and GTT were compared between the two groups using the Wilcoxon Rank Sum test. A p value of less than 0.05, with a two-tail test, was considered statistically significant. Statistical analysis was performed using the R statistical software, version 0.99.893, © 2009–2016 R Studio, Inc.

3. Results

A total of 442 VCE were identified in our capsule endoscopy database, of which 68 were performed in hospitalized patients. Twelve VCE were excluded for the following reasons: 6 patients had endoscopic placements including 2 with previous gastric surgery; 2 had capsule retention; 2 had VCE with technical failure; 1 received linaclotide; 1 patient had prior small bowel resection. In addition, two patients had insufficient data and were excluded. Therefore, 54 VCE were included in the analysis, in which 29 consecutive patients received prucalopride. Twenty-six VCE were performed using Endocapsule (17 in the control and 9 in the prucalopride) and 28 using Pillcam (8 in the control and 20 in the prucalopride). For the entire study population, the mean age was 64.8 years (±15) and 64.8% were male.

The baseline characteristics for patients who received prucalopride versus those who did not receive prucalopride are shown in Table 1. There were no differences between the prucalopride and the control group concerning age, gender, indication for VCE, medical comorbidities, antiplatelets, anticoagulants, nonsteroidal anti-inflammatory drugs, or narcotics use. All patients tolerated the procedure well with no adverse events.

The results of the study are summarized in Table 2. In the entire study population, the median SBTT was 196

TABLE 1: Baseline characteristics of study population, the prucalopride versus the control group.

Patient characteristic	Prucalopride $n = 29$	Control $n = 25$	p value
Age mean, year (SD)	64.4 (13.9)	65.2 (16.4)	0.85
Male	20 (68.9%)	15 (60%)	0.49
Indication			1
Overt OGIB	26 (89.6%)	23 (92%)	
Occult OGIB	1 (3.4%)	1 (4%)	
Abnormal radiology	2 (6.8%)	1 (4%)	
Medical comorbidities			
Cardiac disease	11 (37.9%)	12 (48%)	0.52
Congestive heart failure	5 (17.2%)	7 (28%)	0.37
Valvular heart disease	8 (27.5%)	5 (20%)	0.46
Cerebrovascular disease	3 (10.3%)	5 (20%)	0.45
Chronic kidney disease	4 (13.7%)	1 (4%)	0.35
Chronic lung disease	2 (6.8%)	2 (8%)	1
Liver cirrhosis	3 (10.3%)	0 (0%)	0.23
Diabetes	8 (27.5%)	7 (28%)	0.97
Antiplatelets (ASA and/or plavix)	11 (37.9%)	7 (28%)	0.44
NSAIDS	2 (6.8%)	2 (8%)	1
Anticoagulants	6 (20.6%)	5 (20%)	0.95
Narcotics	3 (10.3%)	1 (4%)	0.61

SD, standard deviation; OGIB, obscure gastrointestinal bleeding; NSAIDS, nonsteroidal anti-inflammatory drugs.

TABLE 2: Transit times and completion rates in the prucalopride versus the control group.

Outcome	Prucalopride	Control	p value
SBTT median, minutes (IQR, range)	92 (63–195, 29–357)	275.5 (263.5–299.5, 152–383)	<0.001
GTT median, minutes (IQR, range)	30 (11–46, 0–116)	27, (13–60, 2–240)	0.61
SB completion rate	93.1%	76%	0.12

SBTT, small bowel transit time; IQR, interquartile range; GTT, gastric transit time; SB, small bowel.

minutes (IQR 78–275.5, range 29–383). The median SBTT was significantly shorter in the prucalopride group (92 versus 275.5 minutes, $p < 0.001$). To exclude any effect related to an unapparent change in our practice during the study period, we reanalyzed the data after excluding all VCE that were performed prior January 2015 (26 VCE). In the remaining 28 VCE included in this analysis, all VCE were performed using the Pillcam VCE. This analysis also revealed a significantly shorter median SBTT in the prucalopride group (85 versus 293 minutes, $p < 0.001$). Figure 1 shows the Kaplan-Meier curves for time to complete small bowel examination for the prucalopride versus the control group. Figure 2 showed the distributions of SBTT before the introduction of prucalopride, during the period of prucalopride use and after the end of prucalopride period.

The capsule remained in the stomach only in 1 patient and this was in the control group. In the entire study population, the median GTT was 30 minutes (IQR 11–54, range 0–240). There was no difference in the median GTT between the prucalopride and the control group (30 versus 27.5, $p = 0.61$). Similarly, there was no difference in the GTT between VCE with complete and incomplete small bowel examination (median GTT was 30 minutes for both, $p = 0.85$). Figure 3 shows the Kaplan-Meier curves for time to gastric passage for the prucalopride versus the control group.

Of the 54 VCE, the cecum was reached in 46 which resulted in an overall completion rate of 85.1%. The completion rate was higher in the prucalopride group (93.1%, 27/29) compared to the control group (76%, 19/25), $p = 0.12$. The overall diagnostic yield was 61.1% (33/54). Positive findings are summarized in Table 3. The diagnostic yield was higher in the prucalopride group (75.8%, 22/29) compared to the control group (44%, 11/25), $p = 0.03$. There was a trend for a higher diagnostic yield in complete VCE (65.2%, 30/46) compared to incomplete VCE (37.5%, 3/8), $p = 0.23$.

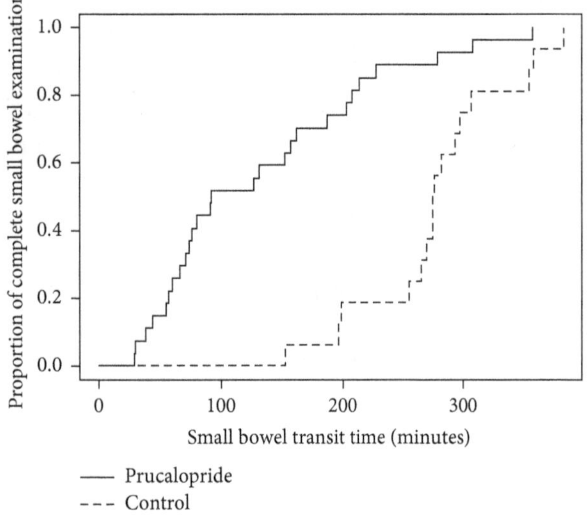

Figure 1: Kaplan-Meier curves for time to complete small bowel examination since the first duodenal image for all VCE that reached cecum. The median SBTT was significantly shorter in the prucalopride group (92, 95% CI: 74, 187) compared to the control group (275.5, 95% CI: 266, 354). *VCE, video capsule endoscopy; SBTT, small bowel transit time; CI, confidence* interval.

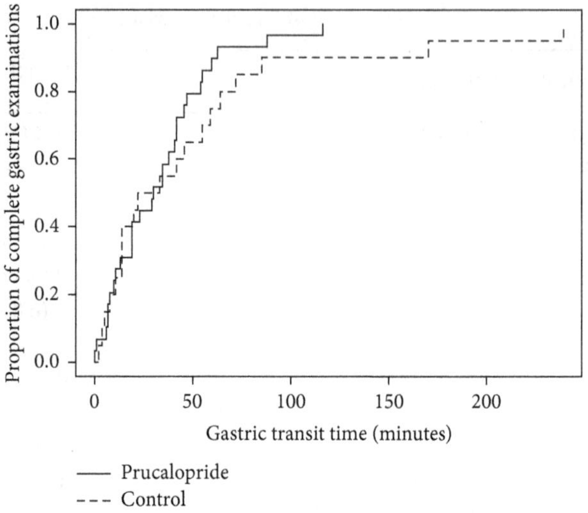

Figure 3: Kaplan-Meier curves for time to capsule passage into duodenum since the first gastric image for all VCE that reached duodenum. The median GTT was not significantly different between the prucalopride group (30, 95% CI: 19, 42) and the control group (27.5, 95% CI: 14, 72). *VCE, video capsule endoscopy; GTT, gastric transit time; CI, confidence* interval.

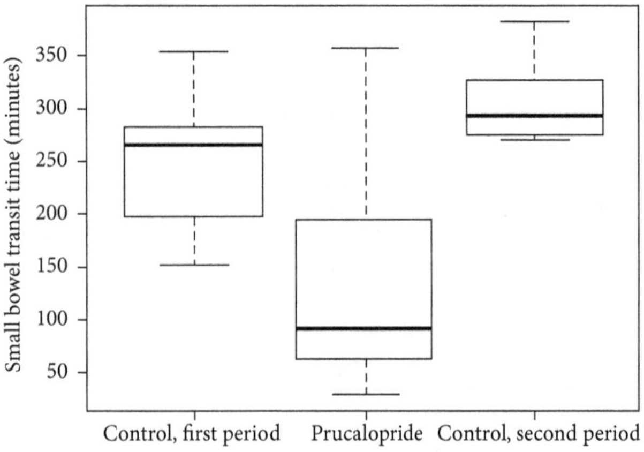

Figure 2: Box plot diagrams showing the distributions of small bowel transit time in the three study periods. Control, first period (October 2011 to March 2014); the period of prucalopride use (from March 2014 to December 2015); control, second period (December 2015 to September 2016).

Table 3: Summary of positive findings.

	Prucalopride (n = 29)	Control (n = 25)
All positive findings	22	11
Angiodysplasia	12	4
Ulcer/erosions	4	3
Fresh blood	6	2
Mass	0	2

4. Discussion

Incomplete small bowel examination is an important limitation for the diagnostic utility of VCE. Several factors have been recognized as potential risk factors for incomplete VCE including the inpatients status, prior small bowel surgery, prolonged gastric passage, older age, diabetes, and poor bowel preparation [7–9, 26]. Hospitalized patients are particularly at risk for incomplete VCE, with a completion rate in the range of 64 to 73% [7–11]. One potential strategy is to accelerate the passage of the capsule through the stomach and small bowel preventing prolonged transit time. The use of purgatives does not appear to affect the transit times or the completion rates [17, 18]. Several prokinetic agents, such as erythromycin and metoclopramide, have been investigated but the evidence remains inconclusive [16, 17]. Magnetic manipulation of the VCE was not successful to shorten the GTT, while limited data suggests that the right lateral position might be of some benefit to increase the completion rate [27, 28]. The alternative strategy is to extend the battery life. However, even when the battery life is extended to 16 hours, 10% of VCE are incomplete [29].

The primary objective of our study was to examine if prucalopride, given at the time of VCE ingestion, decreases small bowel transit time in hospitalized patients. We found that prucalopride significantly decreased small bowel transit time. The median SBTT was 92 minutes in the prucalopride group and 275.5 minutes in the control group, $p < 0.001$. Patients in the prucalopride group were more likely to have complete small bowel examination, 93.1% versus 76%, although this did not reach the level of statistical significance ($p = 0.12$) as our study was not adequately powered to assess a difference in the completion rates.

Our study is the first study to evaluate the effect of prucalopride on SBTT in patients undergoing VCE. While the effect of prucalopride on the colonic motility is well described in humans, its effect on small bowel motility has been less studied. Animal studies suggest that prucalopride stimulates small intestinal motility [19, 20]. Studies in healthy volunteers were limited by small size and revealed mixed results. In a cross-over study that included healthy volunteers, prucalopride significantly decreased the transit time from mouth to cecum [22]. In contrast, in another small study that also included healthy subjects, prucalopride did not significantly affect gastric or small bowel transit time [23]. However, in a randomized controlled trial that included patients with constipation, who are likely to be at a higher risk incomplete VCE studies, prucalopride has been shown to decrease both the gastric and the small bowel transit times [24].

In the present study, the SBTT in the prucalopride group was substantially shorter than the SBTT reported in the literature for both inpatient and outpatient VCE. Furthermore, the completion rate in the prucalopride group was also substantially higher than the completion rate reported in the literature for the inpatient VCE and is comparable to the completion rates for outpatient VCE [9–11]. For the control group, the SBTT and completion rate were similar to what is reported in the literature [7–9, 11]. Therefore, the differences in the SBTT and the completion rates between the two groups in our study did not result from disproportionately longer SBTT and lower completion rate in the control group biasing the results in favor of the prucalopride group. The significant difference in the SBTT persisted after we excluded all VCE that were done prior to January 2015 indicating that the difference was not resulting from an unapparent change in our practice in the five-year period of the study. Furthermore, as shown in Figure 2, the marked decrease in the SBTT after the introduction of prucalopride was followed by a marked increase in the SBTT when prucalopride was no longer used, suggesting a causative effect of prucalopride rather than just an association. The bivariate analysis revealed no differences in the baseline characteristics between the two study groups.

Interestingly, the increase in the completion rate in the prucalopride group resulted from accelerating the small bowel transit rather than the gastric passage, as there was no difference in the GTT between the prucalopride group and the control group. Previous studies evaluating the effect of prucalopride on gastric emptying revealed controversial results [21, 23, 24]. While prucalopride did not significantly affect the GTT in our study, it is unclear if prucalopride would accelerate the passage of the capsule in a subset of patients who have prolonged GTT, such as patients with diabetic gastroparesis. It is worth noting that we administered prucalopride at the time of capsule ingestion, which may not have been the ideal time to influence the GTT as the maximum plasma concentration usually occurs after 2.7 hours of ingestion [30].

The ultimate goal of decreasing SBTT is to increase the rate of complete examinations, thus enhancing the diagnostic utility of VCE by increasing the diagnostic yield and/or eliminating the uncertainty related to incomplete examinations. Two published studies associated higher diagnostic yields with prolonged SBTT raising concerns about the routine use of prokinetic agents [31, 32]. While there are limitations for both studies, including the retrospective design and the absence of strict definitions for positive findings, theoretically there is more opportunity to miss lesions when fewer images are obtained as a result of rapid transit. However, when the prolonged transit is the cause for incomplete examinations, accelerating the slow transit may enhance the diagnostic yield by increasing the completion rate or by having a higher proportion of small bowel examined when the examination is incomplete. Even without an increase in the diagnostic yield, the presence of complete small bowel examination is clinically important, as it decreases the likelihood of small bowel pathology.

We found that the use of prucalopride was associated with an increase in the diagnostic yield, 75.8% versus 44%. This increase in the diagnostic yield is, however, higher than what to be expected by the increase in the completion rate in the prucalopride group, although there was a higher yield in complete VCE versus incomplete VCE examinations (65% versus 37%). Our study was not powered or specifically designed to evaluate for a difference in the diagnostic yield as we could not account for all variables that may affect the diagnostic yield such as the quality of bowel preparation, time from the bleeding event to VCE, and variability in reporting VCE findings. A large prospective study would be required to evaluate the effect of significant shortening of the transit time on the diagnostic yield.

Our study has limitations that should be considered, including the retrospective design and the relatively small sample size. The difference in the SBTT between the prucalopride and the control group was, however, substantial. While we found no differences between the two study groups with regard to the baseline characteristics for the collected variables, we could not collect data on the level of physical activity. At least one previous study correlated the level of physical activity with the completion rate [33]. Since all patients were hospitalized with comparable medical comorbidities, it would be unlikely that a big difference in physical activity existed.

In conclusion, this is the first study to evaluate the effect of prucalopride on SBTT in patients undergoing VCE. Our results suggest that the administration of prucalopride at the time of VCE ingestion is a simple and effective intervention to shorten small bowel transit in hospitalized patients. Future studies, preferably randomized controlled trials, are needed to confirm these results.

Abbreviations

VCE: Video capsule endoscopy
SBTT: Small bowel transit time
GTT: Gastric transit time.

Disclosure

An earlier version of this work was presented as an abstract at Gastrointestinal Endoscopy journal 2017.

Authors' Contributions

Majid Alsahafi was responsible for study concept, design, data acquisition, analysis, interpretation, and drafting the manuscript, Paula Cramer was responsible for study concept and data acquisition, Nazira Chatur was responsible for study concept and design, and Fergal Donnellan was responsible for study concept, design, analysis, and interpretation. All authors reviewed the manuscript for critical revision and approved the final version.

References

[1] A. de Leusse, K. Vahedi, J. Edery et al., "Capsule endoscopy or push enteroscopy for first-line exploration of obscure gastrointestinal bleeding?" *Gastroenterology*, vol. 132, no. 3, pp. 855–862, 2007.

[2] P. M. Dionisio, S. R. Gurudu, J. A. Leighton et al., "Capsule endoscopy has a significantly higher diagnostic yield in patients with suspected and established small-bowel crohn's disease: a meta-analysis," *American Journal of Gastroenterology*, vol. 105, no. 6, pp. 1240–1248, 2010.

[3] A. Mata, J. Llach, A. Castells et al., "A prospective trial comparing wireless capsule endoscopy and barium contrast series for small-bowel surveillance in hereditary GI polyposis syndromes," *Gastrointestinal Endoscopy*, vol. 61, no. 6, pp. 721–725, 2005.

[4] T. Rokkas and Y. Niv, "The role of video capsule endoscopy in the diagnosis of celiac disease: A meta-analysis," *European Journal of Gastroenterology & Hepatology*, vol. 24, no. 3, pp. 303–308, 2012.

[5] L. B. Gerson, J. L. Fidler, D. R. Cave, and J. A. Leighton, "ACG clinical guideline: diagnosis and management of small bowel bleeding," *American Journal of Gastroenterology*, vol. 110, no. 9, pp. 1265–1287, 2015.

[6] Z. Liao, R. Gao, C. Xu, and Z. S. Li, "Indications and detection, completion, and retention rates of small-bowel capsule endoscopy: a systematic review," *Gastrointestinal Endoscopy*, vol. 71, no. 2, pp. 280–286, 2010.

[7] C. Yazici, J. Losurdo, M. D. Brown et al., "Inpatient capsule endoscopy leads to frequent incomplete small bowel examinations," *World Journal of Gastroenterology*, vol. 18, no. 36, pp. 5051–5057, 2012.

[8] J. Westerhof, R. K. Weersma, and J. J. Koornstra, "Risk factors for incomplete small-bowel capsule endoscopy," *Gastrointestinal Endoscopy*, vol. 69, no. 1, pp. 74–80, 2009.

[9] E. Ben-Soussan, G. Savoye, M. Antonietti, S. Ramirez, E. Lerebours, and P. Ducrotté, "Factors that affect gastric passage of video capsule," *Gastrointestinal Endoscopy*, vol. 62, no. 5, pp. 785–790, 2005.

[10] C. A. Robinson, C. Jackson, D. Condon, and L. B. Gerson, "Impact of inpatient status and gender on small-bowel capsule endoscopy findings," *Gastrointestinal Endoscopy*, vol. 74, no. 5, pp. 1061–1066, 2011.

[11] P. Stanich, J. Guido, B. Kleinman, K. Betkerur, K. Porter, and M. Meyer, "Video capsule endoscopy completion and total transit times are similar with oral or endoscopic delivery," *Endoscopy International Open*, vol. 04, no. 02, pp. E228–E232, 2016.

[12] M. Pennazio, R. Santucci, E. Rondonotti et al., "Outcome of patients with obscure gastrointestinal bleeding after capsule endoscopy: report of 100 consecutive cases," *Gastroenterology*, vol. 126, no. 3, pp. 643–653, 2004.

[13] E. J. Carey, J. A. Leighton, R. I. Heigh et al., "A single-center experience of 260 consecutive patients undergoing capsule endoscopy for obscure gastrointestinal bleeding," *American Journal of Gastroenterology*, vol. 102, no. 1, pp. 89–95, 2007.

[14] P. Apostolopoulos, C. Liatsos, I. M. Gralnek et al., "Evaluation of capsule endoscopy in active, mild-to-moderate, overt, obscure GI bleeding," *Gastrointestinal Endoscopy*, vol. 66, no. 6, pp. 1174–1181, 2007.

[15] A. Singh, C. Marshall, B. Chaudhuri et al., "Timing of video capsule endoscopy relative to overt obscure GI bleeding: Implications from a retrospective study," *Gastrointestinal Endoscopy*, vol. 77, no. 5, pp. 761–766, 2013.

[16] A. Koulaouzidis, A. Giannakou, D. E. Yung, K. J. Dabos, and J. N. Plevris, "Do prokinetics influence the completion rate in small-bowel capsule endoscopy? A systematic review and meta-analysis," *Current Medical Research and Opinion*, vol. 29, no. 9, pp. 1171–1185, 2013.

[17] V. S. Kotwal, B. M. Attar, S. Gupta, and R. Agarwal, "Should bowel preparation, antifoaming agents, or prokinetics be used before video capsule endoscopy? A systematic review and meta-analysis," *European Journal of Gastroenterology & Hepatology*, vol. 26, no. 2, pp. 137–145, 2014.

[18] T. Rokkas, K. Papaxoinis, K. Triantafyllou, D. Pistiolas, and S. D. Ladas, "Does purgative preparation influence the diagnostic yield of small bowel video capsule endoscopy?: a meta-analysis," *American Journal of Gastroenterology*, vol. 104, no. 1, pp. 219–227, 2009.

[19] M. R. Briejer, J.-P. Bosmans, P. Van Daele et al., "The in vitro pharmacological profile of prucalopride, a novel enterokinetic compound," *European Journal of Pharmacology*, vol. 423, no. 1, pp. 71–83, 2001.

[20] K. J. Lepard, J. Ren, and J. J. Galligan, "Presynaptic modulation of cholinergic and non-cholinergic fast synaptic transmission in the myenteric plexus of guinea pig ileum," *Neurogastroenterology & Motility*, vol. 16, no. 3, pp. 355–364, 2004.

[21] B. F. Kessing, A. J. P. M. Smout, R. J. Bennink, N. Kraaijpoel, J. M. Oors, and A. J. Bredenoord, "Prucalopride decreases esophageal acid exposure and accelerates gastric emptying in healthy subjects," *Neurogastroenterology & Motility*, vol. 26, no. 8, pp. 1079–1086, 2014.

[22] A. V. Emmanuel, M. A. Kamm, A. J. Roy, and K. Antonelli, "Effect of a novel prokinetic drug, R093877, on gastrointestinal transit in healthy volunteers," *Gut*, vol. 42, no. 4, pp. 511–516, 1998.

[23] E. P. Bouras, M. Camilleri, D. D. Burton, and S. McKinzie, "Selective stimulation of colonic transit by the benzofuran 5HT4 agonist, prucalopride, in healthy humans," *Gut*, vol. 44, no. 5, pp. 682–686, 1999.

[24] E. P. Bouras, M. Camilleri, D. D. Burton, G. Thomforde, S. McKinzie, and A. R. Zinsmeister, "Prucalopride accelerates gastrointestinal and colonic transit in patients with constipation without a rectal evacuation disorder," *Gastroenterology*, vol. 120, no. 2, pp. 354–360, 2001.

[25] J.-C. Saurin, M. Delvaux, J.-L. Gaudin et al., "Diagnostic value of endoscopic capsule in patients with obscure digestive bleeding: blinded comparison with video push-enteroscopy," *Endoscopy*, vol. 35, no. 7, pp. 576–584, 2003.

[26] K. Triantafyllou, C. Kalantzis, A. A. Papadopoulos et al., "Video-capsule endoscopy gastric and small bowel transit time and completeness of the examination in patients with diabetes mellitus," *Digestive and Liver Disease*, vol. 39, no. 6, pp. 575–580, 2007.

[27] M. Hale, K. Drew, R. Sidhu, and M. McAlindon, "Does magnetically assisted capsule endoscopy improve small bowel capsule endoscopy completion rate? A randomised controlled trial," *Endoscopy International Open*, vol. 04, no. 02, pp. E215–E221, 2016.

[28] Z. Liao, F. Li, and Z.-S. Li, "Right lateral position improves complete examination rate of capsule endoscope: A prospective randomized, controlled trial," *Endoscopy*, vol. 40, no. 6, pp. 483–487, 2008.

[29] G. E. Tontini, F. Wiedbrauck, F. Cavallaro et al., "Small-bowel capsule endoscopy with panoramic view: results of the first multicenter, observational study (with videos)," *Gastrointestinal Endoscopy*, vol. 85, no. 2, pp. 401–408.e2, 2017.

[30] S. Flach, G. Scarfe, J. Dragone et al., "A Phase I Study to Investigate the Absorption, Pharmacokinetics, and Excretion of [14C]Prucalopride After a Single Oral Dose in Healthy Volunteers," *Clinical Therapeutics*, vol. 38, no. 9, pp. 2106–2115, 2016.

[31] J. M. Buscaglia, S. Kapoor, J. O. Clarke et al., "Enhanced diagnostic yield with prolonged small bowel transit time during capsule endoscopy," *International Journal of Medical Sciences*, vol. 5, no. 6, pp. 303–308, 2008.

[32] J. Westerhof, J. J. Koornstra, R. A. Hoedemaker, W. J. Sluiter, J. H. Kleibeuker, and R. K. Weersma, "Diagnostic yield of small bowel capsule endoscopy depends on the small bowel transit time," *World Journal of Gastroenterology*, vol. 18, no. 13, pp. 1502–1507, 2012.

[33] T. Shibuya, H. Mori, T. Takeda et al., "The relationship between physical activity level and completion rate of small bowel examination in patients undergoing Capsule endoscopy," *Internal Medicine*, vol. 51, no. 9, pp. 997–1001, 2012.

Permissions

All chapters in this book were first published in CJGH, by Hindawi Publishing Corporation; hereby published with permission under the Creative Commons Attribution License or equivalent. Every chapter published in this book has been scrutinized by our experts. Their significance has been extensively debated. The topics covered herein carry significant findings which will fuel the growth of the discipline. They may even be implemented as practical applications or may be referred to as a beginning point for another development.

The contributors of this book come from diverse backgrounds, making this book a truly international effort. This book will bring forth new frontiers with its revolutionizing research information and detailed analysis of the nascent developments around the world.

We would like to thank all the contributing authors for lending their expertise to make the book truly unique. They have played a crucial role in the development of this book. Without their invaluable contributions this book wouldn't have been possible. They have made vital efforts to compile up to date information on the varied aspects of this subject to make this book a valuable addition to the collection of many professionals and students.

This book was conceptualized with the vision of imparting up-to-date information and advanced data in this field. To ensure the same, a matchless editorial board was set up. Every individual on the board went through rigorous rounds of assessment to prove their worth. After which they invested a large part of their time researching and compiling the most relevant data for our readers.

The editorial board has been involved in producing this book since its inception. They have spent rigorous hours researching and exploring the diverse topics which have resulted in the successful publishing of this book. They have passed on their knowledge of decades through this book. To expedite this challenging task, the publisher supported the team at every step. A small team of assistant editors was also appointed to further simplify the editing procedure and attain best results for the readers.

Apart from the editorial board, the designing team has also invested a significant amount of their time in understanding the subject and creating the most relevant covers. They scrutinized every image to scout for the most suitable representation of the subject and create an appropriate cover for the book.

The publishing team has been an ardent support to the editorial, designing and production team. Their endless efforts to recruit the best for this project, has resulted in the accomplishment of this book. They are a veteran in the field of academics and their pool of knowledge is as vast as their experience in printing. Their expertise and guidance has proved useful at every step. Their uncompromising quality standards have made this book an exceptional effort. Their encouragement from time to time has been an inspiration for everyone.

The publisher and the editorial board hope that this book will prove to be a valuable piece of knowledge for researchers, students, practitioners and scholars across the globe.

List of Contributors

Farzad Shidfar and Samaneh Sadat Bahrololumi
Department of Nutrition, School of Public Health, Iran University of Medical Sciences, Tehran, Iran

Saeid Doaei
Natural Products and Medicinal Plants Research Center, North Khorasan University of Medical Sciences, Bojnurd, Iran

Saeid Doaei
Department of Public Health, School of Health, North Khorasan University of Medical Sciences, Bojnurd, Iran

Assieh Mohammadzadeh
Department of Nutrition Sciences, Student Research Committee, Ahvaz Jundishapur University of Medical Sciences, Ahvaz, Iran

Maryam Gholamalizadeh
Student Research Committee, Cancer Research Center, Shahid Beheshti University of Medical Sciences, Tehran, Iran

Ali Mohammadimanesh
Student Counseling Center, Hamadan University of Medical Sciences, Hamadan, Iran

Irene S. Yu
Division of Medical Oncology, Department of Medicine, British Columbia Cancer Agency, University of British Columbia,Vancouver, BC, Canada

Winson Y. Cheung
Section of Medical Oncology, Department of Oncology, Tom Baker Cancer Centre, University of Calgary, Calgary, AB, Canada

Mohammad Golriz, Omid Ghamarnejad, Elias Khajeh, Mohammadsadegh Sabagh, Markus Mieth, Katrin Hoffmann, Alexis Ulrich, Thilo Hackert, Markus W.Büchler and Arianeb Mehrabi
Department of General, Visceral, and Transplantation Surgery, University of Heidelberg, Heidelberg, Germany

Mohammad Golriz, Katrin Hoffmann, Karl Heinz Weiss, Peter Schirmacher and Arianeb Mehrabi
Liver Cancer Center Heidelberg (LCCH), Heidelberg, Germany

Karl HeinzWeiss
Department of Gastroenterology and Hepatology, University of Heidelberg, Heidelberg, Germany

Peter Schirmacher
Institute of Pathology, University of Heidelberg, Heidelberg, Germany

Samuel H. Sigal
Department of Medicine, Montefiore Medical Center and Albert Einstein College of Medicine, Bronx, New York USA

Alpesh Amin
Department of Medicine, University of California, Irvine, California, USA

Joseph A. Chiodo III
Agile Therapeutics, Inc., Princeton, New Jersey, 08540, USA

Arun Sanyal
Virginia Commonwealth University Medical Center, Richmond, Virginia, USA

Ke Chen, Yu Pan, Bin Zhang, Xiao-long Liu and Xue-yong Zheng
Department of General Surgery, Sir Run Run Shaw Hospital, School of Medicine, Zhejiang University, 3 East Qingchun Road, Hangzhou, Zhejiang 310016, China

Hendi Maher
School of Medicine, Zhejiang University, 866 Yuhangtang Road, Hangzhou, Zhejiang 310058, China

Dawesh P. Yadav, Saurabh Kedia, Sawan Bopanna, Sandeep Goyal, Saransh Jain, Govind K. Makharia and Vineet Ahuja
Department of Gastroenterology and Human Nutrition, All India Institute of Medical Sciences, New Delhi 110029, India

Kumble Seetharama Madhusudhan and Raju Sharma
Department of Radiodiagnosis, All India Institute of Medical Sciences, New Delhi 110029, India

Naval K. Vikram
Department of Medicine, All India Institute of Medical Sciences, New Delhi 110029, India

Yujen Tseng, Tiancheng Luo, Xiaoqing Zeng and Yichao Wei
Department of Gastroenterology, Zhongshan Hospital, Fudan University, Shanghai, China

Lili Ma
Department of Endoscopy Center, Zhongshan Hospital, Fudan University, Shanghai, China

Ling Li
Department of Geriatrics, Zhongshan Hospital, Fudan University, Shanghai, China

Pengju Xu
Department of Radiology, Zhongshan Hospital, Fudan University, Shanghai, China

Shiyao Chen
Department of Gastroenterology, Endoscopy Center and Evidence-Based Medicine Center, Zhongshan Hospital, Fudan University, Shanghai, China

Cristina Dopazo, Ramón Charco, Mireia Caralt, Elizabeth Pando, José Luis Lázaro Concepción Gómez-Gavara and Itxarone Bilbao
Department of HPB Surgery and Transplants, Hospital Universitario Vall d'Hebron,
Universidad Aut´onoma de Barcelona, Barcelona, Spain

Lluis Castells
Hepatology Unit, Department of Internal Medicine, Hospital Vall d'Hebron, CIBERehd,
Universidad Aut´onoma de Barcelona, Barcelona, Spain

Xiaoli Fan, Yongjun Zhu, Ruoting Men, Maoyao Wen, Yi Shen and Li Yang
Department of Gastroenterology and Hepatology, West China Hospital, Sichuan University, Chengdu, Sichuan 610041, China

Changli Lu
Department of Pathology,West China Hospital, Sichuan University, Chengdu, Sichuan 610041, China

Oluwaseun Shogbesan and Anthony Donato
Department of Medicine, Tower Health System, Sixth Avenue and Spruce Street, West Reading, PA 19611, USA

Dilli Ram Poudel and Asad Jehangir
Hospitalist Services, Tower Health System, Sixth Avenue and Spruce Street,West Reading, PA 19611, USA

Samjeris Victor
Department of Biochemistry and Molecular Biology, Pennsylvania State University, State College, PA 16801, USA

Opeyemi Fadahunsi
Division of Cardiology, Dalhousie University, Halifax, NS B3H 4RS, Canada

Gbenga Shogbesan
Department of Internal Medicine, Piedmont Athens Regional Medical Center, Athens, GA 30606,USA

Genevieve Huard, Thomas Schiano, Jang Moon and Kishore Iyer
Intestinal Rehabilitation and Transplantation Program, Recanati/Miller Transplantation Institute, Mount Sinai Medical Center,New York, NY, USA

Genevieve Huard and Thomas Schiano
Division of Liver Diseases, Mount Sinai Medical Center, New York, NY, USA

Genevieve Huard
Division of Liver Diseases, Centre Hospitalier de l'Universit´e de Montr´eal, Montr´eal, QC, Canada

YiMin Zhang, Li Shao, Ning Zhou, JianZhou Li, Juan Lu, Jie Wang, ErMei Chen, ZhongYang Xie and LanJuan Li
State Key Laboratory for Diagnosis and Treatment of Infectious Diseases,
Collaborative Innovation Center for Diagnosis and Treatment of Infectious Diseases, The First Affiliated Hospital, College of Medicine, Zhejiang University, Hangzhou, Zhejiang Province, China

Yu Chen
Department of Experimental Animals, Zhejiang Academy of Traditional Chinese Medicine, Hangzhou, Zhejiang Province, China

Yang Ye, Xue-Rui Wang, Yang Zheng, Jing-Wen Yang, Na-Na Yang, Guang-Xia Shi and Cun-Zhi Liu
Acupuncture and Moxibustion Department, Beijing-Hospital of Traditional Chinese Medicine Affiliated to Capital Medical University, Beijing Key Laboratory of Acupuncture Neuromodulation, Beijing, China

Yang Ye and Na-Na Yang
Beijing University of Chinese Medicine, Beijing, China

Xiaoping Wang, Caifei Shen, Jianjiang Yang, Sen Qin,Haijun Zeng, Xiaoling Wu, Shanhong Tang and Weizheng Zeng
Department of Gastroenterology, Chengdu Military General Hospital, Chengdu, Sichuan, China

Xiaoping Wang, Sen Qin and Shanhong Tang
College of Medicine, Southwest Jiaotong University, Chengdu, Sichuan, China

Xianjun Yang
Chengdu Military Command Disease Prevention and Control Center, Chengdu, Sichuan, China

Wen-xiong Xu, Xiang Zhu, Chao-shuang Lin,You-ming Chen, Hong Deng, Yong-yu Mei, Zhi-xin Zhao,Dong-ying Xie, Zhi-liang Gao, Chan Xie and Liang Peng
Department of Infectious Diseases,Third Affiliated Hospital of Sun Yat-sen University, Guangzhou, Guangdong 510630, China
Guangdong Key Laboratory of Liver Disease Research,Third Affiliated Hospital of Sun Yat-sen University, Guangzhou,Guangdong 510630, China

Qian Zhang
Department of Infectious Diseases, Union Hospital, Tongji Medical College, Huazhong University of Science and Technology,Wuhan, Hubei 430022, China

Bing Li, Chuan Liu, Lang Wang, Yang Li, Yong Du, Chuan Zhang, Xiao-xue Xu and Han Feng Yang
Sichuan Key Laboratory of Medical Imaging, Department of Radiology, Affiliated Hospital of North Sichuan Medical College,Nanchong City, Sichuan Province 637000, China

David Kara, Anna Hüsing-Kabar, Hartmut Schmidt, Gursimran Chandhok, Miriam Maschmeier and Iyad Kabar
Department of Gastroenterology and Hepatology, University Hospital Muenster, 48149 Muenster, Germany

Inga Grünewald
University Hospital Muenster, Gerhard-Domagk-Institute of Pathology, 48149 Muenster, Germany

Gursimran Chandhok
Department of Anatomy and Developmental Biology, and Neuroscience Program, Monash Biomedicine Discovery Institute, Monash University, Clayton, Melbourne, VIC 3800, Australia

Omar Abdel-Rahman
Clinical Oncology Department, Faculty of Medicine, Ain Shams University, Cairo, Egypt

Omar Abdel-Rahman and Winson Y. Cheung
Department of Oncology, University of Calgary, Tom Baker Cancer Centre, Calgary, Alberta, Canada

Helena Magalhães, Mário Fontes-Sousa and Manuela Machado
Medical Oncology Department, Portuguese Institute of Oncology of Porto (IPO Porto), Porto, Portugal

P. Priyanka and Yousaf B. Hadi
Department of Medicine,West Virginia University Hospitals, Morgantown, WV, USA

G. J. Reynolds
Department of Medicine, Section of Digestive diseases, West Virginia University Hospitals, Morgantown, WV, USA

Gang Ning, Yi-ting Li, You-ming Chen, Ying Zhang, Ying-fu Zeng and Chao-shuang Lin
Department of Infectious Diseases,TheThird Affiliated Hospital of Sun Yat-Sen University, Guangzhou 510630, China

Maryam Moini
Gastroenterohepatology Research Center, Shiraz University of Medical Sciences, Nemazee Hospital, Zand Street,Shiraz 71935-1311, Iran

Mitra Yazdani Sarvestani
Department of Internal Medicine, Fasa University of Medical Sciences, Ebne Sina Square, Fasa, Iran

Mesbah Shams
Endocrinology and Metabolism Research Center, Shiraz University of Medical Sciences, Shiraz, Iran

Masood Nomovi
Department of Internal Medicine, Shiraz University of Medical Sciences, Shiraz, Iran

Timna Naftali, Nahum Ruhimovich Fabiana Sklerovsky-Benjaminov and Fred Konikoff
Department of Gastroenterology and Hepatology, Meir Medical Center, affiliated with the Sackler School of Medicine,Tel Aviv University, Tel Aviv, Israel

Adi Eindor-Abarbanel, Shay Matalon, Haim Shirin and Efrat Broide
The Kamila Gonczarowski Institute for Gastroenterology and Liver Diseases, Assaf Harofeh Medical Center,affiliated with the Sackler School of Medicine, Tel Aviv University, Tel Aviv, Israel

Ariella Bar-Gil Shitrit and Yael Milgrom
Digestive Diseases Institute, Shaare Zedek Medical Center, Jerusalem, Israel

Tomer Ziv-Baran
Department of Epidemiology and Preventive Medicine, School of Public Health, Sackler Faculty of Medicine, Tel Aviv University,Tel Aviv, Israel

Bin Zhang, Yu Pan, Ke Chen, Ming-Yu Chen, He-Pan Zhu, Yi-Bin Zhu, Yi Dai, Jiang Chen and Xiu-jun Cai
Department of General Surgery, Sir Run Run Shaw Hospital, School of Medicine, Zhejiang University, 3 East Qingchun Road, Hangzhou, Zhejiang Province 310016, China

Bin Zhang, Yu Pan, Ke Chen, Hendi Maher, Ming-Yu Chen, He-Pan Zhu and Yi-Bin Zhu
School of Medicine, Zhejiang University, 866 Yuhangtang Road, Hangzhou, Zhejiang Province 310058, China

Bogdan Malkowski
Department of Nuclear Medicine, Oncological Center of Bydgoszcz, Bydgoszcz, Poland
Department of PET and Molecular Imaging, Collegium Medicum, University of Nicolaus Copernicus, Bydgoszcz, Poland

Pawel Wareluk and Michal Studniarek
Department of Diagnostic Imaging, Medical University of Warsaw, Warsaw, Poland

Tomasz Gorycki and Katarzyna Skrobisz
Department of Radiology, Medical University of Gdańsk, Gdańsk, Poland

Yan Hu, Xiaoting Chen, Xiaojing Chen, Shuang Zhang, Tianyan Jiang, Jing Chang and Yanhong Gao
Department of Geriatrics, Xinhua Hospital of Shanghai Jiaotong University, School of Medicine, Shanghai 2000092, China

Eva Sticova
Clinical and Transplant Pathology Centre, Institute for Clinical and Experimental Medicine, Prague 4, 140 21, Czech Republic.
Department of Pathology,Third Faculty of Medicine, Charles University, Prague 10, 100 00, Czech Republic

Milan Jirsa
Laboratory of Experimental Hepatology, Experimental Medicine Centre, Institute for Clinical and Experimental Medicine, Prague 4, 140 21, Czech Republic

Joanna PawBowska
Department of Gastroenterology, Hepatology, Nutritional Disorders and Pediatrics,
The Children's Memorial Health Institute (CMHI), Warsaw 04-730, Poland

Jilcha Diribi Feyisa and Hailemichael Desalegn
Department of Internal Medicine, Saint Paul's Hospital Millennium Medical College, Ethiopia

Melka Kenea and Efrem Gashaw
Department of Surgery, Arba Minch General Hospital, Ethiopia

Eskezyiaw Agedew Getahun
Department of Public Health, College of Health Sciences, Arba Minch University, Ethiopia

Barry Leon Hicks
Department of Surgery, Arba Minch University, Ethiopia

Bei Li, Chuan Zhang and Yu-Tao Zhan
Department of Gastroenterology, Beijing Tongren Hospital, Capital Medical University, Beijing 100730, China

Hanan M. Alghamdi
Department of Surgery, King Fahd Hospital of the University, University of Imam Abdulrahman Bin Faisal College of Medicine, Dammam, Saudi Arabia

Afnan F. Almuhanna and Bander F. Aldhafery
Department of Radiology, King Fahd Hospital of the University, University of Imam Abdulrahman Bin Faisal College of Medicine,Dammam, Saudi Arabia

Raed M. AlSulaiman, Ahmed Almarhabi and Abdulaziz AlQurain
Department of Internal Medicine, King Fahd Hospital of the University, University of Imam Abdulrahman Bin Faisal College of Medicine, Dammam, Saudi Arabia

Kyeong-Ah Kwak and and Young-Seok Park
Department of Oral Anatomy, School of Dentistry, Seoul National University and Dental Research Institute, Seoul, Republic of Korea

Hyun-Jae Cho
Department of Preventive and Social Dentistry, School of Dentistry, Seoul National University and Dental Research Institute, Seoul, Republic of Korea

Jin-Young Yang
Department of Dental Hygiene, Daejeon Institute of Science and Technology, Daejeon, Republic of Korea

Majid Alsahafi, Paula Cramer, Nazira Chatur and Fergal Donnellan
Division of Gastroenterology, Vancouver General Hospital, University of British Columbia, Vancouver, BC, Canada

Majid Alsahafi
Department of Medicine, King Abdulaziz University, Jeddah, Saudi Arabia

Index

A
Adipose Tissue, 2, 7, 53, 249, 258-259
Adrenal Dysfunction, 183, 186
Adrenal Function, 183-186
Alanine Aminotransferase, 1, 6-7, 78-79, 106-107, 204
Allograft, 71, 76, 95-101, 103, 205, 228
Alpha-fetoprotein, 126, 128, 130-131, 156, 226, 240
Anesthesia, 66, 118, 142-143
Antibiotic Therapy, 85, 143-144, 184
Aspartate Aminotransferase, 1, 27, 79, 106-107, 204

B
Bile Duct, 78, 80-81, 223, 226, 244-245, 247
Bisphosphonate, 210-211, 214-217, 219-220
Bone Marrow Transplant, 85-86
Bowel Disease, 52, 58-59, 85-86, 89-90, 92-93, 174, 189, 191-193, 210-211, 219-220, 233
Bowel Resection, 210, 267-268

C
Cessation, 132-135, 138-141, 248
Chemotherapy, 8-10, 14-16, 19-24, 85, 92, 158-163, 165-166
Cholangiogram, 244-245
Cholestasis, 78, 81-82, 98, 221, 223-232
Chronic Hepatitis, 126, 128, 130, 132-133, 140-141, 175-176, 178, 181-182, 237, 243, 255, 264-265
Clostridium Difficile, 73, 85-86, 92-93
Coagulation Dysfunction, 105, 108
Crohn's Disease, 52-59, 89, 93, 190-191, 193, 210-211, 219-220, 272

D
Duodenal Polyps, 148, 150-153

E
Esophagogastroduodenoscopy, 167, 170-172

F
Fatty Acid, 98, 103, 209, 223
Fatty Liver, 1-2, 4, 6-7, 27, 126-127, 149, 154, 237-238, 240-243
Fecal Microbiota, 85-86, 92-94
Functional Dyspepsia, 113-115, 121-125

G
Gastric Cancer, 127, 129, 159-163, 165-166
Gastrointestinal Endoscopy, 68-69, 89, 148, 151, 153-154, 174, 271-272
Gastropathy, 148, 150-152, 154
Glutamyl Transferase, 1, 224, 228

H
Hematopoietic Cell Lineage, 105, 108, 110
Hepatectomy, 18-24, 26-28, 37-38, 40-45, 48-51, 194-195, 198-199, 203-205, 250
Hepatic Encephalopathy, 29-30, 32, 35, 61, 78, 97, 105, 108, 111, 127-128, 130, 248
Hepatic Steatosis, 1-2, 7, 243
Hepatocellular Carcinoma, 20-21, 27, 37, 49-51, 127, 133-134, 140, 149, 155, 157-158, 175, 181, 225-226, 239, 241-243, 250, 256
Human Immunodeficiency Virus, 85, 89
Hypertensive Polyposis, 148, 152
Hyponatremia, 29, 31-36, 183, 185-188

I
Ileocecal Valve, 97-98, 103
Immune System, 85, 142, 145, 160, 162, 166
Immunotherapy, 10, 15, 76, 158-160, 162, 165
Inferior Vena Cava, 97, 101, 204
Intestinal Failure, 95-96, 101-103
Intestinal Rehabilitation, 95-98, 101
Intestinal Transplantation, 95-97, 99-104
Intrahepatic, 48, 127, 130, 148, 182, 187, 221, 223-232, 247, 257

J
Jejunoileum, 95, 100-101

L
Laparoscopy, 12, 16, 48, 69, 194-195, 197-199, 203-205, 238
Liver Cirrhosis, 49-51, 69, 84, 127, 133, 148-149, 152-155, 183-185, 187, 241-242, 248-251, 255-256, 260, 262-265
Liver Disease, 1, 6-7, 19-24, 26-28, 30, 32, 34, 50, 68-69, 72, 75, 77, 84, 92, 95-96, 98, 101-104, 110, 128, 131-133, 148-149, 151, 154, 157, 181, 183-187, 194, 226, 229-231, 248, 250, 258, 272
Liver Fibrosis, 95, 97-98, 108, 111-112, 180, 225, 239, 242-243, 248-249, 251, 255-257, 259-261, 264-266
Liver-intestine Transplantation, 95-96, 98-101, 103-104

M
Malabsorption, 52, 210
Mesenteric Artery, 95-96, 101

Metabolic Syndrome, 1-2, 237, 242
Monocytes, 175-177, 179-182, 262
Motility Disorders, 95, 100
Multivisceral Transplantation, 95-96, 100-102, 104

N
Nitric Oxide, 112, 114, 119-120, 122, 124, 148

O
Osteopenia, 210-211, 219
Osteoporosis, 78-79, 210-211, 216, 219-220, 236

P
Pancreatic Adenocarcinoma, 8, 15-17
Pancreatic Cancer, 8-9, 12-17
Pathophysiology, 113, 118-119, 230-231
Polypectomy, 148, 151-153
Polyposis Syndrome, 95, 101
Porcine, 105-107
Portomesenteric Thrombosis, 95, 100-101, 104
Prognostic Biomarker, 10, 13
Pruritus, 221-222, 224, 226-228, 231-232
Pyogenic Liver Abscess, 142, 146-147

R
Radiologist, 3, 53
Rheumatoid Arthritis, 90, 105, 110

S
Steatohepatitis, 1, 7, 72, 78, 225, 228, 238, 241-243, 264
Systemic Therapy, 8, 155-158

T
Thrombocytopenia, 18-19, 21, 25-28, 71-75, 99, 148, 151-152, 162
Transcriptome, 105-111

U
Ulcerative Colitis, 52-55, 57-59, 89, 92-93, 190, 193, 210-211, 219-220
Ultrasound, 3, 12, 66, 78, 133, 143, 239-240, 247, 262

V
Vasodilation, 29, 183, 186

www.ingramcontent.com/pod-product-compliance
Lightning Source LLC
Chambersburg PA
CBHW061315190326
41458CB00011B/3808